Mastering
Healthcare
Terminology

Contents

Mastering

Healthcare Terminology

5TH EDITION

Betsy J. Shiland
MS, RHIA, CCS, CPC, CPHQ, CTR, CHDA, CPB
AHIMA Approved ICD-10-CM/PCS Trainer

Former Assistant Professor
Allied Health Department
Community College of Philadelphia
Philadelphia, Pennsylvania

With 500 illustrations

3251 Riverport Lane
St. Louis, Missouri 63043

International Standard Book Number: 978-0-323-29858-2

Content Strategy Director: Jeanne Olsen
Senior Content Strategist: Linda Woodard
Content Development Manager: Luke Held
Publishing Services Manager: Julie Eddy
Senior Project Manager: Celeste Clingan
Design Direction: Brian Salisbury

Printed in China

Last digit is the print number: 9   8   7   6   5   4   3   2

Working together
to grow libraries in
developing countries

www.elsevier.com • www.bookaid.org

Contributor

Erinn Kao, PharmD, RPh
Pharmacist
GE Healthcare
St. Louis, Missouri

Reviewers

Randal Beard, MEd, RMA
MCI School of Health Science
ECPI University
Virginia Beach, Virginia

Angela R. Campbell, RHIA, AHIMA
Approved ICD-10-CM/PCS Trainer
Medical Insurance Manager
Eastern Illinois University
Charleston, Illinois
Curriculum Designer, Online Instructor
Health Information Technology Program
Northwestern College
Chicago, Illinois

Michele M. Crase, MT (ASCP) MPH
Instructor
Northern Illinois University
DeKalb, Illinois

Lisa Monique Hall, MAEd, RhED, BS
Health Educator, CMA
Allen School of Health Sciences
Jamaica, New York

Sandra Hertkorn, LVN
Reimbursement Specialist
Instructor Advanced Coding-Externship Coordinator
Bryan College Sacramento Campus
Gold River, California

Yvette Kennedy, OD, CBCS
En Visionary I-Care
Garner Charlotte, North Carolina

Ann Lunde, BS, CMT
Waubonsee Community College
Sugar Grove, Illinois

David McBride, BA, MA, RT (R) (CT) (MR)
Program Director
Westmoreland County Community College
Youngwood, Pennsylvania

Barbareta A. Welch McGill, BSN, MSN, DRS, RN
Clinical Instructor
North Carolina Central University
Department of Nursing
Durham, North Carolina

Patricia B. McKeown, AAS, RHIT
Adjunct Instructor
South Plains College
Levelland, Texas

Lisa Mendez, BBE, MEd
Professor
Sheridan College
Oakville, Ontario, Canada

Bharat Mody, MBBS
Instructor
Star Career Academy
Clifton, New Jersey

Teresa Pirone, CNA, LMT
Danbury, Connecticut

Karen K. Smith, MEd, RHIA, CPC
Instructor
University of Arkansas for Medical Sciences
College of Health Professions
Health Information Management Program
Little Rock, Arkansas

Teresa D. Tarkington, CPC, CMRS
Program Lead—Billing and Coding Specialist
Daymar Institute
Murfreesboro, Tennessee

Carole A. Zeglin, MSEd, BS, MT, MA (RMA)
Professor/Director Clinical Laboratory,
    Medical Assisting, and Phlebotomy Programs
Westmoreland County Community College
Youngwood, Pennsylvania

Preface

Beginning a healthcare career is like visiting a foreign country. If you want to converse with the inhabitants, you need to speak their language. If you are interested in a career in healthcare, fluency in its terminology is required. The goal of *Mastering Healthcare Terminology* is to help you learn the large number of terms that describe very specific healthcare conditions or procedures in the easiest, most effective manner possible.

We don't often think about what makes up our language, perhaps because we are so familiar with it. Prefixes, suffixes, and word roots make up both the English language and healthcare language. A student of terminology can develop a sizable vocabulary by learning these decodable word parts and the rules necessary to join them together. Memorizing eponyms, abbreviations, symbols, and nondecodable terms completes a healthcare professional's vocabulary.

ORGANIZATION OF THE BOOK

Mastering Healthcare Terminology has been designed for your success. Each feature has been chosen to help you learn this new language quickly and effectively.

To get you started, Chapters 1 and 2 orient you to the basic concepts necessary to learn healthcare terminology. Chapter 1 is focused on word parts and basic building and decoding skills. Chapter 2 explains the organization of the body, as well as positional and directional terms. You will use the material in both of these chapters throughout the remainder of the text.

Chapters 3 through 14 are body system chapters, each organized in the same way. The function of each system is introduced first, followed by the anatomy and physiology. A summary table of common anatomy and physiology word parts for the system functions as an excellent study tool. Once the terms for normal function are covered, pathologic terms, diagnostic techniques, therapeutic interventions, pharmacologic terms, and common abbreviations are presented.

Chapters 15 and 16 cover specialty terminology. Chapter 15 discusses the terminology for mental and behavioral health. Chapter 16 covers cancer terminology for all the body systems.

The internal structure of each chapter consists of small learning segments or "chunks." Concepts, terms, and abbreviations for a topic are covered and then immediately followed by exercises that reinforce and assess your understanding and retention of the material. Pathology and procedure terms are organized into tables that include phonetic pronunciations followed by the terms' component word parts and their meanings. Special boxes alert you to terminology pitfalls. Electronic healthcare records, case studies, and engaging end-of-chapter exercises provide you the opportunity to practice the terminology you've learned.

FEATURES

We've loaded *Mastering Healthcare Terminology* with special features to help you quickly and correctly learn the medical terminology you need to effectively communicate in the clinical setting.

Be Careful! Boxes remind students of potentially confusing look-alike or sound-alike word parts and terms.

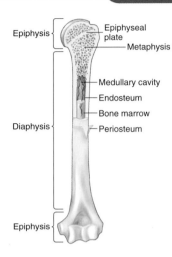

Fig. 3-2 Long bone.

Epiphysis

Epiphyseal plate

Metaphysis

Medullary cavity

Endosteum

Bone marrow

Diaphysis

Periosteum

Epiphysis

⊗ Be Careful!

Remember that the ends of the long bones closest to the points of attachment (hips and shoulders) are described as **proximal,** *whereas those farthest from the points of attachment (feet and hands) are described as* **distal.**

sis) (*pl.* epiphyses). Underneath the epiphyses are the **epiphyseal** (eh pee FIZZ ee ul) **plates,** which are the areas where bone growth normally occurs. Around the ages from 16 to 25, the plates close, and bone growth stops. The epiphysis and epiphyseal plates together form the **metaphysis** (meh TAFF ih sis).

The outer covering of the bone is called the **periosteum** (pair ee OS tee um), and the inner lining of the bone is known as the **endosteum** (en DOS tee um). These two coverings hold the cells responsible for bone remodeling: osteoblasts and osteoclasts. The shape of a bone enables practitioners to speak very specifically about a particular area on that bone. For instance, any groove, opening, or hollow space is called a **depression.** Depressions provide an entrance and exit for vessels and protection for the organs they hold. Raised or projected areas are called **processes.** These are often areas of attachment for ligaments or tendons. The tables that follow give examples of bone depressions and processes.

metaphysis
  meta- = change
  -physis = growth, nature

periosteum
  peri- = surrounding
  oste/o = bone
  -um = structure

endosteum
  endo- = within
  oste/o = bone
  -um = structure

Word parts next to their text mentions in the anatomy and physiology section, to demonstrate the origins of terms.

Bone Depressions

Depression	Combining Form	Meaning/Function	Example
foramen (*pl.* foramina) foh RAY men	foramin/o	An opening or hole	foramen magnum, mental foramina
fossa (*pl.* fossae) FAH sah	foss/o	A hollow or depression, especially on the surface of the end of a bone	olecranal fossa
sinus (*pl.* sinuses) SYE nus	sin/o sinus/o	A cavity or channel lined with a membrane	paranasal sinuses

Decode the following terms below using your knowledge of word parts.

17. submandibular _____

18. costochondral _____

19. lumbosacral _____

20. thoracic _____

21. substernal _____

EXERCISE 5: Bones of the Cranium and Face

Label the diagram using the terms provided.

temporal bone
mandible
ethmoid bone
mastoid process
lacrimal bone
zygomatic bone
maxilla
nasal bones

EXERCISE 6: Bones of the Spine

Label the diagram using the terms provided.

coccyx
cervical vertebrae
lumbar vertebrae
sacrum
thoracic vertebrae

Labeling exercises help students learn anatomy and the accompanying combining forms.

90   Chapter 3

 EXERCISE 16: Congenital Conditions

Build the terms.

1. process of joined fingers/toes _____

> **Case studies** provide students the opportunity to see terminology in use.

nt without cartilage _____

/toes _____

Case Study **LeDanton Bradford**

LeDanton Bradford is a healthy, well-developed infant with six digits on the ulnar side of his right hand and webbing between the third and fourth digits on his left hand. All the phalanges in the other digits appear to be present and normal. At first his parents are reluctant to correct the abnormalities, but when LeDanton is 6 months old, they sign consents for surgery to correct both disorders.

1. What is the term that means a condition of extra fingers or toes? _____

2. What is the term that means a condition of webbed fingers or toes? _____

3. A/an _____ is an individual bone in a finger or toe.

4. The little finger is on the ulnar side of the hand?
    a. true
    b. false

5. What is the prefix that means many? _____

Terms Related to Bone Disease

Term	Word Origin	Definition
osteodynia ahs tee oh DIN ee ah	*oste/o* bone *-dynia* pain	Bone pain.
osteitis deformans ahs tee EYE tis dee FOR menz	*oste/o* bone *-itis* inflammation *deformans* misshapen	Misshaped bone resulting from excessive breakdown and formation of bone tissue. Also known as **Paget disease.**
osteomalacia ahs tee oh mah LAY sha	*oste/o* bone *-malacia* softening	Softening of bone caused by loss of minerals from the bony matrix as a result of vitamin D deficiency. When osteomalacia occurs in childhood, it is called **rickets.**
osteomyelitis ahs tee oh mye eh LYE tis	*oste/o* bone *myel/o* bone marrow *-itis* inflammation	Inflammation and/or infection of the bone and bone marrow.
osteoporosis ahs tee oh poor OH sis	*oste/o* bone *por/o* passage *-osis* abnormal condition	Loss of bone mass, which results in the bones being fragile and at risk for fractures (Fig. 3-11). **Osteopenia** refers to a less severe bone mass loss. (*-penia* = deficiency)

> **Pathology and diagnostic terminology presented in tables** include pronunciation of term, word parts, and definition.

Medical Record Dylan Koldmann

KOLDMANN, DYLAN M. - 507940 Opened by Bradey Oppenheimer, MD

Task   Edit   View   Time Scale   Options   Help

KOLDMANN, DYLAN M.   Age: 7 years   Sex: Male   Loc: ARH
DOB: 01/27/2007   MRN: 507940   FIN: 3506004

Reference Text Browser | Form Browser | Medication Profile

Orders | Last 48 Hours | **ED** | Lab | Radiology | Assessments | Surgery | Clinical Notes | Pt. Info | Pt. Schedule | Task List | I & O | MAR

Flowsheet: ED   Level: ED Record   ◉ Table ○ Group ○ List

Navigator
✓ ED Record

7-year-old sustained injury to right hand when fell off bike. Pain over thenar eminence. Able to bend at his wrist and flex at his DIP and PIP joints and every digit of the hand with exception of first digit.

Exam of right hand is significant for mild protrusion but no ecchymosis and minimal edema overlying thenar eminence of the right hand. Good wrist mobility. X-ray significant for what appears to be a Salter-Harris fracture of the first metacarpal. Immobile and follow-up tomorrow with Ortho for possible cast.

PROD | MAHAFC | 26 March 2014 | 16:10

EXERCISE 15: Emergency Department Report

Use the preceding emergency department record to answer the following questions.

1. Dylan's injury is to the fleshy area of the palm near the thumb, the "thenar eminence." Explain the difference between a DIP and a PIP joint. _____

2. Not being able to "flex" a body part means one is unable to _____

3. "First digit, R hand" means _____

4. The first metacarpal is a bone of the _____

 *Click on **Hear It, Spell It** to practice spelling the anatomy and physiology terms you have learned in this chapter.*

EXERCISE 22: Admission Record

Using the admission record on p. 102, answer the following questions:

1. Which bone did Jean Herold break while exercising? Give both the medical term and the common

   _____

2. _____ *closest to her shoulder* or *farthest from her shoulder?* (Underline one.)

3. _____ ture sustained. _____

4. What other musculoskeletal disorder does she currently have? _____

5. What does "cannot adduct her arm and shoulder without pain" mean? _____

> **Age Matters boxes** highlight important concepts and terminology for both pediatric and geriatric patients.

 Age Matters

Pediatrics

As can be seen from our table of congenital disorders, there are several musculoskeletal conditions that a child may be born with: achondroplasia, MD, two disorders of the phalanges (syndactyly and polydactyly), spina bifida occulta, talipes, and congenital torticollis. Although not exclusive to childhood, pediatric statistics reveal high numbers of children treated each year for the effects of physical trauma. Fractures are common: beginning with clavicular fractures (the result of birth trauma) to fractures of the arms (humerus, radius, and ulna) and the legs (femur, tibia, and fibula). Sprains, strains, dislocations, and subluxations are other pediatric diagnoses that appear with regularity for this system.

Geriatrics

Statistics collected on the geriatric population of patients also report a high number of fractures. These, however, are mainly fractures of the hip and femur and are often preceded by bone loss caused by osteoporosis or cancer. OA, often referred to as "wear and tear disease," is another disorder that afflicts many patients as they age. The high numbers of total knee replacement (TKR) surgeries today are often the result of this disease.

ⓔ *You can review the pathology terms you've learned in this chapter by playing **Medical Millionaire**.*

DIAGNOSTIC PROCEDURES

Terms Related to Imaging

Term	Word Origin	Definition
arthrography ar THRAH gruh fee	*arthr/o* joint *-graphy* process of recording	X-ray recording of a joint.
arthroscopy ar THRAHS kuh pee	*arthr/o* joint *-scopy* process of viewing	Visual examination of a joint, accomplished by use of an arthroscope (Fig. 3-21).
computed tomography (CT) scan	*tom/o* section *-graphy* process of recording	Imaging technology that records transverse planes of the body for diagnostic purposes.
dual energy x-ray absorptiometry (DEXA) scan DECK suh		A procedure that measures the density of bone at the hip and spine. Also called **bone mineral density studies** (Fig. 3-22).

Continued

110   Chapter 3

⊘ EXERCISE 24: Therapeutic Interventions

Match the therapeutic terms with their definitions.

_____ 1. débridement

_____ 2. open reduction (OR)

_____ 3. amputation

_____ 4. myorrhaphy

_____ 5. osteoclasis

_____ 6 arthrodesis

_____ 7. prosthesis

_____ 8. spondylosyndesis

_____ 9. arthrocentesis

_____ 10. closed reduction (CR)

A. suture of muscle
B. intentional fracture of bone
C. alignment of ends of bone with incision
D. alignment of ends of bone without incision
E. surgical puncture of a joint
F. artificial body part
G. removal of a limb
H. removal of debris
I. spinal fusion
J. fixation of a joint

Build a term that means:

11. surgical repair of a joint _____

12. intentional breaking of a bone _____

13. excision of a bunion _____

14. surgical repair of a tendon and muscle _____

15. removal of a meniscus _____

16. surgical repair of a ligament _____

PHARMACOLOGY

analgesics: Reduce pain. Examples include morphine (MS Contin), hydrocodone (Vicodin or Lortab, in combination with acetaminophen), acetaminophen (Tylenol), and NSAIDs such as naproxen (Anaprox).

antiinflammatories: Used to reduce inflammation and pain. Examples include steroidal and nonsteroidal antiinflammatory drugs (NSAIDs). Methylprednisolone (Medrol) is an example of a steroid; ibuprofen (Advil, Motrin) and celecoxib (Celebrex) are examples of NSAIDs.

bisphosphonates: Prevent and sometimes reverse bone loss to treat diseases such as osteoporosis, Paget disease, or bone cancer. Examples include alendronate (Fosamax) and zoledronic acid (Zometa).

disease-modifying antirheumatic drugs (DMARDs): Slow progression of rheumatoid arthritis while also reducing signs and symptoms. Examples include leflunomide (Arava), etanercept (Enbrel), and infliximab (Remicade).

muscle relaxants: Relieve pain caused by muscle spasms by relaxing the skeletal muscles. Examples include cyclobenzaprine (Flexeril) and metaxalone (Skelaxin).

Review exercises encourage word building and practical use of terminology.

116   Chapter 3

Sort the terms below into the correct categories.

Term Sorting

Anatomy and Physiology	Pathology	Diagnostic Procedures	Therapeutic Interventions

arthrocentesis	CTS	MRI	radius
arthrodesis	DEXA	myelogram	ROM
arthrography	diaphysis	myorrhaphy	serum calcium
arthroscopy	digitus	osteoclasis	spondylolisthesis
arthrosis	EMG	osteomyelitis	sternum
articulation	goniometry	osteoplasty	syndactyly
bunion	humerus	osteoporosis	tendinitis
bursitis	laminectomy	osteosarcoma	tenomyoplasty
cartilage	ligament	Phalen test	TKR
costa	meniscectomy	prosthesis	ulna

STUDENT RESOURCES

Electronic assets for students on Evolve include entertaining interactive games and activities that have been designed to test specific areas of knowledge as you prepare for quizzes and exams. Breeze through the challenges of learning healthcare terminology and quickly learn to speak the language of your future career! Included with *Mastering Healthcare Terminology, Fifth Edition,* are a variety of learning aids intended to make your study of healthcare terminology as efficient and enjoyable as possible.

Easily learn the anatomy for each body system with **Body Spectrum Electronic Anatomy Coloring Book** and **Label It**.

Match word parts with their definitions with **Match the Word Parts** and **Electronic Flash Cards**.

Watch **medical animations** to help you visualize pathologic and procedural terms.

Build terms with **Word Shop**.

Learn medical terminology by playing **Medical Millionaire** and **Tournament of Terminology**.

Practice spelling medical terms with **Hear It, Spell It**. Download *iTerms* to listen to all the terms and definitions from the text.

Sort terms into categories with *Term Sorting*.

Practice your retention of terminology with **Quick Quizzes**.

Explore healthcare careers by watching **Career Videos**.

Medical Terminology Online

Medical Terminology Online for Mastering Healthcare Terminology, Fifth Edition, is a great resource to supplement your textbook. This web-delivered course supplement, available for separate purchase, provides a range of visual, auditory, and interactive elements to reinforce your learning and synthesize concepts presented in the text. Interactive lesson reviews at the end of each module provide you with testing tools that are actually fun. Clicking on a bolded term provides you with the pronunciation, definition, and Spanish translation.

This online course supplement is accessible only if you have purchased the access code packaged with your book. If you did not purchase the book/access package, ask your instructor for information or visit http://evolve.elsevier.com/ to purchase.

Instructors interested in *Medical Terminology Online,* please contact your sales rep, call Faculty Support at 1-800-222-9570, or visit http://evolve.elsevier.com/ for more information.

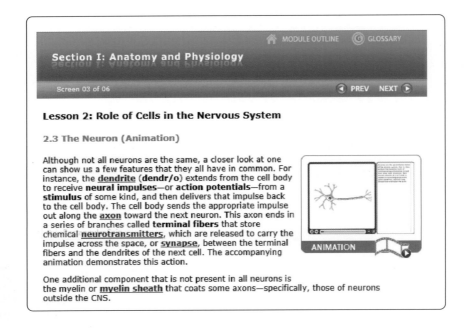

To the Instructor

You are the most important driving force behind your students' mastery of medical terminology. That's why we have provided you with all the resources you will need to teach this new language to your students:

- A **PowerPoint presentation** includes over 1000 slides to make teaching from Shiland a breeze. Slides are enhanced with additional images.
- **A test bank** consists of over 5400 questions. Multiple-choice, fill-in-the-blank, and true/false questions that can be sorted by subject, objective, and type of questions using Examview.
- **Handouts** can be used for classroom quizzes or homework.
- **Emailable, gradable quizzes** on the student site can be used for extra credit.
- **TEACH Lesson Plans** help you prepare for class and make full use of the rich array of ancillaries and resources that come with your textbook.
  TEACH is short for "Total Education and Curriculum Help," which accurately describes how these lesson plans and lecture materials have been providing creative and innovative instructional strategies to both new and experienced instructors to the benefit of their students.
  Each lesson plan contains:
  - 50-minute lessons that correlates chapter objectives with content and teaching resources
  - Convenient lists of key terms for each chapter
  - Classroom activities and critical-thinking questions that engage and motivate students
  Visit http://evolve.elsevier.com/Shiland/Mastering for more information.

From the Author

My greatest joy as a teacher has been to run into students long after they have finished one of my classes: students now practicing the career of their choice that they had begun so many years before. Students tell me how much they have used what they learned, how glad they are that they took the course, and, finally, how much fun it was. Certainly, healthcare terminology is a serious subject, but there is no reason not to have fun while you are learning. The Evolve website that accompanies this text will allow you to practice all aspects of terminology, while playing games that test your knowledge of all that serious stuff. Research shows that you need to be in contact with a new term at least six times to remember it. By attending class, reading the chapters, completing the exercises, and playing the games, you will have easily met that goal.

I am deeply grateful to all the people who have helped me in getting this fifth edition to print. Thanks are due to the following:

- To my past students: for your questions, your enthusiasm, and your drive to accomplish a career in healthcare.
- To **Erinn Kao** for updating the pharmacology information and to **Jeanne Robertson,** who expertly turned my thoughts into beautiful illustrations for the text.
- To my Elsevier cohorts: **Linda Woodard,** for her calm leadership and relentless drive for quality in every aspect of the book; to **Celeste Clingan** for her production expertise, and to **Brian Salisbury** for his beautiful design—thank you all for guiding me once again through the process.
- To my family: brother and sister-in-law, **Thomas** and **Maureen Shiland**, both National Board Certified teachers, who have provided many discussions and resources that helped me solidify my thinking on the structure of the exercises and games. And most important of all: thanks to my son, **Thomas**, who continues to inspire, encourage, and support me.

Betsy Shiland
Betsy.shiland@verizon.net

Contents

Introduction to Healthcare Terminology

1

CHAPTER OUTLINE

OBJECTIVES

- State the derivation of most healthcare terms.
- Use the rules given to build, spell, and pronounce healthcare terms.
- Use the rules given to change singular terms to their plural forms.

- Recognize and recall an introductory word bank of prefixes, suffixes, and combining forms and their respective meanings.

You'll find fun interactive learning on the Shiland Evolve website at http://evolve.elsevier.com/Shiland. The Evolve Student Resources include:

- **Term Sorting**—sort terms into categories.
- **Tournament of Terminology game**—answer questions in a multitude of medical terminology categories.
- **Match the Word Parts**—match word parts with definitions.
- **Medical Millionaire game**—earn a "million dollars" by answering questions about pathology terms.
- **Word Shop**—practice building terms.
- **Label It**—practice labeling anatomy.
- **Hear It, Spell It**—listen to a term, and then spell it correctly.
- **Flash Cards**—learn word parts and their definitions.
- **Body Spectrum Electronic Anatomy Coloring Book**—review anatomy.
- **iTerms Audio**—listen to all of the terms and definitions from the text.
- **Career Videos**—listen to professionals speak about healthcare careers.

DERIVATION OF HEALTHCARE TERMS

Healthcare terminology is a specialized vocabulary derived from Greek and Latin word components. This terminology is used by professionals in the medical field to communicate with each other. By applying the process of "decoding," or recognizing the word components and their meanings and using these to define the terms, anyone will be able to interpret literally thousands of medical terms.

The English language and healthcare terminology share many common origins. This proves to be an additional bonus for those who put forth the effort to learn hundreds of seemingly new word parts. Two excellent and highly relevant examples are the **combining forms** (the "subjects" of most terms) gloss/o and lingu/o, which mean "tongue" in Greek and Latin, respectively. Because the tongue is instrumental in articulating spoken language, Greek and Latin equivalents appear, not surprisingly, in familiar English vocabulary. The table below illustrates the intersection of our everyday English language with the ancient languages of Greek and Latin and can help us to clearly see the connections. **Suffixes** (word parts that appear at the end of some terms) and **prefixes** (word parts that appear at the beginning of some terms) also are presented in this table. Special notice should be given to the pronunciation key that is provided directly under the examples: You will have to use your tongue to say them! *Please remember that terminology is spoken as well as written and read.* You must take advantage of the many resources that this text provides if you wish to fully communicate as a healthcare professional.

Ancient Word Origins in Current English and Healthcare Terminology Usage

Term	Word Origins	Definition
glossary (GLAH sur ee)	*gloss/o* tongue (Greek) *-ary* pertaining to	An English term meaning "an alphabetical list of terms with definitions."
glossitis (glah SYE tiss)	*gloss/o* tongue (Greek) *-itis* inflammation	A healthcare term meaning "inflammation of the tongue."
bi**lingu**al (by LIN gwal)	*bi-* two *lingu/o* tongue (Latin) *-al* pertaining to	An English term meaning "pertaining to two languages."
sub**lingu**al (sub LIN gwal)	*sub-* under *lingu/o* tongue (Latin) *-al* pertaining to	A healthcare term meaning "pertaining to under the tongue."

Did you notice that healthcare terms use the word origins literally, whereas English words are related to word origins but are not exactly the same? Fortunately, most healthcare terms may be assigned a simple definition through the use of their word parts.

TYPES OF HEALTHCARE TERMS

Decodable Terms

Decodable terms are those terms that can be broken into their Greek and Latin word parts and given a working definition based on the meanings of those word parts. Most medical terms are decodable, so learning word parts is important. The word parts are:

- **Combining form:** Word root with its respective combining vowel.
  - **Word root:** Word origin.
  - **Combining vowel:** A letter sometimes used to join word parts. Usually an "o" but occasionally an "a," "e," "i," or "u."
- **Suffix:** Word part that appears at the end of a term. Suffixes are used to indicate whether the term is an anatomic, pathologic, diagnostic, or therapeutic intervention term.
- **Prefix:** Word part that sometimes appears at the beginning of a term. Prefixes are used to further define the absence, location, number, quantity, or state of the term.

In our first examples, gloss/ and lingu/ are word roots with an "o" as their combining vowel. Gloss/o and lingu/o are therefore combining forms; -ary, -al, and -itis are suffixes; and bi- and sub- are prefixes. Figs. 1-1 and 1-2 demonstrate the decoding of the terms **glossitis** and **sublingual**. Throughout the text, we will be using combining forms so that you will learn the appropriate combining vowel for that particular term.

Nondecodable Terms

Not all terms are composed of word parts that can be used to assemble a definition. These terms are referred to as **nondecodable terms** (that is, words used in medicine whose definitions must be memorized without the benefit of word parts). These terms will have a blank space in the word origin tables presented in the text or will include only a partial notation, because the word origins either are not helpful or don't exist. Examples of nondecodable terms include the following:

- **Cataract:** From the Greek term meaning "waterfall." In healthcare language, this means progressive opacification of the lens.
- **Asthma:** From the Greek term meaning "panting." Although this word origin is understandable, the definition is a respiratory disorder characterized by recurring episodes of paroxysmal dyspnea (difficulty breathing).
- **Diagnosis:** The disease or condition that is named after a healthcare professional evaluates a patient's signs, symptoms, and history. Although the term is built from word parts (dia-, meaning "through," "complete;" and -gnosis, meaning "state of knowledge"), using these word parts to form the definition of diagnosis, which is "a state of complete knowledge," really isn't very helpful.
- **Prognosis:** Similar to *diagnosis*, the term *prognosis* can be broken down into its word parts (pro-, meaning "before" or "in front of;" and -gnosis, meaning "state of knowledge"), but this does not give the true definition of the term, which is "a prediction of the probable outcome of a disease or disorder."
- **Sequela** (suh KWELL ah): A condition that results from an injury or disease.
- **Acute:** A term that describes an abrupt, severe onset (acu- means "sharp") to a disease.
- **Chronic:** Developing slowly and lasting for a long time (chron/o means "time"). Diagnoses may be additionally described as being either acute or chronic.
- **Sign:** An objective finding of a disease state (e.g., fever, high blood pressure, rash).
- **Symptom:** A subjective report of a disease (pain, itching).

gloss \\\> itis
word root   suffix
glossitis

Fig. 1-1 Decoding of the term **glossitis.**

sub \\\< lingu \\\> al
prefix   word root   suffix
sublingual

Fig. 1-2 Decoding of the term **sublingual.**

Other types of terms that are not built from word parts include the following:

- **Eponyms:** Terms that are named after a person or place associated with the term.* Examples include:
  - **Alzheimer disease,** which is named after Alois Alzheimer, a German neurologist. The disease is a progressive mental deterioration.
  - **Achilles tendon,** which is a body part named after a figure in Greek mythology whose one weak spot was this area of his anatomy. Tendons are bands of tissue that attach muscles to bone. The Achilles tendon is the particular tendon that attaches the calf muscle to the heel bone (calcaneus). Unlike some eponyms, this one does have a medical equivalent, the calcaneal tendon.

Abbreviations and Symbols

Abbreviations are terms that have been shortened to letters and/or numbers for the sake of convenience. Symbols are graphic representations of a term. Abbreviations and symbols are extremely common in written and spoken healthcare terminology but can pose problems for healthcare workers. The Joint Commission has published a "DO NOT USE" list of dangerously confusing abbreviations, symbols, and acronyms that should be avoided (see Appendix C). The Institute of Safe Medical Practice, Inc., has provided a more extensive list. Each healthcare organization should have an official list, which includes the single meaning allowed for each abbreviation or symbol. Examples of acceptable abbreviations and symbols include the following:

- **Simple abbreviations:** A combination of letters (often, but not always the first of significant word parts) and sometimes numbers
  - IM: Abbreviation for "intramuscular" (pertaining to within the muscles)
  - C2: Second cervical vertebra (second bone in neck)
- **Acronyms:** Abbreviations that are also pronounceable
  - CABG: Coronary artery bypass graft (a detour around a blockage in an artery of the heart)
  - TURP: Transurethral resection of the prostate (a surgical procedure that removes the prostate through the urethra)
- **Symbols:** Graphic representations of terms
  ♂ stands for male
  ♀ stands for female
  ↑ stands for increased
  ↓ stands for decreased
  + stands for present
  − stands for absent

EXERCISE 1: Derivation of Healthcare Terms and Nondecodable Terms

Match the following types of healthcare terms with their examples.

_____ 1. symbol   _____ 4. eponym   A. CABG
                                                  B. Alzheimer disease
_____ 2. decodable term _____ 5. nondecodable term   C. ♀
                                                  D. glossitis
_____ 3. simple abbreviation _____ 6. acronym   E. C2
                                                  F. asthma

*This text presents terms without the possessive 's. This practice is in accordance with the American Medical Association (AMA) and the American Association of Transcriptionists (AAMT).

Many students find that flash cards help them remember word parts. If this is a strategy that could work for you, now is a great place to start, whether the cards are purchased or handmade. One card will be needed for each word part with the part on one side and the definition on the reverse. The Evolve website that accompanies this text provides mobile-optimized flash cards that can be sorted by chapter, by type of word part (prefix, suffix, combining form), and by abbreviation.

DECODING TERMS

Check, Assign, Reverse, and Define Method (CARD Method)

Using Greek and Latin word components to decipher the meanings of healthcare terms requires a simple four step process—the check, assign, reverse, and define (CARD) method. You need to:

- **Check** for the word parts in a term.
- **Assign** meanings to the word parts.
- **Reverse** the meaning of the suffix to the front of your definition.
- **Define** the term.

Using Fig. 1-3, see how this process is applied to your first patient, Alex.

Alex was diagnosed with glossitis, which made it difficult for him to speak.

	glossitis
Check	gloss/itis
Assign	tongue/inflammation
Reverse	tongue/inflammation
Define	inflammation (of the) tongue

Fig. 1-3 How to decode a healthcare term using the **check, assign, reverse, and define (CARD)** method.

Most of the terms presented in this text appear in standardized tables. The term and its pronunciation appear in the first column, the word origin in the second, and a definition in the third. A table that introduces six healthcare terms that include six different combining forms and suffixes is provided on p. 6. (The use of prefixes will be introduced later.) Success in decoding these terms depends on how well you remember the twelve word parts that are covered in the following table. Once you master these twelve word parts, you will be able to recognize and define many other medical terms that use these same word parts—a perfect illustration of how learning a few word parts helps you learn many healthcare terms. The "wheel of terminology" included on Fig. 1-4 demonstrates how the different suffixes in the table on p. 6 can be added to a combining form to make a variety of terms.

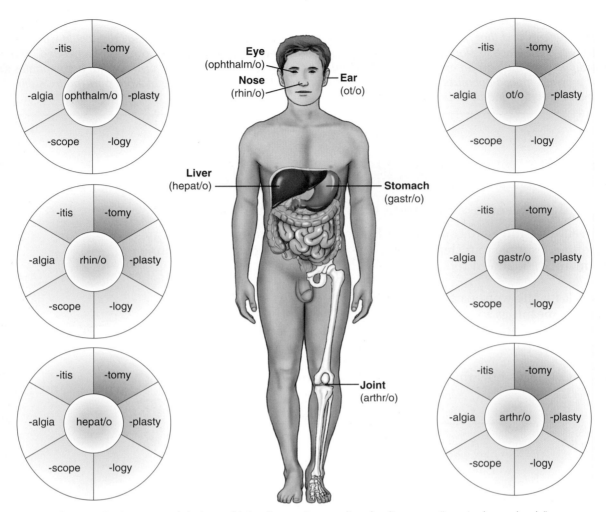

Fig. 1-4 Body parts and their combining forms. Surrounding the figure are "terminology wheels" that show how different suffixes can be added to a combining form to make a variety of terms.

Common Combining Forms and Suffixes

Combining Forms	Suffixes
arthr/o = joint	-algia = pain
gastr/o = stomach	-tomy = incision
ophthalm/o = eye	-scope = instrument to view
ot/o = ear	-logy = study of
rhin/o = nose	-plasty = surgical repair
hepat/o = liver	-itis = inflammation

The following table demonstrates how terms are presented in this book. Notice that the first column includes the term and its pronunciation. The second column breaks the term down into word parts and their meanings. The third column includes the definition of the term and any synonyms.

Samples of Decodable Terms

Term	Word Origins	Definition
arthralgia ar THRAL jah	***arthr/o*** joint ***-algia*** pain of	Pain of a joint. Also called **arthrodynia** (-dynia means pain).
gastrotomy gass TROT uh mee	***gastr/o*** stomach ***-tomy*** incision	Incision of the stomach.
ophthalmoscope off THAL muh skohp	***ophthalm/o*** eye ***-scope*** instrument to view	Instrument used to view the eye.
otology oh TALL uh jee	***ot/o*** ear ***-logy*** study of	Study of the ear.
rhinoplasty RYE noh plass tee	***rhin/o*** nose ***-plasty*** surgical repair	Surgical repair of the nose.
hepatitis heh peh TYE tiss	***hepat/o*** liver ***-itis*** inflammation	Inflammation of the liver.

EXERCISE 2: Combining Forms

Match the combining forms with their meanings.

_____ 1. ear   _____ 4. eye   A. rhin/o

                                              B. arthr/o

_____ 2. stomach   _____ 5. joint   C. ot/o

                                              D. gastr/o

_____ 3. nose   E. ophthalm/o

EXERCISE 3: Suffixes

Match the suffixes with their meanings.

_____ 1. pain   _____ 4. incision   A. -tomy

                                              B. -algia

_____ 2. surgical repair   _____ 5. study of   C. -logy

                                              D. -plasty

_____ 3. instrument to view   E. -scope

EXERCISE 4: Decoding the Terms Using Check, Assign, Reverse, and Define

Using the method shown in Fig. 1-3 and the twelve word parts you have just memorized, decode and define these five new terms.

1. ophthalmology _____

2. otoplasty _____

3. gastralgia _____

4. arthroscope _____

5. rhinotomy _____

BUILDING TERMS

Now that you've seen how terms are decoded, we will discuss how they are built. First, a few rules on how to spell healthcare terms correctly.

Spelling Rules

With a few exceptions, decodable healthcare terms follow five simple rules.

1. If the suffix starts with a vowel, a combining vowel is *not* needed to join the parts. For example, it is simple to combine the combining form **arthr/o** and suffix **-itis** to build the term **arthritis**, which means "an inflammation of the joints." The combining vowel "**o**" is not needed because the suffix starts with the vowel "**i.**"
2. If the suffix starts with a consonant, a combining vowel *is* needed to join the two word parts. For example, when building a term using **arthr/o** and **-plasty**, the combining vowel is retained and the resulting term is spelled **arthroplasty**, which refers to a surgical repair of a joint.
3. If a combining form ends with the same vowel that begins a suffix, one of the vowels is dropped. The term that means "inflammation of the inside of the heart" is built from the suffix **-itis** (inflammation), the prefix **endo-** (inside), and the combining form **cardi/o. Endo-** + **cardi/o** + **-itis** would result in *endocardiitis*. Instead, one of the "i"s is dropped, and the term is spelled **endocarditis**.
4. If two or more combining forms are used in a term, the combining vowel is retained between the two, regardless of whether the second combining form begins with a vowel or a consonant. For example, joining **gastr/o** and **enter/o** (small intestine) with the suffix **-itis**, results in the term **gastroenteritis**. Notice that the combining vowel is *kept* between the two combining forms (even though **enter/o** begins with the vowel "e"), and the combining vowel is *dropped* before the suffix **-itis**.
5. Sometimes when two or more combining forms are used to make a medical term, special notice must be paid to the order in which the combining forms are joined. For example, joining **esophag/o** (which means esophagus), **gastr/o** (which means stomach), and **duoden/o** (which means duodenum, [the first part of the small intestines]) with the suffix **-scopy** (process of viewing), produces the term *esophagogastroduodenoscopy*. An **esophagogastroduodenoscopy (EGD)** is a visual examination of the esophagus, stomach, and duodenum. In this procedure, the examination takes place in a specific sequence (that is, esophagus first, stomach second, and then the duodenum). Thus the term reflects the direction from which the scope travels through the body (Fig. 1-5).

Suffixes

The body system chapters in this text (Chapters 3 through 14) include many combining forms that are used to build terms specific to each system. These combining forms will not be seen elsewhere, except as a sign or symptom of a particular disorder. **Suffixes,** however, are used over and over again throughout the text. Suffixes usually can be grouped according to their purposes. The tables on pages 9 to 15 cover the majog suffix categores.

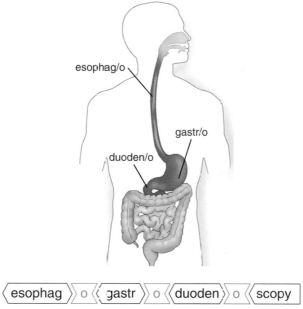

esophag 〉o〈 gastr 〉o〈 duoden 〉o〈 scopy

Fig. 1-5 The decoding of the term **esophagogastroduodenoscopy (EGD).**

Noun-Ending Suffixes

Noun endings are used most often to describe anatomic terms. Noun endings such as -icle, -ole, and -ule describe a diminutive structure.

Noun-Ending Suffixes

Suffix	Meaning	Example	Word Origins	Definition
-icle	small, tiny	cuticle	*cut/o* skin *-icle* small	Small skin (surrounding the nail).
-is	structure, thing	hypodermis	*hypo-* under *derm/o* skin *-is* structure	Structure under the skin.
-ole	small, tiny	arteriole	*arteri/o* artery *-ole* small	Small artery.
-ule	small, tiny	venule	*ven/o* vein *-ule* small	Small vein.
-um	structure, thing, membrane	endocardium	*endo-* within *cardi/o* heart *-um* structure	Structure within the heart.
-y	process of, condition	atrophy	*a-* no, not, without *troph/o* development *-y* process of	Process of no development.

Adjective Suffixes

Adjective suffixes such as those listed in the following table usually mean "pertaining to." For example, when the suffix **-ac** is added to the combining form **cardi/o**, the term *cardiac* is formed, which means "pertaining to the heart." Remember that when you see an adjective term, you need to see what it is describing. For example, cardiac pain is pain of the heart, and cardiac surgery is surgery done on the heart. An adjective tells only half of the story.

Adjective Suffixes

Suffix	Meaning	Example	Word Origins	Definition
-ac	pertaining to	cardiac	*cardi/o* heart *-ac* pertaining to	Pertaining to the heart.
-al	pertaining to	cervical	*cervic/o* neck *-al* pertaining to	Pertaining to the neck.
-ar	pertaining to	valvular	*valvul/o* valve *-ar* pertaining to	Pertaining to a valve.
-ary	pertaining to	coronary	*coron/o** heart, crown *-ary* pertaining to	Pertaining to the heart.
-eal	pertaining to	esophageal	*esophag/o* esophagus *-eal* pertaining to	Pertaining to the esophagus.
-ic	pertaining to	hypodermic	*hypo-* below *derm/o* skin *-ic* pertaining to	Pertaining to below the skin.
-ous	pertaining to	subcutaneous	*sub-* under *cutane/o* skin *-ous* pertaining to	Pertaining to under the skin.

*Coron/o literally means "crown," but is used most frequently to describe the arteries that supply blood to the heart; so the meaning "heart" has been added.

Pathology Suffixes

Pathology suffixes describe a disease process or a sign or symptom. The meanings vary according to the conditions that they describe.

Pathology Suffixes

Suffix	Meaning	Example	Word Origins	Definition
-algia	pain	cephalalgia	*cephal/o* head *-algia* pain	Pain in the head.
-cele	herniation	cystocele	*cyst/o* bladder, sac *-cele* herniation, protrusion	Herniation of the bladder.
-dynia	pain	cardiodynia	*cardi/o* heart *-dynia* pain	Pain in the heart.
-emia	blood condition	hyperlipidemia	*hyper-* excessive *lipid/o* fats *-emia* blood condition	Condition of excessive fats in the blood.
-ia	condition	agastria	*a-* without *gastr/o* stomach *-ia* condition	Condition of having no stomach.
-itis	inflammation	gastroenteritis	*gastr/o* stomach *enter/o* small intestine *-itis* inflammation	Inflammation of the stomach and small intestine.

Pathology Suffixes—cont'd

Suffix	Meaning	Example	Word Origins	Definition
-malacia	softening	chondromalacia	*chondr/o* cartilage *-malacia* softening	Softening of the cartilage.
-megaly	enlargement	splenomegaly (Fig. 1-6)	*splen/o* spleen *-megaly* enlargement	Enlargement of the spleen.
-oma	tumor, mass	osteoma	*oste/o* bone *-oma* tumor, mass	Tumor of a bone.
-osis	abnormal condition	psychosis	*psych/o* mind *-osis* abnormal condition	Abnormal condition of the mind.
-pathy	disease process	gastropathy	*gastr/o* stomach *-pathy* disease process	Disease process of the stomach.
-ptosis	prolapse, drooping, sagging	hysteroptosis	*hyster/o* uterus *-ptosis* prolapse	Prolapse of the uterus.
-rrhage, -rrhagia	bursting forth	hemorrhage	*hem/o* blood *-rrhage* bursting forth	Bursting forth of blood.
-rrhea	discharge, flow	otorrhea	*ot/o* ear *-rrhea* discharge, flow	Discharge from the ear.
-rrhexis	rupture	cystorrhexis	*cyst/o* bladder, sac *-rrhexis* rupture	Rupture of the bladder.
-sclerosis	abnormal condition of hardening	arteriosclerosis	*arteri/o* artery *-sclerosis* abnormal condition of hardening	Abnormal condition of hardening of an artery.
-stenosis	abnormal condition of narrowing	tracheostenosis	*trache/o* trachea, windpipe *-stenosis* abnormal condition of narrowing	Abnormal condition of narrowing of the trachea or windpipe.

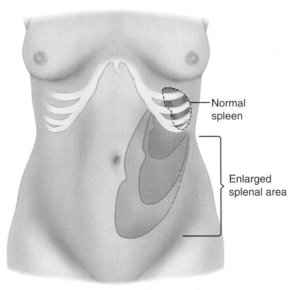

Fig. 1-6 Splenomegaly.

Normal spleen

Enlarged splenal area

⊗ Be Careful!

Don't confuse **-malacia** *meaning softening with* **-megaly** *meaning enlargement.*

⊗ Be Careful!

Don't confuse **-sclerosis** *meaning hardening with* **-stenosis** *meaning narrowing.*

⊗ Be Careful!

Don't confuse **-rrhage** *and* **-rrhagia** *meaning bursting forth with* **-rrhea** *meaning a discharge.*

⟳ EXERCISE 5: Noun-Ending, Adjective, and Pathology Suffixes

Match the suffixes with their meaning.

_____ 1. -icle, -ole, -ule   _____ 6. -malacia   A. softening
                                                          B. abnormal condition of hardening
_____ 2. -megaly   _____ 7. -algia   C. pain
                                                          D. prolapse
_____ 3. -um   _____ 8. -ptosis   E. small, tiny
                                                          F. blood condition
_____ 4. -ic, -al, -ous   _____ 9. -emia   G. enlargement
                                                          H. abnormal condition of herniation, protrusion
_____ 5. -cele   _____ 10. -sclerosis I. pertaining to
                                                          J. structure, thing, membrane

Using the method shown in Fig. 1-3 and the new word parts introduced in the tables above, decode and define these five new terms.

11. cardiomegaly _____

12. osteomalacia _____

13. valvulitis _____

14. cephalic _____

15. gastroptosis _____

Diagnostic Procedure Suffixes

Diagnostic procedure suffixes indicate a procedure that helps to determine the diagnosis. Although a few diagnostic procedures also can help to treat a disease, most are used to establish a particular disease or disorder.

Diagnostic Procedure Suffixes

Suffix	Meaning	Example	Word Origins	Definition
-graphy	process of recording	mammography	*mamm/o* breast *-graphy* process of recording	Process of recording the breast.
-metry	process of measuring	spirometry (Fig. 1-7)	*spir/o* breathing *-metry* process of measuring	Process of measuring breathing.
-opsy	process of viewing	biopsy	*bi/o* living, life *-opsy* process of viewing	Process of viewing living tissue.
-scopy	process of viewing	esophagogastroduodenoscopy	*esophag/o* esophagus *gastr/o* stomach *duoden/o* duodenum *-scopy* process of viewing	Process of viewing the esophagus, stomach, and duodenum.

Therapeutic Intervention Suffixes

Therapeutic intervention suffixes indicate types of treatment. Treatments may be medical or surgical in nature.

Therapeutic Intervention Suffixes*

Suffix	Meaning	Example	Word Origins	Definition
-ectomy	removal, resection, excision	tonsillectomy	*tonsill/o* tonsil *-ectomy* removal, excision	Removal of the tonsils.
-plasty	surgical repair	rhinoplasty	*rhin/o* nose *-plasty* surgical repair	Surgical repair of the nose.
-rrhaphy	suture, repair	splenorrhaphy	*splen/o* spleen *-rrhaphy* suture, repair	Suture of the spleen.
-stomy	new opening	colostomy	*col/o* colon, large intestine *-stomy* new opening	New opening of the colon or large intestine (Fig. 1-8).
-tomy	incision, cutting	osteotomy	*oste/o* bone *-tomy* incision	Incision into the bone.
-tripsy	crushing	lithotripsy	*lith/o* stone *-tripsy* crushing	Crushing of stones.

*In October 2015, the institution of the International Classification of Diseases, 10th revision, Clinical Modification (ICD-10-CM) will change how we define these suffixes. The current definitions of removal, resection, and excision will each have distinctly different meanings. After 2015, using only one of these words in defining a medical term gives it a very specific and potentially misleading meaning.

Fig. 1-7 Spirometry.

Don't confuse **-ectomy** meaning a removal with **-stomy** meaning a new opening or **-tomy** meaning an incision.

Stoma (new, artificial opening)

Fig. 1-8 Colostomy.

Instrument Suffixes

Instruments are indicated by yet another set of suffixes. Note the obvious similarities to their diagnostic and therapeutic "cousins." For example, electrocardiography is a diagnostic procedure that is done to measure the electrical activity in the heart; an electrocardiograph is the instrument that is used to perform electrocardiography.

Instrument Suffixes

Suffix	Meaning	Example	Word Origins	Definition
-graph	instrument to record	electrocardiograph	*electr/o* electricity *cardi/o* heart *-graph* instrument to record	Instrument to record the electricity of the heart.
-meter	instrument to measure	thermometer	*therm/o* temperature, heat *-meter* instrument to measure	Instrument to measure temperature.
-scope	instrument to view	ophthalmoscope	*ophthalm/o* eye *-scope* instrument to view	Instrument to view the eye.
-tome	instrument to cut	osteotome	*oste/o* bone *-tome* instrument to cut	Instrument to cut bone (Fig. 1-9).
-tripter	machine to crush	lithotripter	*lith/o* stone *-tripter* machine to crush	Machine to crush stone.
-trite	instrument to crush	lithotrite	*lith/o* stone *-trite* instrument to crush	Instrument to crush stone (Fig. 1-10).

Fig. 1-9 Osteotome.

Fig. 1-10 Lithotrite.

Specialty and Specialist Suffixes

Specialties and specialists require yet another category of suffixes. Someone who specializes in the study of the heart would be called a *cardiologist*. **Cardi/o** means "heart" and **-logist** means "one who specializes in the study of."

Specialty and Specialist Suffixes

Suffix	Meaning	Example	Word Origins	Definition
-er	one who	polysomnographer	*poly-* many, much, excessive, frequent *somn/o* sleep *graph/o* record *-er* one who	One who records many (aspects of) sleep.
-iatrician	one who specializes in treatment	geriatrician	*ger/o* old age *-iatrician* one who specializes in treatment	One who specializes in treatment of old age (patients).

Specialty and Specialist Suffixes—cont'd

Suffix	Meaning	Example	Word Origins	Definition
-iatrics	treatment	pediatrics	*ped/o* children *-iatrics* treatment	The treatment of children.
-iatrist	one who specializes in treatment	psychiatrist*	*psych/o* mind *-iatrist* one who specializes in treatment	One who specializes in treatment of the mind.
-iatry	process of treatment	psychiatry	*psych/o* mind *-iatry* process of treatment	Process of treatment of the mind.
-ist	one who specializes	dentist	*dent/i* teeth *-ist* one who specializes	One who specializes in the teeth.
-logist	one who specializes in the study of	psychologist†	*psych/o* mind *-logist* one who specializes in the study of	One who specializes in the study of the mind.
-logy	study of	neonatology	*neo-* new *nat/o* born, birth *-logy* study of	The study of the newborn.

*A psychiatrist holds a medical degree.
†A psychologist usually has a master's or a doctoral degree.

EXERCISE 6: Diagnosis, Therapy, Instrument, and Specialty/Specialist Suffixes

Match the suffixes with their meanings.

_____ 1. -tome   _____ 6. -scope

_____ 2. -logy   _____ 7. -scopy

_____ 3. -graphy   _____ 8. -ectomy

_____ 4. -meter   _____ 9. -tomy

_____ 5. -logist   _____ 10. -stomy

A. removal, resection
B. new opening
C. instrument to view
D. process of viewing
E. instrument to cut
F. instrument to measure
G. incision, cutting
H. process of recording
I. study of
J. one who specializes in the study of

Using the method shown in Fig. 1-3 and the new word parts introduced in the preceding tables, decode and define these five new terms.

11. osteologist _____

12. spirometer _____

13. hysteroscopy _____

14. cystoscope _____

15. splenectomy _____

Case Study *Debbie Halloran*

Debbie is a returning student who has decided on health information management (HIM) as a career. She decides to spend her time reviewing suffixes. She quickly learns that -ia means condition and -itis means inflammation, because they are parts of terms she's heard before. However, she has never heard terms that use the suffixes -sclerosis, -malacia, -ptosis, -rrhaphy, or -trite. Can you guess the right answers?

1. What does -sclerosis mean?
   a. abnormal condition of softening
   b. abnormal condition of hardening
   c. prolapse, drooping, sagging
   d. enlargement

2. What does -malacia mean?
   a. abnormal condition of softening
   b. abnormal condition of hardening
   c. prolapse, drooping, sagging
   d. enlargement

3. What does -ptosis mean?
   a. abnormal condition of softening
   b. abnormal condition of hardening
   c. prolapse, drooping, sagging
   d. enlargement

4. What does -rrhaphy mean?
   a. new opening
   b. suture, repair
   c. process of viewing
   d. instrument to crush

5. What does -trite mean?
   a. new opening
   b. suture, repair
   c. process of viewing
   d. instrument to crush

Prefixes

Prefixes modify a medical term by indicating a structure's or a condition's:

- Absence
- Location
- Number or quantity
- State

Sometimes, as with other word parts, a prefix can have more than one meaning. For example, the prefix **hypo-** can mean "below" or "deficient." To spell a term with the use of a prefix, simply add the prefix directly to the beginning of the term. No combining vowels are needed!

Prefixes

Prefix	Meaning	Example	Word Origins	Definition
a-	no, not, without	apneic	*a-* without *pne/o* breathing *-ic* pertaining to	Pertaining to without breathing.
an-	no, not, without	anophthalmia	*an-* without *ophthalm/o* eye *-ia* condition	Condition of without an eye.
ante-	forward, in front of, before	anteversion	*ante-* forward *vers/o* turning *-ion* process of	Process of turning forward.
anti-	against	antibacterial	*anti-* against *bacteri/o* bacteria *-al* pertaining to	Pertaining to against bacteria.

Prefixes—cont'd

Prefix	Meaning	Example	Word Origins	Definition
dys-	abnormal, difficult, bad, painful	dystrophy	*dys-* abnormal *-trophy* process of nourishment	Process of abnormal nourishment
endo-, end-	within	endoscopy	*endo-* within *-scopy* process of viewing	Process of viewing within.
epi-	above, upon	epigastric	*epi-* above *gastr/o* stomach *-ic* pertaining to	Pertaining to above the stomach.
hyper-	excessive, above	hyperglycemia	*hyper-* excessive *glyc/o* sugar, glucose *-emia* blood condition	Blood condition of excessive sugar.
hypo-	below, deficient	hypoglossal	*hypo-* below *gloss/o* tongue *-al* pertaining to	Pertaining to below the tongue.
inter-	between	intervertebral	*inter-* between *vertebr/o* vertebra, backbone *-al* pertaining to	Pertaining to between the backbones.
intra-	within	intramuscular	*intra-* within *muscul/o* muscle *-al* pertaining to	Pertaining to within the muscle.
neo-	new	neonatal	*neo-* new *nat/o* birth, born *-al* pertaining to	Pertaining to a newborn.
par-	near, beside	parotid	*par-* near *ot/o* ear *-id* pertaining to	Pertaining to near the ear.
para-	near, beside, abnormal	paraphilia	*para-* abnormal *phil/o* attraction *-ia* condition	Condition of abnormal attraction.
per-	through	percutaneous	*per-* through *cutane/o* skin *-ous* pertaining to	Pertaining to through the skin, as in a nephrolithotomy (Fig. 1-11).
peri-	surrounding, around	pericardium	*peri-* surrounding *cardi/o* heart *-um* structure	Structure surrounding the heart.
poly-	many, much, excessive, frequent	polyneuritis	*poly-* many *neur/o* nerve *-itis* inflammation	Inflammation of many nerves.
post-	after, behind	postnatal	*post-* after *nat/o* birth, born *-al* pertaining to	Pertaining to after birth.

Continued

Prefixes—cont'd

Prefix	Meaning	Example	Word Origins	Definition
pre-	before, in front of	prenatal	*pre-* before *nat/o* birth, born *-al* pertaining to	Pertaining to before birth.
sub-	under, below	subhepatic	*sub-* under *hepat/o* liver *-ic* pertaining to	Pertaining to under the liver.
trans-	through, across	transurethral	*trans-* through *urethr/o* urethra *-al* pertaining to	Pertaining to through the urethra.

— Skin

Fig. 1-11 Percutaneous nephrolithotomy

 Be Careful!

*Don't confuse **inter-** meaning between with **intra-** meaning within.*

 Be Careful!

*Don't confuse **ante-** meaning forward with **anti-** meaning against.*

Be Careful!

*Don't confuse **per-** meaning through with **peri-** meaning surrounding and **pre-** meaning before.*

 Be Careful!

*Don't confuse **hyper-** meaning excessive or above with **hypo-** meaning below or deficient.*

 EXERCISE 7: Prefixes

Match the prefixes with their meanings.

_____ 1. anti-   _____ 6. dys-

_____ 2. inter-   _____ 7. intra-

_____ 3. poly-   _____ 8. peri-

_____ 4. ante-   _____ 9. sub-

_____ 5. hyper-   _____ 10. per-

A. under, below
B. above, excessive
C. against
D. bad, difficult, painful, abnormal
E. within
F. many
G. through
H. between
I. forward
J. around, surrounding

Using the method shown in Fig. 1-3 and the new word parts introduced in the preceding tables, decode and define these five terms.

11. subhepatic _____

12. pericardium _____

13. dyspneic _____

14. percutaneous _____

15. hypoglycemia _____

Case Study Kate Martin

Kate realizes how important it is to memorize as many prefixes as she can. She concentrates especially hard on those prefixes that are so similar to one another. See if you can get the right answers to these confusing prefixes.

1. What is the prefix that means between?
   a. inter-
   b. intra-
   c. peri-
   d. pre-

2. What is the prefix that means near, beside, abnormal?
   a. par-
   b. para-
   c. per-
   d. peri-

3. What is the prefix that means near, beside (but not abnormal)?
   a. par-
   b. para-
   c. per-
   d. peri-

4. What is the prefix that means above, upon?
   a. endo-
   b. hypo-
   c. sub-
   d. epi-

5. What two prefixes mean within?
   a. endo-, intra-
   b. epi-, inter-
   c. ante-, per-
   d. peri-, trans-

SINGULAR/PLURAL RULES

Because most healthcare terms end with Greek or Latin suffixes, making a healthcare term singular or plural is not always done the same way as it is in English. The following table gives the most common singular/plural endings and the rules for using them. Examples of unusual singular/plural endings and singular/plural exercises will be included throughout the text.

Rules for Using Singular and Plural Endings

If a Term Ends in:	Form the Plural by:	Singular Example	Plural Example	Plural Pronounced as:
-a	dropping the -a and adding -ae	vertebra (a bone in the spine) VUR tuh brah	vertebrae VUR tuh bray	Long a, e, or i, depending on the term
-is	dropping the -is and adding -es	arthrosis (an abnormal condition of a joint) ar THROH sis	arthroses ar THROH seez	seez
-ix or -ex	dropping the -ix or -ex and adding -ices	appendix ap PEN dicks	appendices ap PEN dih seez	seez
-itis	dropping the -itis and adding -itides	arthritis (inflammation of a joint) ar THRY tiss	arthritides ar THRIH tih deez	deez
-nx	dropping the -nx and adding -nges	phalanx (a bone in the fingers or toes) FAY lanks	phalanges fuh LAN jeez	ng (as in sing) and jeez
-um	dropping the -um and adding an -a	endocardium (the structure inside the heart) en doh KAR dee um	endocardia en doh KAR dee ah	ah
-us	dropping the -us and adding an -i	digitus (a finger or toe) DIJ ih tus	digiti DIJ ih tye	eye
-y	dropping the -y and adding -ies	therapy (a treatment) THAIR ah pee	therapies THAIR ah peez	eez

EXERCISE 8: Plurals

Change the singular terms to plural using the rules given in the preceding table.

1. esophagus (the tube joining the throat with the stomach) _____

2. larynx (the voice box) _____

3. fornix (an arched structure) _____

4. pleura (the sac surrounding the lungs) _____

5. diagnosis _____

6. myocardium _____

7. cardiomyopathy _____

8. hepatitis _____

Pronunciation of Unusual Letter Combinations

Spelling	Pronunciation	Term	Meaning
eu	you	**eu**thyroid yoo THIGH royd	Good, healthy thyroid function.
ph	f (fill)	**ph**alanx FAY lanks	One of the bones of the fingers or toes.
pn	n (no)	**pn**eumonitis noo moh NYE tis	Inflammation of the lungs.
ps	s (sort)	**ps**ychology sye KALL uh jee	Study of the mind.
pt	t (top)	**pt**osis TOH sis	Prolapse, drooping.
rh, rrh	r (row)	**rh**initis rye NYE tis	Inflammation of the nose.
x	z (zoo)	**x**eroderma zeer oh DUR mah	Condition of dry skin.

EXERCISE 9: Pronunciation of Unusual Letter Combinations

If you hear a term starting with the sound and it's not under that letter in the dictionary:	Try looking for it under _____ in the dictionary.
z	
f	
n	
u	
t	
s	

Common Combining Forms

Combining Form	Meaning	Combining Form	Meaning
arteri/o	artery	lith/o	stone
arthr/o	joint	mamm/o	breast
bacteri/o	bacteria	muscul/o	muscle
bi/o	living, life	my/o	muscle
cardi/o	heart	nat/o	birth, born
cephal/o	head	neur/o	nerve
cervic/o	neck, cervix	ophthalm/o	eye
chondr/o	cartilage	oste/o	bone
col/o	large intestine, colon	ot/o	ear
coron/o	crown, heart	path/o	disease
cut/o	skin	ped/o	child
cutane/o	skin	phil/o	attraction
cyst/o	bladder, sac	pne/o	breathing
dent/i	tooth	psych/o	mind
derm/o	skin	rhin/o	nose
duoden/o	duodenum	somn/o	sleep
electr/o	electricity	spir/o	breathing
enter/o	small intestine	splen/o	spleen
esophag/o	esophagus	therm/o	heat, temperature
gastr/o	stomach	tonsill/o	tonsil
gloss/o	tongue	trache/o	trachea, windpipe
glyc/o	glucose, sugar	troph/o	nourishment
hem/o	blood	urethr/o	urethra
hepat/o	liver	valvul/o	valve
hyster/o	uterus	ven/o	vein
lingu/o	tongue	vers/o	turning
lipid/o	lipid, fat	vertebr/o	backbone, vertebra

Case Study Harry Chu

Harry is a new healthcare student who thinks he might want to become a physician's assistant. He likes to practice decoding terms. What does the combining form mean in each of the following terms?

1. Cystocele means herniation of the _____.

2. Ophthalmology is the study of the _____.

3. Otalgia is pain in the _____.

4. Osteoma is a tumor in a _____.

5. Hepatitis is inflammation of the _____.
   a. stomach
   b. gallbladder
   c. mouth
   d. liver

Case Study Medical Terminology Class

Jed, Taylor, Alan, and Jessica are enrolled in a hybrid medical terminology course, and they come to the classroom only 1 day a week. Today their instructor has assigned a group activity to practice building terms. Here are some of the terms that they have been assigned to build:

1. Inflammation of a joint _____

2. Study of the heart _____

3. Process of viewing within _____

4. Pertaining to above the stomach _____

5. Pertaining to beside the nose _____

Chapter Review

Match the word parts to their definitions.

Word Part Definitions

Prefixes
a-
anti-
dys-
inter-
intra-
par-
para-
per-
peri-
poly-
pre-
sub-

Definition

1. _____ between
2. _____ through
3. _____ near, beside
4. _____ within
5. _____ against
6. _____ no, not, without
7. _____ surrounding, around
8. _____ abnormal
9. _____ before, in front of
10. _____ many, much, excessive, frequent
11. _____ under, below
12. _____ abnormal, difficult, painful, bad

Suffixes
-ar
-dynia
-ectomy
-graphy
-ia
-itis
-logy
-meter
-oma
-osis
-pathy
-plasty
-rrhage
-rrhaphy
-rrhea
-scopy
-stenosis
-stomy
-tomy
-tripter

Definition

13. _____ pain
14. _____ discharge, flow
15. _____ narrowing
16. _____ tumor, mass
17. _____ instrument to crush
18. _____ inflammation
19. _____ bursting forth
20. _____ process of viewing
21. _____ study of
22. _____ incision, cutting
23. _____ surgical repair
24. _____ removal, resection, excision
25. _____ process of recording
26. _____ instrument to measure
27. _____ suture
28. _____ new opening
29. _____ abnormal condition
30. _____ disease process
31. _____ pertaining to
32. _____ condition

Wordshop

Prefixes	Combining Forms	Suffixes
an-	arteri/o	-al
endo-	cardi/o	-algia
epi-	cephal/o	-ectomy
hypo-	col/o	-graphy
neo-	enter/o	-ia
par-	gastr/o	-ic
per-	hepat/o	-id
peri-	hyster/o	-itis
poly-	nat/o	-logy
pre-	ophthalm/o	-megaly
sub-	ot/o	-scope
trans-	rhin/o	-scopy
	somn/o	-stomy
	splen/o	-um

Build the following terms by combining the earlier word parts. Some word parts may be used more than once. Some may not be used at all. The number in parentheses indicates the number of word parts needed

Definition	Term
1. condition of without an eye (3)	_____
2. pertaining to near the ear (3)	_____
3. pertaining to under the liver (3)	_____
4. inflammation of the stomach and small intestines (3)	_____
5. instrument to view the ear (2)	_____
6. structure surrounding the heart (3)	_____
7. new opening of the colon (2)	_____
8. process of recording an artery (2)	_____
9. process of viewing within (2)	_____
10. removal of the uterus (2)	_____
11. the study of (many) sleep (3)	_____
12. pertaining to before birth (3)	_____
13. pain in the head (2)	_____
14. pertaining to above the stomach (3)	_____
15. enlargement of the spleen (2)	_____

2

Body Structure and Directional Terminology

OBJECTIVES

- Recognize and use terms associated with the organization of the body.
- Recognize and use terms associated with positional and directional vocabulary.
- Recognize and use terms associated with the body cavities.

- Recognize and use terms associated with the abdominopelvic regions and quadrants.
- Recognize and use terms associated with planes of the body.

For interactive learning, go to the Shiland Evolve website, and click on:
- **Match the Word Parts** to review body structure and directional word parts.
- **Word Shop** to practice word building.
- **Tournament of Terminology** to test your knowledge of body structure and directional terminology terms.

*Click on **Chapter at a Glance** for a list of key word parts and terms for this chapter.*

ORGANIZATION OF THE HUMAN BODY

The human body and its general state of health and disease may be understood by studying the various **body systems**, such as the digestive and respiratory systems. Each body system is composed of different **organs**, such as the stomach and lungs. These organs are made up of combinations of **tissues**, such as epithelial and muscular tissue, which in turn are composed of various **cells** that have very specialized functions.

cell = cyt/o, -cyte

All of these levels of organization are involved in a continual process of sensing and responding to conditions in the organism's environment. A negative change at one level of one system may cause a reaction throughout the entire body. **Homeostasis** (hoh mee oh STAY sis) is the normal dynamic process of balance needed to maintain a healthy body. When the body can no longer compensate for trauma or pathogens, disease, disorder, and dysfunction result.

homeostasis
  home/o = same
  -stasis = controlling

Cells

The smallest unit of the human body is the **cell.** Although there are a number of different types of cells, all of them share certain characteristics, one of them being **metabolism** (muh TAB boh lih zum). Metabolism is the act of converting energy by continually building up substances by **anabolism** (an NAB boh lih zum) and breaking down substances by **catabolism** (kuh TAB boh lih zum) for use by the body. Metabolism can be described as an equation:

metabolism
  meta- = change, beyond
  bol/o = throwing
  -ism = state of

anabolism
  ana- = up, apart
  bol/o = throwing
  -ism = state of

Metabolism = Anabolism + Catabolism

See Fig. 2-1 for an illustration of a cell and the corresponding Cell Parts table that follows for a brief description of the pictured organelles and their functions.

catabolism
  cata- = down
  bol/o = throwing
  -ism = state of

— Cell membrane
— Ribosomes
— Nucleus
— Mitochondrion
Lysosome —
Cytoplasm —

Fig. 2-1 The cell.

Cell Parts

Cell Part	Word Origin	Function
cytoplasm SYE toh plaz um	*cyt/o* cell *-plasm* formation	Holds the organelles of the cell.
lysosome LYE soh sohm	*lys/o* dissolving *-some* body	Organelle that serves a digestive function for the cell.
ribosome RYE boh sohm	*rib/o* ribose *-some* body	Site of protein formation; contains ribonucleic acid (RNA).
mitochondrion (*pl.* mitochondria) mye toh KAHN dree un	*mitochondri/o* mitochondria *-on* structure	Converts nutrients to energy in the presence of oxygen.
nucleus (*pl.* nuclei) NOO klee us	*nucle/o* nucleus *-us* structure	Control center of cell; contains deoxyribonucleic acid (DNA), which carries genetic information.

*You can review the cell structure by clicking on **Body Spectrum Electronic Anatomy Coloring Book → Cell Structure.***

Tissues

Tissue is a group of similar cells from the same origin that together carry out a specific function. There are four major categories of **tissue**. Within each type, the tissue either is supportive (**stromal** [STROH mull] tissue), or does the actual work (**parenchymal** [pair EN kuh mull] tissue) of the organ. For example, parenchymal nerve cells are the neurons that conduct the nervous impulse. Neuroglia is stromal nerve cells that enhance and support the functions of the nervous system. The four types of tissue include the following:

Epithelial (eh puh THEE lee ul): Acts as an internal or external covering for organs (for example, the outer layer of the skin or the lining of the digestive tract). Note that the derivation of the term includes a combining form for the nipple (thel/e). Originally the term *epithelium* was used to describe the membrane covering the nipple. Later the usage was expanded to include all of the surface membranes whether they were on the skin or mucosal membrane surfaces that communicate with the outside of the body.

Connective: Includes a variety of types, all of which have an internal structural network. Examples include bone, blood, and fat.

Muscular: Includes three types, all of which share the unique property of being able to contract and relax. Examples include heart muscle, skeletal muscle, and visceral muscle.

Nervous: Includes cells that provide transmission of information to regulate a variety of functions (for example, neurons [nerve cells]).

Organs

Organs, also referred to as **viscera** (VIH sur ah) (*sing.* viscus), are arrangements of various types of tissue that accomplish specific purposes. The heart, for example, is made up of muscle tissue, called **myocardium** (mye oh KAR dee um), and it is lined with epithelial tissue known as **endocardium** (en doh KAR dee um). Organs are grouped within body systems but do have specific terms to describe their parts.

Parts of Organs

Organs can be divided into parts and have a set of terms that describe these various parts. See the table on p. 29.

---

tissue = hist/o

stromal = strom/o

parenchymal
  par- = near
  en- = in
  chym/o = juice
  -al = pertaining to

epithelial
  epi- = upon
  thel/e = nipple
  -al = pertaining to

muscle = my/o

nervous = neur/o

organ = viscer/o

myocardium
  my/o = muscle
  cardi/o = heart
  -um = structure

endocardium
  endo- = within
  cardi/o = heart
  -um = structure

Parts of Organs

	Term	Combining Form	Definition
	apex (*pl.* apices) A pecks	*apic/o*	The pointed extremity of a conical structure.
	body (corporis) KOR por iss	*corpor/o* *som/o* *somat/o*	The largest or most important part of an organ.
	fornix (*pl.* fornices) FOR nicks	*fornic/o*	Any vaultlike or arched structure.
	fundus (*pl.* fundi) FUN dis	*fund/o*	The base or deepest part of a hollow organ that is farthest from the mouth of the organ.
	hilum (*pl.* hila) HYE lum	*hil/o*	Recess, exit, or entrance of a duct into a gland, or of a nerve and vessels into an organ.
	lumen (*pl.* lumina) LOO min	*lumin/o*	The space within an artery, vein, intestine, or tube.
	sinus (*pl.* sinuses) SYE nus	*sin/o, sinus/o*	A cavity or channel in bone, a dilated channel for blood, or a cavity that permits the escape of purulent (pus-filled) material. **Antrum** (*pl.* antra) and **sinus** are synonyms.
	vestibule VES tih byool	*vestibul/o*	A small space or cavity at the beginning of a canal.

EXERCISE 1: Intracellular Functions

Match each cell part with its function.

_____ 1. mitochondria   _____ 4. lysosomes

_____ 2. ribosomes   _____ 5. cytoplasm

_____ 3. nucleus

A. directs and replicates the cell
B. watery solution within cell, holds organelles
C. contain enzymes to digest material
D. responsible for energy production
E. synthesize proteins

EXERCISE 2: Types of Tissue

Match the characteristics of the tissue with its type.

_____ 1. contracts tissue   _____ 3. has an internal structural network   A. nervous
B. epithelial
_____ 2. transmits information   _____ 4. is an internal/external body covering   C. muscular
D. connective

EXERCISE 3: Organ Parts

Match the combining forms with their meanings.

_____ 1. fund/o   _____ 5. vestibul/o   A. cavity/channel in bone/organ
B. pointed extremity of conical structure
_____ 2. lumin/o   _____ 6. fornic/o   C. archlike structure
D. base or deepest part of a hollow organ
_____ 3. sin/o   _____ 7. hil/o   E. entrance/exit/recess for ducts/vessels
F. space within an artery or tube
_____ 4. apic/o   _____ 8. corpor/o   G. largest, most important part of organ, body
H. small space at beginning of a canal

EXERCISE 4: Pertaining to Organ Parts

Fill in the blanks with the definitions of the following terms.

1. intraluminal _____

2. hilar _____

3. periapical _____

4. antral _____

5. nuclear _____

6. cytoplasmic _____

7. extracorporeal _____

8. vestibular _____

9. fundal _____

Fill in the blank with the correct organ part.

10. Fatty deposits may form in the _____ (space within) of the arteries, resulting in atherosclerosis.

11. Hector had a stone that was obstructing urine flow at the level of the _____ (exit/entrance) of the right kidney.

12. The x-rays showed a blunted _____ (tip) of the left lung.

13. The _____ (largest part) of the stomach was described as inflamed.

14. The paranasal _____ (cavities in bone) were completely blocked.

Case Study Samantha Weil

Samantha Weil, a medical terminology student with three teenagers, read the section about naming organ parts with interest and thought, "Wow, I thought this would be really boring, but I think I actually recognize some of these terms:

Fundus—I remember that when I was pregnant, my OB would measure the height of the fundus of my uterus.

Apex—I've seen the term *apex* used when referring to the top of a hill, but I didn't realize that it actually meant a point and could be at the top or the bottom of a structure, like the apex of the heart, which is actually the bottom of the heart.

Vestibule—My grandmother always referred to the vestibule of her house where she kept her umbrellas and we left our boots. It was that little area between the outside and inside doors of her house. I guess I can picture the vestibule of an ear now.

Sinus—Interesting. I thought sinuses were only in the skull, but now I know they are in my heart too.

Corporis—When I read that the body of an organ can also be called its *corporis,* the term sounded like the word "corpse" to me. And that certainly *is* a body!"

1. The base or deepest part of a hollow organ that is farthest from the mouth of an organ is called the _____?

2. A cavity or channel in bone, a dilated channel for blood, or a cavity that permits the escape of purulent material is called a _____?

3. The pointed extremity of a conical structure is the _____?

4. The largest or most important part of an organ is the _____?

5. A small space or cavity at the beginning of a canal is a _____?

Body Systems

The organs of the body systems work together to perform certain defined functions. For example, movement is a function of the musculoskeletal system. Although each system has a number of functions, one must remember that the systems interact, and problems with one system can affect the function of other systems. For example, in the condition called *secondary hypertension,* disease in one body system (usually the lungs) causes a pathologic increase in blood pressure in the cardiovascular system. This hypertensive pressure is secondary to the primary cause (lung disease). Once the disorder of the initial system resolves, the hypertension disappears.

The table on p. 32 lists each body system and its function.

 Be Careful!

Do not confuse **my/o,** *the combining form for muscle, and* **myel/o,** *the combining form for spinal cord or bone marrow.*

Body Systems

Body System	Functions
musculoskeletal muss kyoo loh SKELL uh tul	Support, movement, protection
integumentary in teg yoo MEN tuh ree	Cover and protection
gastrointestinal gass troh in TESS tih nul	Nutrition
urinary YOOR ih nair ee	Elimination of nitrogenous waste
reproductive	Reproduction
blood/lymphatic/immune lim FAT tick	Transportation of nutrients/waste, protection
cardiovascular kar dee oh VASS kyoo lur	Transportation of blood
respiratory RESS pur ah tore ee	Delivers oxygen to cells and removes carbon dioxide
nervous/behavioral NER vus	Receive/process information
special senses	Information gathering
endocrine EN doh krin	Effects changes through chemical messengers

EXERCISE 5: Body Systems and Functions

_____ 1. information gathering

_____ 2. delivers oxygen to cells and removes carbon dioxide

_____ 3. reproduction

_____ 4. cover and protection

_____ 5. transportation of nutrients/waste, protection

_____ 6. effects changes through chemical messages

_____ 7. receive/process information

_____ 8. nutrition

_____ 9. transportation of blood

_____ 10. support, movement, protection

_____ 11. elimination of nitrogenous waste

A. integumentary
B. gastrointestinal
C. male reproductive
D. musculoskeletal
E. endocrine
F. special senses
G. blood, lymphatic, and immune
H. respiratory
I. female reproductive
J. nervous
K. urinary
L. cardiovascular

Combining Forms for Body Organization

Meaning	Combining Form	Adjective Form
blood	hem/o, hemat/o	hematic
bone	oste/o, osse/o	osseous, osteal
breakdown, dissolve	lys/o	lytic
cell	cyt/o, cellul/o	cellular
epithelium	epitheli/o	epithelial
fat	adip/o	adipose
heart	cardi/o	cardiac
heart muscle	myocardi/o	myocardial
juice	chym/o	chymous
muscle	my/o, muscul/o	muscular
nerve	neur/o	neural
nipple	thel/e	thelial
nucleus	kary/o, nucle/o	nuclear
organ, viscera	organ/o, viscer/o	visceral
same	home/o	
stroma	strom/o	stromal
system	system/o	systemic
tissue	hist/o	
to throw, throwing	bol/o	

Prefixes for Body Organization

Prefix	Meaning
ana-	up, apart, away
cata-	down
en-	in
endo-	within
epi-	above, upon
meta-	beyond, change
para-	near, beside, abnormal
supra-	upward, above

Suffixes for Body Organization

Suffix	Meaning
-al, -ous	pertaining to
-ia, -ism	condition, state of
-on	structure
-plasm	formation
-some	body
-stasis	controlling, stopping
-um	structure, thing, membrane
-us	structure

The levels of organization of the body are accompanied by a number of specialties and their associated specialists.

Specialties/Specialists and General Terms

Term	Word Origin	Definition
cytology sye TALL uh jee	*cyt/o* cell *-logy* study of	The study of the cells. A **cytologist** specializes in the study of the cell. The suffix **-logist** means "one who specializes in the study of."
histology his TALL uh jee	*hist/o* tissue *-logy* study of	The study of tissues. A **histologist** specializes in the study of tissues.
anatomy ah NAT uh mee	*ana-* up, apart, away *-tomy* incision, cutting	To cut apart; the study of the structure of the body. An **anatomist** specializes in the structure of the body.
physiology fiz ee ALL uh jee	*physi/o* growth *-logy* study of	The study of growth; the study of the function of the body. A **physiologist** specializes in the study of the function of the body.
pathology pah THOL uh jee	*path/o* disease *-logy* study of	The study of disease. A **pathologist** specializes in the study of disease.
biopsy BYE op see	*bi/o* life, living *-opsy* process of viewing	Process of viewing living tissue that has been removed for the purpose of diagnosis and/or treatment.
necropsy NEH krop see	*necr/o* death, dead *-opsy* process of viewing	Process of viewing dead tissue.
autopsy AH top see	*auto-* self *-opsy* process of viewing	Process of viewing by self; term is commonly used to describe the examination of a dead body to determine cause(s) of death.

EXERCISE 6: Specialties/Specialists/General Terms

_____ 1. physi/o

_____ 2. necr/o

_____ 3. ana-

_____ 4. bi/o

_____ 5. cyt/o

_____ 6. auto-

_____ 7. -opsy

_____ 8. path/o

_____ 9. -logy

_____ 10. -logist

A. up, apart, away
B. disease
C. study of
D. cell
E. self
F. one who specializes in the study of
G. death, dead
H. process of viewing
I. life, living
J. growth

EXERCISE 7: Decoding Terms

Write the meanings of the following terms.

1. cytology _____

2. pathologist _____

3. necropsy _____

4. histologist _____

5. biopsy _____

ANATOMIC POSITION AND SURFACE ANATOMY

Now that you understand the levels of organization of the body, you need the terms that describe locations, positions, and directions on the body. A standard frame of reference, the **anatomic position**, is the position in which the body stands erect with face forward, arms at the sides, palms forward, with toes pointed forward. This position is used to describe the surface anatomy of the body, both front (ventral) and back (dorsal). Fig. 2-2 shows the anatomic position, both front and back, and it is labeled with all the surface anatomy labels that you will encounter throughout this text.

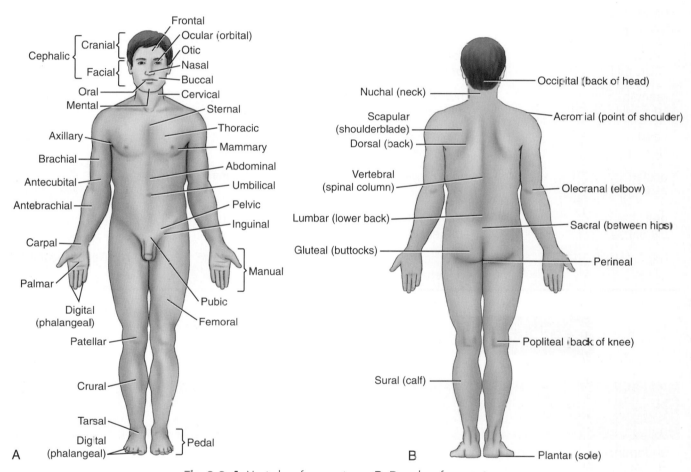

Fig. 2-2 A, Ventral surface anatomy. **B,** Dorsal surface anatomy.

Ventral Surface Anatomy Terms (Head and Neck)

Term	Word Origin	Definition
buccal BUCK uhl	*bucc/o* cheek *-al* pertaining to	Pertaining to the cheek.
cephalic seh FAL ik	*cephal/o* head *-ic* pertaining to	Pertaining to the head.
cervical SUR vik uhl	*cervic/o* neck *-al* pertaining to	Pertaining to the neck. **Collum** is a term that refers to the entire neck.
cranial KRAY nee uhl	*crani/o* skull *-al* pertaining to	Pertaining to the skull.
facial FAY shuhl	*faci/o* face *-al* pertaining to	Pertaining to the face.
frontal FRUN tuhl	*front/o* front *-al* pertaining to	Pertaining to the front, the forehead.
mental MEN tuhl	*ment/o* chin *-al* pertaining to	Pertaining to the chin.
nasal NAY zuhl	*nas/o* nose *-al* pertaining to	Pertaining to the nose.
ocular AHK you lar	*ocul/o* eye *-ar* pertaining to	Pertaining to the eye.
oral OR uhl	*or/o* mouth *-al* pertaining to	Pertaining to the mouth.
otic OH tik	*ot/o* ear *-ic* pertaining to	Pertaining to the ear. Also called **auricular.**

 Be Careful! *The term* **mental** *means pertaining to the chin as well as pertaining to the mind.*

Ventral Surface Anatomy (Trunk)

Term	Word Origin	Definition
abdominal ab DOM ih nuhl	*abdomin/o* abdomen *-al* pertaining to	Pertaining to the abdomen.
axillary AKS ih lay ree	*axill/o* axilla (armpit) *-ary* pertaining to	Pertaining to the armpit.
coxal KOKS uhl	*cox/o* hip *-al* pertaining to	Pertaining to the hip.
deltoid DELL toyd	*delt/o* triangular *-oid* resembling	The triangular muscle covering the shoulder joint. The combining form **om/o** is often used for the shoulder.
inguinal IN gwin uhl	*inguin/o* groin *-al* pertaining to	Pertaining to the groin.
mammary MAM ah ree	*mamm/o* breast *-ary* pertaining to	Pertaining to the breast.

Ventral Surface Anatomy (Trunk)—cont'd

Term	Word Origin	Definition
pelvic PELL vik	*pelv/o, pelv/i* pelvis *-ic* pertaining to	Pertaining to the pelvis.
pubic PEW bik	*pub/o* pubis *-ic* pertaining to	Pertaining to the pubis.
sternal STIR nuhl	*stern/o* sternum (breastbone) *-al* pertaining to	Pertaining to the breastbone.
thoracic thor AS ik	*thorac/o* chest *-ic* pertaining to	Pertaining to the chest. Also called **pectoral**.
umbilical um BILL ih kuhl	*umbilic/o* umbilicus (navel) *-al* pertaining to	Pertaining to the umbilicus.

Ventral Surface Anatomy (Arms and Legs)

Term	Word Origin	Definition
antecubital an tee KYOO bit uhl	*ante-* forward, in front of, before *cubit/o* elbow *-al* pertaining to	Pertaining to the front of the elbow.
brachial BRAY kee uhl	*brachi/o* arm *-al* pertaining to	Pertaining to the arm. **Antebrachial** means pertaining to the forearm.
carpal KAR puhl	*carp/o* wrist *-al* pertaining to	Pertaining to the wrist.
crural KRUR uhl	*crur/o* leg *-al* pertaining to	Pertaining to the leg.
digital DIJ ih tuhl	*digit/o* finger/toe *-al* pertaining to	Pertaining to the finger/toe. **Phalangeal** means pertaining to the bones in the fingers/toes.
femoral FEM or uhl	*femor/o* thigh *-al* pertaining to	Pertaining to the thigh.
manual MAN you uhl	*man/u* hand *-al* pertaining to	Pertaining to the hand.
palmar PALL mar	*palm/o* palm *-ar* pertaining to	Pertaining to the palm. Also termed **volar**.
patellar pah TELL ar	*patell/o, patell/a* kneecap *-ar* pertaining to	Pertaining to the kneecap.
pedal PED uhl	*ped/o* foot *-al* pertaining to	Pertaining to the foot.
tarsal TAR suhl	*tars/o* ankle *-al* pertaining to	Pertaining to the ankle.

Be Careful! Ped/o *means foot in the term pedal, but it can mean child or children in terms such as pediatrics and pedodontics.*

 Be Careful! Man/o *means pressure or scanty, but* **man/u** *and* **man/i** *mean hand.*

Dorsal Surface Anatomy Terms

Term	Word Origin	Definition
acromial ak ROH mee uhl	*acromi/o* acromion *-al* pertaining to	Pertaining to the acromion (highest point of shoulder).
dorsal DOR suhl	*dors/o* back *-al* pertaining to	Pertaining to the back.
gluteal GLOO tee uhl	*glute/o* buttocks *-al* pertaining to	Pertaining to the buttocks.
lumbar LUM bar	*lumb/o* lower back, loin *-ar* pertaining to	Pertaining to the lower back.
nuchal NOO kull	*nuch/o* neck *-al* pertaining to	Pertaining to the neck, especially the back of the neck.
olecranal oh LEK rah nuhl	*olecran/o* elbow *-al* pertaining to	Pertaining to the elbow.
perineal pair ih NEE uhl	*perine/o* perineum *-al* pertaining to	Pertaining to the perineum. The perineum is the space between the external genitalia and the anus.
plantar PLAN tur	*plant/o* sole *-ar* pertaining to	Pertaining to the sole of the foot.
popliteal pop lih TEE uhl	*poplit/o* back of knee *-eal* pertaining to	Pertaining to the back of the knee.
sacral SAY kruhl	*sacr/o* sacrum *-al* pertaining to	Pertaining to the sacrum.
scapular SKAP yoo luhr	*scapul/o* scapula, shoulderblade *-ar* pertaining to	Pertaining to the scapula.
sural SOO ruhl	*sur/o* calf *-al* pertaining to	Pertaining to the calf.
vertebral ver TEE bruhl	*vertebr/o* vertebra, spine *-al* pertaining to	Pertaining to the spine.

EXERCISE 8: Surface Anatomy Terms

Match the word parts with their definitions.

_____ 1. cephal/o

_____ 2. cervic/o

_____ 3. brachi/o

_____ 4. sur/o

_____ 5. ped/o

_____ 6. axill/o

_____ 7. thorac/o

_____ 8. mamm/o

_____ 9. digit/o

_____ 10. carp/o

_____ 11. glute/o

_____ 12. vertebr/o

_____ 13. ot/o

_____ 14. or/o

_____ 15. crani/o

_____ 16. man/u

_____ 17. cubit/o

_____ 18. plant/o

_____ 19. bucc/o

_____ 20. tars/o

A. armpit
B. wrist
C. mouth
D. breast
E. elbow
F. buttocks
G. head
H. cheek
I. backbones
J. arm
K. calf
L. ankle
M. neck
N. hand
O. sole
P. chest
Q. ear
R. foot
S. skull
T. fingers/toes

EXERCISE 9: Surface Anatomy

Label the regions with the surface anatomy terms provided.

pubic
pelvic
brachial
tarsal
manual
cervical
cranial
axillary
inguinal
buccal
femoral
facial
carpal
digital
patellar
abdominal
crural
sternal
otic
pedal
thoracic

 *Click on **Label It** to practice labeling surface anatomy.*

POSITIONAL AND DIRECTIONAL TERMS

Positional and directional terms are used in healthcare terminology to describe up and down, middle and side, and front and back. Because people may be lying down, raising their arms, and so on, standard English terms cannot be used to describe direction. The following table lists directional and positional terms as opposite pairs with their respective combining forms or prefixes and illustrations. For example, x-rays may be taken from the front of the body to the back—an anteroposterior (AP) view—or from the back to the front—a postero-anterior (PA) view (Figs. 2-3 and 2-4). The midline of the body is an imaginary line drawn from the crown of the head down between the eyes, through the chest, and separating the legs.

Fig. 2-3 Patient positioned for anteroposterior (AP) x-ray of the chest.

Fig. 2-4 Patient positioned for posteroanterior (PA) x-ray of the chest.

Positional and Directional Terms

	Term	Word Origin	Definition
	anterior (ant) an TEER ee or **ventral** VEN truhl	*anter/o* front *-ior* pertaining to *ventr/o* belly *-al* pertaining to	Pertaining to the front. Pertaining to the belly side.
	posterior (pos) poss TEER ee or **dorsal** DOR suhl	*poster/o* back *-ior* pertaining to *dors/o* back *-al* pertaining to	Pertaining to the back. Pertaining to the back of the body.
	superior (sup) soo PEER ee or **cephalad** SEFF uhl add	*super/o* upward *-ior* pertaining to *cephal/o* head *-ad* toward	Pertaining to upward. Pertaining toward the head.
	inferior (inf) in FEER ee or **caudad** CAW dad	*infer/o* downward *-ior* pertaining to *caud/o* tail *-ad* toward	Pertaining to downward. Toward the tail.
	medial MEE dee uhl	*medi/o* middle *-al* pertaining to	Pertaining to the middle (midline).
	lateral (lat) LAT ur uhl	*later/o* side *-al* pertaining to	Pertaining to the side.
	ipsilateral ip see LAT er uhl	*ipsi-* same *later/o* side *-al* pertaining to	Pertaining to the same side.
	contralateral kon trah LAT er uhl	*contra-* opposite *later/o* side *-al* pertaining to	Pertaining to the opposite side.

Positional and Directional Terms—cont'd

	Term	Word Origin	Definition
	unilateral you nee LAT er uhl	*uni-* one *later/o* side *-al* pertaining to	Pertaining to one side.
	bilateral bye LAT er uhl	*bi-* two *later/o* side *-al* pertaining to	Pertaining to two sides.
	superficial (external) soo per FISH uhl		On the surface of the body.
	deep (internal)		Away from the surface of the body.
	proximal PROCK sih muhl	*proxim/o* near *-al* pertaining to	Pertaining to near the origin.
	distal DISS tuhl	*dist/o* far *-al* pertaining to	Pertaining to far from the origin.
	dextrad* DEKS trad	*dextr/o* right *-ad* toward	Toward the right.
	sinistrad* SIN is trad	*sinistr/o* left *-ad* toward	Toward the left.
	afferent AF fur ent	*af-* toward *fer/o* to carry *-ent* pertaining to	Pertaining to carrying toward a structure.

*This is the *patient's,* not the reader's, right and left.

Continued

Positional and Directional Terms—cont'd

	Term	Word Origin	Definition
	efferent EF fur ent	**ef-** away from **fer/o** to carry **-ent** pertaining to	Pertaining to carrying away from a structure.
	supine SOO pine		Lying on one's back.
	prone PROHN		Lying on one's belly.

⊗ Be Careful!   *Do not confuse **anter/o** meaning front with **antr/o** meaning a cavity.*

⊗ Be Careful!   *Do not confuse **bi-** meaning two with **bi/o** meaning life.*

EXERCISE 10: Word Parts for Positional and Directional Terms

Match the word parts with their definitions.

_____ 1. bi-   _____ 10. contra-   A. same
                                                   B. side
_____ 2. infer/o   _____ 11. super/o   C. toward (suffix)
                                                   D. upward
_____ 3. anter/o   _____ 12. af-   E. right
                                                   F. opposite
_____ 4. ef-   _____ 13. sinistr/o   G. left
                                                   H. pertaining to
_____ 5. medi/o   _____ 14. ipsi-   I. two
                                                   J. near
_____ 6. proxim/o   _____ 15. dist/o   K. back
                                                   L. away from, out
_____ 7. uni-   _____ 16. dextr/o   M. middle
                                                   N. front
_____ 8. later/o   _____ 17. -ad   O. toward, in (prefix)
                                                   P. downward
_____ 9. poster/o   _____ 18. -icr   Q. far
                                                   R. one

 EXERCISE 11: Positional and Directional Terms

Match the definition with the correct term.

_____ 1. medial   _____ 7. prone   A. pertaining to downward
                                                   B. pertaining to carrying away from a structure
_____ 2. inferior   _____ 8. deep   C. pertaining to the middle
                                                   D. pertaining to the opposite side
_____ 3. distal   _____ 9. contralateral   E. away from the surface of the body
                                                   F. pertaining to far from the origin
_____ 4. anterior   _____ 10. ipsilateral   G. pertaining to carrying toward a structure
                                                   H. pertaining to the same side
_____ 5. dorsal   _____ 11. afferent   I. pertaining to the back of the body
                                                   J. lying on one's back
_____ 6. supine   _____ 12. efferent   K. pertaining to the front
                                                   L. lying on one's belly

Medical Record John Greco

Greco, John J - 759990 Opened by Perez, Raechel, MD

Task   Edit   View   Time Scale   Options   Help

Greco, John J   Age: 33 years   Sex: Male   Loc: CMH-STL
                                     DOB: 01/27/1982   MRN: 759990   FIN: 5411777

Reference Text Browser | Form Browser | Medication Profile

Orders | Last 48 Hours | ED | Lab | Radiology | Assessments | **Surgery** | Clinical Notes | Pt. Info | Pt. Schedule | Task List | I & O | MAR

Flowsheet: Surgery   Level: Operative Report   Table   Group   List

Navigator
✓   Operative Report

Preoperative diagnosis: Esophagitis with stricture
Postoperative diagnosis: Same, along with gastritis
Surgical procedure: Upper GI endoscopy with biopsy

33-year-old male with a long history of gastroesophageal reflux, history of strictures, recommended for GI endoscopy. The patient was taken to the endoscopy suite, and under topical anesthetic, the endoscope was inserted without difficulty. The **proximal** and midesophagus were normal. The **distal** esophagus showed signs of reflux with circumferential stricture. Upon entering the stomach, it was filled with bile. No **proximal** lesions. A biopsy was performed on the antrum for *Helicobacter*. Pyloric channel and duodenum were clean. J-maneuver revealed no fundic abnormalities. The endoscope was withdrawn, and the patient then was dilated with a #42 French with Hurst dilators. The patient tolerated the procedure well and returned to the recovery room in stable condition.

PROD | MAHAFC | 26 March 2015 | 12:11

EXERCISE 12: Operative Report

Using the operative report above, answer the following questions.

1. Which organ was described as inflamed before the operation? _____

2. After the operation, which organ/organs were described as inflamed? _____

3. Translate: "The proximal and midesophagus were normal." _____

4. Which end of the esophagus was farthest from the point of origin? Circle one. *(proximal esophagus, midesophagus, distal esophagus)* _____

BODY CAVITIES

The body is divided into five cavities (Fig. 2-5). Two of these five cavities are in the back of the body and are called the **dorsal** (DOOR sul) **cavities**. The other three cavities are in the front of the body and are called the **ventral** (VEN trul) **cavities**. Most of the body's organs are in one of these five body cavities.

Dorsal Cavities

The **cranial** (KRAY nee ul) **cavity** contains the brain and is surrounded and protected by the cranium, or skull. The **spinal** (SPY nul) **cavity** contains the spinal cord and is surrounded and protected by the bones of the spine, or vertebrae.

Ventral Cavities

The **thoracic** (thoh RASS ick) cavity contains the heart, lungs, esophagus, and trachea (windpipe) and is protected by the ribs, the **sternum** (breastbone), and the **vertebrae** (backbones). This chest cavity is further divided into the two **pleural** (PLOOR ul) **cavities** that contain the lungs; the **mediastinum** (mee dee uh STY num), the space between the lungs; and the **pericardial** (pair ih KAR dee ul) **cavity** that holds the heart.

The pleura is a double-folded serous (watery) membrane that serves to provide a small amount of lubrication that allows the lungs to contract and expand with minimal friction. The side of the membrane that is closest to the lung is called the **visceral pleura**, and the side that is closest to the body wall is called the **parietal pleura**.

The pericardial cavity shares a similar structure to the pleural cavity, again having a double-folded serous membrane designed to avoid friction on the organ that it encloses. In this case, the inner membrane is termed the **visceral pericardium**, and the outer membrane is called the **parietal pericardium**.

The **abdominopelvic** (ab DOM ih noh FELL vick) **cavity** is composed of two cavities (abdominal and pelvic) that are not separated by any physical structure. Because nothing physically separates the abdominal and pelvic cavities, they are often collectively referred to as the *abdominopelvic cavity*.

The abdominal cavity contains the stomach, liver, gallbladder, pancreas, spleen, and intestines, whereas the pelvic cavity contains the bladder and reproductive organs. The skin and muscles provide the only anterior protection for

dorsal = dors/o	
ventral = ventr/o	
cranial = crani/o	
spinal = spin/o	
thoracic = thorac/o	
sternum = stern/o	
vertebrae = vertebr/o	
pleural = pleur/o	
mediastinum = mediastin/o	
abdomen = abdomin/o, celi/o, lapar/o	

Be Careful!

*The term **abdomen** refers to a region, whereas the **stomach** is an organ.*

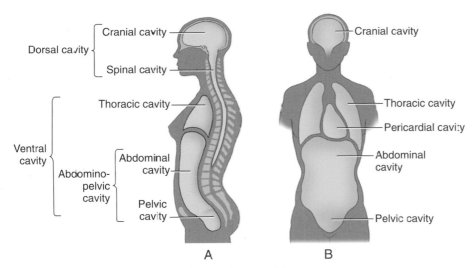

Fig. 2-5 Body cavities.

diaphragm = diaphragmat/o, diaphragm/o, phren/o	
pelvis = pelv/o, pelv/i	
peritoneum = peritone/o	
organ = viscer/o	
wall = pariet/o	
retroperitoneum retro- = behind peritone/o = peritoneum	

the abdominal cavity, and the vertebrae provide the only posterior protection. The abdominal cavity is separated from the thoracic cavity by a broad dome-shaped muscle called the **diaphragm** (DYE uh fram).

The **pelvic** (PELL vick) **cavity** contains the bladder and reproductive organs. These organs are cradled on the sides and in the back by the pelvic bones.

The entire abdominopelvic cavity is lined with yet another serous membrane called the **peritoneum** (pair ih tih NEE um) (Fig. 2-6, *A*). The **parietal** (puh RYE uh tul) layer of the peritoneum lines the abdominopelvic cavity, whereas the **visceral** (VISS er ul) layer surrounds its organs. The term *parietal* is derived from a Latin term for wall, hence this layer is always the one closest to the body wall. The visceral layer of the peritoneum (or pericardium) is the one that is closest to the organ or organs that it encloses. The greater and lesser **omenta** (oh MEN tah) are extensions of the visceral peritoneum that hold and support the cavity's organs (see Fig. 2-6, *B*). The fold of the peritoneum that joins the parietal and visceral layers and attaches it to the posterior wall of the abdominal cavity is called the **mesentery** (MEZ eh tair ee). The **retroperitoneum** is the space in the abdominal cavity behind the peritoneum, which contains the kidneys and other organs.

Fig. 2-6 The peritoneum. **A,** The parietal layer of the peritoneum that lines the abdominopelvic cavity and the visceral layer that lines the organs. **B,** The greater omentum and mesentery.

EXERCISE 13: Body Cavities

Match the organ with the appropriate body cavity.

_____ 1. cranial   _____ 4. spinal   A. spinal cord
                                               B. bladder

_____ 2. abdominal   _____ 5. thoracic   C. stomach
                                                D. brain

_____ 3. pelvic   E. heart

ABDOMINOPELVIC REGIONS

The **abdominopelvic regions** are the nine regions that lie over the abdominopelvic cavity (Fig. 2-7). The area in the center of the abdominopelvic region is called the **umbilical** (um BILL ih kul) area. Laterally, to the left and right of this area, are the **lumbar** (LUM bar) regions. They are called the *lumbar regions* because they are bound by the lumbar vertebrae. Superior to the lumbar regions, and below the ribs, are the **hypochondriac** (hye poh KON dree ack) regions. Medial to the hypochondriac regions, and superior to the umbilical region, is the **epigastric** (eh pee GASS trick) region. Inferior to the umbilical region is the **hypogastric** (hye poh GASS trick) region, and lateral to the sides of the hypogastric region are, respectively, the right and left **iliac** (ILL ee ack) regions, sometimes referred to as the **inguinal** (ING gwih nul) regions.

ABDOMINOPELVIC QUADRANTS

A simpler method of naming a location in the abdominopelvic area is to divide the area into quadrants, using the navel as the intersection. These quadrants are referred to as either right or left, upper or lower (Fig. 2-8). In the right upper quadrant (RUQ) lies the liver. In the left upper quadrant (LUQ) lie the stomach and the spleen. The appendix is in the right lower quadrant (RLQ). If a patient complains of pain in the area of **McBurney's point**, the area that is approximately two-thirds of the distance between the navel and the hip bone in the RLQ, appendicitis is suspected. Except for the appendix, the left lower quadrant (LLQ) contains organs similar to the lower right. In the LLQ, halfway between the navel and the hip bone, is **Munro's point**. This is a standard site of entrance for surgeons who perform laparoscopic surgery.

 Be Careful! *Do not confuse **ile/o** meaning ileum (part of the intestine) with **ili/o** meaning ilium (part of the hip).*

abdominopelvic
    abdomin/o = abdomen
    pelv/o = pelvis
    -ic = pertaining to

umbilical = umbilic/o, omphal/o

lumbar = lumb/o

hypochondriac
    hypo- = under
    chondr/o = cartilage
    -iac = pertaining to

epigastric
    epi- = upon, above
    gastr/o = stomach
    -ic = pertaining to

hypogastric
    hypo- = under
    gastr/o = stomach
    -ic = pertaining to

iliac = ili/o

inguinal = inguin/o

⊗ **Be Careful!**

*Do not confuse **hypo-** meaning under or deficient with **hyper-** meaning above or excess.*

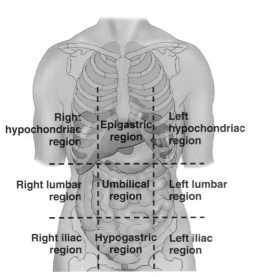

Right hypochondriac region | Epigastric region | Left hypochondriac region

Right lumbar region | Umbilical region | Left lumbar region

Right iliac region | Hypogastric region | Left iliac region

Fig. 2-7 Abdominopelvic regions.

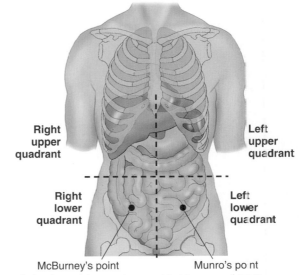

Right upper quadrant | Left upper quadrant

Right lower quadrant | Left lower quadrant

McBurney's point | Munro's point

Fig. 2-8 Abdominopelvic quadrants with Munro and McBurney points.

PLANES OF THE BODY

Another way of describing the body is by dividing it into planes, or flat surfaces, that are imaginary cuts or sections through the body. The use of plane terminology is common when imaging of internal body parts by computed tomography (CT) scans, magnetic resonance imaging (MRI), positron emission tomography (PET) scans, or other imaging techniques. Figs. 2-9 to 2-11 show the three body planes and corresponding views of the brain.

Sagittal (SAJ ih tul) **planes** are vertical planes that separate the sides from each other (see Fig. 2-9). A **midsagittal plane**, also termed the **median plane**, separates the body into equal right and left halves. The **frontal** (or **coronal** [koh ROH nul]) **plane** divides the body into front and back portions (see Fig. 2-10). The **transverse plane** (also called **cross-sectional**) divides the body horizontally into an upper part and a lower part (see Fig. 2-11). A fourth plane, the **oblique plane**, not as commonly used as the first three, divides the body at a slanted angle.

sagittal = sagitt/o

mid- = middle

frontal = front/o

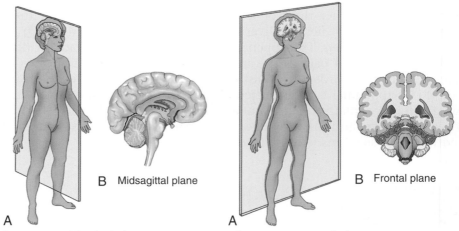

Fig. 2-9 A, Midsagittal plane.
B, Midsagittal section of the brain.

Fig. 2-10 A, Frontal plane.
B, Frontal section of the brain.

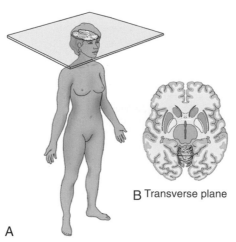

Fig. 2-11 A, Transverse plane.
B, Transverse section of the brain.

Combining and Adjective Forms for Body Cavities, Abdominopelvic Quadrants and Regions, and Planes

Meaning	Combining Form	Adjective Form
abdomen	abdomin/o, celi/o, lapar/o	abdominal, celiac
back	dors/o	dorsal
cartilage	chondr/o	chondral
cranium (skull)	crani/o	cranial
diaphragm	diaphragmat/o, diaphragm/o, phren/o	diaphragmatic, phrenic
front, belly side	front/o, ventr/o	frontal, ventral
groin	inguin/o	inguinal
ileum	ile/o	ileal
ilium	ili/o	iliac
lower back, loin	lumb/o	lumbar
mediastinum	mediastin/o	mediastinal
organ	viscer/o, organ/o	visceral
pelvis	pelv/i, pelv/o	pelvic
peritoneum	peritone/o	peritoneal
pleura	pleur/o	pleural
spine	spin/o	spinal, spinous
sternum	stern/o	sternal
stomach	gastr/o	gastric
thorax (chest)	thorac/o	thoracic
umbilicus (navel)	umbilic/o, omphal/o	umbilical, omphalic
vertebra	vertebr/o	vertebral
wall	pariet/o	parietal

Prefixes for Body Cavities, Abdominopelvic Quadrants and Regions, and Planes

Prefix	Meaning
epi-	above, upon
hyper-	excessive, above
hypo-	deficient, below, under
mid-	middle
trans-	through, across

Suffixes for Body Cavities, Abdominopelvic Quadrants and Regions, and Planes

Suffix	Meaning
-ant, -iac, -ic	pertaining to
-verse	to turn

Click on *Hear It, Spell It* to practice spelling the body structure and directional terms that you have learned in this chapter.

 EXERCISE 14: Abdominopelvic Regions

Using your knowledge of directional terms and the nine abdominopelvic regions, answer the following questions.

1. Superior to the umbilical region is the _____ region.

2. Lateral to the umbilical region are the left and right _____ regions.

3. Medial to the left and right inguinal regions is the _____ region.

4. Inferior to the lumbar regions are the left and right _____ regions.

5. Lateral to the epigastric region are the right and left _____ regions.

 EXERCISE 15: Abdominopelvic Regions

Label the abdominopelvic regions using the terms provided.

right iliac
left lumbar
epigastric
hypogastric
right hypochondriac
left hypochondriac
umbilical
right lumbar
left iliac

 EXERCISE 16: Planes of the Body

1. Which plane divides the body into superior and inferior portions? _____

2. Which plane divides the body into equal left and right sections? _____

3. Which plane divides the body into anterior and posterior sections? _____

Medical Record **Elise Duncan**

Duncan, Elise M - 554427 Opened by Andersen, Michelle J

Task   Edit   View   Time Scale   Options   Help

| Duncan, Elise M | Age: 17 years | Sex: Female | Loc: CMH-STL |
| | DOB: 01/21/1997 | MRN: 554427 | FIN: 5411777 |

Reference Text Browser   Form Browser   Medication Profile

Orders | Last 48 Hours | ED | Lab | Radiology | Assessments | **Surgery** | Clinical Notes | Pt. Info | Pt. Schedule | Task List | I & O | MAR

Flowsheet: Surgery   Level: Operative Report   ⦿ Table ○ Group ○ List

Navigator

✔ Operative Report

The patient was brought to the operating room, given a spinal anesthetic, and placed in the supine position. The right ankle then was prepped and draped in the usual sterile manner. The operation was performed under tourniquet control.

(1) <u>An incision was made laterally over the distal fibula.</u> Initial incision went through skin and subcutaneous tissue. Bleeders throughout the procedure were treated, clamped, and electrocoagulated. The fascia then was incised, and the fracture was identified. The fracture ends were cleared and clamped in anatomic position. A 6-hole, ⅓ semitubular plate was placed posterolaterally and transfixed with the screws. Anatomic position was achieved.

We then proceeded medially, (2) <u>where a short incision was made over the medial malleolus.</u> Initial incision went through skin and subcutaneous tissue. Bleeders throughout the procedure were treated, clamped, and electrocoagulated. The fascia was incised, and a large medial malleolar fracture fragment was identified. The fracture was freshened and then clamped. Three 3-M staples then were used to transfix the fracture. (3 and 4) <u>Intraoperative x-rays then were taken, AP and lateral, which showed anatomic position of all fractures with the ankle joint in anatomic position.</u>

The wound was thoroughly irrigated. Both sides were closed with 3-0 Dexon, subcutaneous tissue with 2-0 Dexon, and the skin with skin clips. A compressive dressing was applied, followed by the application of a short leg cast.

PROD | MAHAFC | 8 June 2014 | 07:32

EXERCISE 17: Operative Report

Refer to the preceding operative report to answer the following questions. Circle the correct answer.

1. "The incision (that) was made laterally over the distal fibula." If you know that the fibula is one of the lower lateral leg bones, the distal end is *(closer to the hip/closer to the toes)*.

2. The malleoli are processes at the distal ends of the fibula and tibia. The medial malleolus is on the *(inner surface/outer surface)* of the leg.

3. The "intraoperative x-rays" were taken *(before/during/after)* the operation.

4. The AP view of the ankle joint fracture was taken from *(back to front/front to back)*.

Abbreviations

Abbreviation	Definition	Abbreviation	Definition
ant	anterior	PA	posteroanterior
AP	anteroposterior	PET	positron emission tomography
CT	computed tomography	pos	posterior
inf	inferior	RLQ	right lower quadrant
lat	lateral	RUQ	right upper quadrant
LLQ	left lower quadrant	sup	superior
LUQ	left upper quadrant		

EXERCISE 18: Abbreviations

1. Which abbreviation means pertaining to the back? _____

2. Which abbreviation means pertaining to upward? _____

3. Which abbreviation means pertaining to the front? _____

4. Which abbreviation means pertaining to the side? _____

5. Which abbreviation means pertaining to downward? _____

Case Study   *Elena Novoyenko*

Elena Novoyenko immigrated to the US from Russia 5 years ago and is still in the process of learning English. However, she decided that she would enjoy a career in healthcare, so she signed up for an online medical terminology class. She realizes how important learning word parts is to understanding the meanings of terms that are built from word parts. For example she was able to remember some of the abdominopelvic regions by memorizing their prefixes.

Epigastric region—The region that is *above/upon* (**epi**-) the stomach.

Hypogastric region—The region *below* (**hypo**-) the stomach.

She was able to figure out the difference between afferent and efferent by remembering that:

Afferent—The prefix **af**- means *toward*, so the word afferent means toward a structure.

Efferent—The prefix **ef**- means *away from*, so the word efferent means away from a structure.

She was also able to memorize the difference between contralateral and ipsilateral by remembering that:

Contralateral—The prefix **contra**- means *opposite*, so the term contralateral means pertaining to the opposite side.

Ipsilateral—The prefix **ipsi**- means *same*, so the term ipsilateral means pertaining to the same side.

1. Which abdominopelvic region is located above the stomach? _____

2. Which abdominopelvic region is located below the stomach? _____

3. Which term means "pertaining to the opposite side?"
   a. ipsilateral
   b. contralateral

4. Which term means "pertaining to the same side?"
   a. ipsilateral
   b. contralateral

5. Which prefix means "toward?"
   a. ef-
   b. af-

6. Which prefix means "away from?"
   a. ef-
   b. af-

Chapter Review

Match the word parts to their definitions.

Word Part Definitions

Prefix		Definition
af-	1. _____	above, upon
bi-	2. _____	beyond, change
contra-	3. _____	one
ef-	4. _____	within
endo-	5. _____	two
epi-	6. _____	toward
ipsi-	7. _____	same
meta-	8. _____	opposite
uni-	9. _____	away from

Combining Form		Definition
anter/o	10. _____	organ
axill/o	11. _____	downward
brachi/o	12. _____	front
caud/o	13. _____	far
cephal/o	14. _____	middle
cervic/o	15. _____	armpit
corpor/o	16. _____	upward
crani/o	17. _____	near
cyt/o	18. _____	left
dextr/o	19. _____	arm
dist/o	20. _____	tail
hist/o	21. _____	abdomen
infer/o	22. _____	side
inguin/o	23. _____	right
lapar/o	24. _____	back
later/o	25. _____	tissue
medi/o	26. _____	body
poster/o	27. _____	head
proxim/o	28. _____	skull
super/o	29. _____	cell
sinistr/o	30. _____	groin
thorac/o	31. _____	neck
viscer/o	32. _____	chest

Wordshop

Prefixes	Combining Forms	Suffixes
bi-	abdomin/o	-ad
contra-	anter/o	-al
hyper-	crani/o	-ar
hypo-	cyt/o	-ic
in-	dextr/o	-ia
inter-	gastr/o	-ior
intra-	hist/o	-logy
ipsi-	inguin/o	-oid
mid-	later/o	-plasm
supra–	lumb/o	
	pelv/o	
	poster/o	
	sagitt/o	
	super/o	
	thorac/o	

Build the following terms by combining the preceding word parts. Some word parts may be used more than once. Some may not be used at all. The number in parentheses is the number of word parts needed.

Definition	Term
1. pertaining to the middle of the sagittal plane (3)	_____
2. pertaining to two sides (3)	_____
3. toward the right (2)	_____
4. pertaining to back to front (3)	_____
5. pertaining to the chest (2)	_____
6. pertaining to the abdomen and pelvis (3)	_____
7. pertaining to the lower back (2)	_____
8. pertaining to the opposite side (3)	_____
9. formation of cells (2)	_____
10. pertaining to upward (2)	_____
11. pertaining to above the chest (3)	_____
12. the study of tissue (2)	_____
13. pertaining to under the stomach (3)	_____
14. pertaining to the same side (3)	_____
15. pertaining to within the skull (3)	_____

Sort the terms below into the correct categories.

Term Sorting

Organization of the Body	Positional and Directional Terms	Body Cavities and Planes	Abdominal Regions and Quadrants

afferent	hilum	nucleus	supine
anterior	hypochondriac	organ	system
apex	hypogastric	pleural	thoracic
coronal	iliac	posterior	transverse
cranial	inguinal	prone	umbilical
cytoplasm	lateral	sagittal	ventral
distal	lumbar	sinus	vestibule
efferent	lumen	spinal	viscera
epigastric	midsagittal	superior	

Replace the highlighted words with the correct terms.

Translations

1. Susie was being treated for a cut on the **pertaining to the sole of the foot** surface of her foot and a wart on **the pertaining to the palm** surface of her hand.

2. Maureen located a vein in the **pertaining to the front of the elbow** space of the patient's left arm for a blood draw.

3. The patient described her leg pain as **pertaining to two sides,** although occasionally it seemed to be only on the right.

4. Sam had cancer sores on his **pertaining to the cheek** membrane.

5. The patient had a **process of viewing living tissue that has been removed for the purpose of diagnosis** of a mole that had recently increased in size.

6. The **space within an artery, vein, intestine, or tube** of one of the patient's coronary arteries was completely blocked.

7. The paralyzed patient had fractured one of the bones in his **pertaining to the chest** spine.

8. Nora had a fracture of the **pertaining to far from the origin** phalanx of her right index finger.

9. A tumor growing in the patient's **the space between the lungs** pressed on his esophagus.

10. The damage caused by the patient's right hemispheric stroke was **pertaining to the opposite side.**

11. The patient was in a **lying on one's back** position so that the physician could examine her abdomen.

12. Jeremy complained of pain resulting from a **lateral to the sides of the hypogastric region** hernia.

13. The man had **pertaining to the chest** and **pertaining to the hip** contusions.

14. Mr. Jones had **pertaining to above the stomach** pain.

RADIOLOGY REPORT

Using the radiology report above, answer the following questions.

1. Which end of the radius was fractured? The end closest to the wrist or the end nearest the elbow?

2. Was the bone displaced backward or forward?

3. The term *articular* means "pertaining to the _____."

4. What does *dorsal* mean?

5. A PA view means _____.

Musculoskeletal System

3

CHAPTER OUTLINE

Functions of the Musculoskeletal
  System
Specialties/Specialists
Anatomy and Physiology
Axial Skeleton
Appendicular Skeleton
  Medical Record: Dylan Koldmann

Pathology
  Case Study: LeDanton Bradford
  Case Study: Vic Vandonberg
  Case Study: Monica Washington
  Case Study: Tyro Londoff
  Medical Record: Jean Herold
Diagnostic Procedures

Therapeutic Interventions
Pharmacology
  Case Study: Consuela Esteban
  Case Study: Pia Romana
  Case Study: Barbara Eversole
Chapter Review
  Medical Record: Evelyn Auden

OBJECTIVES

- Recognize and use terms related to the anatomy and physiology of the musculoskeletal system.
- Recognize and use terms related to the pathology of the musculoskeletal system.

- Recognize and use terms related to the diagnostic procedures for the musculoskeletal system.
- Recognize and use terms related to the therapeutic interventions for the musculoskeletal system.

For interactive learning go to the Shiland Evolve website and click on:
- **Match the Word Parts** to review musculoskeletal word parts.
- **Word Shop** to practice building musculoskeletal terms.
- **Tournament of Terminology** to test your knowledge of the musculoskeletal system.
- **Term Sorting** to sort musculoskeletal terms into categories.
*Click on **Chapter at a Glance** to print off a list of key terms and word parts for this chapter.*

musculoskeletal
muscul/o = muscle
skelet/o = skeleton

bone = oste/o, oss/i, osse/o

joint = arthr/o, articul/o

muscle = muscul/o, my/o, myos/o

ligament = ligament/o, syndesm/o

tendon = tendin/o, tend/o, ten/o

fascia = fasci/o

cartilage = chondr/o, cartilag/o

hematopoiesis
hemat/o = blood
-poiesis = formation

 Be Careful!

*Do not confuse the combining form **fasci/o** meaning fascia with the combining form **faci/o** meaning face.*

orthopedist
orth/o = straight
ped/o = child
-ist = one who specializes

rheumatology
rheumat/o = watery flow
-logy = study of

physiatry
physi/o = nature
-iatry = process or treatment

FUNCTIONS OF THE MUSCULOSKELETAL SYSTEM

The **musculoskeletal** (muss skyoo loh SKELL uh tul) **system (MS)** consists of three interrelated parts: **bones, joints (articulations),** and **muscles.** Bones are connected to one another by fibrous bands of tissue called **ligaments** (LIH gah ments). Muscles are attached to the bone by bands of tissue called **tendons** (TEN duns). The tough fibrous covering of the muscles (and some nerves and blood vessels) is called the **fascia** (FASH ee ah). **Cartilage** (KAR tih lij) is a flexible form of connective tissue that covers the ends of many bones, gives form to the external ear and tip of the nose, and provides support and protection to many other sites in the body.

Imagine a body without bones and muscles! Where would the organ systems be placed? What would protect the vital organs? How would a person move? The musculoskeletal system meets these needs by:

- Acting as a framework for the organ systems
- Protecting many of the body's organs
- Providing the organism with the ability to move

Along with these functions, some bones are responsible for storage of minerals (calcium [Ca] and phosphorus [P]) and the continual formation of blood, a process called **hematopoiesis** (hee mah toh poh EE sis), in the bone marrow.

 Be Careful!   *The combining form **ped/o** can mean child or foot.*

SPECIALTIES/SPECIALISTS

Orthopedics is the healthcare specialty that deals with the majority of musculoskeletal disorders. Historically, the word **orthopedics** comes from **orth/o** (straight) and **ped/o** (child), because corrective procedures for disorders like knock-knees and bowlegs were most successful with the softer bones of children. The specialist is called an **orthopedist.**

Rheumatology is a specialty that deals with disorders of connective tissue, including bone and cartilage. The origin of the term is derived from the Greeks who believed that many joint disorders were caused by an effusion (outpouring) of fluid into the joint space. The specialist is called a **rheumatologist.**

Physiatry, also called *physical medicine,* concerns diagnosis and treatment of disease or injury with the use of physical agents, such as exercise, heat, massage, and light. The specialist is called a **physiatrist.**

 Be Careful!   *Don't confuse a **physiatrist** with a **psychiatrist**.*

EXERCISE 1: Combining Forms for the Musculoskeletal System

Match the musculoskeletal combining forms with their meanings. More than one answer may be correct.

_____ 1. joint   _____ 5. ligament   A. fasci/o   G. tendin/o
                                                 B. hemat/o   H. ligament/o
_____ 2. bone   _____ 6. fascia   C. oste/o   I. myos/o
                                                 D. osse/o   J. articul/o
_____ 3. muscle   _____ 7. cartilage   E. arthr/o   K. syndesm/o
                                                 F. chondr/o   L. ten/o
_____ 4. tendon   _____ 8. blood

Decode the following terms using your knowledge of musculoskeletal word parts and suffixes that you learned in Chapter 1.

9. articular _____

10. tendinous _____

11. muscular _____

12. syndesmal _____

13. chondral _____

14. osseous _____

ANATOMY AND PHYSIOLOGY

Bones

Types of Bones

Most adult bodies contain 206 bones. These bones are categorized as belonging either to the **axial** (ACK see ul) **skeleton,** which consists of the skull, rib cage, and spine, or the **appendicular** (ap pen DICK yoo lur) **skeleton,** which consists of the shoulder bones, collar bones, pelvic bones, arms, and legs (Fig. 3-1). Human bones appear in a variety of shapes that suit their function in the body. See Fig. 3-1 and the following table for the locations and descriptions of these bones.

appendicular = appendic/o

skeleton = skelet/o

Shapes of Human Bones

Types	Examples
long bones	humerus (upper arm bone), femur (thigh bone)
short bones	carpal (wrist bone), tarsal (ankle bone)
flat bones	sternum (breastbone), scapula (shoulder blade)
irregular bones	vertebra (backbone), stapes (a bone of the ear)
sesamoid (SEH sah moyd) bones	patella (kneecap)

Fig. 3-1 Axial and appendicular skeleton. The structures that comprise the axial skeleton are in blue.

osteocyte
oste/o = bone
-cyte = cell

osteoblast
oste/o = bone
-blast = embryonic

osteoclast
oste/o = bone
-clast = breaking down

bone marrow = myel/o

diaphysis
dia- = through
-physis = growth, nature

epiphysis
epi- = above
-physis = growth, nature

Bone Structure

All bones are composed of mature bone cells, which is called **osteocytes** (OS tee oh sytes), and the material between the cells, which is called the **matrix** (MAY tricks). The matrix stores calcium (Ca) and phosphorus (P) for the body to use as needed in the form of mineral salts. Other types of bone cells include **osteoblasts,** cells that build bone, and **osteoclasts,** cells that break down bone cells to transform them as needed. The osteocytes and matrix together make up the hard, outer layer of bone known as **compact bone.** Within the compact bony tissue is a second layer of bone tissue called **spongy** or **cancellous** (KAN seh lus) **bone.** This spongy bone is composed of the same osteocytes and matrix, but, as its name implies, it is less dense. Within the spongy layer lie the medullary cavity and the red **bone marrow,** which produces all of the blood cells needed by the body.

Each long bone (Fig. 3-2) is composed mainly of a long shaft called the **diaphysis** (dye AFF ih sis). Each end of the bone is called an **epiphysis** (eh PIFF ih

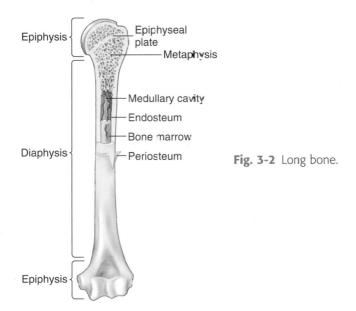

Epiphysis
Epiphyseal plate
Metaphysis
Medullary cavity
Endosteum
Bone marrow
Periosteum
Diaphysis
Epiphysis

Fig. 3-2 Long bone.

Be Careful!

Remember that the ends of the long bones closest to the points of attachment (hips and shoulders) are described as **proximal,** *whereas those farthest from the points of attachment (feet and hands) are described as* **distal.**

sis) (*pl.* epiphyses). Underneath the epiphyses are the **epiphyseal** (eh pee FIZZ ee ul) **plates,** which are the areas where bone growth normally occurs. Around the ages from 16 to 25, the plates close, and bone growth stops. The epiphysis and epiphyseal plates together form the **metaphysis** (meh TAFF ih sis).

The outer covering of the bone is called the **periosteum** (pair ee OS tee um), and the inner lining of the bone is known as the **endosteum** (en DOS tee um). These two coverings hold the cells responsible for bone remodeling: osteoblasts and osteoclasts. The shape of a bone enables practitioners to speak very specifically about a particular area on that bone. For instance, any groove, opening, or hollow space is called a **depression.** Depressions provide an entrance and exit for vessels and protection for the organs they hold. Raised or projected areas are called **processes.** These are often areas of attachment for ligaments or tendons. The tables that follow give examples of bone depressions and processes.

metaphysis
  meta- = change
  -physis = growth, nature

periosteum
  peri- = surrounding
  oste/o = bone
  -um = structure

endosteum
  endo- = within
  oste/o = bone
  -um = structure

Bone Depressions

Depression	Combining Form	Meaning/Function	Example
foramen (*pl.* foramina) foh RAY men	foramin/o	An opening or hole	foramen magnum, mental foramina
fossa (*pl.* fossae) FAH sah	foss/o	A hollow or depression, especially on the surface of the end of a bone	olecranal fossa
sinus (*pl.* sinuses) SYE nus	sin/o sinus/o	A cavity or channel lined with a membrane	paranasal sinuses

Bone Processes			
Process	Combining Form	Meaning/Function	Example
condyle KON dyle	condyl/o	A rounded projection at the end of a bone that anchors the ligaments and articulates with adjacent bones	medial condyle of the femur
crest		A narrow elongated elevation	iliac crest
epicondyle eh pee KON dyle	epicondyl/o	A projection on the surface of the bone above the condyle	lateral epicondyle of the humerus
head		A rounded, usually proximal portion of some long bones	femoral head, humeral head
spine	spin/o	A thornlike projection	spinous process of a vertebra
trochanter troh KAN tur	trochanter/o	One of two bony projections on the proximal ends of the femurs that serve as points of attachment for muscles	greater trochanter
tubercle TOO bur kuhl	tubercul/o	A nodule or small raised area	costal tubercle
tuberosity too bur OSS ih tee		An elevation or protuberance, larger than a tubercle	ischial tuberosity

EXERCISE 2: Bone Basics

Match the bone word parts with their meanings.

_____ 1. myel/o

_____ 2. -physis

_____ 3. peri-

_____ 4. condyl/o

_____ 5. spin/o

_____ 6. sin/o

_____ 7. foramin/o

_____ 8. -um

_____ 9. -blast

_____ 10. epi-

_____ 11. foss/o

_____ 12. endo-

_____ 13. trochanter/o

_____ 14. -cyte

_____ 15. -clast

A. trochanter
B. foramen, hole
C. above, upon
D. cell
E. bone marrow
F. surrounding, around
G. embryonic
H. spine
I. breaking down
J. growth
K. hollow, depression
L. condyle, knob
M. within
N. sinus, cavity
O. structure

Fill in the blank.

16. Osteoblasts _____ bone, whereas osteoclasts _____ bone.

17. The shaft of a long bone is called the _____; the ends of a long bone are
    called _____ (plural!).

18. The outer covering of bone is the _____, whereas the inner lining is the
    _____.

19. A foramen, a sinus, and a fossa are examples of bone _____. A condyle,
    a trochanter, and a tuberosity are examples of bone _____.

20. A synonym for a sinus is a/an _____.

EXERCISE 3: Long Bone

Label the long bone with the terms provided.

diaphysis
epiphysis
bone marrow
periosteum
endosteum
medullary cavity
epiphyseal plate

AXIAL SKELETON

The axial skeleton includes the skull, spine, and rib cage (see Fig. 3-1).

Skull

The skull is made up of two parts: the **cranium** (KRAY nee um) that encloses and protects the brain and the **facial bones** (Fig. 3-3).

Cranium
Frontal bone: Forms the anterior part of the skull and the forehead.
Parietal (puh RYE uh tul) **bones:** Form the sides of the cranium.
Occipital (ock SIP ih tul) **bone:** Forms the back of the skull. Notable is a large hole at the ventral surface in this bone, the foramen magnum (meaning *large*), which allows brain communication with the spinal cord.
Temporal (TEM poor ul) **bones:** Form the lower two sides of the cranium. The **mastoid process** is the posterior part of the bone behind the ear.
Ethmoid (EHTH moyd) **bone:** Forms the roof and walls of the nasal cavity.
Sphenoid (SFEE noyd) **bone:** Anterior to the temporal bones and the basilar part of the occipital bone.
Paranasal sinuses: Air-filled cavities that are named for the bones in which they are located. Each is lined with a mucous membrane (see Fig 3-3, *B*).

---

skull, cranium = crani/o

face = faci/o

frontal = front/o

parietal = pariet/o

occipital = occipit/o

temporal = tempor/o

mastoid = mastoid/o

ethmoid = ethmoid/o

sphenoid = sphenoid/o

paranasal
   para- = near
   nas/o = nose
   -al = pertaining to

Fig. 3-3 A, Skull and facial bones. **B,** Paranasal sinuses, frontal view.

A

B

The last three bones of the skull, the ossicles, are tiny bones within the ear. These will be discussed in Chapter 13.

Facial Bones

Use Fig. 3-3 to locate the names and locations of the majority of the following facial bones:

Zygoma (zye GOH mah): Cheekbone. Also called the **zygomatic** (zye goh MAT tick) **bone.**

Lacrimal (LACK rih mul) **bones:** Paired bones at the corner of each eye that cradle the tear ducts.

Maxilla (MACK sill ah): Upper jaw bone. Also called the **maxillary bone.**

Mandible (MAN dih bul): Lower jaw bone. Also called the **mandibular bone.**

Vomer (VOH mur): Bone that forms the posterior/inferior part of the nasal septal wall between the nostrils.

Palatine (PAL eh tyne) **bones:** Shell-shaped structures that make up part of the roof of the mouth.

Nasal turbinates (conchae) (KON kee): Make up part of the interior of the nose

Nasal bones: Pair of small bones that make up the bridge of the nose.

Rib Cage

The **ribs** consist of twelve pairs of thin, flat bones attached to the thoracic vertebrae in the back and to **costochondral** (kost toh KON drul) tissue in the front (see Fig. 3-4, C). The ribs can be categorized as follows:

* **True ribs:** Seven pairs attached directly to the breastbone (sternum) in the front of the body.
* **False ribs:** Five pairs attached to the sternum by cartilage. Two of the false ribs are called *floating ribs* because they are not attached in the front of the body at all.

In addition to ribs, the rib cage includes the **sternum** (STUR num), also known as the *breastbone*. The sharp point at the most inferior aspect of the sternum is called the **xiphoid** (ZIH foyd) **process.** The combining form *xiph/o* derives from the Greek word for sword, which the xiphoid resembles.

Spine

The **spinal,** or **vertebral,** column is divided into five regions from the neck to the tailbone. It is composed of 26 bones called the **vertebrae** (VUR teh bray) (Fig. 3-4, A). The following table lists and illustrates the bones in the spine. Fig. 3-4, B, illustrates a vertebra with the **laminae** (*sing.* lamina), **spinous** and **transverse processes,** and **facets.** Laminae are thin, platelike arches in the vertebrae. Facets are processes that articulate between vertebrae.

Bones of the Spine	
Region	Type and Abbreviation
cervical (SUR vih kul)	Neck bones (C1-C7)
thoracic (thoh RAS ick)	Upper back (T1-T12)
lumbar (LUM bar)	Lower back (L1-L5)
sacral (SAY krul)	Sacrum (S1-S5) (five bones, fused)
coccygeal (kock sih JEE ul)	Coccyx (KOCK sicks) or tailbone

zygoma = zygom/o, zygomat/o

lacrimal = lacrim/o

maxilla = maxill/o

mandible = mandibul/o

vomer = vomer/o

palatine = palat/o

nasal = nas/o

costochondral
  cost/o = rib
  chondr/o = cartilage
  -al = pertaining to

sternum = stern/o

xiphoid = xiph/o

spine = spin/o

vertebra = vertebr/o, spondyl/o

lamina = lamin/o

neck = cervic/o

thorax (chest) = thorac/o

lumbar (lower back) = lumb/o

sacrum = sacr/o

coccyx = coccyg/o

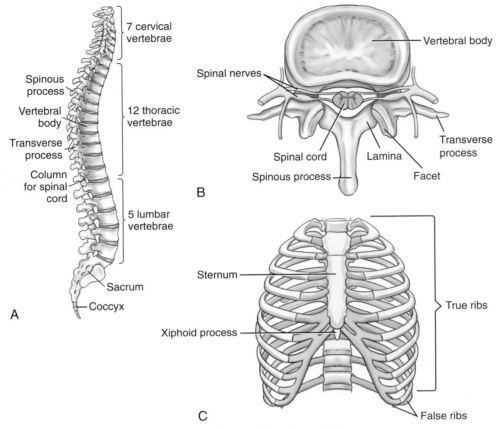

Fig. 3-4 **A,** Spine. **B,** Vertebra. **C,** Ribs.

EXERCISE 4: Axial Skeletal Combining Forms

Match each axial skeletal term with its correct combining form.

_____ 1. cervic/o

_____ 2. lamin/o

_____ 3. ethmoid/o

_____ 4. chondr/o

_____ 5. thorac/o

_____ 6. crani/o

_____ 7. occipit/o

_____ 8. cost/o

_____ 9. zygomat/o

_____ 10. lumb/o

_____ 11. mandibul/o

_____ 12. coccyg/o

_____ 13. vertebr/o

_____ 14. palat/o

_____ 15. maxill/o

_____ 16. stern/o

A. lower jaw bone
B. rib
C. backbone
D. lower back
E. cheekbone
F. roof and walls of nasal cavity
G. cartilage
H. roof of mouth
I. neck
J. skull
K. lamina of vertebra
L. upper jaw bone
M. back of skull
N. chest
O. tailbone
P. breastbone

Decode the following terms below using your knowledge of word parts.

17. submandibular _____

18. costochondral _____

19. lumbosacral _____

20. thoracic _____

21. substernal _____

 EXERCISE 5: Bones of the Cranium and Face

Label the diagram using the terms provided.

temporal bone
mandible
ethmoid bone
mastoid process
lacrimal bone
zygomatic bone
maxilla
nasal bones

 EXERCISE 6: Bones of the Spine

Label the diagram using the terms provided.

coccyx
cervical vertebrae
lumbar vertebrae
sacrum
thoracic vertebrae

EXERCISE 7: Rib Cage

Label the diagram using the terms provided.

xiphoid process
true ribs
sternum
false ribs

 EXERCISE 8: Vertebra

Label the diagram using the terms provided.

transverse process
lamina
spinal nerves
vertebral body
spinal cord
facet

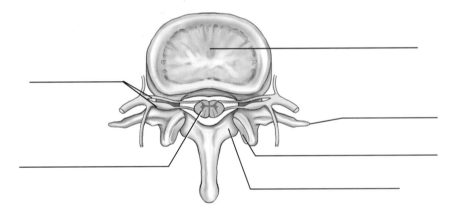

APPENDICULAR SKELETON

The appendicular skeleton is composed of the upper appendicular and lower appendicular skeletons.

Upper Appendicular

The upper appendicular skeleton (Fig. 3-5) includes the shoulder girdle, which is composed of the **scapula, clavicle,** and **upper extremities.** Refer to Fig. 3-1 for a correlation of each bone's description with its location.

Scapula (SKAP yoo lah): The scapulae, or shoulder blades, are flat bones that help to support the arms. The **acromion** (ack ROH mee un) **process** is the lateral protrusion of the scapula that forms the highest point of the shoulder.

Clavicle (KLA vih kul): The clavicle, or collarbone, is one of a pair of long, curved horizontal bones that attach to the upper sternum at one end and the acromion process of the scapula at the other. These bones help to stabilize the shoulder anteriorly. A "wishbone" is composed of the fused clavicles of a bird.

scapula = scapul/o

clavicle = clavicul/o, cleid/o

acromion = acromi/o

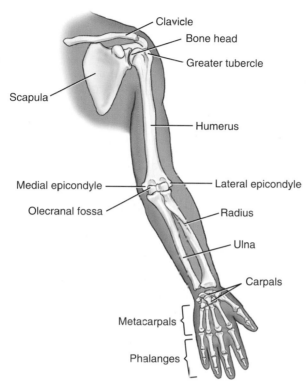

Fig. 3-5 Upper appendicular.

The upper extremities (see Fig. 3-5) consist of the following:

Humerus (HYOO mur us): Upper arm bone.
Radius (RAY dee us): Lower lateral arm bone parallel to the ulna. The distal end articulates with the thumb side of the hand.
Ulna (UL nuh): Lower medial arm bone. The distal end articulates with the little finger side of the hand. The **olecranon** (oh LECK ruh non) is a proximal projection of the ulna that forms the tip of the elbow. Commonly known as the *funny bone,* this structure is actually a process.
Carpus (KAR pus): One of eight wrist bones.
Metacarpus (meh tuh KAR pus): One of the five bones that form the middle part of the hand.
Phalanx (FAY lanks) (*pl.* phalanges): One of the 14 bones that constitute the fingers of the hand, two in the thumb and three in each of the other four fingers. The three bones in each of the four fingers are differentiated as proximal, medial, and distal. The joints between these are referred to as *proximal* and *distal interphalangeal (PIP, DIP) joints.* When one is referring to a whole finger (or toe), the term **digitus** is used.

Lower Appendicular

The lower half of the appendicular skeleton can be divided into the **pelvis** and the **lower extremities.** The **acetabulum** (*pl.* acetabula) is the socket into which the femoral head fits. The pelvic bones (also called the *pelvic girdle*) consist of the following three bones:

Ilium (ILL ee um): The superior and widest bone of the pelvis.
Ischium (ISS kee um): The lower portion of the pelvic bone.
Pubis (PYOO bis) **or pubic bone:** The lower anterior part of the pelvic bone.

humerus	= humer/o
radius	= radi/o
ulna	= uln/o
olecranon	= olecran/o
carpus (wrist)	= carp/o
metacarpus	= metacarp/o
phalanx	= phalang/o
digitus	= digit/o, dactyl/o
pelvis	= pelv/i, pelv/o
ilium	= ili/o
ischium	= ischi/o
pubis	= pub/o

Fig. 3-6 Lower appendicular.

 Be Careful! *Do not confuse **ilium** with its homonym, **ileum**, which is a part of the digestive system.*

The lower extremities (Fig. 3-6) include the following:

Femur (FEE mur): Thigh bone, upper leg bone.
Patella (puh TELL uh): Kneecap.
Tibia (TIB ee uh): Shin bone, lower medial leg bone.
Fibula (FIB yuh luh): Smaller, lower lateral leg bone.
Malleolus (mah LEE oh lus): Process on the distal ends of tibia and fibula.
Tarsus (TAR sus): One of the seven bones of the ankle, hindfoot, and midfoot. The **calcaneus** is the heel bone.
Metatarsus (met uh TAR sus): One of the five foot bones between the tarsals and the phalanges.
Phalanx: One of 14 toe bones, two in the great toe and three in each of the other four toes.

femur = femor/o

patella = patell/o, patell/a

tibia = tibi/o

fibula = fibul/o, perone/o

malleolus = malleol/o

tarsal = tars/o

calcaneus = calcane/o

metatarsal = metatars/o

 Be Careful! *Do not confuse **perone/o** meaning fibula with **peritone/o** meaning the lining of the abdomen.*

EXERCISE 9: The Appendicular Skeleton

Match the upper appendicular combining forms with their meanings.

Combining Forms

_____ 1. humer/o

_____ 2. scapul/o

_____ 3. uln/o

_____ 4. olecran/o

_____ 5. clavicul/o, cleid/o

_____ 6. metacarp/o

_____ 7. digit/o

_____ 8. phalang/o

_____ 9. radi/o

_____ 10. carp/o

Upper Appendicular Meanings

A. collarbone, clavicle
B. wrist bone
C. finger, toe
D. one of the finger or toe bones
E. lower lateral arm bone
F. upper arm bone
G. lower medial arm bone
H. elbow
I. shoulder blade
J. hand bone

Match the lower appendicular combining forms with their meanings.

Combining Forms

_____ 11. patell/o

_____ 12. pub/o

_____ 13. metatars/o

_____ 14. tibi/o

_____ 15. ili/o

_____ 16. malleol/o

_____ 17. pelv/o, pelv/i

_____ 18. ischi/o

_____ 19. fibul/o, perone/o

_____ 20. femor/o

_____ 21. tars/o

_____ 22. calcane/o

Lower Appendicular Meanings

K. foot bone
L. lower portion of pelvic bone
M. ankle bone
N. lower anterior pelvic bone
O. shin bone
P. kneecap
Q. superior, widest bone of pelvis
R. processes on distal tibia and fibula
S. thigh bone
T. pelvis
U. lower, lateral leg bone
V. heel bone

Decode the terms.

23. interphalangeal _____

24. humeroulnar _____

25. infrapatellar _____

26. femoral _____

27. supraclavicular _____

EXERCISE 10: Upper Appendicular Skeleton

Label the diagram using the terms provided.

radius
carpals
scapula
clavicle
metacarpals
humerus
ulna
phalanges

 EXERCISE 11: Lower Appendicular Skeleton

Label the diagram using the terms provided.

femur
metatarsals
fibula
pubis
tarsals
malleolus
tibia
phalanges
patella
ischium
ilium

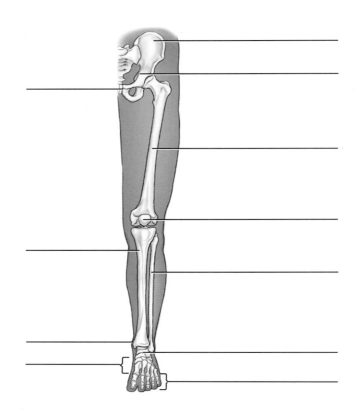

Joints

Joints, or *articulations* as they are sometimes called, are the parts of the body where two or more bones of the skeleton join. Examples of joints include the knee, which joins the tibia and the femur, and the elbow, which joins the humerus with the radius and ulna. Joints provide **range of motion (ROM),** the range through which a joint can be extended and flexed. Different joints have different ROM, ranging from no movement at all to full range of movement. Categorized by ROM, they are as follows:

No ROM: Most **synarthroses** (sin ar THROH sees) are immovable joints held together by fibrous cartilaginous tissue. The suture lines of the skull are examples of synarthroses.

Limited ROM: Amphiarthroses (am fee ar THROH sees) are joints joined together by cartilage that are slightly movable, such as the vertebrae of the spine or the pubic bones.

Full ROM: Diarthroses (dye ar THROH sees) are joints that have free movement. The most commonly known are ball-and-socket joints (such as, the hip) and hinge joints (such as, the knees). Other examples of diarthroses include the elbows, wrists, shoulders, and ankles. See Fig. 3-7 for an illustration of a knee joint that shows the bones, muscles, tendons, bursae, synovial membrane, and cavity in the knee.

Diarthroses, or **synovial** (sih NOH vee ul) **joints,** as they are frequently called, are the most complex of the joints. Because these joints help a person move around for a lifetime, they are designed to efficiently cushion the jarring of the bones and to minimize friction between the surfaces of the bones. Many of the synovial joints have **bursae** (BURR see) (*sing.* bursa), which are sacs of fluid that are located between the bones of the joint and the tendons that hold the muscles in place. Bursae help cushion the joints when they move. Synovial joints also have joint capsules that enclose the ends of the bones, a synovial membrane that lines the joint capsules and secretes fluid to lubricate the joint, and articular cartilage that covers and protects the bone. The **menisci** (*sing.* meniscus) consist of crescent-shaped cartilage in the knee joint that additionally cushions the joint. **Ligaments** are strong bands of white fibrous connective tissue that connect one bone to another at the joints.

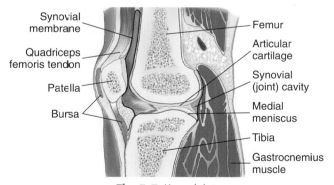

Fig. 3-7 Knee joint.

Muscles

A **muscle** is a tissue that is composed of cells with the ability to contract and relax. Because of those two specialized actions, the body is able to move. The muscles in the human body are specialized into three different functions:

* **Skeletal muscle** is striated (striped in appearance) and allows the skeleton to move voluntarily.

joint = articul/o, arthr/o

synarthrosis
  syn- = together
  arthr/o = joint
  -sis = condition

amphiarthrosis
  amphi- = both
  arthr/o = joint
  -sis = condition

diarthrosis
  dia- = through
  arthr/o = joint
  -sis = condition

synovial = synovi/o

bursa = burs/o

meniscus = menisc/o

muscle = my/o, myos/o, muscul/o

skeletal muscle = rhabdomy/o

smooth muscle = leiomy/o

heart muscle = myocardi/o

tendon = tend/o, tendin/o, ten/o

- **Smooth muscle** is responsible for involuntary movement of the organs.
- **Heart muscle** pumps blood to the circulatory system.

Muscles are attached to bones by strong fibrous bands of connective tissue called **tendons.** The bone that is at the end of the attachment that does not move and is nearest to the trunk is termed the *origin (O);* the bone that is at the end that does move and is farthest from the trunk is termed the *insertion (I).* The function of a muscle is its *action (A).* For example, a flexor muscle bends a joint, and an extensor muscle stretches out a joint. These muscle pairs are termed *antagonistic* muscles. *Synergistic* muscles work together to refine a movement.

The illustrations in Fig. 3-8 show posterior and anterior views of the major skeletal muscles of the body. Although the naming of all the muscles in the body is too much to cover in this text, there are a few helpful conventions that can

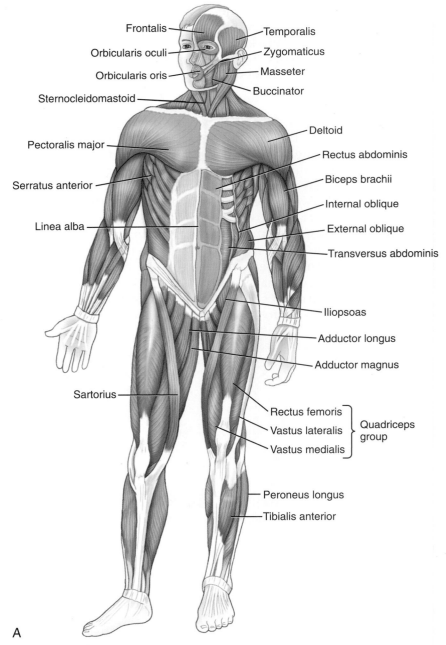

Fig. 3-8 Major muscles of the body. **A,** Anterior view.

Trapezius

Deltoid

Triceps brachii

Latissimus dorsi

Gluteus medius

Gluteus maximus

Adductor magnus

Biceps femoris

Gracilis

Semitendinosus

Semimembranosus

} Hamstring
group

Gastrocnemius

Soleus

Achilles tendon
(calcaneal tendon)

B

Mastoid
process

Insertion

Sternocleidomastoid
muscle

Clavicle

Origin

Sternum

C

Fig. 3-8, cont'd B, Posterior view. **C,** Close-up of the sternocleidomastoid muscle.

sternocleidomastoid
  stern/o = sternum
  cleid/o = clavicle
  mastoid/o = mastoid

chest = pector/o

be followed. Refer to the following table for examples of how muscles are named by their location, number of insertions, size, shape, and muscle action. Some muscles get their names from their general location. For instance the pectoris muscle is a large muscle in the chest (pector/o). The final convention is to name a muscle by its origins and insertion. For example, the **sternocleidomastoid** (stur noh kly doh MASS toyd) muscle (see Fig. 3-8, *C*) attaches to the sternum, the clavicle, and the mastoid process.

Muscle Naming Conventions

Naming Device	Name of Muscle	Word Origin	Definition
location	zygomaticus	*zygomatic/o* zygoma *-us* noun ending	Cheek muscle.
number of insertions	biceps brachii	*bi-* two **ceps* heads *brachi/o* arm *-i* plural noun ending	Muscle that flexes upper arm.
size	gluteus maximus	*glute/o* buttock *-us* noun ending *maxim/o* large *-us* noun ending	Large buttock muscle.
shape	deltoid	*delt/o* triangle *-oid* like	Triangular muscle in upper back.
muscle action	adductor longus	*ad-* toward *duct/o* carrying *-or* one who *long/o* long *-us* noun ending	Upper leg muscle that carries one leg back to the midline.
origin/insertion	sternocleidomastoid (see Fig. 3-8, *C*)	*stern/o* breastbone *cleid/o* collarbone *mastoid/o* mastoid process	Muscle that originates in the sternum and collarbone and inserts on the mastoid process.

*ceps is a variation of *cephal/o,* the combining form for head. These word parts are used for "the head" or the beginning of a structure and also are used for bones (bone heads), as well as muscle heads.

EXERCISE 12: Joints and Muscles

Match the joint and muscle combining forms with their meanings.

_____ 1. arthr/o, articul/o   _____ 7. my/o, myos/o, muscul/o
_____ 2. myocardi/o   _____ 8. leiomy/o
_____ 3. delt/o   _____ 9. tendin/o, ten/o, tend/o
_____ 4. rhabdomy/o   _____10. burs/o
_____ 5. synovi/o   _____11. glute/o
_____ 6. menisc/o

A. smooth muscle
B. triangle
C. sac of fluid to cushion joints
D. skeletal muscle
E. joint
F. crescent-shaped cartilage
G. heart muscle
H. synovial
I. muscle
J. connects bone to muscle
K. buttock

Build the terms.

12. pertaining to within the muscle _____

13. pertaining to buttocks _____

14. pertaining to the synovium _____

Muscle Actions

	Action	Word Origin	Description
	extension ecks TEN shun	*ex-* out *tens/o* stretching *-ion* process of	Process of stretching out; increasing the angle of a joint.
	flexion FLEK shun	*flex/o* bending *-ion* process of	Process of decreasing the angle of a joint.
	abduction ab DUK shun	*ab-* away from *duct/o* carrying *-ion* process of	Process of carrying away from the midline.
	adduction ad DUK shun	*ad-* toward *duct/o* carrying *-ion* process of	Process of carrying toward the midline.
	supination soo pin NAY shun		Turning the palm upward.
	pronation proh NAY shun		Turning the palm downward.
	dorsiflexion DOOR sih flek shun	*dors/i* back *flex/o* bending *-ion* process of	Process of bending back.
	plantar flexion PLAN tar FLEK shun	*plant/o* sole *-ar* pertaining to *flex/o* bending *-ion* process of	Lowering the foot; pointing the toes away from the shin.

Muscle Actions—cont'd

	Action	Word Origin	Description
	eversion ee VER shun	*e-* out *vers/o* turning *-ion* process of	Process of turning out.
	inversion n VER shun	*in-* in *vers/o* turning *-ion* process of	Process of turning in.
	protraction proh TRAK shun	*pro-* forward *tract/o* pulling *-ion* process of	Process of pulling forward; the forward movement of a muscle.
	retraction ree TRAK shun	*re-* backward *tract/o* pulling *-ion* process of	Process of backward pulling; the backward movement of a muscle.
	rotation roh TAY shun	*rot/o* wheel *-ation* process of	Process of a bone turning on its axis (like a wheel).
	circumduction sir cum DUK shun	*circum-* around *duct/o* carrying *-ion* process of	Process of carrying around; the circular movement of the distal end of a limb around its point of attachment.

EXERCISE 13: Muscle Actions

Label each illustration with the muscle action indicated.

_____

_____

_____

_____

_____

_____

_____

_____

 EXERCISE 14: Muscle Actions

Match the muscle action with the correct definition.

_____ 1. plantar flexion   _____ 8. rotation

_____ 2. circumduction   _____ 9. supination

_____ 3. pronation   _____ 10. eversion

_____ 4. inversion   _____ 11. dorsiflexion

_____ 5. adduction   _____ 12. abduction

_____ 6. extension   _____ 13. flexion

_____ 7. protraction   _____ 14. retraction

A. process of turning in
B. process of bending
C. process of bone turning on its axis
D. process of bending back
E. process of pulling backward
F. turning the palm downward
G. process of carrying away from (the midline)
H. turning the palm upward
I. process of turning out
J. process of pulling forward
K. process of stretching out
L. process of carrying around
M. process of carrying toward (the midline)
N. lowering the foot

*You can review the anatomy of the musculoskeletal system by clicking on **Body Spectrum Electronic Anatomy Coloring Book → Muscular** and **Skeletal**.*
*Click on **Label It** to practice labeling the musculoskeletal system.*

Medical Record Dylan Koldmann

KOLDMANN, DYLAN M. - 507940 Opened by Bradley Oppenheimer, MD

Task   Edit   View   Time Scale   Options   Help

KOLDMANN, DYLAN M.

	Age: 7 years	Sex: Male	Loc: ARH
	DOB: 01/27/2007	MRN: 507940	FIN: 3506004

Reference Text Browser   Form Browser   Medication Profile

Orders | Last 48 Hours | ED | Lab | Radiology | Assessments | Surgery | Clinical Notes | Pt. Info | Pt. Schedule | Task List | I & O | MAR

Flowsheet: ED   Level: ED Record   ⊙ Table ○ Group ○ List

Navigator

✓ ED Record

7-year-old sustained injury to right hand when fell off bike. Pain over thenar eminence. Able to bend at his wrist and flex at his DIP and PIP joints and every digit of the hand with exception of first digit.

Exam of right hand is significant for mild protrusion but no ecchymosis and minimal edema overlying thenar eminence of the right hand. Good wrist mobility. X-ray significant for what appears to be a Salter-Harris fracture of the first metacarpal. Immobile and follow-up tomorrow with Ortho for possible cast.

PROD MAHA-C   26 March 2014   16:10

EXERCISE 15: Emergency Department Report

Use the preceding emergency department record to answer the following questions.

1. Dylan's injury is to the fleshy area of the palm near the thumb, the "thenar eminence." Explain the difference between a DIP and a PIP joint. _____

   _____

2. Not being able to "flex" a body part means one is unable to _____.

3. "First digit, R hand" means _____.

4. The first metacarpal is a bone of the _____.

*Click on **Hear It, Spell It** to practice spelling the anatomy and physiology terms you have learned in this chapter.*

Combining and Adjective Forms for the Anatomy of the Musculoskeletal System

Meaning	Combining Form	Adjective Form
bone	oste/o, osse/o, oss/i	osseous, osteal
bone marrow	myel/o	
bursa	burs/o	bursal
calcaneus (heel bone)	calcane/o	calcaneal
carpal bone	carp/o	carpal
cartilage	chondr/o, cartilag/o	cartilaginous, chondral
clavicle (collarbone)	clavicul/o, cleid/o	clavicular, cleidal
coccyx (tailbone)	coccyg/o	coccygeal
condyle	condyl/o	condylar
elbow (olecranon)	olecran/o	olecranal
epicondyle	epicondyl/o	epicondylar
ethmoid	ethmoid/o	ethmoidal
fascia	fasci/o	fascial
femur (thigh bone)	femor/o	femoral
fibula (lower lateral leg bone)	fibul/o, perone/o	fibular, peroneal
finger, toe, (whole), digitus	dactyl/o, digit/o	digital
foramen	foramin/o	foraminal
frontal bone	front/o	frontal
humerus (upper arm bone)	humer/o	humeral
ilium	ili/o	iliac
ischium	ischi/o	ischial
jaw	gnath/o	
joint (articulation)	arthr/o, articul/o	articular
lacrima	lacrim/o	lacrimal
lamina	lamin/o	laminar
ligament	ligament/o, syndesm/o	ligamentous, syndesmal
lower back	lumb/o	lumbar
malleolus	malleol/o	malleolar
mandible (lower jaw bone)	mandibul/o	mandibular
mastoid process	mastoid/o	mastoid
maxilla (upper jaw bone)	maxill/o	maxillary
meniscus	menisc/o	meniscal
metacarpus (hand bone)	metacarp/o	metacarpal

Combining and Adjective Forms for the Anatomy of the Musculoskeletal System—cont'd

Meaning	Combining Form	Adjective Form
metatarsus (foot bone)	metatars/o	metatarsal
muscle	my/o, myos/o, muscul/o	muscular
muscle (heart)	myocardi/o, cardiomy/o	myocardial
muscle (skeletal)	rhabdomy/o	
muscle (smooth)	leiomy/o	
neck	cervic/o	cervical
occiput	occipit/o	occipital
palatine bone	palat/o	palatine
parietal bone	pariet/o	parietal
patella (kneecap)	patell/o, patell/a	patellar
pelvis	pelv/i, pelv/o	pelvic
phalanx (one of the bones of the fingers or toes)	phalang/o	phalangeal
pubis (pubic bone)	pub/o	pubic
radius (lower lateral arm bone)	radi/o	radial
rib (costa)	cost/o	costal
sacrum	sacr/o	sacral
scapula (shoulderblade)	scapul/o	scapular
skeleton	skelet/o	skeletal
skull (cranium)	crani/o	cranial
sole	plant/o	plantar
sphenoid	sphenoid/o	sphenoidal
spinal column, spine	spin/o, rachi/o, vertebr/o	spinal, vertebral, rachial
sternum, breastbone	stern/o	sternal
tarsus (anklebone)	tars/o	tarsal
temporal bone	tempor/o	temporal
tendon	tendin/o, tend/o, ten/o	tendinous
thorax (chest)	thorac/o	thoracic
tibia (shinbone)	tibi/o	tibial
ulna	uln/o	ulnar
vertebra (backbone)	vertebr/o, spondyl/o	vertebral
vomer	vomer/o	
xiphoid process	xiph/o	xiphoid
zygoma (cheekbone)	zygomat/o	zygomatic

Prefixes for the Anatomy of the Musculoskeletal System

Prefix	Meaning
ab-	away from
ad-	toward
amphi-	both
bi-	two
circum-	around
dia-	through, complete
endo-, end-	within
epi-	above, upon
ex-, e-	out
in-	in
inter-	between
intra-	within
peri-	surrounding, around
pro-	forward
re-	back
syn-	together, joined

Suffixes for the Anatomy of the Musculoskeletal System

Suffix	Meaning
-ar, -al, -ic, -ous, -eal	pertaining to
-blast	embryonic
-clast	breaking down
-cyte	cell
-oid	full of, like
-physis	growth
-poiesis	formation
-sis	condition
-um	structure

PATHOLOGY

Terms Related to Congenital Conditions

Term	Word Origin	Definition
achondroplasia a kon droh PLAY zha	*a-* without *chondr/o* cartilage *-plasia* condition of development	Disorder of the development of cartilage at the epiphyses of the long bones and skull, resulting in dwarfism.
muscular dystrophy (MD) MUSS kyoo lur DISS troh fee	*muscul/o* muscle *-ar* pertaining to *dys-* bad, abnormal *-trophy* process of nourishment, development	Group of disorders characterized as an inherited progressive atrophy of skeletal muscle without neural involvement (Fig. 3-9).

Terms Related to Congenital Conditions—cont'd

Term	Word Origin	Definition
polydactyly pall ee DACK tih lee	*poly-* many, much *dactyl/o* fingers, toes *-y* condition	Condition of more than five fingers or toes on each hand or foot (Fig. 3-10, *A*).
spina bifida occulta SPY nah BIFF ih dah ah KULL tah	*spin/o* spine *bi-* two *-fida* to split *occulta* hidden	Congenital malformation of the bony spinal canal without involvement of the spinal cord.
syndactyly sin DACK tih lee	*syn-* joined, together *dactyl/o* fingers, toes *-y* condition	Condition of the joining of the fingers or toes, giving them a webbed appearance (see Fig. 3-10, *B*).
talipes TALL ih peez		Deformity resulting in an abnormal twisting of the foot. Also called **clubfoot**. May also be acquired.
torticollis tore tih KOLL lis	*tort/i* twist *coll/o* neck *-is* noun ending	Prolonged congenital or acquired condition that manifests itself as a contraction of the muscles of the neck. Also called **wryneck**

Fig. 3-9 Muscular dystrophy (MD). These brothers show typical stance, lumbar lordosis, and forward thrusting of the abdomen.

Fig. 3-10 A, Polydactyly. **B,** Syndactyly.

EXERCISE 16: Congenital Conditions

Build the terms.

1. process of joined fingers/toes _____

2. condition of development without cartilage _____

3. process of many fingers/toes _____

Case Study LeDanton Bradford

LeDanton Bradford is a healthy, well-developed infant with six digits on the ulnar side of his right hand and webbing between the third and fourth digits on his left hand. All the phalanges in the other digits appear to be present and normal. At first his parents are reluctant to correct the abnormalities, but when LeDanton is 6 months old, they sign consents for surgery to correct both disorders.

1. What is the term that means a condition of extra fingers or toes? _____

2. What is the term that means a condition of webbed fingers or toes? _____

3. A/an _____ is an individual bone in a finger or toe.

4. The little finger is on the ulnar side of the hand?
   a. true
   b. false

5. What is the prefix that means many? _____

Terms Related to Bone Disease

Term	Word Origin	Definition
osteodynia ahs tee oh DIN ee ah	*oste/o* bone *-dynia* pain	Bone pain.
osteitis deformans ahs tee EYE tis dee FOR menz	*oste/o* bone *-itis* inflammation *deformans* misshapen	Misshaped bone resulting from excessive breakdown and formation of bone tissue. Also known as **Paget disease.**
osteomalacia ahs tee oh mah LAY sha	*oste/o* bone *-malacia* softening	Softening of bone caused by loss of minerals from the bony matrix as a result of vitamin D deficiency. When osteomalacia occurs in childhood, it is called **rickets.**
osteomyelitis ahs tee oh mye eh LYE tis	*oste/o* bone *myel/o* bone marrow *-itis* inflammation	Inflammation and/or infection of the bone and bone marrow.
osteoporosis ahs tee oh poor OH sis	*oste/o* bone *por/o* passage *-osis* abnormal condition	Loss of bone mass, which results in the bones being fragile and at risk for fractures (Fig. 3-11). **Osteopenia** refers to a less severe bone mass loss. (*-penia* = deficiency)

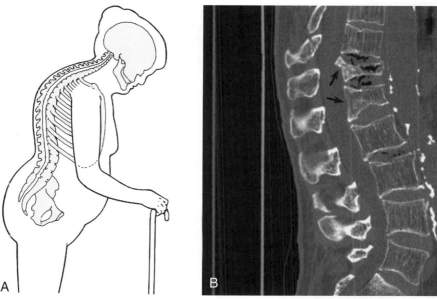

Fig. 3-11 A, The hallmark of osteoporosis: the dowager hump. Affected persons lose height, have a bent spine, and appear to sink into their hips. **B,** X-ray showing a compression fracture of T12 and L1 subsequent to osteoporosis.

Terms Related to Chondropathies

Term	Word Origin	Definition
chondromalacia kon droh mah LAY see ah	*chondr/o* cartilage *-malacia* softening	Softening of the cartilage.
costochondritis kahs toh kon DRY tis	*cost/o* rib *chondr/o* cartilage *-itis* inflammation	Inflammation of the cartilage of the ribs.

Terms Related to Arthropathies and Related Disorders

Term	Word Origin	Definition
arthrosis ar THROH sis	*arthr/o* joint *-osis* abnormal condition	Abnormal condition of a joint; may be **hemarthrosis, hydrarthrosis,** or **pyarthrosis** (blood, fluid, or pus, respectively, in a joint cavity).
Baker cyst BAY kur sist	*cyst/o* sac, bladder	Cyst of synovial fluid in the poplitea area of leg; often associated with rheumatoid arthritis (RA).
bunion BUN yun	*bunion/o* bunion	Fairly common, painful enlargement and inflammation of the first metatarsophalangeal joint (the base of the great toe).
bursitis bur SYE tis	*burs/o* bursa *-itis* inflammation	Inflammation of a bursa.
carpal tunnel syndrome (CTS) KAR pul TUN ul	*carp/o* wrist bone *-al* pertaining to *syn-* joined together *-drome* to run	Compression injury that manifests itself as fluctuating pain, numbness, and paresthesias of the hand caused by compression of the median nerve at the wrist (Fig. 3-12).
crepitus KREP ih tus	*crepit/o* crackling *-us* thing	Crackling sound heard in joints.

Continued

Terms Related to Arthropathies and Related Disorders—cont'd

Term	Word Origin	Definition
osteoarthritis (OA) ahs tee oh arth RYE tis	*oste/o* bone *arthr/o* joint *-itis* inflammation	Joint disease characterized by degenerative articular cartilage and a wearing down of the bones' edges at a joint; considered a "wear and tear" disorder. Also called **degenerative joint disease (DJD)** (Fig. 3-13).
osteophytosis ahs tee oh fye TOH sis	*oste/o* bone *phyt/o* growth nature *-osis* abnormal condition	Abnormal bone growth in a joint. **Heberden nodes** are osteophytes of the interphalangeal joints in RA (Fig. 3-14).
polyarthralgia pah lee ar THRAL gee uh	*poly-* many *arthr/o* joint *-algia* pain	Condition in which there is pain in several joints simultaneously.
rheumatoid arthritis (RA) ROO mah toyd arth RYE tis	*rheumat/o* watery flow *-oid* full of, like *arthr/o* joint *-itis* inflammation	Inflammatory joint disease believed to be autoimmune in nature; occurs in a much younger population (ages 20 to 45) than OA (see Fig. 3-14).
scleroderma SKLAIR oh dur mah	*scler/o* hard *derm/o* skin *-a* noun ending	Connective tissue disorder that causes hardening and thickening of the skin.
systemic lupus erythematosus (SLE) siss TEM ick LOO pus eh rith mah TOH sis	*system/o* system *-ic* pertaining to *erythemat/o* red *-osus* noun ending	Chronic, systemic inflammation of unknown etiology (cause). Characterized by arthritis and a distinctive red, butterfly-like rash on nose and cheeks. Also called **disseminated lupus erythematosus (DLE).**
temporomandibular joint disorder (TMJ) tem pore oh man DIB byoo lur	*tempor/o* temporal bone *mandibul/o* lower jaw *-ar* pertaining to	Dysfunctional temporomandibular joint, accompanied by gnathalgia, or jaw pain.
tendinitis ten din EYE tis	*tendin/o* tendon *-itis* inflammation	Inflammation of a tendon.

Fig. 3-12 Carpal tunnel syndrome (CTS).

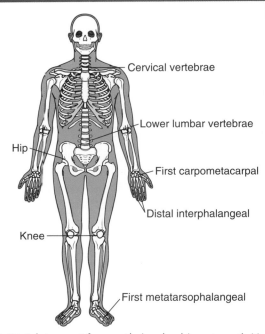

Fig. 3-13 Joints most frequently involved in osteoarthritis (OA).

Fig. 3-14 A, Bouchard nodes seen in rheumatoid arthritis (RA) of the hands. Moderate involvement. **B,** Arthrogram of wrist showing RA and resultant osteophytosis.

EXERCISE 17: Bone, Cartilage, and Joint Disorders

Match the bone, cartilage, or joint disorders with their definitions.

_____ 1. chondromalacia

_____ 2. crepitus

_____ 3. bunion

_____ 4. temporomandibular joint disorder (TMJ)

_____ 5. osteitis deformans

_____ 6. rheumatoid arthritis (RA)

_____ 7. costochondritis

_____ 8. Baker cyst

_____ 9. osteoarthritis (OA)

_____ 10. osteomyelitis

_____ 11. carpal tunnel syndrome (CTS)

_____ 12. osteophytosis

A. softening of the cartilage
B. inflammation of the bone and bone marrow
C. crackling sound in a joint
D. autoimmune inflammatory joint disease
E. compression injury of median nerve of wrist
F. enlargement of first metatarsophalangeal joint
G. also known as Paget disease
H. degenerative joint disease (DJD)
I. fluid-filled sac behind knee
J. inflammation of cartilage of ribs
K. abnormal bony growths around joints
L. dysfunctional joint in jaw bone

Build the terms.

13. pain in a bone _____

14. inflammation of a bursa _____

15. inflammation of a tendon _____

16. abnormal condition of passages in bone _____

17. softening of bone _____

Case Study Vic Vandonberg

Vic Vandonberg presents with jaw pain and reports a "clicking" sound when he opens his mouth. He says that sometimes it feels like his jaw is going to get stuck open. He admits that he grinds and clenches his teeth, especially at night. His physician assistant suspects TMJ disorder. He recommends analgesics and bite guards.

1. What is TMJ? _____ _____

2. The mandible is the lower _____ bone.

3. Gnathalgia means _____ in the jaw.

4. What is the medical term for the sound a joint makes when the bones rub together? _____

Spinal Malcurvatures

Back pain accounts for the greatest number of musculoskeletal complaints in the United States. In healthcare terminology, those complaints are classified as **dorsalgia** (door SAL zsa) (**dors/o** = back + **-algia** = pain), upper back pain, and **lumbago** (lum BAY goh) (**lumb/o** = lumbar + **-ago** = disease), lower back pain.

The spine has natural curves that allow support and flexibility; however, sometimes these curves become exaggerated and cause pain and disfigurement. The following are the most common types of disorders and malcurvatures of the spine. Occasionally, combinations of these disorders occur.

Terms Related to Deforming Dorsopathies and Spondylopathies

Term	Word Origin	Definition
ankylosing spondylitis ang kih LOH sing spon dill LYE tis	*ankyl/o* stiffening *spondyl/o* vertebra *-itis* inflammation	Chronic inflammatory disease of idiopathic origin, which causes a fusion of the spine.
herniated intervertebral disk	*inter-* between *vertebr/o* vertebra *-al* pertaining to	Protrusion of the central part of the disk that lies between the vertebrae, resulting in compression of the nerve root and pain.
kyphosis kye FOH sis	*kyph/o* round back *-osis* abnormal condition	Extreme posterior curvature of the thoracic area of the spine (Fig. 3-15, *A*).
lordosis lore DOH sis	*lord/o* swayback *-osis* abnormal condition	Swayback; exaggerated anterior curve of the lumbar vertebrae (lower back) (see Fig. 3-15, *B*).
scoliosis skoh lee OH sis	*scoli/o* curvature *-osis* abnormal condition	Lateral **S** curve of the spine that can cause an individual to lose inches in height (see Fig. 3-15, *C*).
spinal stenosis SPY nul steh NOH sis	*spin/o* spine *-al* pertaining to stenosis abnormal condition of narrowing	Abnormal condition of narrowing of the spinal canal with attendant pain, sometimes caused by OA or spondylolisthesis (Fig. 3-16).
spondylolisthesis spon dih loh liss THEE sis	*spondyl/o* vertebra *-listhesis* slipping	Condition resulting from the partial forward dislocation of one vertebra over the one beneath it.
spondylosis spon dih LOH sis	*spondyl/o* vertebra *-osis* abnormal condition	An abnormal condition characterized by stiffening of the vertebral joints.

Lordosis   **Kyphosis**   **Scoliosis**

Fig. 3-15 A, Kyphosis. **B,** Lordosis. **C,** Scoliosis.

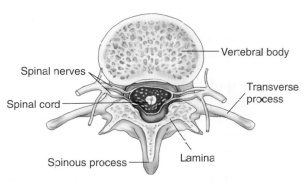

Fig. 3-16 Spinal stenosis. Bony overgrowth has narrowed the spinal canal and pinched the spinal nerves. Compare with normal vertebra in Fig. 3-4, *B.*

Terms Related to Muscle Disorders

Term	Word Origin	Definition
contracture kun TRACK chur	*con-* together *tract/o* pulling *-ure* condition	Chronic fixation of a joint in flexion (such as, a finger) caused by atrophy and shortening of muscle fibers after a long period of disuse.
fibromya gia fye broh mye AL jah	*fibr/o* fiber *my/o* muscle *-algia* pain	Disorder characterized by musculoskeletal pain, fatigue, muscle stiffness and spasms, and sleep disturbances. **Myalgia** is a general term that means muscle pain.
myasthenia gravis mye ah STHEE nee ah GRAV us	*my/o* muscle *a-* without, no *-sthenia* condition of strength *gravis* severe	Usually severe condition characterized by fatigue and progressive muscle weakness, especially of the face and throat.
plantar fasciitis plan tur fass ee EYE tis	*plant/o* sole *-ar* pertaining to *fasci/o* fascia *-itis* inflammation	Inflammation of the fascia on the sole of the foot. The chronic form is called **plantar fasciosis.**
polymyositis pahl ee mye oh SYE tis	*poly-* many *myos/o* muscle *-itis* inflammation	Chronic, idiopathic inflammation of a number of voluntary muscles.
postlaminectomy syndrome post lam in ECK tuh mee	*post-* after *lamin/o* lamina *-ectomy* removal	Group of symptoms that occur together after the removal of a lamina to correct a spinal disorder.
rhabdomyolysis rab doh mye AL ih sis	*rhabdomy/o* striated muscle *-lysis* breakdown, destruction	Breakdown of striated/skeletal muscle.

EXERCISE 18: Spinal and Muscle Disorders

Match the muscle and spinal disorders with their definitions.

_____ 1. ankylosing spondylitis

_____ 2. spinal stenosis

_____ 3. herniated intervertebral disk

_____ 4. plantar fasciitis

_____ 5. postlaminectomy syndrome

_____ 6. lumbago

_____ 7. contracture

_____ 8. fibromyalgia

_____ 9. lordosis

_____ 10. scoliosis

_____ 11. dorsalgia

_____ 12. myasthenia gravis

A. upper back pain
B. inflammation of the fascia of the foot
C. chronic flexion of a joint caused by muscle atrophy
D. muscle disorder characterized by musculoskeletal pain, fatigue, and sleep disorders
E. lateral S curve of the spine
F. protrusion of the central part of the vertebral disk
G. narrowing of the spinal canal
H. chronic inflammatory disease of idiopathic origin, which causes fusion of the spine
I. usually severe disease characterized by muscular weakness
J. symptoms that occur after removal of the lamina
K. swayback
L. lower back pain

Build the terms.

13. condition of slipping of the vertebrae _____

14. abnormal condition of the vertebra _____

15. abnormal condition of curvature _____

16. pertaining to inflammation of the fascia of the sole _____

17. breakdown of striated muscle _____

18. inflammation of many muscles _____

Case Study Monica Washington

Monica Washington is a personal shopper at a high-end department store. She is on her feet 8 hours a day, usually in 4-inch heels. To keep in shape, she runs several miles every weekend. She visits her family doctor with complaints of sharp pain on the bottom of her right foot. Her doctor diagnoses Monica with plantar fasciitis and tells her to take nonsteroidal antiinflammatory drugs (NSAIDs) as needed and see if she can get relief with stretching exercises and a foot splint that she wears at night. If these measures don't work, then Monica will be referred for orthotics, much to Monica's distress.

1. Where does plantar fasciitis occur?
   a. top of foot   b. side of foot
   c. bottom of foot

2. What is the chronic form of plantar fasciitis called?
   _____

3. Plantar fasciitis causes pain in the heel. What is the medical term that means heel? _____

4. Fascia is a sheath that covers:
   a. bone   b. muscle
   c. ligaments   d. tendons

Trauma

Fractures

Put simply, a fracture is a broken bone. However, there are a number of types of breaks, each with its own name. Most fractures occur as a result of trauma, but some can result from an underlying disease, such as osteoporosis or cancer; these **pathologic fractures** are also sometimes called *spontaneous fractures*. All fractures may be classified as simple (closed) or compound (open) fractures. The break in a simple fracture does not rupture the skin, but a compound fracture splits open the skin, which allows more opportunity for infection to take place. See the following table for different types of fractures.

Sprain/Strain and Dislocation/Subluxation

A **sprain** is a traumatic injury to a joint involving the ligaments. Swelling, pain, and discoloration of the skin may be present. The severity of the injury is measured in grades:

Grade I sprain is a stretching of a ligament.
Grade II sprain is a partial tearing of a ligament.
Grade III sprain is a complete tear of a ligament.

A **strain** is a lesser injury, usually described as overuse or overstretching of a muscle or tendon.

A bone that is completely out of its place in a joint is called a **dislocation.** If the bone is partially out of the joint, it is considered to be a **subluxation** (sub luck SAY shun). This can be a congenital or an acquired condition.

Compartment syndrome is a potentially serious medical condition that is a result of swelling within the fascia. The increased pressure limits the blood supply, which in turn may lead to nerve and muscle damage.

Colles   Comminuted

Complicated   Compression

Greenstick   Hairline

Impacted   Salter-Harris

Fig. 3-17 Fractures.

Terms Related to Trauma	
Type	**Definition**
Fractures* (Fig. 3-17)	
Colles	Fracture at distal end of the radius at the epiphysis. Often occurs when patient has attempted to break his/her fall.
comminuted	Bone is crushed and/or shattered into multiple pieces.
complicated	Bone is broken and pierces an internal organ.
compression	Fractured area of bone collapses on itself.
greenstick	Partially bent and partially broken. Relatively common in children.
hairline	Minor fracture appearing as a thin line on x-ray. May not extend through bone.
impacted	Broken bones with ends driven into each other.
Salter-Harris	Fracture of epiphyseal plate in children.
Other Trauma (Figs. 3-18 and 3-19)	
dislocation	Bone that is completely out of its joint socket.
subluxation	Partial dislocation.
sprain	Traumatic injury to ligaments of a joint, including tearing of a ligament.
strain	Overstretching or tear of muscle or a tendon.

*All fracture examples are coded as closed fractures.

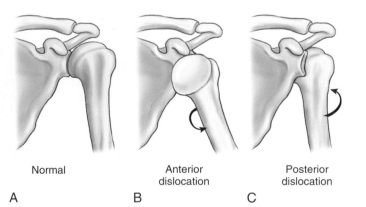

Normal   Anterior   Posterior
                  dislocation   dislocation

A   B   C

Fig. 3-18 A, Normal shoulder. Dislocated shoulder, anterior
(B) and posterior **(C).**

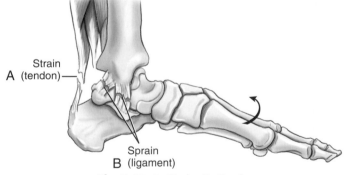

Strain
A (tendon)

Sprain
B (ligament)

Fig. 3-19 A, Strain. **B,** Sprain.

EXERCISE 19: Fractures

Match the fractures with their definitions.

_____ 1. complicated

_____ 2. greenstick

_____ 3. Colles

_____ 4. impacted

_____ 5. comminuted

_____ 6. simple/closed

_____ 7. compound/open

_____ 8. hairline

_____ 9. pathologic

A. broken bone pierces internal organ
B. broken bone pierces skin
C. spontaneous fracture as a result of disease
D. bone is partially bent and partially broken
E. bone is broken, skin is closed
F. distal end of radius is broken
G. ends of broken bone are driven into each other
H. fracture appears as a line on the bone and fracture may
    not be completely through bone
I. bone is crushed

EXERCISE 20: Other Trauma

1. A partial displacement of a bone at a joint is a _____;

    full displacement is a _____.

2. An injury that can be described in grades and involves the soft tissue of a joint is a

    _____.

3. An overstretching of a muscle is a _____.

4. Swelling within the confines of a muscle fascia can lead to _____.

Terms Related to Benign Neoplasms

Term	Word Origin	Definition
chondroma kon DROH mah	*chondr/o* cartilage *-oma* tumor, mass	Benign tumor of the cartilage, usually occurring in children and adolescents.
exostosis eck sahs TOH sis	*ex-* out *oste/o* bone *-osis* abnormal condition	Abnormal condition of bony growth. Also called **hyperostosis** and **osteochondroma.**
leiomyoma lye oh mye OH mah	*leiomy/o* smooth muscle *-oma* tumor, mass	Benign tumor of smooth muscle. The most common leiomyoma is in the uterus and is termed a *fibroid.*
osteoma ahs tee OH mah	*oste/o* bone *-oma* tumor, mass	Benign bone tumor, usually of compact bone.
rhabdomyoma rab doh mye OH mah	*rhabdomy/o* skeletal muscle *-oma* tumor, mass	Benign tumor of striated/voluntary/skeletal muscle.

Terms Related to Malignant Neoplasms

Term	Word Origin	Definition
chondrosarcoma kon droh sar KOH mah	*chondr/o* cartilage *-sarcoma* connective tissue cancer	Malignant tumor of the cartilage. Occurs most frequently in adults (Fig. 3-20).
leiomyosarcoma lye oh mye oh sar KOH mah	*leiomy/o* smooth muscle *-sarcoma* connective tissue cancer	Malignant tumor of smooth muscle. Most commonly appearing in the uterus.
osteosarcoma ahs tee oh sar KOH mah	*oste/o* bone *-sarcoma* connective tissue cancer	Malignant tumor of bone. Also called **Ewing sarcoma.** Most common children's bone cancer.
rhabdomyosarcoma rab doh mye oh sar KOH mah	*rhabdomy/o* skeletal muscle *-sarcoma* connective tissue cancer	Highly malignant tumor of skeletal muscle. Also called **rhabdosarcoma** or **rhabdomyoblastoma.**

Fig. 3-20 A, Chondrosarcoma of femur. **B,** X-ray showing prominent dense calcification in a large chondrosarcoma.

EXERCISE 21: Neoplasms

Match the neoplasms with their definitions.

_____ 1. rhabdomyosarcoma

_____ 2. osteosarcoma

_____ 3. leiomyosarcoma

_____ 4. chondrosarcoma

A. connective tissue cancer of bone
B. connective tissue cancer of cartilage
C. connective tissue cancer of skeletal muscle
D. connective tissue cancer of smooth muscle

Build the term.

5. benign tumor of skeletal muscle _____

6. benign bone tumor _____

7. benign tumor of smooth muscle _____

8. benign tumor of cartilage _____

9. an abnormal condition of out(growth) of bone _____

ⓔ *Click on **Hear It, Spell It** to practice spelling the pathology terms that you have learned in this chapter.*

Case Study **Tyro Londoff**

Eighteen-year-old high school soccer player, Tyro Londoff, has severe knee pain, swelling, and a mass on the proximal end of the right tibia. He reports that he has played soccer since he was 6 years old, and he has had a few injuries to his right leg over the years. On Saturday, he twisted his knee during a playoff game, and the swelling and pain have not gone away. He reports that last year he had badly fractured his shinbone, which required a pin to repair the break. Radiographs and a magnetic resonance imaging (MRI) scan of the knee show a Grade I sprain of the anterior collateral ligaments and what appears to be an osteochondroma on the proximal end of the tibia.

The previous repair remains intact with no signs of osteomyelitis. Treatment consists of analgesics, rest, and prolonged absence from playing soccer. The osteochondroma will be monitored for change over time.

1. Osteomyelitis is decoded to mean an inflammation of the bone and _____.

2. Osteochondroma is decoded to mean a tumor or mass of the bone and _____.

3. The proximal end of the tibia is ____ the hip.
   a. closer to
   b. farther from

4. The word part oste/o means _____.

5. A Grade I sprain is the _____ severe type of sprain?
   a. least
   b. most

Herold, Jean F - 12438 Opened by Landrey, Melissa, PA

Task   Edit   View   Time Scale   Options   Help

As Of 09:19

Herold, Jean F

Age: 54 years   Sex: Female   Loc: AR-OC
DOB: 07/23/1960   MRN: 12438   FIN: 8425633

Reference Text Browser | Form Browser | Medication Profile

Orders | Last 48 Hours | ED | Lab | Radiology | **Assessments** | Surgery | Clinical Notes | Pt. Info | Pt. Schedule | Task List | I & O | MAR

Flowsheet: Assessments   Level: History & Physical   ⦿ Table   ○ Group   ○ List

Navigator

✓   History & Physical

CHIEF COMPLAINT:	Right shoulder pain/fracture
HISTORY OF PRESENT ILLNESS:	Patient is a 54-year-old female who works as a health-care worker. While out exercising last night, she fell on her right shoulder. She has a comminuted fracture of the proximal humerus involving the humeral head, extending into the joint space. Admitted for observation and analgesia. CT of shoulder reveals the need for a humeral prosthesis. Some discomfort with deep inspiration. Unclear whether this is in the shoulder or possible right chest wall.
PAST MEDICAL HISTORY:	Cholecystectomy 1986. ORIF left forearm, fracture same forearm, age 9. Has some dependent edema and takes Lasix 80 mg daily for it. Does not wear compression stockings as they make her feet feel cold. Also diagnosis of fibromyalgia in 2008.
FAMILY HISTORY:	Mother died age 64 post surgical pulmonary embolus.
REVIEW OF SYSTEMS:	Negative.
PHYSICAL EXAM:	Pleasant, uncomfortable, overweight female appearing her stated age and in no distress. HEENT normal, neck supple, thyroid normal. No JVD, carotids normal. Lungs decreased breath sounds at bases. Heart regular rate and rhythm. Extremities: normal range of motion of lower extremities. Motor sensory deep tendon reflexes are normal in arm. Trace pretibial edema bilaterally without venostasis changes. Excellent peripheral pulses. Cannot adduct her arm and shoulder without pain. X-ray of shoulder and CT show comminuted fracture.
ASSESSMENT:	Comminuted right proximal humeral fracture involving humeral head.
PLAN:	Admit for analgesia, IV fluids. Has a little nausea probably from analgesics. Won't have surgery until tomorrow. Preoperative labs, EKG, and chest x-ray will be obtained before that time.

PROD MAHAFC   22 Jan 2015   09:19

EXERCISE 22: Admission Record

Using the admission record on p. 102, answer the following questions:

1. Which bone did Jean Herold break while exercising? Give both the medical term and the common name. _____

2. Did she fracture the area *closest to her shoulder* or *farthest from her shoulder?* (Underline one.)

3. Describe the type of fracture sustained. _____

4. What other musculoskeletal disorder does she currently have? _____

5. What does "cannot adduct her arm and shoulder without pain" mean? _____

 Age Matters

Pediatrics

As can be seen from our table of congenital disorders, there are several musculoskeletal conditions that a child may be born with: achondroplasia, MD, two disorders of the phalanges (syndactyly and polydactyly), spina bifida occulta, talipes, and congenital torticollis. Although not exclusive to childhood, pediatric statistics reveal high numbers of children treated each year for the effects of physical trauma. Fractures are common: beginning with clavicular fractures (the result of birth trauma) to fractures of the arms (humerus, radius, and ulna) and the legs (femur, tibia, and fibula). Sprains, strains, dislocations, and subluxations are other pediatric diagnoses that appear with regularity for this system.

Geriatrics

Statistics collected on the geriatric population of patients also report a high number of fractures. These, however, are mainly fractures of the hip and femur and are often preceded by bone loss caused by osteoporosis or cancer.

OA, often referred to as "wear and tear disease," is another disorder that afflicts many patients as they age. The high numbers of total knee replacement (TKR) surgeries today are often the result of this disease.

 *You can review the pathology terms you've learned in this chapter by playing **Medical Millionaire.***

DIAGNOSTIC PROCEDURES

Terms Related to Imaging

Term	Word Origin	Definition
arthrography ar THRAH gruh fee	*arthr/o* joint *-graphy* process of recording	X-ray recording of a joint.
arthroscopy ar THRAHS kuh pee	*arthr/o* joint *-scopy* process of viewing	Visual examination of a joint, accomplished by use of an arthroscope (Fig. 3-21).
computed tomography (CT) scan	*tom/o* section *-graphy* process of recording	Imaging technology that records transverse planes of the body for diagnostic purposes.
dual energy x-ray absorptiometry (DEXA) scan DECK suh		A procedure that measures the density of bone at the hip and spine. Also called **bone mineral density studies** (Fig. 3-22).

Continued

Terms Related to Imaging—cont'd

Term	Word Origin	Definition
electromyography (EMG) ee leck troh mye AH gruh fee	*electr/o* electricity *my/o* muscle *-graphy* process of recording	Procedure that records the electrical activity of muscles.
magnetic resonance imaging (MRI)		Procedure that uses magnetic properties to record detailed information about internal structures.
myelogram MYE eh loh gram	*myel/o* spinal cord *-gram* record, recording	X-ray of spinal canal done after injection of contrast medium.
x-ray (radiograph)		Imaging technique using electromagnetic radiation for recording internal structures.

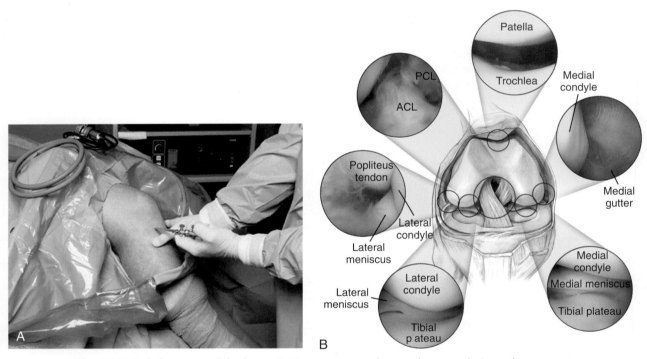

Fig. 3-21 A, Arthroscopy of the knee. **B,** Knee structures that can be seen during arthroscopy at six different points *(circles).*

Fig. 3-22 Dual energy x-ray absorptiometry (DEXA) scan. **A,** DEXA system. **B,** Scan of lumbar vertebrae.

Other Diagnostic Tests

Term	Word Origin	Definition
goniometry goh nee AH meh tree	*goni/o* angle *-metry* process of measuring	The process of measuring a joint's ROM. The instrument used is called a **goniometer** (Fig. 3-23).
Phalen test FAY lin		A diagnostic test where the back (dorsal surfaces) of the patient's hands are pressed together to elicit the symptoms of CTS (Fig. 3-24).
range of motion (ROM) testing		An assessment of the degree to which a joint can be extended and flexed.
rheumatoid factor (RF) test ROO mah toyd	*rheumat/o* watery flow *-oid* resembling	Lab test that looks for RF present in the blood of those who have RA.
serum calcium (Ca)		Test to measure the amount of calcium in the blood.

Fig. 3-23 Goniometry using a goniometer.

Fig. 3-24 Phalen test.

EXERCISE 23: Diagnostic Procedures

Match the diagnostic tests to their definitions.

_____ 1. MRI scan   _____ 5. RF   A. test for RA
                                            B. imaging technique using electromagnetic radiation
_____ 2. DEXA scan   _____ 6. serum   C. imaging of a plane of the body
                               calcium   D. blood test for calcium (Ca)
_____ 3. x-ray   E. test to measure bone density, using dual energy x-ray
                       _____ 7. EMG   F. imaging using magnetic resonance
_____ 4. ROM   G. range of motion
                       _____ 8. CT scan   H. electromyography

Build the terms.

9.   process of viewing a joint _____

10. process of recording a joint _____

11. process of recording the electrical (activity) of a muscle _____

12. process of recording the spinal cord _____

THERAPEUTIC INTERVENTIONS

Setting Fractures

Broken bones must be "set"—that is, aligned and immobilized; the most common method is with a plaster cast. If a bone does not mend and realign correctly, it is said to be a **malunion.** If no healing takes place, it is a **nonunion.** A piece of bone that does not have a renewed blood supply will die; this tissue then is called a **sequestrum** (seh KWES trum). Removal of dirt, damaged tissue, or foreign objects from a wound is one of the first steps in repairing an open fracture. This removal of debris is called **débridement** (de breed MON). Methods of fixation and alignment are described as follows:

External fixation (EF): Noninvasive stabilization of broken bones in which no opening is made in the skin; instead, the stabilization takes place mainly through devices external to the body that offer traction (Fig. 3-25, *A*).
Internal fixation (IF): Stabilization of broken bones in their correct position, using pins, screws, plates, and so on, which are fastened to the bones to maintain correct alignment (see Fig. 3-25, *B*).
Reduction: Alignment and immobilization of the ends of a broken bone. Also referred to as **manipulation.** *Open reduction (OR)* requires incision of the skin; *closed reduction (CR)* does not require incision.

An **ORIF** is an **o**pen **r**eduction using **i**nternal **f**ixation. A **CREF** is a **c**losed **r**eduction using **e**xternal **f**ixation.

Fig. 3-25 Fixation. **A,** External. **B,** Internal.

Terms Related to Therapeutic Interventions

Term	Word Origin	Definition
amputation am pyoo TAY shun		Removal of a limb when there are no feasible options to save it.
arthrocentesis ar throh sen TEE sis	*arthr/o* joint *-centesis* surgical puncture	Surgical puncture of a joint to remove fluid.
arthrodesis ar throh DEE sis	*arthr/o* joint *-desis* binding	Binding or stabilization of a joint by operative means.
arthroplasty ar throh plas tee	*arthr/o* joint *-plasty* surgical repair	General term meaning surgical repair of a joint.
bunionectomy bun yun ECK tuh mee	*bunion/o* bunion *-ectomy* excision, resection	Removal of a bunion (Fig. 3-26).
kyphoplasty KYE foh plas tee	*kyph/o* round back *-plasty* surgical repair	Minimally invasive procedure designed to address the pain of fractured vertebrae resulting from osteoporosis or cancer (Fig. 3-27). A balloon is used to inflate the area of fracture before a cement-like substance is injected. The substance hardens rapidly, and pain relief is immediate in most patients.
laminectomy lam ih NECK tuh mee	*lamin/o* lamina *-ectomy* excision, resection	Removal of the bony arches of one or more vertebrae to relieve compression of the spinal cord (Fig. 3-28).
meniscectomy men iss ECK tuh mee	*menisc/o* meniscus *-ectomy* removal	Removal of a meniscus, such as in the knee.
myorrhaphy mye ORE rah fee	*my/o* muscle *-rrhaphy* suture	Suture of a muscle.

Continued

Terms Related to Therapeutic Interventions—cont'd

Term	Word Origin	Definition
operative ankylosis AH pur ah tiv ang kih LOH sis	*ankyl/o* stiffening *-osis* abnormal condition	Procedure used in the treatment of spinal fractures or after diskectomy or laminectomy for the correction of a herniated vertebral disk; also used to describe surgical fixation of a joint. Also called **arthrodesis.**
osteoclasis AHS tee oh klay sis	*oste/o* bone *-clasis* intentional breaking	Refracture of a bone; usually done if a bone has a malunion.
osteoplasty AHS tee oh plas tee	*oste/o* bone *-plasty* surgical repair	Surgical repair of a bone.
prosthesis (*pl.* prostheses) prahs THEE sis	*prosth/o* addition *-is* thing	An artificial body part that is constructed to replace missing limbs, eyes, and other body parts.
spondylosyndesis spon dih loh sin DEE sis	*spondyl/o* vertebra *syn-* together *-desis* binding	Fixation of an unstable segment of the spine by skeletal traction, immobilization of the patient in a body cast, or stabilization with a bone graft or synthetic device. Also called **spinal fusion** and **spondylodesis.**
syndesmoplasty sin DEZ moh plas tee	*syndesm/o* ligament *-plasty* surgical repair	Surgical repair of a ligament.
tenomyoplasty ten oh MYE oh plas tee	*ten/o* tendon *my/o* muscle *-plasty* surgical repair	Surgical repair of a muscle and a tendon.
total hip replacement (THR)		Replacement of the femoral head and the acetabulum of the hip with either plastic or metal appliances (Fig. 3-29, *A*).
total knee replacement (TKR)		Extensive surgical procedure that involves the replacement of the entire knee joint, either unilaterally or bilaterally (see Fig. 3-29, *B*).
traction	*tract/o* pulling *-ion* process of	The process of pulling a body part into correct alignment, as to correct a dislocation.

Fig. 3-26 Bunionectomy.

Medial eminence of metatarsal bone is removed

Fig. 3-27 Kyphoplasty.

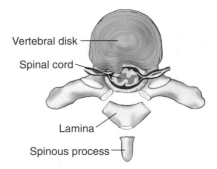

Vertebral disk

Spinal cord

Lamina

Spinous process

Fig. 3-28 Laminectomy.

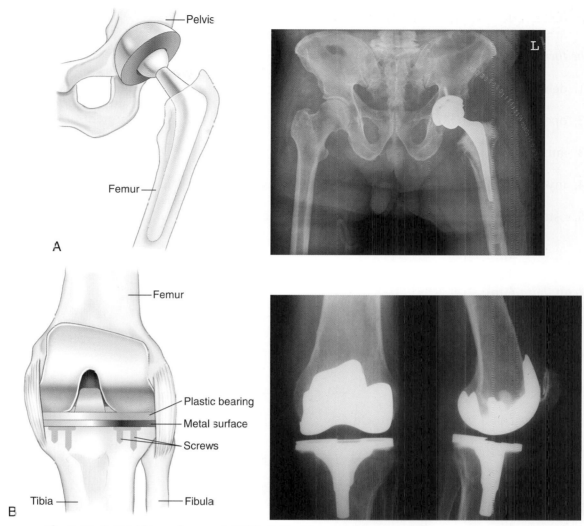

Fig. 3-29 A, Total hip replacement (THR). **B,** Total knee replacement (TKR).

EXERCISE 24: Therapeutic Interventions

Match the therapeutic terms with their definitions.

_____ 1. débridement

_____ 2. open reduction (OR)

_____ 3. amputation

_____ 4. myorrhaphy

_____ 5. osteoclasis

_____ 6. arthrodesis

_____ 7. prosthesis

_____ 8. spondylosyndesis

_____ 9. arthrocentesis

_____ 10. closed reduction (CR)

A. suture of muscle
B. intentional fracture of bone
C. alignment of ends of bone with incision
D. alignment of ends of bone without incision
E. surgical puncture of a joint
F. artificial body part
G. removal of a limb
H. removal of debris
I. spinal fusion
J. fixation of a joint

Build a term that means:

11. surgical repair of a joint _____

12. intentional breaking of a bone _____

13. excision of a bunion _____

14. surgical repair of a tendon and muscle _____

15. removal of a meniscus _____

16. surgical repair of a ligament _____

PHARMACOLOGY

analgesics: Reduce pain. Examples include morphine (MS Contin), hydroco-done (Vicodin or Lortab, in combination with acetaminophen), acetamino-phen (Tylenol), and NSAIDs such as naproxen (Anaprox).

antiinflammatories: Used to reduce inflammation and pain. Examples include steroidal and nonsteroidal antiinflammatory drugs (NSAIDs). Meth-ylprednisolone (Medrol) is an example of a steroid; ibuprofen (Advil, Motrin) and celecoxib (Celebrex) are examples of NSAIDs.

bisphosphonates: Prevent and sometimes reverse bone loss to treat diseases such as osteoporosis, Paget disease, or bone cancer. Examples include alen-dronate (Fosamax) and zoledronic acid (Zometa).

disease-modifying antirheumatic drugs (DMARDs): Slow progression of rheumatoid arthritis while also reducing signs and symptoms. Examples include leflunomide (Arava), etanercept (Enbrel), and infliximab (Remicade).

muscle relaxants: Relieve pain caused by muscle spasms by relaxing the skeletal muscles. Examples include cyclobenzaprine (Flexeril) and metaxalone (Skelaxin).

EXERCISE 25: Pharmacology

1. What class of drugs may prevent osteoporosis? _____ .

2. RA progression may be treated with _____ .

3. NSAIDs are used to treat what kinds of symptoms? _____

4. _____ are used to treat muscle spasms.

 Click on **Hear It, Spell It** to practice spelling the diagnostic and therapeutic terms you have learned in this chapter.

Case Study Consuela Esteban

Nine-year-old Consuela Esteban fell off her skateboard, injuring her leg. Pain, swelling, bruising, and crepitus are all present by the time her father gets her to the emergency department (ED). Radiographs confirm a closed fracture of the distal tibia. The ED physician performs reduction on the fracture and puts a plaster cast on Consuela's leg. She is sent home with analgesics.

1. Which term indicates a grating sound? _____
   _____

2. How do you know the bone did not pierce the skin?
   _____

3. Which term means that the ends of the bone are realigned before being casted? _____

4. Analgesics were prescribed to reduce Consuela's _____ .

Case Study Pia Romana

Pia Romana, a 54-year-old administrative assistant, has been suffering cervicalgia for a month. Myelography and MRI of her upper spine reveal an intervertebral herniated disk in C3. Because this is the third time that Pia has experienced herniation of this particular disk, her physician refers her to an orthopedic surgeon, who performs a laminectomy.

1. The suffix -*algia* means _____
   _____ .

2. Which region of the spine is C3 located in? _____
   _____

3. The prefix *inter-* means _____ .

4. The record that is created when myelography is performed is called a/an _____ .

5. Laminectomy is the _____ of the lamina of the vertebra.
   a. cutting
   b. removal
   c. repair
   d. new opening

Case Study   Barbara Eversole

Barbara Eversole visits her orthopedic surgeon complaining of pain and stiffness in her left knee. She says that the knee is especially stiff when she gets up in the morning, but that it "works better" after she is up and about for a while. Upon examination, the knee is swollen and ROM is limited. Barbara's family history includes OA on the maternal side but no RA. Barbara's mobility has become increasingly limited, and NSAIDS have had little effect on the pain. Her orthopedic surgeon plans on sending her to physical therapy, and if there is no improvement, may consider TKR.

1. What does OA stand for? _____
   _____

2. Barbara does not have RA. What does RA stand for?
   _____

3. What does ROM stand for? _____
   _____

4. What does TKR stand for? _____
   _____

5. What type of drug is an NSAID? _____
   _____

Abbreviations

Abbreviation	Meaning
A	action
C1-C7	first cervical through seventh cervical vertebrae
CR	closed reduction
CREF	closed reduction external fixation
CT	computed tomography
CTS	carpal tunnel syndrome
DEXA	dual energy x-ray absorptiometry
DIP	distal interphalangeal joint
DJD	degenerative joint disease
EF	external fixation
EMG	electromyography
Fx, #	fracture
I	insertion
L1-L5	first lumbar through fifth lumbar vertebrae
MD	muscular dystrophy

Abbreviation	Meaning
MRI	magnetic resonance imaging
NSAID	nonsteroidal antiinflammatory drug
O	origin
OA	osteoarthritis
OR	open reduction
ORIF	open reduction internal fixation
PIP	proximal interphalangeal joint
RA	rheumatoid arthritis
RF	rheumatoid factor
ROM	range of motion
S1-S5	first sacral through fifth sacral segments
SLE	systemic lupus erythematosus
T1-T12	first thoracic through twelfth thoracic vertebrae
THR	total hip replacement
TKR	total knee replacement

EXERCISE 26: Abbreviations

Explain the meanings of the abbreviations used in the following examples.

1. Greta is an 83-year-old white female with a compression Fx of L5. A DEXA scan revealed loss of bone mass.

   _____

2. The patient had been self-medicating her DJD with NSAIDs.

   _____

3. EMG was used to diagnose Ryan's MD.

   _____

4. Which of the following is not an imaging procedure—CT, CTS, MRI?

   _____

Chapter Review

Match the word parts to their definitions.

Word Part Definitions

Prefix/Suffix

Prefix/Suffix
-centesis
-clasis
-desis
-listhesis
-malacia
-osis
peri-
-physis
-plasia
syn-

Definition

1. _____ binding
2. _____ condition of development
3. _____ surgical puncture
4. _____ together, joined
5. _____ softening
6. _____ slipping
7. _____ surrounding, around
8. _____ intentional breaking
9. _____ growth
10. _____ abnormal condition

Combining Form

Combining Form
arthr/o
carp/o
cervic/o
chondr/o
cleid/o
coccyg/o
cost/o
dactyl/o
femor/o
gnath/o
humer/o
mandibul/o
my/o
myel/o
olecran/o
oste/o
patell/a
phalang/o
rhabdomy/o
scapul/o
spondyl/o
zygomat/o

Definition

11. _____ collarbone
12. _____ bone
13. _____ jaw (entire)
14. _____ skeletal muscle
15. _____ upper arm bone
16. _____ wrist
17. _____ cheekbone
18. _____ thigh bone
19. _____ neck
20. _____ vertebra
21. _____ cartilage
22. _____ spinal cord
23. _____ finger/toe (whole)
24. _____ finger/toe bone
25. _____ rib
26. _____ muscle
27. _____ elbow
28. _____ tailbone
29. _____ kneecap
30. _____ joint
31. _____ lower jaw
32. _____ shoulder blade

Word Shop

Prefixes	Combining Forms	Suffixes
a-	arthr/o	-desis
an-	chondr/o	-itis
inter-	cost/o	-lysis
peri-	dactyl/o	-malacia
poly-	my/o	-oma
syn-	myos/o	-osis
	oste/o	-plasia
	phyt/o	-plasty
	rhabdomy/o	-rrhaphy
	spin/o	-um
	spondyl/o	-y
	syndesm/o	
	ten/o	

Build the following terms by combining the preceding word parts. Some word parts may be used more than once. Some may not be used at all. The number in parentheses indicates the number of word parts needed.

Definition	Term
1. structure surrounding bone (3)	_____
2. inflammation of many muscles (3)	_____
3. inflammation surrounding a joint (3)	_____
4. softening of the cartilage (2)	_____
5. condition of many fingers/toes (3)	_____
6. destruction of skeletal muscle (2)	_____
7. abnormal condition of bone growth (3)	_____
8. binding of a joint (2)	_____
9. suture of a muscle (2)	_____
10. condition of joined fingers/toes (3)	_____
11. tumor of cartilage (2)	_____
12. binding of vertebrae together (3)	_____
13. surgical repair of a ligament (2)	_____
14. no formation of cartilage (3)	_____
15. surgical repair of a tendon and a muscle (3)	_____

Sort the terms below into the correct categories.

Term Sorting

Anatomy and Physiology	Pathology	Diagnostic Procedures	Therapeutic Interventions

arthrocentesis	CTS	MRI	radius
arthrodesis	DEXA	myelogram	ROM
arthrography	diaphysis	myorrhaphy	serum calcium
arthroscopy	digitus	osteoclasis	spondylolisthesis
arthrosis	EMG	osteomyelitis	sternum
articulation	goniometry	osteoplasty	syndactyly
bunion	humerus	osteoporosis	tendinitis
bursitis	laminectomy	osteosarcoma	tenomyoplasty
cartilage	ligament	Phalen test	TKR
costa	meniscectomy	prosthesis	ulna

Replace the highlighted words with the correct terms.

Translations

1. Ms. Alston was diagnosed with **softening of the cartilage** of her knee and a **cyst of synovial fluid in the popliteal area of her leg.**

2. After a crushing injury to her leg, the physician performed **removal of the limb** and replaced it with a/an **artificial body part.**

3. The surgeon performed a **suture of a muscle** to correct Mr. Adams' injury.

4. The patient had a **surgical puncture of a joint** to correct **an abnormal condition of blood in the joint** of Jason's left hip.

5. Dr. Matthews performed **an alignment and immobilization** of the right **collarbone** of 5-year-old Caitlin, who had fallen while jumping on her bed.

6. The student had a **diagnostic test where the dorsal surfaces of the hands are pressed together** to diagnose **compression injury of the median nerve at the wrist.**

7. Sarah Henderson had **abnormal bone growths** in the **joints between the bones of her fingers.**

8. The patient had **an extreme posterior curvature of the thoracic area of the spine** that was a result of her **loss of bone mass.**

9. The patient was admitted for **inflammation of the bone and bone marrow** of his **lower lateral arm bone.**

10. The patient complained of **inflammation of the fascia on the sole of the foot** and **inflammation of a tendon.**

11. **A procedure that records the electrical activity of muscles** was used to confirm the child's **group of disorders characterized as an inherited progressive atrophy of skeletal muscle.**

12. An x-ray revealed **a partially bent and partially broken** fracture of the child's right **upper arm bone.**

13. The baby was diagnosed with **condition of more than five fingers on her hand** and **condition of the joining of the toes.**

14. Mrs. Anderhub had **a removal of a bunion** to correct her **painful enlargement and inflammation of the first metatarsophalangeal joint.**

Medical Record Evelyn Auden

Auden, Evelyn E - 29202 Opened by Chong, Mae-Li (surgeon)

Task   Edit   View   Time Scale   Options   Help

Auden, Evelyn E   Age: 72 years   Sex: Female   Loc: ARH-ANC
                                DOB: 09/02/1942   MRN: 29202   FIN: 8425633

Reference Text Browser | Form Browser | Medication Profile

Orders | Last 48 Hours | ED | Lab | Radiology | Assessments | **Surgery** | Clinical Notes | Pt. Info | Pt. Schedule | Task List | I & O | MAR

Flowsheet: Surgery   Level: Operative Report   ⦿ Table ○ Group ○ List

Navigator ✕
✓ Operative Report

Preoperative Diagnosis: Degenerative Joint
    Disease, Right Knee
Postoperative Diagnosis: Degenerative Joint
    Disease, Right Knee
Name of Operation: Total Knee Replacement

Anesthesia: Spinal
Estimated Blood Loss: 150 cc
Antibiotics: Vancomycin 1 gm
Tourniquet: 350 mm Hg
Complications: none

Components: Zimmer NextGen LPS
Femur: size G
Tibia: 6
Articulating Surface: 10 mm
Patella: 38

Procedure
The patient was properly identified in the OR, and the leg was prepped and draped in the
routine fashion. The leg was exsanguinated, and the tourniquet inflated. A standard anterior
approach was made along with the median parapatellar arthrotomy. The patella was everted.
The fat pad was partially removed, the knee flexed, and all joint surfaces prepared in the
conventional manner to the size needed. The surfaces were prepared with pulse irrigating
system followed by antibiotic irrigation. They were then dried. All components were cemented
simultaneously. Any excess cement was removed with curettes and/or osteotomes.
    The knee was placed in full extension, if not slight hyperextension, while the cement cured.
The patient tolerated the procedure well and left the operating room in stable condition.

PROD | MAHAFC | 12 April 2015 | 11:11

⟳ OPERATIVE REPORT

Using the operative report on p. 118, answer the following questions.

1. A synonym for the preoperative diagnosis of degenerative joint disease is _____

   _____.

2. An "anterior approach" to the knee would be through which part of the knee? _____

   _____

3. What is the "patella?" _____

4. To what does the term *parapatellar* refer? _____

5. What is an "arthrotomy?" _____

6. If the patella was everted, how would it be placed? _____

7. What is an "osteotome?" _____

8. What would "hyperextension" be? _____

4 Integumentary System

OBJECTIVES

- Recognize and use terms related to the anatomy and physiology of the integumentary system.
- Recognize and use terms related to the pathology of the integumentary system.
- Recognize and use terms related to the diagnostic procedures for the integumentary system.
- Recognize and use terms related to the therapeutic interventions for the integumentary system.

For more interactive learning, go to the Shiland Evolve website and click on:
- **Match the Word Parts** to review integumentary word parts.
- **Word Shop** to practice word building.
- **Tournament of Terminology** to test your knowledge of integumentary terms.
- **Term Sorting** to practice sorting integumentary terms.

*Click on **Chapter at a Glance** for a list of key word parts and terms for this chapter.*

FUNCTIONS OF THE INTEGUMENTARY SYSTEM

The most important function of the **skin** (integument) is that it acts as the first line of defense in protecting the body from disease by providing an external barrier. It also helps regulate the temperature of the body, provides information about the environment through the sense of touch, assists in the synthesis of vitamin D (essential for the normal formation of bones and teeth), and helps eliminate waste products from the body. It is the largest organ of the body and accomplishes its diverse functions with assistance from its accessory structures, which include the **hair, nails,** and two types of **glands: sebaceous (oil)** and **sudoriferous (sweat).** Any impairment of the skin has the potential to lessen its ability to carry out these functions, which can lead to disease.

SPECIALTIES/SPECIALISTS

The study of the skin, hair, and nails is called *dermatology.* A **dermatologist** is one who specializes in this area.

ANATOMY AND PHYSIOLOGY

Skin

The skin is composed of two layers: the **epidermis** (eh pih DUR mis), which forms the outermost layer, and the **dermis** or **corium** (KORE ee um), the inner layer (Fig. 4-1). The dermis is attached to a layer of connective tissue called the **hypodermis** or the **subcutaneous** (sub kyoo TAY nee us) layer, which is mainly composed of fat (adipose tissue).

skin = derm/o, dermat/o, cut/o, cutane/o

hair = trich/o, pil/o

nail = onych/o, ungu/o

oil, sebum = seb/o, sebac/o

sweat = hidr/o, sudor/i

dermatologist
dermat/o = skin
-logist = one who specializes in the study of

epidermis
epi- = above, upon
derm/o = skin
-is = structure

hypodermis
hypo- = under, below
derm/o = skin
-is = structure

subcutaneous
sub- = under, below
cutane/o = skin
-ous = pertaining to

fat = adip/o

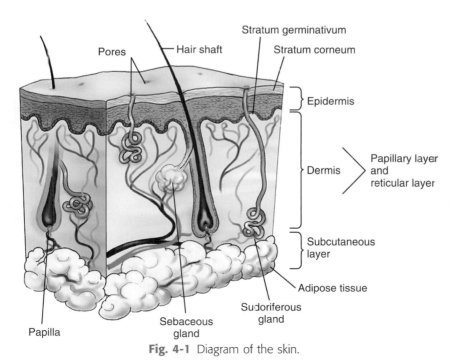

Fig. 4-1 Diagram of the skin.

scaly = squam/o

keratinocyte
kerat/o = hard, horny
-in = substance
-cyte = cell

avascular
a- = without
vascul/o = vessel
-ar = pertaining to

basal = bas/o

melanocyte
melan/o = black
-cyte = cell

sudoriferous
sudor/i = sweat
-ferous = pertaining to carrying

sebaceous
sebac/o = oil
-ous = pertaining to

sebum = seb/o

hair = trich/o, pil/o

follicle = follicul/o

papilla = papill/o

⊗ Be Careful!

Don't confuse **strata** *meaning layers with* **striae** *meaning stretch marks.*

Free edge
Lunula
Cuticle
Nail body
Nail bed
Bone
Nail root

Fig. 4-2 The nail.

Epidermis

The top layer, the epidermis, is composed of several different layers, or strata, (*sing.* stratum) of epithelial (eh pih THEE lee ul) tissue. Epithelial tissue covers many of the external and internal surfaces of the body. Because the type of epithelial tissue that covers the body has a microscopic **scaly** appearance, it is referred to as **stratified squamous epithelium** (SKWAY muss eh pih THEE lee um) (squamous means scaly).

Although there is a limited blood supply to the epidermis (it is **avascular** [a VAS kyoo lur]—that is, it contains no blood vessels), constant activity is taking place. New skin cells are formed in the **basal** (BAY sul) (bottom) layer of the epidermis, the **stratum germinativum** (STRAY tum jur mih nuh TIH vum). This layer is also the site where **melanin** (pigment) is produced by cells called **melanocytes.** When the skin is exposed to ultraviolet (UV) light, the melanocytes secrete more melanin. Birthmarks, age spots, and freckles result from the clumping of melanin. Individuals have different skin colors because of varying numbers of melanocytes in the basal layer of the skin. The new cells move outward toward the **stratum corneum** (top layer). During the transition from the lowest layer to the outer layer, these cells are then called **keratinocytes** because they are filled with **keratin** (KAIR ah tin), which is a hard protein material. The nature of the keratin adds to the protective nature of the skin, giving it a waterproof property that helps retain moisture within the body.

Dermis

The **dermis,** or corium, is the thick, underlying layer of the skin that is composed of vascular connective tissue arranged in two layers. The **papillary layer** is the upper thin layer composed of fibers made from protein and collagen that serves to regulate blood flow through its extensive vascular supply. The **reticular layer** is the lower, thicker layer, which also is composed of collagen fibers. This layer holds the **hair follicles, sweat,** and **sebaceous glands,** which are the glands that produce oil.

Accessory Structures

Glands

The **sudoriferous** (soo dur IF uh rus) glands, also called the sweat glands, are located in the dermis and provide one means of thermoregulation for the body. They secrete sweat through tiny openings in the surface of the skin called **pores.** The secretion of sweat is called **perspiration.** These glands are present throughout the body but are especially abundant in the following areas: the soles of the feet, the palms of the hands, the armpits or axillae (*sing.* axilla), the upper lip, and the forehead.

The **sebaceous** (seh BAY shus) **glands** secrete an oily, acidic substance called **sebum** (SEE bum), which helps to lubricate hair and the surface of the skin. The acidic nature of sebum is key in inhibiting the growth of bacteria.

Hair

Hair has its roots in the dermis; these roots, together with their coverings, are called **hair follicles** (FALL ih kuls). The visible part is called the **hair shaft.** Underneath the follicle is a nipple-shaped structure that encloses the capillaries called the **papilla** (pah PILL ah) (*pl.* papillae). Epithelial cells on top of the papilla are responsible for the formation of the hair shaft. When these cells die, hair can no longer regenerate, and hair loss occurs. The main function of hair is to assist in thermoregulation by holding heat near the body. When it is cold, hair stands on end, holding a layer of air as insulation near the body (piloerection).

Nails

Nails cover and thus protect the dorsal surfaces of the distal bones of the fingers and toes (Fig. 4-2). The part that is visible is the **nail body** (also called the *nail* *plate*), whereas the **nail root** is in a groove under a small fold of skin at the base of the nail. The **nail bed** is the highly vascular tissue under the nail that appears pink when the blood is oxygenated or blue/purple when it is oxygen deficient. The moonlike white area at the base of the nail is called the **lunula** (LOON yoo lah), beyond which new growth occurs. The small fold of skin above the lower part of the nail is called the **cuticle** (KYOO tih kul) or **eponychium** (eh puh NICK ee um). The **paronychium** (pair ih NICK ee um) is the fold of skin that is near the sides of the nail.

eponychium
  epi- = above
  onych/o = nail
  -ium = structure

paronychium
  par- = near
  onchy/o = nail
  -ium = structure

Don't confuse papill/o meaning papilla or "nipple" with papul/o meaning pimple.

You can review the anatomy of the integumentary system by clicking on **Body Spectrum Electronic Anatomy Coloring Book → Integumentary.**

 EXERCISE 1: Anatomy and Physiology

Match the integumentary term to its combining form.

_____ 1. follicle

_____ 2. fat

_____ 3. black

_____ 4. scaly

_____ 5. sweat

_____ 6. hard, horny

_____ 7. skin

_____ 8. oil, sebum

_____ 9. hair

_____ 10. nail

A. squam/o
B. follicul/o
C. trich/o, pil/o
D. sudor/i, hidr/o
E. kerat/o
F. melan/o
G. derm/o, cutane/o
H. adip/o
I. sebac/o, seb/o
J. onych/o, ungu/o

Decode the terms.

11. avascular _____

12. subungual _____

13. hypodermic _____

⟳ EXERCISE 2: The Skin

Label the structures of the skin using the terms provided.

pores
sebaceous gland
stratum corneum
papilla
epidermis
sudoriferous gland
hair shaft
subcutaneous layer
dermis
stratum
germinativum

   *Click on **Label It** to practice labeling the structures of the skin.*

Medical Record **Todd Feldman**

Feldman, Todd T - 555422 Opened by Dover, Scott MD

Task   Edit   View   Time Scale   Options   Help

| Feldman, Todd T | Age: 38 years | Sex: Male | Loc: WHC-SMMC |
| | DOB: 01/27/1978 | MRN: 555422 | FIN: 3506004 |

Reference Text Browser | Form Browser | Medication Profile

Orders | Last 48 Hours | ED | Lab | Radiology | Assessments | **Surgery** | Clinical Notes | Pt. Info | Pt. Schedule | Task List | I & O | MAR

Flowsheet: Surgery   Level: Operative Report   ○ Table ○ Group ○ List

Navigator

✓ Operative Report

Preoperative Diagnosis: Nail bed deformity and nail plate deformity, right middle finger
Postoperative Diagnosis: Nail bed deformity and nail plate deformity, right middle finger
Operation: Nail bed and nail plate ablation and shortening of distal phalanx
                          and primary flap coverage, tip, right middle finger

Patient was brought into the operating suite and middle carpal block was induced into the right middle finger. The right upper extremity was then prepped with Betadine and draped in a sterile fashion. Digital tourniquet was applied and with 43 magnification loupes, we ablated the nail plate with rongeurs. We then excised the nail bed, elliptically excising this and excising it directly off the distal phalanx. The underlying distal phalanx was extremely rough and pitted. After complete ablation of the nail bed, we removed the tuft of the distal phalanx with the rongeurs. This freed up enough volar skin so that we could close this flap up primarily. We sutured this with 5-0 nylon and then excised dog ears and both radial and ulnar sides and closed with 5-0 nylon suture. Appearance was excellent. Xeroform was applied, the digital tourniquet was removed and good circulation returned to the finger. Tube gauze dressing was then applied.

Patient will be dismissed as an outpatient and arrangements made for follow-up in 2 weeks for suture removal.

| PROD | MAHAFC | 30 Dec 2016 | 16:24 |

EXERCISE 3: Operative Report

Using the preceding operative report, answer the following questions:

1. What are the two structures (nail bed and nail plate) that are being removed (ablated)? _____

   _____

2. Where is the "volar skin" located? (Refer to Chapter 2 if you've forgotten.) _____

3. What is a "digital tourniquet," and why do you think it was used? _____

4. From your knowledge of the anatomy of a nail, what, if any, parts of the nail do you think remain?

   _____

*Click on **Hear It, Spell It** to practice spelling the anatomy and physiology terms that you have learned in this chapter.*

Combining and Adjective Forms for the Anatomy of the Integumentary System

Meaning	Combining Form	Adjective Form
base, bottom	bas/o	basal
black, dark	melan/o	melanotic
fat	adip/o	adipose
follicle	follicul/o	follicular
gland	aden/o	adenal
hair	trich/o, pil/o	pilar
hard, horny	kerat/o	keratic
nail	ungu/o, onych/o	ungual, onychia
papilla	papill/o	papillary
scaly	squam/o	squamous
sebum, oil	seb/o, sebac/o	sebaceous
skin	derm/o, dermat/o, cut/o, cutane/o	cutaneous, dermic, dermatic
sudoriferous gland	hidraden/o	
sweat	hidr/o, sudor/i	hidrotic, sudorous
vessel	vascul/o	vascular

Prefixes for the Anatomy of the Integumentary System

Prefix	Meaning
a-	no, not, without
epi-	above
hypo-, sub-	under, below

Suffixes for the Anatomy of the Integumentary System

Suffix	Meaning
-al, -ar, -ous, -ic	pertaining to
-cyte	cell
-ferous	pertaining to carrying
-is	structure

PATHOLOGY

Skin Lesions

A skin **lesion** (LEE zhun) is any visible, localized abnormality of skin tissue. It can be described as either primary or secondary. **Primary lesions** (Fig. 4-3) are early skin changes that have not yet undergone natural evolution or change caused by manipulation. **Secondary lesions** (Fig. 4-4) are the result of natural evolution or manipulation of a primary lesion.

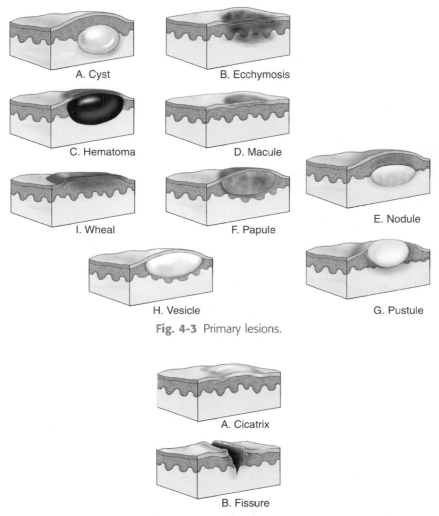

A. Cyst

B. Ecchymosis

C. Hematoma

D. Macule

I. Wheal

F. Papule

E. Nodule

H. Vesicle

G. Pustule

Fig. 4-3 Primary lesions.

A. Cicatrix

B. Fissure

Fig. 4-4 Secondary lesions.

Terms Related to Primary Skin Lesions

Term	Word Origin	Definition
cyst sist	*cyst/o* sac, bladder	Nodule filled with a semisolid material, such as a keratinous or sebaceous cyst (see Fig. 4-3, *A*).
ecchymosis (*pl.* ecchymoses) eck ih MOH sis	*ec-* out *chym/o* juice *-osis* abnormal condition	Hemorrhage or extravasation (leaking) of blood into the subcutaneous tissue. The resultant darkening is commonly described as a **bruise** (see Fig. 4-3, *B*).

Continued

Terms Related to Primary Skin Lesions—cont'd

Term	Word Origin	Definition
hematoma hee mah TOH mah	*hemat/o* blood *-oma* mass	Collection of extravasated blood trapped in the tissues and palpable to the examiner, such as on the ear (see Fig. 4-3, *C*).
macule MACK yool	*macul/o* spot	Flat blemish or discoloration less than 1 cm, such as a freckle, port-wine stain, or tattoo (see Fig. 4-3, *D*).
nodule NOD yool	*nod/o* knot *-ule* small	Palpable, solid lesion less than 2 cm, such as a very small lipoma (see Fig. 4-3, *E*).
papule PAP yool	*papul/o* pimple	Raised solid skin lesion raised less than 1 cm, such as a pimple (see Fig. 4-3, *F*).
patch		Large, flat, nonpalpable macule, larger than 1 cm.
petechia (*pl.* petechiae) peh TEEK ee ah		Tiny ecchymosis within the dermal layer.
plaque plack		Raised plateaulike papule greater than 1 cm, such as a psoriatic lesion or seborrheic keratosis.
purpura PUR pur ah	*purpur/o* purple *-a* noun ending	Massive hemorrhage into the tissues under the skin.
pustule PUS tyool	*pustul/o* pustule	Superficial, elevated lesion containing pus that may be the result of an infection, such as acne (see Fig. 4-3, *G*).
telangiectasia tell an jee eck TAY zsa	*tel/e* far *angi/o* vessel *-ectasia* dilation	Permanent dilation of groups of superficial capillaries and venules. Also know as **spider veins.**
tumor TOO mur		Nodule more than 2 cm; any mass or swelling, including neoplasms.
vesicle VESS ih kul	*vesicul/o* blister or small sac	Circumscribed, elevated lesion containing fluid and smaller than $\frac{1}{2}$ cm, such as an insect bite. If larger than $\frac{1}{2}$ cm, it is termed a **bulla.** Commonly called a **blister** (see Fig. 4-3, *H*).
wheal wheel		Circumscribed, elevated papule caused by localized edema, which can result from a bug bite. Urticaria, or hives, results from an allergic reaction.

Terms Related to Secondary Skin Lesions

Term	Word Origin	Definition
atrophy AT troh fee	*a-* no, not, without *troph/o* development *-y* process	Paper-thin, wasted skin often occurring in the aged or as stretch marks (**striae,** STRY ay) from rapid weight gain.
cicatrix (*pl.* cicatrices) SICK ah tricks		A **scar**—an area of fibrous tissue that replaces normal skin after destruction of some of the dermis (see Fig. 4-4, *A*).
eschar ES kar	*eschar/o* scab	Dried serum, blood, and/or pus. May occur in inflammatory and infectious diseases, such as impetigo, or as the result of a burn. Also called a **scab** (Fig. 4-5).

Terms Related to Secondary Skin Lesions—cont'd

Term	Word Origin	Definition
fissure FISH ur		Crack-like lesion of the skin, such as an anal fissure (see Fig. 4-4, *B*).
keloid KEE loyd		Type of scar that is an overgrowth of tissue at the site of injury in excess of the amount of tissue necessary to repair the wound. The extra tissue is partially due to an accumulation of collagen at the site (Fig. 4-6).
ulcer UL sur		Circumscribed craterlike lesion of the skin or mucous membrane resulting from **necrosis** (neck KROH sis), or tissue death, that can accompany an inflammatory, infectious, or malignant process. An example is a **decubitus ulcer** (deh KYOO bih tus) seen sometimes in bedridden patients (see Fig 4-17).

Fig. 4-5 Cutaneous anthrax eschar.

Fig. 4-6 Keloid caused by ear piercing.

EXERCISE 4: Skin Lesions

Match the primary lesions with their definitions.

_____ 1. vesicle _____ 4. ecchymosis

_____ 2. papule _____ 5. macule

_____ 3. wheal _____ 6. pustule

A. extravasated blood into subcutaneous tissue caused by trauma
B. flat blemish or discoloration
C. circumscribed, raised papule
D. superficial, elevated lesion containing pus
E. circumscribed, raised lesion containing fluid
F. solid, raised skin lesion

Match the smaller version of a primary skin lesion with the larger version.

_____ 7. petechia   _____ 10. macule

_____ 8. vesicle   _____ 11. nodule

_____ 9. papule

A. plaque
B. tumor
C. ecchymosis
D. bulla
E. patch

Match the secondary lesions with their definitions.

_____ 12. ulcer   _____ 15. atrophy

_____ 13. cicatrix   _____ 16. eschar

_____ 14. fissure

A. paper-thin, wasted skin
B. scab
C. crack-like lesion
D. circumscribed, craterlike lesion
E. scar

Terms Related to Dermatitis and Bacterial Infections

Term	Word Origin	Definition
atopic dermatitis a TOP ick dur mah TYE tis	*a-* no, not, without *top/o* place, location *-ic* pertaining to *dermat/o* skin *-itis* inflammation	Chronic, pruritic superficial inflammation of the skin usually associated with a family history of allergic disorders.
cellulitis sell yoo LYE tis	*cellul/o* cell *-itis* inflammation	Diffuse, spreading, acute inflammation within solid tissues. The most common cause is a *Streptococcus pyogenes* infection (Fig. 4-7).
contact dermatitis	*dermat/o* skin *-itis* inflammation	Irritated or allergic response of the skin that can lead to an acute or chronic inflammation (Fig. 4-8).
eczema ECK suh muh		Superficial inflammation of the skin, characterized by vesicles, weeping, and pruritus. Also called **dermatitis**.
folliculitis foh lick yoo LYE tis	*follicul/o* follicle *-itis* inflammation	Inflammation of the hair follicles, which may be superficial or deep and acute or chronic.
furuncle FYOOR ung kul		Localized, suppurative staphylococcal skin infection originating in a gland or hair follicle and characterized by pain, redness, and swelling. If two or more furuncles are connected by subcutaneous pockets, it is called a **carbuncle** (Fig. 4-9).

Fig. 4-7 Cellulitis of the lower leg.

Fig. 4-8 Contact dermatitis caused by allergy to metal snap on pants.

Terms Related to Dermatitis and Bacterial Infections—cont'd

Term	Word Origin	Definition
impetigo im peh TYE goh		Superficial vesiculopustular bacterial skin infection, normally seen in children, but possible in adults (Fig. 4-10).
pilonidal cyst pye loh NYE duhl	*pil/o* hair *nid/o* nest *-al* pertaining to	Growth of hair in a cyst in the sacral region.
pruritus proo RYE tuss		Itching. The marks that result from intense scratching are called **excoriations**.
seborrheic dermatitis seh boh REE ick	*seb/o* sebum *-rrheic* pertaining to discharge *dermat/o* skin *-itis* inflammation	Inflammatory scaling disease of the scalp and face. In newborns, this is known as **cradle cap**.

Fig. 4-9 Furuncle.

Fig. 4-10 Impetigo.

EXERCISE 5: Dermatitis and Bacterial Infections

Fill in the blank.

1. Another term for dermatitis is _____.

2. A chronic, pruritic superficial inflammation of the skin associated with a family history of allergic disorders is called _____.

3. An irritated or allergic response of the skin that can lead to an acute or chronic inflammation is called

   _____.

4. An inflammatory scaling disease of the scalp and face is termed _____.

5. A superficial vesiculopustular skin infection normally seen in children is called _____.

6. A localized, suppurative staphylococcal skin infection in a gland or hair follicle is called a

   _____.

7. Growth of hair in a cyst in the sacral region of the skin is a _____.

Build the terms.

8. inflammation of the hair follicles _____

9. inflammation of the (skin) cells _____

Case Study **Devin Doughtery**

Devin Doughtery is a 6-year-old boy with reddened, crusty, weeping lesions around his mouth, nose, and eyes. He complains that his face is itchy, and his mother reports that several children in the class have the same rash. Devin is given an antibacterial medication and told to resist scratching the lesions as much as possible.

1. Small, circumscribed elevated lesions filled with fluid are _____.

2. Superficial elevated lesions that contain pus are _____.

3. What is the medical term that means itchy? _____

4. Devin is diagnosed with _____.

5. What kind of infection does Devin have?
   a. viral
   b. fungal
   c. bacterial
   d. parasitic

Terms Related to Yeast and Fungal Infections

Term	Word Origin	Definition
candidiasis kan dih DYE ah sis		Yeast infection in moist, occluded areas of the skin (armpits, inner thighs, underneath pendulous breasts) and mucous membranes. Also called **moniliasis** (mah nih LYE ah sis).
dermatomycosis dur muh toh mye KOH sis	*dermat/o* skin *myc/o* fungus *-osis* abnormal condition	Fungal infection of the skin. Also called **dermatophytosis.**
tinea capitis TIN ee ah KAP ih tis	*capit/o* head *-is* structure	Fungal infection of the scalp; also known as **ringworm.**
tinea corporis TIN ee ah KOR poor is	*corpor/o* body *-is* structure	Ringworm of the body, manifested by pink to red papulosquamous annular (ringlike) plaques with raised borders; also known as **ringworm** (Fig. 4-11).
tinea cruris TIN ee ah KROO ris	*crur/o* leg *-is* structure	A fungal infection that occurs mainly on external genitalia and upper legs in males, particularly in warm weather; also known as **jock itch.**
tinea pedis TIN ee ah PEH dis	*ped/o* foot *-is* structure	Fungal infection of the foot; also known as **athlete's foot.**

Fig. 4-11 Tinea corporis.

Fig. 4-12 Lice in hair (pediculosis).

Terms Related to Parasitic Infestations

Term	Word Origin	Definition
pediculosis peh dick yoo LOH sis	*pedicul/i* lice *-osis* abnormal condition	Parasitic infestation with lice, involving the head, body, or genital area (Fig. 4-12).
scabies SKAY bees		Parasitic infestation caused by mites; characterized by pruritic papular rash.

Terms Related to Viral Infections

Term	Word Origin	Definition
exanthematous diseases eks an THEM ah tus	*exanthemat/o* rash *-ous* pertaining to	Generally, viral diseases characterized by a specific type of rash **(exanthem)**. The main ones are measles, rubella, fifth disease, roseola, and chickenpox.
herpes simplex virus (HSV) HUR peez SIM plecks		Viral infection characterized by clusters of small vesicles filled with clear fluid on raised inflammatory bases on the skin or mucosa. HSV-1 causes fever blisters **(herpetic stomatitis)** and **keratitis,** an inflammation of the cornea. HSV-2 is more commonly known as **genital herpes.**
herpes zoster HUR peez ZAH stur		Acute, painful rash caused by reactivation of the latent varicella-zoster virus. Also known as **shingles** (Fig. 4-13).
verruca (*pl.* verrucae) veh ROO kah		Common, contagious epithelial growths usually appearing on the skin of the hands, feet, legs, and face; can be caused by any of 60 types of the human papillomavirus (HPV) (Fig. 4-14). Also called **warts.**

Fig. 4-13 Herpes zoster.

Fig. 4-14 Verrucae (warts).

⊗ Be Careful!

The combining form **stomat/o** *in the term* stomatitis *means mouth, not stomach.*

EXERCISE 6: Yeast, Fungal, Parasitic, and Viral Infections

Match these fungal or yeast infections with their definitions or synonyms.

_____ 1. athlete's foot

_____ 2. ringworm of scalp

_____ 3. moniliasis

_____ 4. jock itch

_____ 5. rash

_____ 6. ringworm of body

_____ 7. shingles

_____ 8. warts

A. tinea corporis
B. tinea cruris
C. tinea capitis
D. tinea pedis
E. verrucae
F. candidiasis
G. herpes zoster
H. exanthem

Build the term.

9. infestation with lice _____.

10. fungal infection of the skin _____.

Case Study **Zander Woo**

Six-month-old Zander Woo is brought to the clinic by his mother. The baby is fussy and has been so for several days. On examination, there appear to be patches of inflammation in the folds of the skin and on his tongue. Zander is diagnosed with a yeast infection and prescribed an antifungal cream.

1. What was Zander's diagnosis? _____ _____

2. Another term for candidiasis is _____.

3. Candidiasis is a type of _____ infection.
   a. viral
   b. fungal
   c. bacterial
   d. parasitic

4. A fungal infection of the skin is called _____ _____.

Terms Related to Disorders of Hair Follicles and Sebaceous Glands

Term	Word Origin	Definition
acne vulgaris ACK nee vul GARE us	*vulgar/o* common *-is* noun ending	Inflammatory disease of the sebaceous glands characterized by papules, pustules, inflamed nodules, and **comedones** (kah mih DOH neez) (*sing.* comedo), which are plugs of sebum that partially or completely block a pore. Blackheads are open comedones, and whiteheads are closed comedones.
alopecia al oh PEE shee ah		Hair loss, resulting from genetic factors, aging, or disease (Fig. 4-15).
hypertrichosis hye pur trih KOH sis	*hyper-* excessive *trich/o* hair *-osis* abnormal condition	Abnormal excess of hair; also known as **hirsutism** (HER soo tih zum).
keratinous cyst kur AT tin us	*kerat/o* hard, horny *-in* substance *-ous* pertaining to	Benign cavity lined by keratinizing epithelium and filled with sebum and epithelial debris. Also called a **sebaceous cyst**.
milia MILL ee ah		Tiny superficial keratinous cysts caused by clogged oil ducts.

Fig. 4-15 Alopecia.

Fig. 4-16 Psoriasis.

Term Related to Scaling Papular Diseases

Term	Word Origin	Definition
psoriasis sohr EYE ah sis		Common chronic skin disorder characterized by circumscribed, salmon-red patches covered by thick, dry, silvery scales that are the result of excessive development of epithelial cells (Fig. 4-16).

Terms Related to Cornification and Pressure Injuries

Term	Word Origin	Definition
callus KAL us		Common painless thickening of the stratum corneum at locations of external pressure or friction.
corn		Horny mass of condensed epithelial cells overlying a bony prominence as the result of pressure or friction; also referred to as a **clavus** (KLA vus).
decubitus ulcer (decub) deh KYOO bih tus		Inflammation, ulcer, or sore in the skin over a bony prominence. Most often seen in aged, debilitated, cachectic (wasted), or immobilized patients; pressure sores or ulcers are graded by stages of severity. The highest stage, stage 4, involves muscles, fat, and bone. Also known as a **bedsore, pressure ulcer,** or **pressure sore** (Fig. 4-17).
ichthyosis ick thee OH sis	*ichthy/o* fish *-osis* abnormal condition	Category of dry skin that has the scaly appearance of a fish. It ranges from mild to severe. The mild form is known as **xeroderma** (zir uh DUR mah). *Xer/o* means "dry."

Fig. 4-17 Decubitus ulcers. **A,** Stage 1. **B,** Stage 2. **C,** Stage 3. **D,** Stage 4.

EXERCISE 7: Disorders of Hair Follicles and Sebaceous Glands, Scaling Papular Diseases, and Pressure Injuries

Fill in the blanks with the correct terms from the following list.

acne vulgaris, alopecia, clavus, decubitus ulcer, hypertrichosis, keratinous cyst, milia, pressure sore, psoriasis, xeroderma

1. What is a disorder of circumscribed salmon-red patches covered with thick, silvery scales? _____

    _____

2. What is another name for hirsutism? _____

3. What is the term for hair loss? _____

4. What is the term for a benign cavity filled with sebum and epithelial debris and lined with keratinized

    epithelium? _____

5. What is the common inflammatory disease of the sebaceous glands characterized by comedones,

    papules, pustules, and inflamed nodules? _____

6. What is another term for a corn? _____

7. What are two alternative terms for bedsores? _____

8. What are tiny, superficial keratinous cysts? _____

9. What is the term for mildly dry skin? _____

Case Study Keisha Landerson

Fifty-year-old Keisha Landerson complains of circumscribed salmon-red patches on her skin that are covered by thick, dry, silvery scales. These occur on her face and scalp, causing her a great deal of self-consciousness and distress. She says she has tried a "never-ending parade" of over-the-counter (OTC) creams and ointments and medicated shampoos, but nothing has had much effect.

1. Keisha exhibits symptoms that are consistent with a description of the chronic skin disorder _____ _____.

2. Keisha's disorder occurs as a result of excessive development of _____ cells.

3. As the physician describes what has caused Keisha's condition, he explains that the _____ prevents excessive loss of water, salts, and heat from the body.

4. How do you pronounce *psoriasis*?
   a. puh sohr EYE uh sis
   b. sohr EYE uh sis
   c. SOHR us sis
   d. psss ORE ih sis

Terms Related to Pigmentation Disorders

Term	Word Origin	Definition
albinism AL bih niz um	*albin/o* white *-ism* condition	Complete lack of melanin production by existing melanocytes, resulting in pale skin, white hair, and pink irides (*sing.* iris).
dyschromia diss KROH mee ah	*dys-* abnormal *chrom/o* color *-ia* condition	Abnormality of skin pigmentation. **Hyperchromia** is abnormally increased pigmentation. **Hypochromia** is abnormally decreased pigmentation.
vitiligo vih tih LYE goh		Benign acquired disease of unknown origin, consisting of irregular patches of various sizes lacking in pigment (Fig. 4-18).

 Be Careful!

Hidr/o *with an* **i** *means sweat;* **hydr/o** *with a* **y** *means water. Both are pronounced* HYE droh.

 Be Careful!

Don't confuse **milia,** *a condition resulting from oil-filled ducts, with* **miliaria,** *a condition resulting from sweat-filled ducts.*

Fig. 4-18 Vitiligo.

Terms Related to Disorders of Sweating

Term	Word Origin	Definition
anhidrosis an hye DROH sis	*an-* no, not, without *hidr/o* sweating *-osis* abnormal condition	A condition in which a person produces little or no sweat.
hidradenitis hye drah din EYE tis	*hidraden/o* sweat gland *-itis* inflammation	Inflammation of the sweat glands (Fig. 4-19).
hyperhidrosis hye pur hye DROH sis	*hyper-* excessive *hidr/o* sweat *-osis* abnormal condition	Excessive perspiration caused by heat, strong emotion, menopause, hyperthyroidism, or infection.
miliaria mill ee AIR ee uh		Minute vesicles and papules, often with surrounding **erythema** (redness), caused by occlusion of sweat ducts during times of exposure to heat and high humidity.

Fig. 4-19 Hidradenitis.

EXERCISE 8: Pigmentation Disorders and Disorders of Sweating

Build the terms.

1. abnormal condition of excessive sweat _____

2. abnormal condition of pigmentation _____

3. inflammation of the sweat glands _____

4. abnormal condition of no sweat _____

Fill in the blank.

5. An acquired disorder of irregular patches of various sizes lacking in pigment is _____.

6. A patient whose body produces no melanin has a condition of _____.

7. Minute vesicles and papules caused by occlusion of sweat ducts are called _____.

Terms Related to Disorders of the Nails

Term	Word Origin	Definition
onychia ah NICK ee ah	*onych/o* nail *-ia* condition	Inflammation of the fingernail. Also called **onychitis**.
onychocryptosis ah nick oh krip TOH sis	*onchy/o* nail *crypt-* hidden *-osis* abnormal condition	Abnormal condition of hidden (ingrown) nail. It can cause pain, swelling, and **erythema** (redness).
onycholysis ah nick AHL ih sis	*onych/o* nail *-lysis* loosening	Separation of the nail plate from the nail bed (Fig. 4-20).
onychomalacia ah nick oh mah LAY shah	*onych/o* nail *-malacia* softening	Softening of the nails.
onychomycosis ah nick oh my KOH sis	*onych/o* nail *myc/o* fungus *-osis* abnormal condition	Abnormal condition of nail fungus. Also called **tinea unguium** (Fig. 4-21).
paronychia pair uh NICK ee ah	*par-* beside, near *onych/o* nail *-ia* condition	Infection of the skin beside the nail.

⊗ Be Careful!

Paronychium *is the structure that surrounds the nail.* **Paronychia** *is an infection of the nail.*

Fig. 4-20 Onycholysis.

Fig. 4-21 Onychomycosis (tinea unguium). Early changes show subungual debris at the distal end of the nail plate.

EXERCISE 9: Disorders of the Nails

Match the word parts to their definitions.

_____ 1. loosening

_____ 2. fungus

_____ 3. hidden

_____ 4. softening

_____ 5. condition

A. -ia
B. crypt-
C. -lysis
D. myc/o
E. -malacia

Build the terms.

6. softening of the nail _____

7. abnormal condition of fungus of the nail _____

8. abnormal condition of hidden nail _____

9. loosening of the nail _____

Case Study Angela Trova

Angela Trova is a 35-year-old biller and coder who says she has "an ingrown nail" on her right index finger. On examination, the finger is tender, swollen, and erythematous. Angela says that she had this problem a couple of years ago, and the nail was removed.

1. What is the medical term for an ingrown nail? _____

2. Crypt/o means _____.

3. Erythematous means pertaining to _____ _____.

4. What is the part of the nail that is visible called? _____

Burns

Burns are injuries to tissues that result from exposure to thermal, chemical, electrical, or radioactive agents. They may be classified into four different degrees of severity, depending on the layers of the skin that are damaged. Coders must categorize burns higher than second degree according to the "rule of nines" (Fig. 4-22) that divides the body into percentages that are, for the most part, multiples of nine: the head and neck equal 9%, each upper limb 9%, each lower limb 18%, the front and back of the torso 36%, and the genital area 1%. Fig. 4-23 is an illustration of the different degrees of burns.

- **Superficial burn:** Burn in which only the first layer of the skin, the epidermis, is damaged; also known as a *first-degree burn.* Characterized by redness (erythema), tenderness, and hyperesthesia, with no scar development.
- **Partial-thickness burn:** Burn in which only the first and second layers of the skin (epidermis and part of the dermis) are affected; sometimes called a

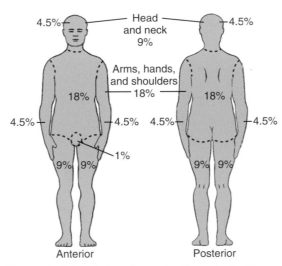

Fig. 4-22 Rule of nines for estimating extent of burns.

Fig. 4-23 Degrees of burns and depth of tissue involvement.

second-degree burn. If the burn extends to the papillary level, it is classified as a *superficial partial-thickness burn.* If it extends farther, to the reticular layer, it is classified as a *deep partial-thickness burn.* Characterized by redness, blisters, and pain, with possible scar development.

- **Full-thickness burn:** Burn that damages the epidermis, dermis, and subcutaneous tissue; also known as a *third-degree burn.* Pain is not present because the nerve endings in the skin have been destroyed. Skin appearance may be deep red, pale gray, brown, or black. Scar formation is likely.

- **Deep full-thickness burn:** Although not a universally accepted category, some burn specialists use this category to describe a rare burn that extends beyond the subcutaneous tissue into the muscle and bone. Also called a *fourth-degree burn.*

EXERCISE 10: Burns

Match the characteristics of the burns listed with their degree.

_____ 1. superficial

_____ 2. partial thickness

_____ 3. full thickness

_____ 4. deep full thickness

A. Ironing a blouse for work, Rhonda burned her hand, resulting in blisters and erythema.

B. John suffered burns over two-thirds of his body with many areas of tissue burned to the bone.

C. Because Kristin forgot to reapply her sunblock, she sustained a sunburn that resulted in painful reddened skin.

D. Smoking in bed resulted in burns that destroyed the epidermis and dermis and extended through the hypodermis on the victim's chest and shoulders.

Terms Related to Benign (Noncancerous) Skin Growths

Term	Word Origin	Definition
angioma an jee CH mah	*angi/o* vessel *-oma* tumor, mass	Localized vascular lesion that includes hemangiomas (Fig. 4-24), vascular nevi, and lymphangiomas.
dermatofibroma dur mat toh fye BROH mah	*dermat/o* skin *fibr/o* fiber *-oma* tumor, mass	Fibrous tumor of the skin that is painless, round, firm, and usually found on the extremities.
dysplastic nevus (*pl.* nevi) dis PLAS tick NEE vus	*dys-* abnormal *plast/o* formation *-ic* pertaining to *nev/o* birthmark *-us* structure, thing	A nevus is a pigmented lesion often present at birth. It is also called a **mole**. Various abnormal changes of a pigmented congenital skin blemish give rise to concern for progression to malignancy. Changes of concern are categorized as ABCDE. **a**symmetry **b**orders, irregular **c**olors, changes or uneven pigmentation **d**iameter, increasing size or more than 6 mm **e**levation
lipoma lih POH mah	*lip/o* fat *-oma* tumor, mass	Fatty tumor that is a soft, movable, subcutaneous nodule (Fig. 4-25).
seborrheic keratosis seh boh REE ick kair ah TOH sis	*seb/o* sebum *-rrheic* pertaining to discharge *kerat/o* hard, horny *-osis* abnormal condition	Benign, circumscribed, pigmented, superficial warty skin lesion. An **actinic keratosis** is a lesion caused by sun exposure.
skin tags		Small, soft, pedunculated (with a stalk) lesions that are harmless outgrowths of epidermal and dermal tissue, usually occurring on the neck, eyelids, armpits, and groin; usually occur in multiples. Also known as **acrochordons** (ack roh KORE dons).

Fig. 4-24 Hemangioma.

Fig. 4-25 Lipoma.

EXERCISE 11: Benign Skin Growths

Matching the benign skin growths to their definitions.

_____ 1. pigmented lesion   _____ 4. benign warty skin lesion   A. skin tag
                                                                          B. lipoma
_____ 2. acrochordon   _____ 5. vascular nevus   C. seborrheic keratosis
                                                                          D. mole
_____ 3. fatty tumor   E. angioma

Decode the terms.

6. dermatofibroma _____

7. angioma _____

8. seborrheic keratosis _____

Terms Related to Malignant Neoplasms

Term	Word Origin	Definition
basal cell carcinoma (BCC) BAY suhl kar sih NOH mah	*bas/o* base *-al* pertaining to carcinoma cancer of epithelial origin	The most common form of skin cancer, it originates in the basal layer of the epidermis. It usually occurs on the face as a result of sun exposure and rarely metastasizes (spreads to distant sites).
Kaposi sarcoma (KS) KAP uh see sar KOH mah	*sarcoma* connective tissue cancer	A rare form of skin cancer that takes the form of red/blue/brown/purple nodules, usually on the extremities. One form appears most often in patients with deficient immune systems, such as acquired immunodeficiency syndrome (AIDS).
malignant melanoma mell uh NOH mah	*melan/o* black, dark *-oma* tumor, mass	This cancerous tumor arises from mutated melanocytes. This particular cancer is the leading cause of death from all skin diseases (Fig. 4-26).
squamous cell carcinoma (SCC) SKWAY muss	*squam/o* scaly *-ous* pertaining to carcinoma cancer of epithelial origin	The second most common type of skin cancer, also caused by sun exposure, but developing from squamous cells (Fig. 4-27).

Fig. 4-26 Malignant melanoma on arm.

Fig. 4-27 Squamous cell carcinoma (SCC) on the ear.

EXERCISE 12: Malignant Neoplasms

Match the malignant neoplasms to their definitions.

_____ 1. squamous cell carcinoma (SCC)

_____ 2. Kaposi sarcoma (KS)

_____ 3. basal cell carcinoma (BCC)

_____ 4. malignant melanoma

A. most common type of skin cancer, derived from base level of epidermis; rarely metastasizes
B. cancer arising from mutated pigment cells
C. malignancy of squamous skin cells
D. rare form of skin cancer that appears most often in patients with deficient immune systems, such as AIDS

Click on **Hear It, Spell It** to practice spelling the pathology terms you have learned in this chapter.

Age Matters

Pediatrics

Children routinely appear at physician offices with skin disorders. Some of the most common are impetigo, acne, seborrheic dermatitis, cellulitis, and pediculosis. Although none of these are serious disorders, impetigo and pediculosis are highly contagious. Also seen are the different degrees of burns, usually accidental, but potentially life threatening.

Geriatrics

Elderly patients have a completely different set of diagnoses. The disorders categorized as those related to cornification, especially corns and calluses, are seen routinely in medical offices. These masses or thickenings of the skin are formed as a defensive response to constant friction, usually within shoes. Pressure sores (also called *bedsores* or *decubitus ulcers*) are seen most often in bedridden patients whose skin may already be atrophied and thin. Eczema, actinic keratoses, cellulitis, and fungal infections are also common complaints. The last category of skin disorders often seen in the elderly is the area of neoplasms. Although younger patients with skin cancers are often seen, older patients, by definition, have had a longer time to be exposed to the sun and develop malignancies.

DIAGNOSTIC PROCEDURES

Terms Related to Biopsies

Term	Word Origin	Definition
excisional biopsy		Biopsy (Bx) in which the entire tumor may be removed with borders as a means of diagnosis and treatment (Fig. 4-28).
exfoliation ecks foh lee A shun		Scraping or shaving off samples of friable (easily crushed) lesions for a laboratory examination called **exfoliative cytology.**
incisional biopsy		Biopsy in which larger tissue samples may be obtained by excising a wedge of tissue and suturing the incision (see Fig. 4-28).
needle aspiration		Aspiration of fluid from lesions to obtain samples for culture and examination.
punch biopsy		Biopsy in which a tubular punch is inserted through to the subcutaneous tissue and the tissue is cut off at the base (Fig. 4-29).

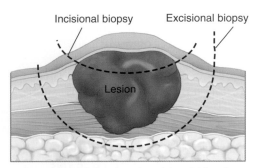

Fig. 4-28 Incisional and excisional biopsies.

Fig. 4-29 Punch biopsy.

Terms Related to Laboratory Tests

Term	Word Origin	Definition
bacterial analyses		Culture and serology of lesions to help diagnose such disorders as impetigo.
fungal tests		Cultures of scrapings of lesions used to identify fungal infections, such as tinea pedis, tinea capitis, and tinea cruris.
sweat tests		Laboratory test for abnormally high levels of sodium and chloride present in the perspiration of persons with cystic fibrosis.
tuberculosis (TB) skin tests		Intradermal test (e.g., Mantoux test) using purified protein derivative (PPD) to test for either dormant or active TB; this is a much more accurate test than the multiple puncture tine test, which had been used for screening purposes (Fig. 4-30).
Tzanck test tzahnk		Microscopic examination of lesions for the purpose of diagnosing herpes zoster and HSV.
viral culture		Sampling of vesicular fluid for the purpose of identifying viruses.

Terms Related to Laboratory Tests—cont'd

Term	Word Origin	Definition
Wood's light examination		Method used to identify a variety of skin infections through the use of a Wood's light, which produces UV light; tinea capitis and pseudomonas infections in burns are two of the disorders that it can reveal (Fig. 4-31).
wound and abscess cultures		Lab samplings that can identify pathogens in wounds, such as diabetic or decubitus ulcers, postoperative wounds, or abscesses.

Fig. 4-30 Mantoux test. The technician is in the process of correctly placing a Mantoux tuberculin skin test in the recipient's forearm, which will cause a 6 mm to 10 mm wheal (i.e., a raised area of skin surface) to form at the injection site.

Fig. 4-31 Wood's light.

 EXERCISE 13: Diagnostic Procedures

Fill in the blanks with the correct terms from the following list.

excisional, exfoliation, incisional, needle aspiration, punch

1. An entire tumor is removed in a/an _____ biopsy.

2. Fluid from a lesion is aspirated to obtain samples for culture in a/an _____ biopsy.

3. A wedge of tissue is removed and the incision is sutured in a/an _____ biopsy.

4. Samples of friable lesions are scraped or shaved off in _____.

5. A cylindrical punch is inserted into the subcutaneous tissue layer, and the tissue is cut off at the base

    in a/an _____ biopsy.

Match the following disorders with the tests that may be used to diagnose them.

_____ 6. ringworm	_____ 10. herpes zoster, herpes simplex virus (HSV)	A. Wood's light examination
_____ 7. impetigo		B. Mantoux test
		C. bacterial analysis
_____ 8. cystic fibrosis	_____ 11. tinea capitis, pseudomonas	D. wound abscess culture
		E. sweat test
		F. fungal test
_____ 9. tuberculosis (TB)	_____ 12. bedsore, infection	G. Tzanck test

Medical Report   Angelina Herrara

HERRARA, ANGELINA S - 77603

Task   Edit   View   Time Scale   Options   Help

HERRARA, ANGELINA S.   Age: 9 years   Sex: Female   Loc: SMOC
                                  DOB: 03/20/2007   MRN: 77603   FIN: 201376

| Reference Text Browser | Form Browser | Medication Profile |

| Orders | Last 48 Hours | ED | Lab | Radiology | **Assessment** | Surgery | Clinical Notes | Pt. Info | Pt. Schedule | Task List | I & O | MAR |

Flowsheet: Surgery   Level: History and Physical   ● Table ○ Group ○ List

Navigator
✓ History and Physical

Patient presents for her initial evaluation complaining of severe pruritic rash on her left and right antecubital fossa × 4 days. Mother reports the rash began on her daughter's arms but has also erupted on her forearms and lower extremities. Also has multiple lesions across her chest. Mother denies any new lotions, soaps, detergents, clothes, pets. No different foods or exposure to poison ivy. Has no previous history of dermatitis.

Denies current fever, chills; other than rash all other systems are unremarkable.

PHYSICAL EXAMINATION: Diffuse vesicular lesions across the upper torso, forearms, and thighs.
Erythematous area of vesicular lesions in her right and left popliteal fossa.
Vesicular diffuse lesions, cause unclear.

ASSESSMENT: Most likely this represents a viral exanthem. She is given topical hydrocortisone cream and advised to use Benadryl for itching.

PROD | MAHAFC | 26 March 2016 | 9:35

 EXERCISE 14: Progress Note

Review the preceding progress note, and answer the following questions:

1. How do we know that her rash is itchy?

_____

2. What phrase tells us that she has had no skin inflammations diagnosed in the past?

_____

3. What characteristic would "vesicular" lesions have?

_____

4. "Exanthem" is a medical term for what?

_____

THERAPEUTIC INTERVENTIONS

Terms Related to Grafting Techniques and Other Therapies

Term	Word Origin	Definition
allograft AL oh graft	*all/o* other	Harvest of skin from another human donor for temporary transplant until an autograft is available. Also called a **homograft.**
autograft AH toh graft	*auto-* self	Harvest of the patient's own skin for transplant (Fig. 4-32).
dermatome DUR mah tohm	*dermat/o* skin *-tome* instrument to cut	Instrument used to remove split-thickness skin grafts (Fig. 4-33).
flap		Section of skin transferred from one location to an immediately adjacent one. Also called a **skin graft (SG).**
laser therapy		Procedure to repair or destroy tissue, particularly in the removal of tattoos, warts, port wine stains, and psoriatic lesions.
occlusive therapy	*occlus/o* to close *-ive* pertaining to	Use of a nonporous occlusive dressing to cover a treated area to enhance the absorption and effectiveness of a medication; used to treat psoriasis, lupus erythematosus, and chronic hand dermatitis.
psoralen plus ultraviolet A (PUVA) therapy SORE ah lin		Directing a type of UV light onto psoriatic lesions.
skin graft (SG)		Skin transplant performed when normal skin cover has been lost as a result of burns, ulcers, or operations to remove cancerous tissue.
full-thickness graft		Skin graft in which full portions of both the epidermis and the dermis are used.
split-thickness skin graft (STSG)		Skin graft in which the epidermis and parts of the dermis are used.
xenograft ZEE noh graft	*xen/o* foreign	Temporary skin graft from another species, often a pig, used until an autograft is available. Also called a **heterograft.**

Fig. 4-32 Epithelial autografts. Thin sheets of skin are attached to gauze backing.

Fig. 4-33 Dermatome.

Terms Related to Tissue Removal

Term	Word Origin	Definition
cauterization kah tur ih ZAY shun	*cauter/i* burn *-zation* process of	Destruction of tissue by burning with heat.
cryosurgery KRY oh sur juh ree	*cry/o* extreme cold	Destruction of tissue through the use of extreme cold, usually liquid nitrogen.
curettage kyoo ruh TAJZ		Scraping of material from the wall of a cavity or other surface to obtain tissue for microscopic examination; this is done with an instrument called a **curette** (Fig. 4-34).
débridement dah breed MON		First step in wound treatment, involving removal of dirt, foreign bodies (FBs), damaged tissue, and cellular debris from the wound or burn to prevent infection and to promote healing.
escharotomy ess kar AH tuh mee	*eschar/o* scab *-tomy* incision	Surgical incision into necrotic tissue resulting from a severe burn. This may be necessary to prevent edema leading to ischemia (loss of blood flow) in underlying tissue.
incision and drainage (I&D)		Cutting open and removing the contents of a wound, cyst, or other lesion.
Mohs surgery MOHZ		Repeated removal and microscopic examination of layers of a tumor until no cancerous cells are present (Fig. 4-35).
shaving (paring)		Slicing of thin sheets of tissue to remove lesions.
onychectomy ah nick ECK tuh mee	*onych/o* nail *-ectomy* removal, excision	Removal of a fingernail or toenail because of trauma or disease.

CURETTAGE

A   B

Fig. 4-34 Curettage.

Tumor sliced with scalpel and cut into quadrants before frozen; dark areas represent tumor

Tumor

Maps of tumor

Level 1

Tumor

Level
1
2
3
4
5
6

Basal cell carcinoma with finger-like projections of tumor in the dermis

Frozen section specimens

2

3

4

5

6

Maps of tumor location drawn from frozen section specimens, indicating areas of remaining tumor that must be removed

Fig. 4-35 Mohs surgery.

Terms Related to Cosmetic Procedures

Term	Word Origin	Definition
blepharoplasty BLEF ar oh plas tee	*blephar/o* eyelid *-plasty* surgical repair	Surgical repair of the eyelid.
chemical peel		Use of a mild acid to produce a superficial burn; normally done to remove wrinkles (Fig. 4-36)
dermabrasion dur mah BRAY zhun	*derm/o* skin *-abrasion* scraping of	Surgical procedure to resurface the skin; used to remove acne scars, nevi, wrinkles, and tattoos.
dermatoplasty DUR mat tuh plas tee	*dermat/o* skin *-plasty* surgical repair	Transplant of living skin to correct effects of injury, operation, or disease.
lipectomy lih PECK tuh mee	*lip/o* fat *-ectomy* removal, excision	Removal of fatty tissue.
liposuction LYE poh suck shun	*lip/o* fat	Technique for removing adipose tissue with a suction pump device (Fig. 4-37).
rhytidectomy rih tih DECK tuh mee	*rhytid/o* wrinkle *-ectomy* removal, excision	Surgical operation to remove wrinkles. Commonly known as a "face-lift."

Fig. 4-36 Application of a chemical peel.

Fig. 4-37 Liposuction of the neck.

EXERCISE 15: Therapeutic Interventions

1. Explain the differences among the following:

   A. autograft _____

   B. allograft _____

   C. xenograft _____

2. Which type of graft includes the epidermis and the dermis? _____

3. What instrument is used to cut skin for grafting? _____

Fill in the blanks with the correct terms from the list below.

cauterization, cryosurgery, curettage, débridement, incision and drainage, laser therapy, occlusive therapy, shaving, Mohs surgery

4. _____ is used to destroy tattoos.

5. Removing dirt, foreign bodies (FBs), damaged tissue, and cellular debris from a wound is called

   _____.

6. The destruction of tissue by burning with heat is called _____.

7. The destruction of tissue through the use of extreme cold is called _____.

8. Scraping of material from the wall of a cavity is called _____.

9. I&D is _____.

10. Another term for "paring" is _____.

11. Use of a dressing to cover a treated area is called _____.

12. Removal of a tumor by layers is called _____.

Build the term.

13. removal of wrinkles _____

14. removal of fat _____

15. surgical repair of the eyelid _____

16. scraping of skin _____

17. surgical repair of the skin _____

Case Study **Anthony Xavier**

Anthony Xavier is a truck driver carrying load of factory parts from Indiana to Pennsylvania when a driver cuts him off suddenly. When he swerves to avoid hitting the car, his truck tips over on the highway. Anthony loses consciousness and the engine catches fire, but fortunately, other drivers who stop are able to pull him from the truck. Although they have saved his life, Anthony does sustain burns—some more serious than others.

1. Anthony's burns vary in their severity. He has burns around his eyes and forehead that involve the epidermis only; these are called _____ burns.

2. The fingers that hurt Anthony the most have burns that involve both the epidermis and dermis, making this a _____ burn.

3. The surgeon attempts to repair the damage done to Anthony's leg by harvesting skin to be grafted for the burn. If Anthony's own skin is used, this will be a/an _____.

4. While Anthony's skin cells are developing, a temporary skin transplant is needed. Skin from a human donor is used; this is called a/an_____.

5. For some burns on Anthony's forearm, a nurse scrapes the wound to remove dirt, cellular debris, and FBs to prevent infection and promote healing. This procedure is called _____.

6. For burns on his left thigh, Anthony is taken to surgery where an incision is made into the necrotic burn tissue to prevent edema and loss of blood flow. This surgical procedure is called a/an _____.

hypodermic
   hypo = under
   derm/o = skin
   -ic = pertaining to

intradermal
   intra- = within
   derm/o = skin
   -al = pertaining to

subcutaneous
   sub- = under
   cutane/o = skin
   -ous = pertaining to

transdermal
   trans- = through
   derm/o = skin
   -al = pertaining to

PHARMACOLOGY

Routes of Administration

Several medications are administered on, within, or through the skin. The most common of these routes of administration include the following:

hypodermic (H): General term that refers to any injection under the skin.
intradermal (ID): Route of injection within the dermis (Fig. 4-38, *A*). Also called **intracutaneous.**
subcutaneous: Route of injection into the fat layer beneath the skin (see Fig. 4-38, *B*).
topical: Type of drug applied directly onto the skin as a cream, gel, lotion, or ointment.
transdermal therapeutic system (TTS): Use of a transdermal patch; involves placing medication in a gel-like material that is applied to the skin, allowing for a specified timed release of the medicine (Fig. 4-39). Examples are nitroglycerin for angina pectoris and the nicotine patch (NicoDerm) for smoking cessation.

 *Click on **Hear It, Spell It** to practice spelling the diagnostic and therapeutic terms you have learned in this chapter.*

Fig. 4-38 A, Intradermal (ID) injection. **B,** Subcutaneous injection.

Fig. 4-39 Transdermal patch.

Dermatologic Drugs

Traditional Pharmacology

anesthetic agents: Reduce pain and discomfort; some can be given topically on an affected area. Examples include lidocaine (Xylocaine) and benzocaine (Orajel).

antibacterials: Prevent and treat bacterial growth. Topical agents such as erythromycin (Ery 2% Pads) and clindamycin (BenzaClin) are used to treat acne. Triple antibiotic ointment containing bacitracin, polymixin B, and neomycin (Neosporin), silver sulfadiazine (Silvadene), and mupirocin (Bactroban) are used to prevent and treat skin or wound infections. Oral agents for the treatment of acne include erythromycin (Ery-Tab), tetracycline (Sumycin), and minocycline (Minocin).

antifungals: Treat fungal infections. Topical agents include nystatin (Nystop), butenafine (Lotrimin Ultra), ciclopirox (Loprox), and econazole (Ecoza).

antihistamines: Lessen itching by reducing an allergic response. Diphenhydramine (Benadryl) is available in oral and topical formulations. Other oral agents include chlorpheniramine (Chlor-Trimeton), cetirizine (Zyrtec), and loratadine (Claritin).

antiinflammatories: Reduce inflammation and pain. Oral agents include prednisone and aspirin; topical agents include hydrocortisone (Cortizone), fluocinonide (Vanos), and triamcinolone (Kenalog).

antipsoriatics: Treat psoriasis. Examples include anthralin (Drithocreme) and calcipotriene (Dovonex).

antiseptics: Topical agents used to prevent infection by destroying microbials. Examples include iodine and chlorhexidine (Peridex).

antivirals: Reduce the effect of viruses. Examples include valacyclovir (Valtrex) and acyclovir (Zovirax) for the treatment of HSV (cold sores or genital herpes) and herpes zoster (shingles).

emollients (ih MOLL yents): Topical substances that soften and moisturize the skin. Emollients come in the form of lotions, creams, ointments, and bath additives. A couple of well-known OTC products containing emollients are Aveeno and Eucerin.

immunomodulators or **immunosuppressants:** Agents that suppress the body's immune system. Topical agents such as pimecrolimus (Elidel) and tacrolimus (Protopic) are used to treat atopic dermatitis and eczema.

keratolytics (kair ah toh LIT icks): Topical substances used to break down hardened skin and shed the top layer of dead skin to treat warts, calluses, corns, acne, rosacea, and psoriasis. Examples include salicylic acid, cantharidin, and podofilox (Condylox).

pediculicides: Destroy lice. Examples include malathion (Ovide), lindane (Kwell), and permethrin (Nix).

protectives: Topical substances with sun protection factors (SPFs) that protect the skin against UV A and B in sunlight. A wide variety of these are available OTC.

retinoids: Derived from vitamin A, retinoids alter the growth of the top layer of skin and may be used to treat acne, reduce wrinkles, and treat psoriasis. Examples include tretinoin (Retin-A), isotretinoin (Claravis), and tazarotene (Tazorac).

scabicides: Destroy mites and scabies. Examples include permethrin (Elimite) and crotamiton (Eurax).

---

anesthetic
an- = not, without
-esthetic = pertaining to feeling

Be Careful!

ID *means intradermal;*
I&D *means incision and drainage.*

keratolytics
kerat/o = hard, horny
-lytic = pertaining to breaking down

pediculicide
pedicul/i = lice
-cide = killing

scabicides
scab/i = mites
-cide = killing

Complementary and Alternative Methods of Treatment

herbal medicine: Drugs from minimally altered plant sources, such as aloe vera (to treat sunburn and stomach ulcers) or tea tree oil (used for its antibacterial, antiviral, and antifungal properties to treat boils, wound infections, and acne). Also, therapeutic use of essential oils is helpful in treating dry flaky skin, decubitus ulcers, diabetic ulcers, herpes zoster, and herpes simplex virus 1 (HSV-1).

EXERCISE 16: Pharmacology

Fill in the blanks.

1. Medication injected "within the dermis" is given by the _____ route.

2. Medications applied directly to the skin are given by the _____ route.

3. A general term meaning "under the skin" is _____.

4. Medications delivered via a patch through the skin are given by _____.

5. Medication applied to an affected area to reduce pain and discomfort is called a/an

   _____.

6. A topical agent that breaks down hardened skin is called a/an _____.

7. Medications that treat fungal skin infections are called _____.

8. Medications that target bacteria are called _____.

9. Scabies and mites can be killed by using a/an _____.

10. A type of medication that is used to treat inflammation of the skin is _____.

Match the following pharmaceutical agents with their actions.

_____ 11. softens the skin

_____ 12. alters the growth of the outer layer of skin

_____ 13. lessens itching

_____ 14. prevents infection

_____ 15. treats HSV

_____ 16. treats lice

_____ 17. suppresses the immune system

A. antihistamine
B. antiseptic
C. retinoid
D. emollient
E. antiviral
F. immunomodulator
G. pediculicide

Case Study Helena Freeman

Twelve-year-old Helena Freeman is seen with intense itching and scratches on her arms, legs, and scalp. She points to many flattened and raised humps and small white "things" in her hair. Her father says that the school sent home a letter notifying families to be on the lookout for lice. He thinks that is what Helena has.

1. A small, flattened blemish or discoloration is called a/an _____.

2. A small, raised solid skin lesion is a/an _____ _____.

3. The term for the scratches that result from intense scratching are called _____.

4. The medical term for an infestation of lice is _____.

5. The pharmaceutical treatment for lice is a/an _____ _____.

Abbreviations

Abbreviation	Meaning	Abbreviation	Meaning
BCC	basal cell carcinoma	KS	Kaposi sarcoma
Bx	biopsy	PPD	purified protein derivative
FB	foreign body	PUVA	psoralen plus ultraviolet A
H	hypodermic	SCC	squamous cell carcinoma
HPV	human papillomavirus	SG	skin graft
HSV-1	herpes simplex virus 1	STSG	split-thickness skin graft
HSV-2	herpes simplex virus 2	TB	tuberculosis
I&D	incision and drainage	TTS	transdermal therapeutic system
ID	intradermal		

EXERCISE 17: Abbreviations

Write the abbreviation for each of the following.

1. route of administration within the dermis: _____

2. radiation from sunlight: _____

3. skin graft: _____

4. pressure ulcer: _____

5. example of material removed from a wound during débridement: _____

6. incision and drainage: _____

7. biopsy: _____

8. purified protein derivative: _____

9. patch to deliver medicine: _____

10. tuberculosis: _____

Chapter Review

Match the word parts to their definitions.

Word Part Definitions

Prefix/Suffix		Definition
-cide	1. _____	excessive
crypt-	2. _____	abnormal condition
hyper-	3. _____	through
intra-	4. _____	within
-itis	5. _____	kill
-lytic	6. _____	under
-osis	7. _____	hidden
par-	8. _____	inflammation
sub-	9. _____	near
trans-	10. _____	pertaining to destruction

Combining Form		Definition
adip/o	11. _____	sweat
chrom/o	12. _____	black, dark
cutane/o	13. _____	nail
eschar/o	14. _____	color
exanthemat/o	15. _____	wrinkle
follicul/o	16. _____	follicle
hemat/o	17. _____	vessel
hidraden/o	18. _____	papule, pimple
hidr/o	19. _____	macule
kerat/o	20. _____	blood
macul/o	21. _____	foreign
melan/o	22. _____	rash
myc/o	23. _____	hard, horny
onych/o	24. _____	sweat gland
papul/o	25. _____	skin
pedicul/o	26. _____	lice
pil/o	27. _____	oil
rhytid/o	28. _____	scab
seb/o	29. _____	scaly
squam/o	30. _____	hair
vascul/o	31. _____	fat
xen/o	32. _____	fungus

Word Shop

Prefixes	Combining Forms	Suffixes
a-	blephar/o	-ectomy
an-	chrom/o	-desis
dys-	crypt/o	-ia
hyper-	cutane/o	-ic
hypo-	dermat/o	-itis
par-	fibr/o	-lysis
sub-	follicul/o	-malacia
trans-	hidr/o	-oma
	myc/o	-osis
	onych/o	-ous
	rhytid/o	-plasty
	seb/o	-rrheic
	trich/o	-y
	troph/o	

Build the following terms by combining the preceding word parts. Some word parts may be used more than once. Some may not be used at all. The number in parentheses is the number of word parts needed to build the term.

Definition	Term
1. abnormal condition of excessive hair (3)	_____
2. condition of no development (3)	_____
3. removal of wrinkle (2)	_____
4. pertaining to a discharge of oil (2)	_____
5. condition of near the nail (3)	_____
6. abnormal condition of no sweat (3)	_____
7. surgical repair of the eyelids (2)	_____
8. softening of the nails (2)	_____
9. inflammation of a hair follicle (2)	_____
10. condition of abnormal color (3)	_____
11. pertaining to under the skin (3)	_____
12. abnormal condition of fungus of the skin (3)	_____
13. fibrous tumor of the skin (3)	_____
14. destruction/loosening of a nail (2)	_____
15. abnormal condition of "hidden" nail (3)	_____

Sort the terms below into the correct categories.

Term Sorting

Anatomy and Physiology	Pathology	Diagnostic Procedures	Therapeutic Interventions

allograft	dermatoplasty	lunula	sebaceous gland
alopecia	epidermis	Mantoux test	sebum
bacterial analysis	eponychium	melanocyte	strata
blepharoplasty	escharotomy	onychomycosis	tinea pedis
cauterization	excisional Bx	papilla	Tzanck test
curettage	ecchymosis	perspiration	verruca
débridement	eczema	plaque	vesicle
dermabrasion	follicle	punch biopsy	Wood's light
dermatomycosis	hyperhidrosis	rhytidectomy	xenograft

Replace the underlined text with the correct terms.

Translations

1. John was treated for **athlete's foot** after a positive fungal test.

2. Mr. Hassan complained of intense **itching** caused by **parasitic infestation caused by mites.**

3. Melanie said she had **an abnormal condition of excessive perspiration** as the reason for her appointment with her physician.

4. Stephanie went to see her podiatrist to treat her **ingrown toe nail** and asked if he could also treat the **infection beside her nail.**

5. Josh developed an **overgrowth of tissue** where his ear was pierced.

6. When Mia developed **a superficial vesicopustular skin infection,** her mom noticed small **raised solid skin lesions** as well as **tiny blisters** that were characteristic of the disorder.

7. When Laura came home with **an infestation of lice,** her doctor treated it with a **medication that kills lice.**

8. The patient was treated for **an inflammatory disease of the sebaceous glands** with a **drug derived from vitamin A.**

9. The patient was prescribed **topical substances that soften the skin** for her **dry skin.**

10. The patient had **a contagious epithelial growth caused by HPV** on his hand removed with **destruction of tissue through the use of extreme cold.**

11. The burn patient was in for **surgical incision into necrotic tissue** and a consultation for a possible **harvest of skin from another human donor for temporary transplant.**

12. Mrs. Mooreland had **a surgical operation to remove wrinkles** and **a surgical repair of the eyelids.**

13. Mr. Kleinfelter was hospitalized for **a sore in the skin over a bony prominence.**

Medical Record Ben Warner

WARNER, BENJAMIN R - 607231 Opened by O'BRIAN, JENNIFER A.

Task   Edit   View   Time Scale   Options   Help

WARNER, BENJAMIN R

Age: 11 months   Sex: Male   Loc: WHC-SMMC
DOB: 01/20/2014   MRN: 607231   FIN: 3506004

Reference Text Browser | Form Browser | Medication Profile

Orders | Last 48 Hours | ED | Lab | Radiology | Assessment | Surgery | Clinical Notes | Pt. Info | Pt. Schedule | Task List | I & O | MAR

Flowsheet: ED   Level: ED record   ○ Table ○ Group ○ List

Navigator
☑ ED record

Chief Complaint: Second-degree burns on forearm of 11-month-old male. Father states that child pulled hot coffee off table onto arm. Denies other injuries.

Physical Exam:
HEENT: Oropharynx pink and moist, neck supple without adenopathy; no evidence of burns found on face.
CV: RRR with no murmur.
Lungs: Clean bilaterally without adventitious sounds.
ABD: BS throughout, no organomegaly.
Skin: Large area of erythematous skin involving the back of the right hand and extending down the forearm in a splattering pattern. Tissue blanched well with good capillary refill. A large vesicle that had formed on the dorsal side of the hand broke during examination.
Assessment: Superficial partial-thickness burn of the right hand/forearm less than 10%.
Treatment: Wound cleansed with cool sterile water and dressed with Silvadene cream and a telfa dressing. Children's Tylenol administered with homecare discharge. Dressing instructions given.

PROD | MAHAFC | 22 Dec 2014 | 07:08

EMERGENCY DEPARTMENT RECORD

Using the medical record above, answer the following questions.

1. What type of burn is described?

    A. Superficial
    B. Partial thickness
    C. Full thickness

2. What are the characteristics that make this a second-degree burn?

    _____

3. Ben's burn produced a large vesicle. What is a vesicle?

    _____

5

Gastrointestinal System

OBJECTIVES

- Recognize and use terms related to the anatomy and physiology of the gastrointestinal system.
- Recognize and use terms related to the pathology of the gastrointestinal system.

- Recognize and use terms related to the diagnostic procedures for the gastrointestinal system.
- Recognize and use terms related to the therapeutic interventions for the gastrointestinal system.

For more interactive learning, click on:
- **Match the Word Parts** to review gastrointestinal word parts.
- **Word Shop** to practice word building.
- **Tournament of Terminology** to test your knowledge of gastrointestinal terms.
- **Term Sorting** to practice sorting gastrointestinal terms into categories.

*Click on **Chapter at a Glance** for a list of key word parts and terms for this chapter.*

FUNCTIONS OF THE GASTROINTESTINAL SYSTEM

The digestive system (Fig. 5-1) provides the nutrients needed for cells to replicate themselves continually and build new tissue. This is done through several distinct processes: **ingestion,** the intake of food; **digestion,** the breakdown of food; **absorption,** the process of extracting nutrients; and **elimination,** the excretion of any waste products. Other names for this system are the **gastrointestinal (GI) tract,** which refers to the two main parts of the system, and the **alimentary** (al in MEN tair ee) **canal,** which refers to the tubelike nature of the digestive system, starting at the mouth and continuing in varying diameters to the anus.

The digestive system begins in the oral cavity, progresses through the mediastinum and the **abdominal** and pelvic cavities, and finally exits at the anus. The stomach and intestines lie within the peritoneal cavity and are attached to the body wall by a rich vascular membrane termed the *mesentery.* Internally, the alimentary canal is composed of three layers, or tunics. The inner layer is the tunica **mucosa,** which secretes gastric juices, absorbs nutrients, and protects the tissue through the production of mucus. The submucosa, the next tunic, holds the blood, lymphatic, and nervous tissue. The deepest layer is the tunica muscularis, which contracts and relaxes around the tube in a wavelike movement termed **peristalsis,** to move food through the tract.

SPECIALTIES/SPECIALISTS

The main digestive system specialty is called **gastroenterology,** and the specialist is called a **gastroenterologist. Proctologists** treat disorders of the rectum and anus.

While **dentists** diagnose and treat disorders of the teeth, there are subspecialists who extract **(exodontists)** and straighten **(orthodontists)** teeth, as well as those who treat children **(pedodontists),** gum disorders **(periodontists),** and replace missing teeth **(prosthodontists).**

gastrointestinal
  gastr/o = stomach
  intestin/o = intestines
  -al = pertaining to

abdomen = abdomin/o,
lapar/o, celi/o

mucus, mucosa =
mucos/o, myx/o

peristalsis
  peri- = surrounding
  -stalsis = contraction

gastroenterologist
  gastr/o = stomach
  enter/o = small intestine
  -logist = one who
  specializes

exodontist
  exo- = outside
  odont/o = teeth
  -ist = one who specializes

peri- = surrounding

ped/o = child

orth/o = straight

prosth/o = addition

proct/o = rectum and anus

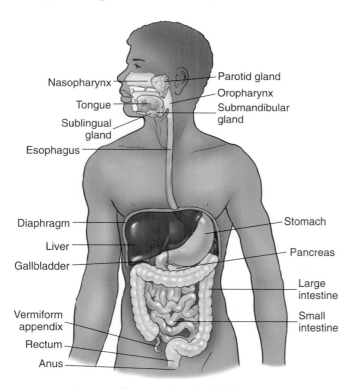

Nasopharynx
Tongue
Sublingual gland
Esophagus
Parotid gland
Oropharynx
Submandibular gland

Diaphragm
Liver
Gallbladder
Vermiform appendix
Rectum
Anus
Stomach
Pancreas
Large intestine
Small intestine

Fig. 5-1 The gastrointestinal (GI) system.

mouth, oral cavity = or/o, stomat/o, stom/o
lips = cheil/o, labi/o
cheek = bucc/o
tongue = gloss/o, lingu/o
palate = palat/o
teeth = dent/i, odont/o
gums = gingiv/o
salivary gland = sialaden/o
saliva = sial/o

parotid
    par- = near
    ot/o = ear
    -id = pertaining to

submandibular
    sub- = under
    mandibul/o = lower jaw, mandible
    -ar = pertaining to

sublingual
    sub- = under
    lingu/o = tongue
    -al = pertaining to

upper jaw = maxill/o
lower jaw = mandibul/o
throat, pharynx = pharyng/o

nasopharynx
    nas/o = nose
    pharyng/o = throat, pharynx

below = hypo-
larynx, voice box = laryng/o

ANATOMY AND PHYSIOLOGY

Oral Cavity

Food normally enters the body through the mouth, or **oral cavity** (Fig. 5-2, *A*). The function of this cavity initially is to break down the food mechanically by chewing **(mastication)** and lubricate the food to make swallowing **(deglutition;** dee gloo TIH shun) easier.

The oral cavity begins at the **lips,** the two fleshy structures surrounding its opening. The inside of the mouth is bounded by the **cheeks,** the **tongue** at the floor, and an anterior **hard palate** (PAL it) and posterior **soft palate,** which form the roof of the mouth. The upper and lower jaws hold 32 permanent **teeth** that are set in the flesh of the **gums,** also called the **gingivae.** The **uvula** (YOO vyoo lah) is the tag of flesh that hangs down from the medial surface of the soft palate. The three pairs of **salivary** (SAL ih vair ee) **glands** provide **saliva,** a substance that moistens the oral cavity, initiates the digestion of starches, and aids in chewing and swallowing. The glands are named for their locations: **parotid** (pair AH tid), near the ear; **submandibular** (sub man DIB yoo lur), under the lower jaw; and **sublingual** (sub LEENG gwul), under the tongue. The upper jaw is called the **maxilla,** and the lower is called the **mandible.**

Throat

The throat, or **pharynx** (FAIR inks), is a tube that connects the oral cavity with the esophagus. It can be divided into three main parts: the nasopharynx, the oropharynx, and the hypopharynx. The **nasopharynx** (nay soh FAIR inks) is the most superior part of the pharynx, located behind the nasal cavity. The **oropharynx** (oh roh FAIR inks) is the part of the throat directly adjacent to the oral cavity, and the **hypopharynx** (hye poh FAIR inks) (also called the **laryngopharynx**) is the part of the throat directly below the oropharynx (see Fig. 5-2, *B*).

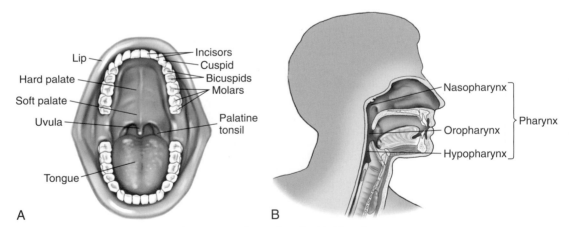

Fig. 5-2 A, The oral cavity. **B,** The pharynx.

Esophagus

The **esophagus** (eh SAH fah gus) is a muscular, mucus-lined tube that extends from the throat to the stomach. It carries a masticated lump of food, a **bolus** (BOH lus), from the oral cavity to the stomach by means of peristalsis. The glands in the lining of the esophagus produce mucus, which aids in lubricating and easing the passage of the bolus to the stomach. The muscle that must relax before the food enters the stomach is known by three names: the **lower esophageal** (eh sah fah JEE ul) **sphincter** (SFINK tur) **(LES)**, the **gastroesophageal sphincter,** or the **cardiac sphincter,** which gets its name because of its proximity to the heart. Sphincters are ringlike muscles that appear throughout the digestive and other body systems.

| **esophagus** = esophag/o |
| **bolus** = bol/o |

EXERCISE 1: Oral Cavity, Throat, and Esophagus

Match the combining forms with the following definitions. There may be more than one combining form for a given definition.

_____ 1. teeth

_____ 2. gums

_____ 3. roof of mouth

_____ 4. tongue

_____ 5. mouth

_____ 6. lips

_____ 7. cheek

_____ 8. salivary gland

_____ 9. saliva

_____ 10. throat

_____ 11. esophagus

A. esophag/o
B. bucc/o
C. cheil/o
D. or/o, stom/o, stomat/o
E. lingu/o
F. palat/o
G. labi/o
H. gingiv/o
I. gloss/o
J. sial/o
K. stomat/o
L. pharyng/o
M. dent/i, odont/o
N. sialaden/o

Decode the following terms using your knowledge of gastrointestinal word parts.

12. perioral _____

13. gingival _____

14. periodontal _____

15. submandibular _____

16. nasopharyngeal _____

EXERCISE 2: Oral Cavity, Throat, and Esophagus

Label the figures below using the terms provided.

lip	bicuspids	hypopharynx
molars	tongue	oropharynx
palatine tonsil	incisors	nasopharynx
hard palate	soft palate	
uvula		

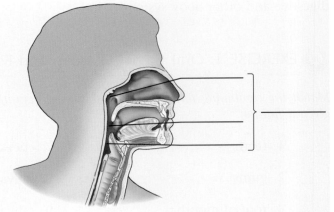

Stomach

stomach = gastr/o

fundus = fund/o

body, corporis = corpor/o

pylorus = pylor/o

rugae = rug/o

The **stomach,** where digestion begins, is an expandable vessel, which is divided into three sections: the top, or **fundus** (FUN dus); the **body;** and the muscle between the stomach and first part of the small intestine, or **pylorus** (pye LORE us) (also called the **gastric antrum**) (Fig. 5-3). The portion of the stomach that surrounds the esophagogastric connection is the **cardia** (KAR dee ah). The **fundus** is the area of the stomach that abuts the diaphragm. This section of the stomach has no acid-producing cells, unlike the remainder of the stomach. The body, or **corporis,** is the central part of the stomach, and the pylorus (*pl.* pylori) is at the distal end of the stomach, where the small intestine begins. A small muscle, the **pyloric sphincter,** regulates the gentle release of food from the stomach into the small intestine. When the stomach is empty, it has an appearance of being lined with many ridges. These ridges, or wrinkles, are called **rugae** (ROO jee) (*sing.* ruga).

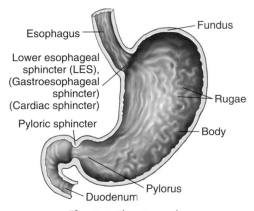

Fig. 5-3 The stomach.

The function of the stomach is to temporarily store the chewed food that it receives from the esophagus. This food is mixed with gastric juices and hydrochloric acid to further the digestive process chemically. This mixture is called **chyme** (kyme). The smooth muscles of the stomach contract to aid in the mechanical digestion of the food. A continual coating of mucus protects the stomach and the rest of the digestive system from the acidic nature of the gastric juices.

Small Intestine

Once the chyme has been formed in the stomach, the pyloric sphincter relaxes a bit at a time to release portions of it into the first part of the **small intestine,** called the **duodenum** (doo AH deh num). The small intestine gets its name, not because of its length (it is about 20 feet long), but because of the diameter of its **lumen** (LOO mun) (a tubular cavity within the body). The second section of the small intestine is the **jejunum** (jeh JOO num), and the distal part of the small intestine is the **ileum** (ILL ee um).

Multiple circular folds in the small intestines, called **plicae** (PLY see), contain thousands of tiny projections called **villi** (VILL eye) (*sing.* villus), which contain blood capillaries that absorb the products of carbohydrate and protein digestion. The villi also contain lymphatic vessels, known as **lacteals** (LACK tee uls), that absorb **lipid** (LIH pid) substances from the chyme. A lipid is a fatty substance.

The suffix -*ase* is used to form the name of an enzyme. It is added to the name of the substance upon which the enzyme acts: for example, **lipase,** which acts on lipids, or amylase, which acts on starches. -*ose* is a chemical suffix indicating that a substance is a carbohydrate, such as *glucose.*

Large Intestine

In contrast to the small intestine, the **large intestine** or **colon** (Fig. 5-4) is only about 5 feet long, but it is much wider in diameter. The primary function of the large intestine is the elimination of waste products from the body. Some synthesis of vitamins occurs in the large intestine, but unlike the small intestine, the large intestine has no villi and is not well suited for absorption of nutrients. The **ileocecal** (ILL ee oh SEE kul) valve is the exit from the small intestine and the entrance to the colon. The first part of the large intestine, the **cecum** (SEE kum), has a wormlike appendage, called the **vermiform appendix** (VUR mih form ah PEN dicks) (*pl.* appendices), dangling from it. Although this organ does not seem to have any direct function related to the digestive system, it is thought to have a possible immunologic defense mechanism.

No longer called chyme, whatever has not been absorbed by the small intestines is now called **feces** (FEE sees). The feces pass from the cecum to the **ascending colon** (KOH lin), through the **transverse colon,** the **descending colon,** the **sigmoid colon** (the S-shaped part of the large intestine), and on to the **rectum** (the last straight part of the colon), where they are held until released from the body completely through the **anus** (the final sphincter in the GI tract.) The process of releasing feces from the body is called **defecation,** or a bowel movement (BM).

Do not confuse -*cele*, the suffix meaning herniation, with *celi/o,* a combining form for abdomen.

Do not confuse **an/o,** the combining form for anus; **ana-,** the prefix meaning up or apart; and **an-,** the prefix meaning no, not, or without.

small intestine	= enter/o
duodenum	= duoden/o
lumen	= lumin/o
jejunum	= jejun/o
ileum	= ile/o
fold, plica	= plic/o
villus	= vill/o
lipid, fat	= lipid/o, lip/o
large intestine, colon	= col/o, colon/o

The combining form **gastr/o** *refers only to the stomach. The combining forms* **abdomin/o, lapar/o,** *and* **celi/o** *refer to the abdomen.*

ileocecal
   ile/o = ileum
   cec/o = cecum
   -al = pertaining to

cecum	= cec/o
appendix	= appendic/o, append/o
feces	= fec/a
sigmoid colon	= sigmoid/o
rectum, straight	= rect/o
anus	= an/o
rectum and anus	= proct/o

Don't confuse the term **ilium** *meaning part of the hip bone with* **ileum** *meaning part of the small intestine.*

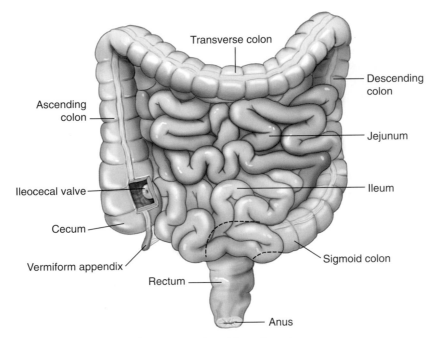

Fig. 5-4 Small and large intestines.

EXERCISE 3: The Stomach, Small Intestine, and Large Intestine

Match the following combining forms and body parts with their terms.

_____ 1. lip/o	_____ 9. gastr/o	A. rectum and anus
		B. first part of large intestines
_____ 2. plic/o	_____ 10. cec/o	C. structure hanging from cecum
		D. small intestines
_____ 3. col/o	_____ 11. sigmoid/o	E. tubular cavity
		F. stomach
_____ 4. jejun/o	_____ 12. lumin/o	G. second part of small intestines
		H. a fatty substance, fat
_____ 5. ile/o	_____ 13. enter/o	I. folds
		J. first part of small intestines
_____ 6. rect/o	_____ 14. pylor/o	K. muscle between stomach and first part of small intestines
_____ 7. an/o	_____ 15. proct/o	L. last straight part of colon
		M. large intestines
_____ 8. duoden/o	_____ 16. appendic/o	N. distal part of small intestines
		O. final sphincter in GI tract
		P. S-shaped part of large intestine

Decode the terms.

17. perirectal _____

18. intraluminal _____

19. epigastric _____

EXERCISE 4: Stomach and Intestines

Label the figures below using the terms provided.

esophagus
pylorus
rugae
pyloric sphincter
fundus
LES
body
duodenum

ascending colon
sigmoid colon
rectum
vermiform appendix
transverse colon
jejunum
anus
ileum
cecum
descending colon

Accessory Organs (Adnexa)

The accessory organs are the **gallbladder** (GALL blad ur) **(GB),** a small sac found on the underside of the right lobe of the liver; liver; and pancreas (Fig. 5-5). These organs secrete fluid into the GI tract but are not a direct part of the tube itself. Sometimes accessory structures are referred to as **adnexa** (ad NECK sah).

The two **lobes** that form the **liver** (LIH vur) virtually fill the right upper quadrant of the abdomen and extend partially into the left upper quadrant directly inferior to the **diaphragm.** The liver filters and stores blood and forms a substance called **bile,** which **emulsifies** (ee MUL sih fyez), or mechanically breaks down, fats into smaller particles so that they can be chemically digested. Bile is composed of **bilirubin** (BILL ee roc bin), the waste product formed by the normal breakdown of hemoglobin in red blood cells at the end of their life spans, and **cholesterol** (koh LESS tur all), a fatty substance found only in animal tissues. Bile is released from the liver through the right and left hepatic ducts, which join to form the **hepatic** (heh PAT ick) **duct.** The **cystic** (SISS tick) **duct** carries bile to and from the GB. When the hepatic and cystic ducts

gallbladder = cholecyst/o
accessory = adnex/o
lobe = lob/o
liver = hepat/o
diaphragm = diaphragmat/o, phren/o
bile = chol/e, bil/i
cholesterol = cholesterol/o

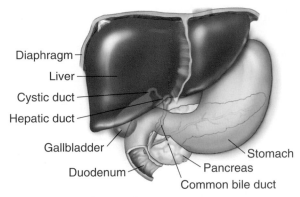

Fig. 5-5 Accessory organs.

common bile duct = choledoch/o

bile vessel = cholangi/o

cholecystokinin
  cholecyst/o = gallbladder
  -kinin = movement
  substance

pancreas = pancreat/o

exocrine
  exo- = outside
  -crine = to secrete

endocrine
  endo- = within
  -crine = to secrete

merge, they form the **common bile duct,** which empties into the duodenum. Collectively, all of these ducts are termed **bile vessels.** Bile is stored in the GB. When fatty food enters the duodenum, a hormone called **cholecystokinin** (koh lee sis toh KYE nin) is secreted, causing a contraction of the GB to move bile out into the cystic duct, then the common bile duct, and finally into the duodenum.

The **pancreas** (PAN kree us) is a gland located in the upper left quadrant. It is involved in the digestion of the three types of food molecules: carbohydrates, proteins, and lipids. The pancreatic enzymes are carried through the pancreatic duct, which empties into the common bile duct. Pancreatic involvement in food digestion is an **exocrine** (ECK soh krin) function because the secretion is into a duct. Pancreatic **endocrine** (EN doh krin) functions (secretion into blood and lymph vessels) are discussed in Chapter 14.

 EXERCISE 5: Accessory Organs

Match the combining forms with their terms.

_____ 1. pancreas

_____ 2. gallbladder (GB)

_____ 3. lobe

_____ 4. liver

_____ 5. bile

_____ 6. bile vessels

_____ 7. common bile duct

A. lob/o
B. chol/e, bil/i
C. hepat/o
D. cholecyst/o
E. cholangi/o
F. choledoch/o
G. pancreat/o

Decode the terms.

8. pancreatic _____

9. biliary _____

10. subhepatic _____

Label the figure below using the terms provided.

common bile duct
liver
stomach
hepatic duct
pancreas
cystic duct
gallbladder
diaphragm
duodenum

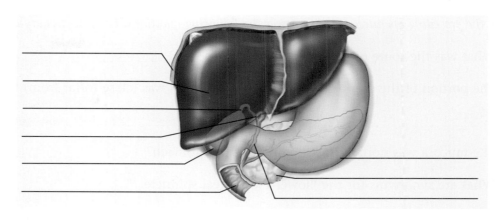

ⓔ *You can review the anatomy of the GI system by clicking on **Body Spectrum Electronic Anatomy Coloring Book → Digestive.***

Medical Record Peter Jacobs

JACOBS, PETER E - 613446 Opened by JEROME, ALAN MD   _ 🗗 ☒

Task   Edit   View   Time Scale   Options   Help

As Of 06:15

JACOBS, PETER E   Age: 61   Sex: Male   Loc: WHC-SMMC
    DOB: 08/20/1952   MRN: 613446   FIN: 3506004

Reference Text Browser | Form Browser | Medication Profile

Orders | Last 48 Hours | ED | Lab | Radiology | Assessment | **Surgery** | Clinical Notes | Pt. Info | Pt. Schedule | Task List | I & O | MAR

Flowsheet Surgery ▼ ...   Level: Operative Report ▼   ⦿ Table ◯ Group ◯ List

Navigator ☒

✓ Operative Report

PREOPERATIVE DIAGNOSIS: Rule out GI pathology
POSTOPERATIVE DIAGNOSIS: SEE "Impression" below
OPERATION: Upper GI endoscopy

Patient was brought into the endoscopy suite where continuous oximetry, blood pressure, and ECG monitoring was placed. He was given 50 mg of fentanyl before procedure. The GIF Olympus 150 video endoscope was introduced through the pharynx without difficulty. Proximal portion of the esophagus appeared normal. At approximately midesophagus, there were noted streaks of erythema extending up into the esophagus. The squamocolumnar junction was 33 cm where there was a smooth concentric narrowing of the esophagus. There was mild friability of this tissue and distally was a moderate hiatal hernia. The scope was advanced through this into the gastric fundus, which was visualized in both the forward and retroflexed manner. Mucosa appeared quite normal. Distally, there was marked erythema of the antrum, particularly surrounding the pylorus. Biopsy was taken for *H. pylori*. The duodenum was difficult to intubate but appeared normal. Scope was withdrawn again to the level of the lower esophageal sphincter at 36 cm. Biopsies were taken from that area and circumferentially up to approximately 32 cm. There was minimal bleeding. Patient tolerated the procedure well.

IMPRESSION:
  1. Reflux esophagitis with stricture at 33 cm
  2. Moderate hiatal hernia
  3. Probably Barrett's esophagus
  4. Diffuse antral gastritis, biopsy pending

PROD MAHAFC 23 July 2014 06:15

EXERCISE 7: Operative Report

Using the preceding operative report, answer the following questions. Use a dictionary as needed for this exercise.

1.   What was the route of the endoscope? _____

2.   The portion of the esophagus that appeared normal was (close to/far from) the mouth. Circle one.

_____

3.   The mucosa was normal in which part of the stomach? _____

4.   What are synonyms for the "lower esophageal sphincter?" _____

> (e) Choose **Hear It, Spell It** to practice spelling the anatomy and physiology terms that you have
> learned in this chapter.

Combining and Adjective Forms for the Anatomy of the Gastrointestinal System

Meaning	Combining Form	Adjective Form
abdomen	abdomin/o, celi/o, lapar/o	abdominal, celiac
accessory	adnex/o	adnexal
anus	an/o	anal
appendix	appendic/o, append/o	appendicular
bile	chol/e, bil/i	biliary
bile vessel	cholangi/o	
bolus	bol/o	
cecum	cec/o	cecal
cheek	bucc/o	buccal
cholesterol	cholesterol/o	
common bile duct	choledoch/o	choledochal
corporis, body	corpor/o	corporeal
duodenum	duoden/o	duodenal
epiglottis	epiglott/o	epiglottal
esophagus	esophag/o	esophageal
fat, lipid	lip/o, lipid/o	lipid
feces	fec/a	fecal
fold, plica	plic/o	plical
fundus	fund/o	fundal
gallbladder	cholecyst/o	cholecystic
glucose, sugar	gluc/o	
gums	gingiv/o	gingival
ileum	ile/o	ileal
intestines	intestin/o	intestinal
jejunum	jejun/o	jejunal

Combining and Adjective Forms for the Anatomy of the Gastrointestinal System—cont'd

Meaning	Combining Form	Adjective Form
large intestine, colon	col/o, colon/o	colonic
lips	cheil/o, labi/o	labial
liver	hepat/o	hepatic
lobe	lob/o	lobular
lower jaw	mandibul/o	mandibular
lumen	lumin/o	luminal
mouth, oral cavity	or/o, stom/o, stomat/o	oral, stomal, stomatic
nose	nas/o, rhin/o	nasal
nutrition	aliment/o	alimentary
palate	palat/o	palatine
pancreas	pancreat/o	pancreatic
pharynx, throat	pharyng/o	pharyngeal
pylorus	pylor/o	pyloric
rectum	rect/o	rectal
rectum and anus	proct/o	
rugae	rug/o	rugous
saliva	sial/o	salivary
salivary gland	sialaden/o	
sigmoid colon	sigmoid/o	sigmoidal
small intestine	enter/o	enteral
starch	amyl/o	
stomach	gastr/o	gastric
teeth	dent/i, odont/o	dental
tongue	gloss/o, lingu/o	lingual, glossal
upper jaw	maxill/o	maxillary
uvula	uvul/o	uvular
villus	vill/o	villous

Prefixes for the Anatomy of the Gastrointestinal System

Prefix	Meaning
endo-	within
exo-	outside
hypo-	below
par-	near
peri-	surrounding
sub-	under

Suffixes for the Anatomy of the Gastrointestinal System

Suffix	Meaning
-al, -ar, -eal, -ic, -id, -ine, -ous	pertaining to
-crine	to secrete
-kinin	movement substance
-stalsis	contraction

 *Click on **Label It** to practice labeling GI structures.*

PATHOLOGY

Terms Related to Upper Gastrointestinal Complaints

Term	Word Origin	Definition
dyspepsia dis PEP see ah	*dys-* abnormal, bad *-pepsia* digestion condition	Feeling of epigastric discomfort that occurs shortly after eating. The discomfort may include feelings of nausea, fullness, heartburn, and/or bloating. Also called *indigestion.*
eructation ee ruck TAY shun		Release of air from the stomach through the mouth. Eructation may be caused by rapid eating or by intentionally or unintentionally swallowing air (aerophagia). Also called **burping** or **belching.**
halitosis hal ih TOH sis	*halit/o* breath *-osis* abnormal condition	Bad-smelling breath.
hematemesis hee mah TEM ah sis	*hemat/o* blood *-emesis* vomiting	Vomiting of blood.
hiccup HICK up		Involuntary contraction of the diaphragm, followed by a rapid closure of the glottis (which in turn causes the characteristic sound of a hiccup). Also known as **hiccough** or **singultus.**
nausea NAH see ah		Sensation that accompanies the urge to vomit but does not always lead to vomiting. The abbreviation N&V refers to nausea and vomiting. The term is derived from a Greek word meaning seasickness.
pyrosis pye ROH sis	*pyr/o* fire *-osis* abnormal condition	Painful burning sensation in esophagus, usually caused by reflux of stomach contents, hyperactivity, or peptic ulcer. Also known as **heartburn.**
regurgitation ree gur jih TAY shun		Return of swallowed food to the mouth. Regurgitation may, however, describe any backward flow in the body, not just that of a GI nature.
vomiting VAH mih ting		Forcible or involuntary emptying of the stomach through the mouth. The material expelled is called **vomitus** or **emesis.**

Terms Related to Lower Gastrointestinal Complaints

Term	Word Origin	Definition
constipation kon stih PAY shun		Infrequent, incomplete, or delayed BMs. **Obstipation** is intractable (difficult to manage) constipation or intestinal obstruction.
diarrhea dye ah REE ah	*dia-* through, complete *-rrhea* discharge, flow	Abnormal discharge of watery, semisolid stools.
flatus FLAY tus		Gas expelled through the anus.
hematochezia hee mat oh KEE zee ah	*hemat/o* blood *-chezia* condition of stools	Bright red, frank lower GI bleeding from the rectum that may originate in the distal colon. Passage of bloody stools.
irritable bowel syndrome (IBS)		Diarrhea, gas, and/or constipation resulting from stress with no underlying disease.
melena mah LEE nah	*melan/o* black, dark	Black, tarry stools caused by the presence of partially digested blood.

EXERCISE 8: Upper and Lower Gastrointestinal Complaints

Match the GI complaints to their definitions.

_____ 1. diarrhea

_____ 2. obstipation

_____ 3. flatus

_____ 4. melena

_____ 5. halitosis

_____ 6. irritable bowel syndrome (IBS)

_____ 7. constipation

_____ 8. nausea

_____ 9. regurgitation

A. bad breath
B. delayed defecation
C. feeling of need to vomit
D. gas passed through the anus
E. backward flow to mouth
F. black, tarry stools
G. loose, watery stools
H. extremely delayed defecation
I. diarrhea/gas/constipation resulting from stress with no underlying disease

Match the synonyms.

_____ 10. indigestion

_____ 11. singultus

_____ 12. pyrosis

_____ 13. eructation

_____ 14. emesis

A. vomit
B. hiccup
C. burping
D. dyspepsia
E. heartburn

Build the terms.

15. condition of blood in the stools _____

16. vomiting of blood _____

17. abnormal condition of digestion _____

Terms Related to Congenital Disorders

Term	Word Origin	Definition
cleft palate kleft PAL it		Failure of the palate to close during embryonic development, creating an opening in the roof of the mouth. **Cleft palate** often is accompanied by a cleft lip (Fig. 5-6).
esophageal atresia eh soff uh JEE ul ah TREE zsa	*esophag/o* esophagus *-eal* pertaining to *a-* without *-tresia* condition of an opening	Esophagus that ends in a blind pouch and therefore lacks an opening into the stomach (Fig. 5-7).
Hirschsprung disease HERSH sprung		Congenital absence of normal nervous function in part of the colon, which results in an absence of peristaltic movement, accumulation of feces, and an enlarged colon. Also called **congenital megacolon.**
pyloric stenosis pye LORE ick sten OH sis	*pylor/o* pylorus *-ic* pertaining to *stenosis* narrowing	Condition in which the muscle between the stomach and the small intestine narrows or fails to open adequately to allow partially digested food into the duodenum.

Fig. 5-6 Cleft palate and cleft lip.

Fig. 5-7 Esophageal atresia.

Fig. 5-8 Aphthous stomatitis.

 EXERCISE 9: Congenital Disorders

Fill in the blank with the correct term.

pyloric stenosis, cleft palate, esophageal atresia, Hirschsprung disease, congenital megacolon

1. The term that refers to the lack of an opening in the tube that extends from the throat to the stomach is _____.

2. A congenital fissure in the roof of the mouth is called _____.

3. If the patient has a lack of normal nervous function in part of the large intestine, which results in an accumulation of feces, he or she may be diagnosed with _____.

4. Another name for the answer to question 3 is _____.

5. A narrowing of the muscle between the stomach and the duodenum is called _____.

Terms Related to Oral Cavity Disorders

Term	Word Origin	Definition
aphthous stomatitis AFF thus stoh mah TYE tis	*aphth/o* ulceration *-ous* pertaining to *stomat/o* mouth *-itis* inflammation	Recurring condition characterized by small erosions (ulcers), which appear on the mucous membranes of the mouth. Also called a **canker sore** (Fig. 5-8).
cheilitis kye LYE tis	*cheil/o* lip *-itis* inflammation	Inflammation of the lips.
cheilosis kye LOH sis	*cheil/o* lip *-osis* abnormal condition	Abnormal condition of the lips present in riboflavin (a B vitamin) deficiency (Fig. 5-9).
dental caries KARE ees	*dent/i* teeth *-al* pertaining to	Plaque disease caused by an interaction between food and bacteria in the mouth, leading to tooth decay. Also called **cavities.**
dental plaque plack	*dent/i* teeth *-al* pertaining to	Film of material that coats the teeth and may lead to dental decay if not removed.
gingivitis jin jih VYE tis	*gingiv/o* gums *-itis* inflammation	Inflammatory disease of the gums characterized by redness, swelling, and bleeding (Fig. 5-10).
herpetic stomatitis hur PET ick stoh man TYE tis	*stomat/o* mouth *-itis* inflammation	Inflammation of the mouth caused by the herpes simplex virus (HSV). Also known as a **cold sore** or **fever blister.**
leukoplakia loo koh PLAY kee ah	*leuk/o* white *-plakia* condition of patches	Condition of white patches that may appear on the lips, tongue, and buccal mucosa (Fig. 5-11). It usually is associated with tobacco use and may be precancerous.
malocclusion mal oh KLOO zhun	*mal-* bad, poor *-occlusion* condition of closure	Condition in which the teeth do not touch properly when the mouth is closed (abnormal bite).
periodontal disease pair ee oh DON tul	*peri-* surrounding *odont/o* tooth *-al* pertaining to	Pathologic condition of the tissues surrounding the teeth.
pyorrhea pye or REE yah	*py/o* pus *-rrhea* flow, discharge	Purulent discharge from the tissue surrounding the teeth; often seen with gingivitis.

Fig. 5-9 Cheilosis.

Fig. 5-10 Gingivitis.

Fig. 5-11 Leukoplakia.

EXERCISE 10: Oral Cavity Disorders

Match the oral cavity disorders to their definitions.

_____ 1. dental caries
_____ 2. cheilosis
_____ 3. aphthous stomatitis
_____ 4. herpetic stomatitis

_____ 5. dental plaque
_____ 6. malocclusion
_____ 7. periodontal disease

A. tooth decay
B. disorder of tissue surrounding teeth
C. abnormal bite
D. canker sore
E. cold sore
F. abnormal condition of lips
G. material that coats teeth

Build the terms.

8. inflammation of the gums _____

9. discharge of pus _____

10. condition of white patches _____

Case Study   Robert Mifflin

Seventeen-year-old Robert Mifflin is seen for complaints of "painful sores in his mouth" and difficulty swallowing. He says that the orange juice he had for breakfast was especially painful. Upon examination, he is diagnosed with herpetic stomatitis and given a prescription for acyclovir and lidocaine. He is told to drink cool, nonacidic beverages and limit his solid food intake until his swallowing is less painful.

1. What is the medical term for difficulty swallowing?
   _____

2. What is the common name for herpetic stomatitis?
   _____

3. Stomatitis is inflammation of the _____.

4. What is the condition called in which small erosions appear on the mucous membranes of the mouth?
   _____

Terms Related to Disorders of the Esophagus

Term	Word Origin	Definition
achalasia ack uh LAY zsa	*a-* without *-chalasia* condition of relaxation	Impairment of esophageal peristalsis along with the LES's inability to relax. Also called **cardiospasm, esophageal aperistalsis** (a per rih STALL sis), and **megaesophagus.**
dysphagia dis FAY jee ah	*dys-* difficult, bad *-phagia* condition of swallowing, eating	Difficulty with swallowing that may be due to an obstruction (e.g., a tumor) or a motor disorder (e.g., a spasm).
gastroesophageal reflux disease (GERD) gass troh eh sah fah JEE ul	*gastr/o* stomach *esophag/o* esophagus *-eal* pertaining to *re-* back *-flux* flow	Flowing back, or return, of the contents of the stomach to the esophagus caused by an inability of the LES to contract normally; characterized by pyrosis with or without regurgitation of stomach contents to the mouth (Fig. 5-12). **Barrett esophagus** is a condition caused by chronic reflux from the stomach. It is associated with an increased risk of cancer.

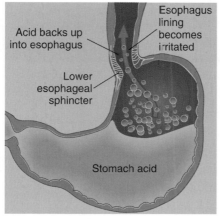

Fig. 5-12 Gastroesophageal reflux disease (GERD).

Fig. 5-13 Chronic peptic ulcer.

Terms Related to Disorders of the Stomach

Term	Word Origin	Definition
gastralgia gass TRAL zsa	*gastr/o* stomach *-algia* pain	Gastric pain. Also called **gastrodynia** (gass troh DIH nee ah).
gastritis gass TRY tis	*gastr/o* stomach *-itis* inflammation	Acute or chronic inflammation of the stomach that may be accompanied by anorexia, nausea and vomiting, or indigestion.
peptic ulcer disease (PUD)		An erosion of the protective mucosal lining of the stomach or duodenum (Fig. 5-13). Also called a **gastric** or **duodenal ulcer**.

EXERCISE 11: Esophageal and Stomach Disorders

Matching. More than one answer may be correct.

_____ 1. peptic ulcer disease (PUD)

_____ 2. gastralgia

_____ 3. gastritis

_____ 4. achalasia

_____ 5. dysphagia

_____ 6. gastroesophageal reflux disease (GERD)

A. cardiospasm
B. difficulty swallowing
C. inflammation of the stomach
D. stomach pain
E. gastrodynia
F. erosion of the gastric mucosa
G. return of the contents of the stomach to the esophagus
H. megaesophagus
I. esophageal aperistalsis

Terms Related to Intestinal Disorders

Term	Word Origin	Definition
anal fissure A null FISH ur	*an/o* anus *-al* pertaining to	Crack-like lesion of the skin around the anus.
anorectal abscess an oh RECK tul AB sess	*an/o* anus *rect/o* rectum *-al* pertaining to	Circumscribed area of inflammation in the anus or rectum, containing pus.

Continued

Terms Related to Intestinal Disorders—cont'd

Term	Word Origin	Definition
appendicitis ah pen dih SYE tis	*appendic/o* appendix *-itis* inflammation	Inflammation of the vermiform appendix (Fig. 5-14).
colitis koh LYE tis	*col/o* colon *-itis* inflammation	Inflammation of the large intestine.
Crohn disease krohn		Inflammation of the ileum or the colon that is of idiopathic origin. Also called **regional** or **granulomatous enteritis.**
diverticulitis dye vur tick yoo LYE tis	*diverticul/o* diverticulum *-itis* inflammation	Inflammation occurring secondary to the occurrence of diverticulosis.
diverticulosis dye vur tick yoo LOH sis	*diverticul/o* diverticulum *-osis* abnormal condition	Development of diverticula, pouches in the lining of the small or large intestines (Fig. 5-15).
fistula FIST yoo lah		Abnormal channel between organs or from an internal organ to the surface of the body.

Fig. 5-14 Appendicitis. Note the darker pink color of the appendix, indicating the inflammation.

Fig. 5-15 A, Diverticulosis. Diverticulosis can lead to diverticulitis **(B)** and subsequent complications.

Terms Related to Intestinal Disorders—cont'd

Term	Word Origin	Definition
hemorrhoid HEM uh royd		Varicose vein in the lower rectum or anus.
ileus ILL ee us		Obstruction. **Paralytic ileus** is lack of peristaltic movement in the intestinal tract. Also called **adynamic ileus.**
inflammatory bowel disease (IBD)		Chronic inflammation of the lining of the intestine characterized by bleeding and diarrhea.
intussusception in tuh suh SEP shun		Inward telescoping of the intestines (Fig. 5-16).
mucositis myoo koh SYE tis	*mucos/o* mucus *-itis* inflammation	Inflammation of the mucous membranes. GI mucositis may be an adverse effect of chemotherapy and can occur throughout the GI tract.
peritonitis pair ih tuh NYE tis	*periton/o* peritoneum *-itis* inflammation	Inflammation of the peritoneum that most commonly occurs when an inflamed appendix ruptures.
polyp PAH lip		Benign growth that may occur in the intestines.
proctitis prock TYE tis	*proct/o* rectum and anus *-itis* inflammation	Inflammation of the rectum and anus. Also called **rectitis.**
pruritus ani proo RYE tis A nye		Common chronic condition of itching of the skin surrounding the anus. Note that pruritus is spelled with a *u,* not an *i.*
ulcerative colitis UL sur uh tiv koh LYE tis	*col/o* colon *-itis* inflammation	Chronic inflammation of the colon and rectum manifesting with bouts of profuse watery diarrhea. A form of IBD.
volvulus VAWL vyoo lus		Twisting of the intestine.

⊗ Be Careful!

The correct spelling is **pruritus,** *not pruritis.*

⊗ Be Careful!

Don't confuse **peritone/o,** *which is the membrane that lines the abdominal cavity, with* **perone/o,** *which is a combining form for the fibula, and* **perine/o,** *the space between the anus and external reproductive organs.*

Fig. 5-16 Intussusception.

EXERCISE 12: Intestinal Disorders

Match the intestinal disorders to their definitions.

_____ 1. polyp

_____ 2. colitis

_____ 3. anal fissure

_____ 4. volvulus

_____ 5. paralytic ileus

_____ 6. fistula

_____ 7. intussusception

_____ 8. peritonitis

_____ 9. pruritus ani

_____ 10. ulcerative colitis

_____ 11. Crohn disease

_____ 12. hemorrhoids

_____ 13. inflammatory bowel disease (IBD)

_____ 14. diverticulitis

_____ 15. anorectal abscess

_____ 16. ileus

A.   general term for an obstruction
B.   a twisting of the intestines
C.   inward telescoping of the intestines
D.   idiopathic inflammation of ileum or colon
E.   profuse watery diarrhea accompanies this condition
F.   ruptured appendix puts a patient at risk for this
G.   growth on mucous membranes
H.   inflammation of pouches in GI tract
I.   inflammation of the large intestine
J.   itching of the skin around the anus
K.   varicosities around the anus and rectum
L.   crack-like lesion in the skin around the anus
M.   abnormal channel that forms between organs or to the outside of the body
N.   circumscribed area of purulent material in the distal end of the digestive tract
O.   lack of peristaltic movement in intestines
P.   erosion of intestinal lining accompanied by bleeding and diarrhea

Build the terms.

17.   inflammation of the appendix _____

18.   abnormal condition of diverticula _____

19.   inflammation of the rectum and anus _____

Terms Related to Gastrointestinal Accessory Organ Disorders

Term	Word Origin	Definition
cholangitis koh lan JYE tis	*cholangi/o* bile vessel *-itis* inflammation	Inflammation of the bile vessels.
cholecystitis koh lee sis TYE tis	*cholecyst/o* gallbladder *-itis* inflammation	Inflammation of the GB, either acute or chronic. May be caused by choledocholithiasis or cholelithiasis.
choledocholithiasis koh lee doh koh lih THY ih sis	*choledoch/o* common bile duct *lith/o* stones *-iasis* presence of	Presence of stones in the common bile duct.

Case Study   Elizabeth Frankfort

Elizabeth Frankfort, who is 68 years old, calls for an appointment for problems with her bowels. She says that she has been constipated for a month and has had a lot of gas. Two days ago, she began to be nauseous and lost her appetite. She says that when she does have a BM, there is blood on the toilet paper. Upon examination, she has a tender abdomen, and she has a temperature of 100.8° F. A review of her record shows diverticulosis that was documented by a previous family doctor in 2008, and it is suspected that she may currently have diverticulitis. A computed tomography (CT) scan of the abdomen and a colonoscopy confirm the diagnosis of inflamed diverticula in the sigmoid colon. Treatment consists of antibiotics, rest, and a liquid diet for the next few days. She is counseled that if the symptoms do not resolve in the next few days, she will need to have the offending diverticula removed surgically.

1. The medical term for "gas" is _____.

2. The term for her delayed, difficult bowel movements is _____.

3. An inflamed abnormal pouch in the digestive tract is called _____.

4. The suffix -osis in the term diverticulosis means _____.

5. The suffix -itis in the term diverticulitis means _____.

Terms Related to Gastrointestinal Accessory Organ Disorders—cont'd

Term	Word Origin	Definition
cholelithiasis koh lee lih THY ih sis	*chol/e* gall, bile *lith/o* stones *-iasis* presence of	Presence of stones (**calculi**) in the GB, sometimes characterized by right upper quadrant pain (**biliary colic**) with nausea and vomiting (Fig. 5-17).
cirrhosis sur OH sis	*cirrh/o* orange-yellow *-osis* abnormal condition	Chronic degenerative disease of the liver, commonly associated with alcohol abuse, chronic liver disease, and biliary tract disorders (Fig. 5-18).
hepatitis heh pah TYE tis	*hepat/o* liver *-itis* inflammation	Inflammation of the liver that is caused by an increasing number of viruses, alcohol, and drugs. Currently named by letter, **hepatitis A to G**, the means of viral transmission is not the same for each form. The most common forms, A to C, are discussed below.
hepatitis A	*hepat/o* liver *-itis* inflammation	Virus transmitted through direct contact with food or water that has been contaminated with fecal matter.
hepatitis B	*hepat/o* liver *-itis* inflammation	Virus transmitted through contaminated blood or sexual contact.
hepatitis C	*hepat/o* liver *-itis* inflammation	Virus transmitted through blood transfusion, percutaneous inoculation, or sharing of infected needles.
jaundice JAHN diss		Yellowing of the skin and sclerae (whites of the eyes) caused by elevated levels of bilirubin. Also called **icterus**.
pancreatitis pan kree uh TYE tis	*pancreat/o* pancreas *-itis* inflammation	Inflammation of the pancreas, which may be acute or chronic.

Fig. 5-17 Cholelithiasis (stones in the gallbladder [GB]).

Fig. 5-18 A, Normal liver. **B,** Cirrhosis of the liver is indicated by nodules on the surface.

EXERCISE 13: Gastrointestinal Accessory Organ Disorders

Fill in the blanks using the following terms.

pancreatitis, hepatitis, cholangitis, choledocholithiasis, jaundice, cholelithiasis, cirrhosis, cholecystitis

1. What is a chronic degenerative disorder of the liver, usually caused by alcohol abuse?

    _____

2. What is the term for the presence of stones in the GB? _____

3. What is the term for inflammation of the bile vessels? _____

4. What is the term for the presence of stones in the common bile duct? _____

5. What is the term for an inflammation of the pancreas? _____

6. What is an inflammatory disease of the liver that is named by letter? _____

7. What is the term for an inflammation of the GB? _____

8. Elevated level of bilirubin resulting in yellowing of the skin is termed _____.

Case Study Andrew Stockhausen

Andrew Stockhausen, who is 37 years old, has a low grade fever, N&V, jaundice, anorexia, and pale, clay-colored stools. He says he had just returned from vacation and thought that he was tired from several days of "partying." Examination of his abdomen reveals an enlarged, tender liver and liver function tests (LFTs) show abnormally high transaminase levels. A diagnosis of hepatitis A is made, and he is told to avoid irritants to the liver, including alcohol, nonsteroidal antiinflammatory drugs (NSAIDs), and fatty foods. He is told to rest, and the expectation is that recovery will occur in 2 to 3 weeks.

1. What does the abbreviation N&V mean? _____ _____

2. Which term refers to an abnormal yellow color? _____

3. Hepatitis is an inflammation of the _____.

4. Hepatitis __ is a virus transmitted through food or water that is contaminated with fecal matter.

Terms Related to Hernias

Term	Word Origin	Definition
femora hernia FEM uh rull HER nee ah	*femor/o* femur *-al* pertaining to	Protrusion of a loop of intestine through the femoral canal into the groin. Also called a **crural hernia.**
hiatal hernia hye A tull HER nee ah	*hiat/o* an opening *-al* pertaining to	Protrusion of a portion of the stomach through the diaphragm. Also known as a **diaphragmatic hernia** and **diaphragmatocele** (dye uh frag MAT oh seel) (Fig. 5-19).
incarcerated hernia in KAR sih ray tid HER nee ah		Loop of bowel with ends occluded (blocked) so that solids cannot pass; herniated bowel can become strangulated. Also called an **irreducible hernia.**
inguinal hernia IN gwin null HER nee ah	*inguin/o* groin *-al* pertaining to	Protrusion of a loop of intestine into the inguinal canal. May be **indirect** (through a normal internal passage) or **direct** (through a muscle wall).
strangulation		Constriction of a tubular structure, including intestines, leading to impedance of circulation and resulting in a lack of blood supply (**ischemia**) and possible tissue death.
umbilical hernia um BILL ih kull HER nee ah	*umbilic/o* umbilicus *-al* pertaining to	Protrusion of the intestine and omentum through a weakness in the abdominal wall (Fig. 5-20). Also known as an **omphalocele** (AHM fah loh seel).

Fig. 5-19 Hiatal hernia.

Fig. 5-20 Umbilical hernia.

EXERCISE 14: Hernias

Match the hernias to their definitions.

_____ 1. hiatal hernia _____ 4. incarcerated hernia   A. diaphragmatocele
                                                        B. protrusion of part of the intestines and
_____ 2. umbilical hernia _____ 5. inguinal hernia   omentum through the abdominal wall
                                                        C. irreducible hernia
_____ 3. strangulation _____ 6. femoral hernia   D. protrusion of intestine in the inguinal
                                                           canal
                                                        E. protrusion of intestine through the
                                                           femoral canal
                                                        F. constriction of a tubular structure

Terms Related to Benign Neoplasms

Term	Word Origin	Definition
cystadenoma sist aden OH mah	*cyst/o* bladder, cyst *aden/o* gland *-oma* tumor, mass	Glandular tumors that are filled with cysts; these are the most common benign tumors in the pancreas.
leiomyoma lye oh mye OH mah	*leiomy/o* smooth muscle *-oma* tumor, mass	Smooth muscle tumor that may occur in the digestive tract.
odontogenic tumor oh don toh JEN ick	*odont/o* tooth *-genic* pertaining to, produced by	Benign tumors that arise around the teeth and jaw (Fig. 5-21).
polyps, adenomatous or hyperplastic POLL ups ad eh noh MAH tuss hye per PLASS tick	*aden/o* gland *-oma* tumor *-ous* pertaining to *hyper-* excessive *plas/o* formation, growth *-tic* pertaining to	Adenomatous (growths that arise from glandular tissue and have potential to become malignant) or hyperplastic (generally, small growths that have no tendency to become malignant) tumors occurring throughout the digestive tract. Polyps may be **sessile** (flat) or **pedunculated** (having a stalk) (Fig. 5-22).

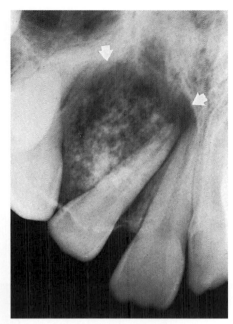

Fig. 5-21 Odontogenic tumor in the region of the right maxillary canine and lateral incisor.

Fig. 5-22 Multiple adenomatous polyps of the large intestine.

Terms Related to Malignant Neoplasms

Term	Word Origin	Definition	
adenocarcinoma ad en noh kar seh NOH mah	*aden/o* gland *-carcinoma* cancerous tumor of epithelial origin	A malignant tumor of epithelial origin that either originates from glandular tissue or has a glandular appearance.	Adenocarcinomas occur throughout the GI tract, but especially in the esophagus, stomach, pancreas, and colon.
hepatocellular carcinoma/ hepatoma heh pat oh SELL you lur kar seh NOH mah heh puh TOH mah	*hepat/o* liver *cellul/o* cell *-ar* pertaining to	Malignant tumors of epithelial origin that originate in the liver cells.	Hepatocellular carcinoma (also called **hepatoma**) is the most common type of primary liver cancer worldwide.
squamous cell carcinoma SKWAY muss	*squam/o* scaly *-ous* pertaining to	Cancers that have a scalelike appearance.	Squamous cell carcinomas arise from the cells that cover the surfaces of the body. These occur throughout the digestive system.

Please note: Metastatic carcinoma is the most common form of liver cancer. The liver is the most common site of all metastases. This is not a primary tumor but one that has spread from another site.

EXERCISE 15: Neoplasms

Fill in the blank.

1. What type of benign growth is described as either sessile or pedunculated? _____

2. What is the most common type of primary liver cancer? _____

3. Which type of cancer occurs throughout the GI tract, but especially in the esophagus, stomach, pancreas, and colon? _____

4. What is the term for a benign tumor that arises from around the teeth and jaw?

_____

 Case Study   **Bill Worth**

Bill Worth is a 59-year-old patient with an extensive medical history. He has been treated for hepatitis C, cirrhosis, and a variety of other ailments in the past 5 years. Today he is being seen for URQ pain, jaundice, and unexplained bruises that have been appearing on his arms and legs. He says that he thinks that his abdomen has gotten larger also, despite the fact that he has lost weight in the past few months. Physical examination reveals hepatomegaly; and further LFTs, an abdominal ultrasound, and subsequent liver biopsy yield a diagnosis of hepatocellular carcinoma.

1. Hepatitis C can be transmitted through blood or blood products, through sexual contact, or from sharing infected _____.

2. Cirrhosis is most commonly caused by _____ abuse.

3. What does the abbreviation URQ mean? _____
_____

4. Hepatomegaly is _____ of the liver.

5. Is the diagnosis a benign or malignant cancer? _____

 Age Matters

Pediatrics

GI congenital disorders are cleft palate, esophageal atresia, Hirschsprung disease, and pyloric stenosis. Although none of these are common, they do require medical intervention. Gastroenteritis and appendicitis—with their possible complications, respectively, of dehydration and peritonitis—are the most common reasons for hospital admissions of children.

Geriatrics

An aging digestive system is more likely to develop new dysfunctional cell growths (both benign and malignant), so statistics for polyps and colorectal cancer are high for the senior age group. Other diagnoses that appear more often are GERD and dysphagia, hemorrhoids, and type 2 diabetes mellitus.

---

e To practice spelling the pathology terms that you have learned in this chapter. click on **Hear It, Spell It.** To review the pathology terms in this chapter, play **Medical Millionaire.**

DIAGNOSTIC PROCEDURES

Visualizing the internal workings of the digestive system can be achieved through a wide variety of techniques but is usually accomplished through either radiographic imaging or endoscopy, or a combination of the two. Most of the procedures listed in the following table are a form of radiography, or "taking x-rays." However, because the tissues of the digestive system are soft (as opposed to bone), a radiopaque contrast medium may be necessary to outline the digestive tract. This substance may be introduced into the body through the oral or anal opening, or it may be injected. Fluoroscopy provides instant visual access to deep tissue structures.

Terms Related to Imaging

Term	Word Origin	Definition
barium enema (BE) BAIR ee um EN nuh mah		Introduction of a barium sulfate suspension through the rectum for imaging of the lower digestive tract to detect obstructions, tumors, and other abnormalities.
barium swallow (BaS)		Radiographic imaging done after oral ingestion of a barium sulfate suspension; used to detect abnormalities of the esophagus and stomach (Fig. 5-23).
cholecystography koh lee sis TAH gruh fee	*cholecyst/o* gallbladder *-graphy* process of recording	Contrast study in which iodine is ingested orally. The GB is then imaged at different time intervals to assess its functioning; this procedure is used to diagnose cholecystitis, cholelithiasis, tumors, and other abnormalities of the GB (Fig. 5-24).
computed tomography (CT) scan	*tom/o* section, cutting *-graphy* process of recording	Radiographic technique that produces detailed images of "slices," or cross sections of the body; used in the digestive system to diagnose tumors or abnormal accumulations of fluid.

Continued

Fig. 5-23 Barium swallow (BaS).

Fig. 5-24 Cholangiography.

Terms Related to Imaging—cont'd

Term	Word Origin	Definition
endoscopic retrograde cholangiopancreatography (ERCP) en doh SKAH pik REH troh grade koh LAN jee oh pan kree ah TAH grah fee	*endo-* within *-scopic* pertaining to process of viewing *cholangi/o* bile vessels *pancreat/o* pancreas *-graphy* process of recording	Radiographic imaging of the bile and pancreatic ducts through the placement of a duodenoscope in the common bile duct and injection of a contrast medium into the common bile duct. A series of x-rays are then taken to show the backward flow (retrograde) of dye into the bile vessels (Fig 5-25).
endoscopy en DAH skuh pee	*endo-* within *-scopy* process of viewing	General term for any internal visualization of the body with an instrument called an **endoscope,** which has its own fiberoptic light source. The endoscope enters the GI tract through the oral cavity (**esophagoscopy, gastroscopy,** and **esophagogastroduodenoscopy [EGD]**), through the anus (**proctoscopy, colonoscopy,** or **sigmoidoscopy**), or through an incision in the abdominal wall (**laparoscopy** or **lap**).
manometry mah NAH met tree	*man/o* scanty *-metry* process of measurement	Test that measures the motor function (muscle pressure) of the esophagus. A **manometer** is used to measure pressure.
percutaneous transhepatic cholangiography (PTC) pur kyoo TAY nee us trans heh PAT ick koh lan jee AH gruh fee	*trans-* through *hepat/o* liver *-ic* pertaining to *cholangi/o* bile vessel *-graphy* process of recording	Radiographic procedure to image the bile vessels using a contrast medium introduced into the hepatic duct by an approach through the skin (Fig 5-26).
sonography soh NAH gruh fee	*son/o* sound *-graphy* process of recording	Use of high-frequency sound waves to image deep structures of the body; used in the digestive system to detect gallstones and tumors.

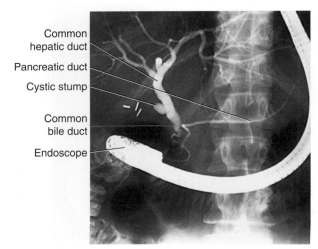

Common hepatic duct
Pancreatic duct
Cystic stump
Common bile duct
Endoscope

Fig. 5-25 Endoscopic retrograde cholangiopancreatography (ERCP).

Fig. 5-26 Percutaneous transhepatic cholangiography (PTC) demonstrating stenosis *(arrow)* of common hepatic duct caused by trauma.

Terms Related to Laboratory Tests

Term	Word Origin	Definition
biopsy BYE op see	*bi/o* life, living *-opsy* process of viewing	Removal and examination of living tissue from the body for diagnostic purposes.
gamma-glutamyl transferase (GGT) GAM uh-GLOO tah mil TRANS fur ace		Blood test to detect increased enzymes that can indicate cirrhosis, hepatitis, acute pancreatitis, acute cholecystitis, or nephrosis, and to test for *Helicobacter pylori* antibodies.
stool culture		Fecal exam to test for microorganisms in the feces, such as worms, amoebae, bacteria, and protozoa.
stool guaiac, hemoccult test GWEYE ack HEEM oh kult	*hem/o* blood *-occult* secret	Fecal specimen exam to detect hidden blood, which may indicate GI bleeding.
total bilirubin BILL lee roo bin		Blood test to detect possible jaundice (yellowing of the skin), cirrhosis, or hepatitis.

 EXERCISE 16: Diagnostic Procedures

Fill in the blanks with the appropriate terms from the following list.

stool culture, hemoccult, total bilirubin, CT scan, barium swallow, guaiac, biopsy, gamma-glutamyl transferase, transhepatic cholangiography, sonography, manometry, barium enema

1. High-frequency sound waves detect a tumor. The imaging technique is called _____.

2. The patient ingests a contrast medium, after which imaging of the esophagus is done. This is called

   _____.

3. A cross-sectional image of the abdomen is taken. This is called a/an _____.

4. A contrast medium was introduced into the patient's rectum, and studies were done of the lower

   digestive tract. This is called a/an _____.

5. What test measures the motor function of the esophagus? _____

6. A fecal examination that tests for microorganisms is called a/an _____.

7. Examination for blood in the stool is done by performing a stool _____

   or _____ test.

8. Removal of living tissue for diagnostic reasons is called _____.

9. What type of test is done to test for jaundice, cirrhosis, or hepatitis? _____

10. What is the test for elevated enzymes of *H. pylori* antibodies? _____

11. What is the x-ray procedure that images the bile vessels through an injection of contrast medium

    into the hepatic duct? _____

Decode the following diagnostic terms.

12. cholecystography _____

13. proctoscopy _____

14. cholangiography _____

15. colonoscopy _____

Case Study   Mai Tang

Mai Tang is a 44-year-old woman who has steady pain in her right upper quadrant that radiates to her right shoulder. She reports being nauseous, has a fever of 101.4° F, and has jaundice. She mentions that her BMs are lighter colored than normal. Laboratory testing includes LFTs, total bilirubin, blood tests, along with amylase and lipase levels.

Cholecystography is done, and all the tests confirm a diagnosis of acute cholecystitis due to an obstruction of the cystic duct. Mai is scheduled for a cholecystectomy immediately.

1. Cholecystitis is _____ of the GB.

2. What color is the skin and eyes of someone who has jaundice? _____

3. Cholecystography is the process of _____ the GB.

4. A cholecystectomy is removal of the _____.

Medical Record Regina Kao

KAO, REGINA N. - 161712

Task   Edit   View   Time Scale   Options   Help

KAO, REGINA N   Age: 54 years   Sex: Female   Loc: SYN
                           DOB: 6/30/1957   MRN: 442791   FIN: 765423

Reference Text Browser | Form Browser | Medication Profile

Orders | Last 48 Hours | ED | Lab | Radiology | Assessment | **Surgery** | Clinical Notes | Pt. Info | Pt. Schedule | Task List | I & O | MAR

Flowsheet: Surgery   ...   Level: Operative Report   ⦿ Table ○ Group ○ List

Navigator
✓ Operative Report

Preoperative Diagnosis: Mucous bloody stools
Postoperative Diagnosis: Diverticula
Surgical procedure: Colonoscopy

Patient is experiencing change in bowel habits, intermittent rectal bleeding, and some mucus. The procedure was described in detail to the patient, and she seemed to understand the risks, alternative treatments.

The patient was taken to the endoscopy suite, and in the left lateral position, the long colonoscope was inserted without incident. The perirectal area was normal. The rectal ampulla was normal. There were scattered diverticula of the left colon. The left colon, transverse colon, and right colon were otherwise normal. The colonoscope was removed, and the patient returned to the recovery room in satisfactory condition.

PROD | MAHAFC | 12 Sept 2014 | 15:22

EXERCISE 17: Operative Report

Using the preceding operative report, answer the following questions.

1. What diagnostic procedure was performed? _____

2. What instrument was used? _____

3. What diagnosis was determined from the procedure? _____

4. What is the "perirectal" area? _____

THERAPEUTIC INTERVENTIONS

When building a therapeutic intervention term that includes the creation of a stoma, the anatomic structures must be named in the order they appear in the body system. For example, a **duodenoileostomy** is an example of an **anastomosis**, a new opening between the duodenum and the ileum. The duodenum is listed first because it occurs before the ileum in the digestive system. Other examples are **esophagogastrostomy** and **jejunocecostomy.**

Terms Related to Therapeutic Interventions

Term	Word Origin	Definition
anastomosis ah nas tih MOH sis		New connection created between two (usually hollow) structures (Fig. 5-27).
bariatric surgery bair ee AT rick	*bar/o* weight *-iatric* pertaining to treatment	A variety of surgical procedures done to control morbid obesity by reducing the size of the stomach and/or by rerouting the small intestine to reduce the absorption of nutrients. These procedures include gastric stapling (gastroplasty), gastric banding (Lap-Band), and gastric bypass (Roux-en-Y).
cholecystectomy koh lee sis TECK tuh mee	*cholecyst/o* gallbladder *-ectomy* removal	Surgical removal of the GB (Fig. 5-28).
colostomy koh LOSS tuh mee	*col/o* colon *-stomy* new opening	Surgical redirection of the bowel to a **stoma** (STOH mah), an artificial opening on the abdominal wall (Fig. 5-29).
enema EH nih mah		Method of introducing a solution into the rectum for therapeutic (relief of constipation) or hygienic (preparation for surgery) reasons.

Fig. 5-27 Anastomosis. Part of the stomach has been cut out, and the duodenum has been anastomosed to the remaining stomach.

Fig. 5-28 Four-part laparoscopic cholecystectomy. **A,** A lensed telescope with camera and long instruments are introduced into small incisions. **B,** The camera image is projected to central monitors.

Terms Related to Therapeutic Interventions—cont'd

Term	Word Origin	Definition
feeding tubes		**Enteral nutrition**—introduced through a digestive structure (Fig. 5-30). **Parenteral nutrition**—introduced through a structure outside of the alimentary canal, usually intravenously.
gastrectomy gass TRECK tuh mee	*gastr/o* stomach *-ectomy* removal	Surgical removal of all or part of the stomach.
gastric gavage gah VAHZH		Feeding through a tube in the stomach.

hemorrhoidectomy
heh moh roy DECK
  tuh mee
	hemorrhoid/o
	  hemorrhoid
	-ectomy removal
		Surgical excision of hemorrhoids.

herniorrhaphy hur nee OR rah fee	*herni/o* hernia *-rrhaphy* suture	Hernia repair; suture of a hernia.
hyperalimentation hye pur al ih men TAY shun	*hyper-* excessive *aliment/o* nutrition *-ation* process of	The therapeutic use of nutritional supplements that exceed recommended daily requirements.

Continued

— Stoma

Fig. 5-29 A, Colostomy. **B,** Stoma.

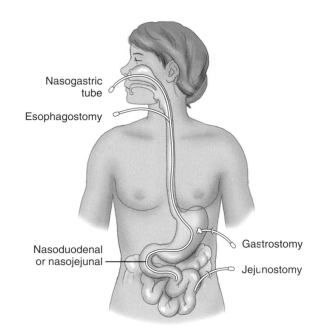

Fig. 5-30 Common placement locations for enteral feeding tubes.

Terms Related to Therapeutic Interventions—cont'd

Term	Word Origin	Definition
laparoscopic surgery lap uh roh SCAH pick	*lapar/o* abdomen *-scopic* pertaining to viewing	Surgery done through several small incisions in the abdominal wall with the aid of an instrument called a **laparoscope**. A **laparoscopic cholecystectomy** is the removal of the GB (see Fig. 5-28).
laparotomy lap uh RAH tuh mee	*lapar/o* abdomen *-tomy* incision	Any surgical incision in the abdominal wall for the purpose of an operative approach or for exploratory purposes.
ligation lye GAY shun	*ligat/o* tying *-tion* the process of	Tying off of a blood vessel or duct (e.g., the cystic duct is ligated when the GB is removed during a cholecystectomy).
lysis of adhesions LYE sis	*lys/o* breakdown *-is* noun ending	Surgical destruction of adhesions (scar tissue that binds two anatomic surfaces) (e.g., in the peritoneal cavity).
nasogastric intubation nay soh GASS trick in too BAY shun	*nas/o* nose *gastr/o* stomach *-ic* pertaining to	Placement of a tube from the nose, down the back of the throat, then into the stomach, for the purpose of enteral feeding or removing gastric contents. The tube is sometimes called an **NG tube**.
odontectomy oh don TECK tuh mee	*odont/o* teeth *-ectomy* removal	Surgical excision of a tooth.
paracentesis pair ah sen TEE sis	*para-* near, beside *-centesis* surgical puncture	Procedure for withdrawing fluid from a body cavity, most commonly to remove fluid accumulated in the abdominal cavity.

Terms Related to Therapeutic Interventions—cont'd

Term	Word Origin	Definition
percutaneous endoscopic gastrostomy (PEG) pur kew TAY nee us en doh SKOP ick gass TROSS tuh mee	*per-* through *cutane/o* skin *-ous* pertaining to *endo-* within *-scopic* pertaining to viewing *gastr/o* stomach *-stomy* new opening	A new opening of the stomach through the skin that allows the surgeon to place a tube for the purpose of enteral feeding.
polypectomy poll ih PECK tuh mee	*polyp/o* polyp *-ectomy* removal	Surgical removal of a sessile or pedunculated polyp.
pyloromyotomy pye lor oh mye AH tuh mee	*pylor/o* pylorus *my/o* muscle *-tomy* incision	An incision of the pyloric sphincter to correct an obstruction, such as pyloric stenosis.
stomatoplasty STOH mat toh plass tee	*stomat/o* mouth *-plasty* surgical repair	Surgical repair of the mouth.
trocar TROH kar		A surgical instrument that is a sharp rod inside of a tube used to puncture a body cavity. Each access point formed is called a "port" (Fig 5-31).

Fig. 5-31 Trocar.

EXERCISE 18: Therapeutic Interventions

Match the therapeutic interventions.

_____ 1. removal of fluid from a body cavity

_____ 2. surgical incision in the abdominal wall

_____ 3. joining of two hollow tubes or organs

_____ 4. introduction of a solution into the rectum for cleansing or therapeutic purposes

_____ 5. tying off of a vessel or a duct

_____ 6. destruction of binding scar tissue

_____ 7. inserting a tube from the nose to the stomach

_____ 8. artificial opening

_____ 9. hernia repair

_____ 10. name of the instrument used to view the interior of the abdominal cavity

_____ 11. removal of hemorrhoids

_____ 12. removal of half of the stomach

_____ 13. opening of large intestine to the wall of the abdomen

_____ 14. surgery done through incisions on abdominal wall with aid of laparoscope

_____ 15. removal of a tooth

A. anastomosis
B. paracentesis
C. laparoscopic surgery
D. hemorrhoidectomy
E. laparotomy

F. enema
G. herniorrhaphy
H. ligation
I. hemigastrectomy
J. nasogastric intubation

K. colostomy
L. laparoscope
M. stoma
N. lysis of adhesions
O. odontectomy

Decode the following therapeutic terms.

16. pyloromyotomy _____

17. colostomy _____

18. herniorrhaphy _____

19. gastrectomy _____

20. polypectomy _____

*Click on **Hear It, Spell It** to practice spelling the diagnostic and therapeutic terms that you have learned in this chapter.*

PHARMACOLOGY

anorexiants (an nor RECK see unts): Appetite suppressants designed to aid in weight control, often in an attempt to treat **morbid obesity** (an amount of body fat that threatens normal health). Examples of anorexiants are phendimetrazine (Bontril) and phentermine (Adipex-P).

antacids: A buffer (neutralizer) of hydrochloric acid in the stomach to temporarily relieve symptoms of GERD, pyrosis, and ulcers. Examples include calcium carbonate (Tums, Rolaids) and aluminum hydroxide with magnesium hydroxide (Maalox).

antidiarrheals: Provide relief from diarrhea by reducing intestinal motility, inflammation, or loss of fluids and nutrients. Examples include loperamide (Imodium), bismuth subsalicylate (Pepto-Bismol), and diphenoxylate with atropine (Lomotil).

antiemetics: Prevent or alleviate nausea and vomiting. Examples include scopolamine (Scopace), ondansetron (Zofran), and promethazine (Phenergan).

gastrointestinal stimulants: Promote motility of smooth muscles in gastrointestinal tract. An example is metoclopramide (Reglan).

histamine-2 receptor antagonists (H2RAs): Reduce hydrochloric acid production in the stomach for moderate-lasting acid suppression. Examples include famotidine (Pepcid) and ranitidine (Zantac).

laxatives: Promote evacuation of the bowel by increasing the bulk of the feces, softening the stool, or lubricating the intestinal wall. Examples include fiber and docusate (Colaces). Simulant laxatives cause more direct bowel evacuation by stimulating peristalsis. Examples include senna (Ex-Lax) and bisacodyl (Dulcolax).

proton pump inhibitors: Reduce production of hydrochloric acid in the stomach for long-lasting acid suppression of disorders like GERD. Examples include omeprazole (Prilosec) and pantoprazole (Protonix).

> **antiemetic**
> anti- = against
> -emetic = pertaining to vomiting

 EXERCISE 19: Pharmacology

Match each disorder with the type of drug that is used to treat it.

_____ 1. nausea and vomiting

_____ 2. chronic GERD

_____ 3. short-term dyspepsia

_____ 4. excessive weight gain

_____ 5. constipation

_____ 6. intestinal cramping and loose, watery stools

A. laxative
B. antidiarrheal
C. proton pump inhibitor
D. antacid
E. antiemetic
F. anorexiant

Case Study   Emmaline Jones

One-day-old Emmaline Jones is seen in the nursery to be evaluated for a cleft palate and lip. The immediate concern, however, is that she is cyanotic, listless, and dehydrated. The mother says that the baby would not take any formula that was introduced with a modified bottle. An attempt to insert a feeding tube is unsuccessful. X-rays show an air-filled pouch in the esophagus and air in the stomach and intestines. A diagnosis of esophageal atresia is given,

the baby is rehydrated, and an emergency esophago-gastrostomy is performed.

1. Given the diagnosis of cleft palate, there is an opening between the oral and _____ cavity.

2. An esophagogastrostomy means that a new _____ has been formed between the esophagus and the stomach?

3. Esophageal atresia means that there is no opening between the esophagus and the _____.

4. What condition does a cheiloplasty correct? _____

5. What is the surgery that needs to be performed for the cleft palate? _____

Case Study   Andre Jordon

Andre Jordon, a 19-year-old student, arrives with a friend at the clinic with bloody, mucus-filled diarrhea. He says that the diarrhea has been present for approximately a day and a half, and he is weak, fatigued, and in pain with severe cramping. Blood tests reveal anemia, and a colonoscopy shows multiple ulcerations in the sigmoid colon. Andre's diagnosis is ulcerative colitis. Counseling includes the possible necessity of a partial colectomy if the disease cannot be controlled with medication.

1. The suffix in colonoscopy means _____.
   a. incision, cutting
   b. process of viewing
   c. process of recording
   d. removal, excision

2. The sigmoid colon is between which two sections of the colon?
   a. descending colon and rectum
   b. cecum and transverse
   c. ascending and descending

3. The suffix in the term colectomy means_____.
   a. incision, cutting
   b. fixation
   c. process of recording
   d. removal, excision

4. What type of disease is ulcerative colitis? _____.

Abbreviations

Abbreviation	Definition	Abbreviation	Definition
BaS	barium swallow	HBV	hepatitis B virus
BE	barium enema	IBD	inflammatory bowel disease
BM	bowel movement	IBS	irritable bowel syndrome
CT scan	computed tomography scan	Lap	laparoscopy, laparotomy
EGD	esophagogastroduodenoscopy	LES	lower esophageal sphincter
ERCP	endoscopic retrograde cholangiopancreatography	N&V	nausea and vomiting
GB	gallbladder	PEG	percutaneous endoscopic gastrostomy
GERD	gastroesophageal reflux disease	PTC	percutaneous transhepatic cholangiography
GGT	gamma-glutamyl transferase		
GI	gastrointestinal	PUD	peptic ulcer disease
HAV	hepatitis A virus		

EXERCISE 20: Abbreviations

Spell out the abbreviations used in the following examples.

1. The 76-year-old patient complained of no BM in the last week. He had not had a/an

   _____ .

2. The patient was admitted for suspected GB disease. _____

3. The nurse recorded the patient's symptoms as N&V, without a fever.

   _____

4. Constant heartburn for Phyllis may have been a result of GERD. _____

5. Stressful situations were made even more so for Bill when his IBS flared up.

   _____

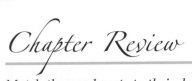

Chapter Review

Match the word parts to their definitions.

Word Part Definitions

Suffix
-chezia
-emesis
-pepsia
-phagia
-rrhaphy
-rrhea
-scopy
-stalsis
-stomy
-tresia

Definition

1. _____ flow, discharge
2. _____ process of viewing
3. _____ condition of an opening
4. _____ new opening
5. _____ suture, repair
6. _____ vomiting
7. _____ condition of stools
8. _____ condition of eating, swallowing
9. _____ contraction
10. _____ digestion condition

Combining Form
an/o
bucc/o
cholangi/o
cholecyst/o
choledoch/o
col/o
enter/o
esophag/o
gastr/o
gingiv/o
inguin/o
hepat/o
labi/o
lingu/o
lumin/o
odont/o
pharyng/o
phren/o
proct/o
py/o
sial/o
stomat/o

Definition

11. _____ tongue
12. _____ gums
13. _____ groin
14. _____ diaphragm
15. _____ esophagus
16. _____ saliva
17. _____ bile vessel
18. _____ common bile duct
19. _____ mouth
20. _____ pus
21. _____ stomach
22. _____ rectum and anus
23. _____ lips
24. _____ liver
25. _____ cheek
26. _____ tooth
27. _____ anus
28. _____ gallbladder
29. _____ throat
30. _____ lumen
31. _____ large intestine
32. _____ small intestines

Word Shop

Prefixes	Combining Forms	Suffixes
a-	cheil/o	-al
an-	chol/e	-eal
dys-	cholecyst/o	-ectomy
peri-	choledoch/o	-ia
pre-	col/o	-iasis
syn-	esophag/o	-ic
trans-	gastr/o	-itis
	hepat/o	-pepsia
	lapar/o	-phagia
	lith/o	-plasty
	nas/o	-rrhea
	odont/o	-stomy
	py/o	-tomy
	stomat/o	-tresia

Build the following terms by combining the preceding word parts. Some word parts may be used more than once. Some won't be used at all. The number in parentheses indicates the number of word parts needed to build the term.

Definition	Term
1. pertaining to the stomach and esophagus (3)	_____
2. condition of no opening (2)	_____
3. pertaining to surrounding the teeth (3)	_____
4. pertaining to the nose and stomach (3)	_____
5. new opening of the colon (2)	_____
6. inflammation of the gallbladder (2)	_____
7. new opening between the stomach and esophagus (3)	_____
8. removal of the gallbladder (2)	_____
9. discharge of pus (2)	_____
10. condition of difficult/painful swallowing (2)	_____
11. condition of bad digestion (2)	_____
12. condition of gallstones (3)	_____
13. condition of stones in the common bile duct (3)	_____
14. incision of the abdomen (2)	_____
15. surgical repair of the mouth (2)	_____

Sort the following terms into their correct categories.

Term Sorting

Anatomy and Physiology	Pathology	Diagnostic Procedures	Therapeutic Interventions

achalasia

anastomosis

barium enema

BaS

cheilitis

cholecystectomy

cholecystography

cholecystokinin

colostomy

CT scan

cystadenoma

deglutition

dyspepsia

ERCP

esophagus

gastric gavage

GGT

halitosis

hematemesis

hematochezia

herniorrhaphy

jaundice

jejunum

laparotomy

LES

leukoplakia

ligation

lipid

manometry

mastication

oropharynx

paracentesis

PEG

peristalsis

PTC

pyrosis

rugae

stomatoplasty

stool guaiac

total bilirubin

Replace the highlighted words with the correct terms.

Translations

1. After having a viewing of the large intestine, the patient needed a removal of a polyp.

2. The patient was tested for an inflammation of the liver due to a yellowing of the skin and sclerae.

3. The patient's protrusion of a loop of the intestine into the inguinal canal was corrected with a suture (repair) of the hernia.

4. The patient's impairment of esophageal peristalsis was diagnosed through the use of a measurement of pressure.

5. A fecal exam to detect hidden blood was used to determine if the patient had bleeding in his gastrointestinal tract.

6. The patient underwent a tying off of a blood vessel or duct during his surgical removal of the gallbladder.

7. Ross underwent surgical redirection of the bowel to a stoma when his inflammation of the ileum or the colon that is of idiopathic origin became too severe.

8. Miriam took a mild medication that causes evacuation of the bowel when she had infrequent, incomplete, or delayed bowel movements.

9. The patient had gas expelled through the anus and an abnormal discharge of watery, semisolid stools.

10. Delay in treating the patient's inflammation of the appendix led to a nearly fatal case of inflammation of the peritoneum.

11. The dentist told Ava she had inflammatory disease of the gums and a condition in which the teeth do not touch properly when the mouth is closed.

12. The infant was born with a failure of the palate to close during embryonic development. Her twin was born with congenital absence of normal nervous function in part of the colon.

13. The newborn experienced return of swallowed food to the mouth of his formula because of esophagus that ends in a blind pouch.

14. Bright red, frank lower GI bleeding from the rectum was one of the symptoms of Frank's varicose vein in the lower rectum.

OPERATIVE REPORT

1. How do you know that Ms. Hopkins has gallstones? _____

    _____.

2. Which term tells you that her gallbladder was inflamed? _____

    _____.

3. Her gallbladder was removed through an endoscopic procedure called a/an _____

    _____.

4. To say that the patient was in a supine position means that she was lying on her _____

    _____.

5. To ligate a structure means to _____.

Urinary System

6

OBJECTIVES

- Recognize and use terms related to the anatomy and physiology of the urinary system.
- Recognize and use terms related to the pathology of the urinary system.

- Recognize and use terms related to the diagnostic procedures for the urinary system.
- Recognize and use terms related to the therapeutic interventions for the urinary system.

For interactive learning, go to the Shiland Evolve website and click on:
- **Match the Word Parts** to review urinary word parts.
- **Word Shop** to practice word building.
- **Tournament of Terminology** to test your knowledge of urinary terms.
- **Term Sorting** to practice sorting urinary terms into categories.

*Click on **Chapter at a Glance** for a list of key word parts and terms for this chapter.*

extracellular
extra = outside
cellul/o = cell
-ar = pertaining to

urination
urin/o = urine, urinary
system
-ation = process of

 Be Careful!

*-uria is a suffix that
means urinary condition;
urea is a chemical
waste product.*

urology
ur/o = urine, urinary
system
-logy = study of

 Be Careful!

*Don't confuse **ureters**
with the **urethra**.*

kidney = nephr/o, ren/o

parenchymal
par- = near
en- = in
chym/o = juices
-al = pertaining to

ureter = ureter/o

bladder = cyst/o, vesic/o

urethra = urethr/o

meatus = meat/o

trigone = trigon/o

stromal tissue = strom/o

retroperitoneal
retro- = backward
peritone/o = peritoneum
-al = pertaining to

renal cortex = cortic/o

renal medulla = medull/o

renal pelvis = pyel/o

renal calyx = calic/o,
cali/o, calyc/o

FUNCTIONS OF THE URINARY SYSTEM

The major function of the urinary system is to continually maintain a healthy balance of the amount and content of **extracellular fluids** within the body. Biologists use the term *homeostasis* to describe this important process. The process of metabolism changes food and liquid (with its requisite fats, carbohydrates, and proteins) into building blocks, energy sources, and waste products. To operate efficiently, the body constantly needs to monitor and rebalance the amounts of these substances in the bloodstream. The breakdown of proteins and amino acids in the liver leaves chemical wastes, such as urea, creatinine, and uric acid, in the bloodstream. These wastes are toxic nitrogenous substances that must be excreted in the urine. The act of releasing urine is called **urination, voiding,** or **micturition** (mick ter RIH shun).

Succinctly phrased by Homer William Smith in 1939, "It is no exaggeration to say that the composition of the blood is determined not by what the mouth ingests but by what the kidneys keep; they are the master chemists of our internal environment, which, so to speak, they synthesize in reverse."

SPECIALTIES/SPECIALISTS

The medical specialist for the diagnosis, treatment, and study of urinary disorders in both sexes is called an **urologist.** Urologists also treat most disorders of the male reproductive system. The specialty is referred to as **urology.**

ANATOMY AND PHYSIOLOGY

The urinary system is composed of two kidneys, two ureters, a urinary bladder, and a urethra (Figs. 6-1 and 6-2). The work of the urinary system is done by a specialized tissue in the **kidneys** called **parenchymal** (pair EN kuh mul) **tissue.** The kidneys function to filter the blood and eliminate waste through the passage of urine. The **ureters** (YOOR eh turs) are thin, muscular tubes that move urine in peristaltic waves from the kidneys to the bladder. The urinary **bladder** is the sac that stores the urine until it is excreted. The bladder is lined with an epithelial mucous membrane of transitional cells. Underneath, a layer termed the *lamina propria* is composed of connective tissue that holds the blood vessels and nerves. The detrusor muscle is the final coat; it normally contracts to expel urine. The **urethra** (yoo REE thrah) is the tube that conducts the urine out of the bladder. The opening of the urethra is called the **urinary meatus** (YOOR in nair ee mee ATE us). The triangular area in the bladder between the ureters' entrance and the urethral outlet is called the **trigone** (TRY gohn). The ureters, bladder, and urethra are all **stromal** (STROH mul) **tissue,** which is a supportive tissue.

The Kidney

Because the kidneys are primarily responsible for the functioning of the urinary system, it is helpful to look at them in greater detail. Each of the two kidneys is located high in the abdominal cavity, tucked under the ribs in the back and behind the lining of the abdominal cavity (**retroperitoneal**). The normal human kidney is about the size of a fist. The term **renal** means *pertaining to the kidneys*. If a kidney were sliced open, the outer portion, the **renal cortex** (KORE tecks) (*pl.* cortices), and the inner portion, called the **renal medulla** (muh DOO lah) (*pl.* medullae), would be visible (Fig. 6-3). The **renal pelvis** and **renal calyces** (KAL ih seez) (*sing.* calyx) are an extension of the ureter inside of the kidney.

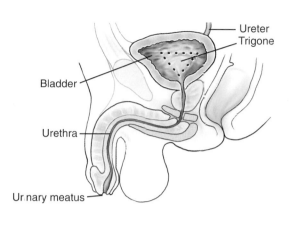

Male

Fig. 6-1 Male urinary system.

Female

Fig. 6-2 Female urinary system.

Fig. 6-3 Cross-section of a kidney.

The **hilum** (HYE lum) (*pl.* hila) is the location on the kidney where the ureter and renal vein leave the kidney and the renal artery enters. The cortex contains tissue with millions of microscopic units called **nephrons** (NEFF rons) (Fig. 6-4). Here in the tiny nephrons, blood passes through a continuous system of urinary filtration, reabsorption, and secretion that measures, monitors, and adjusts the levels of substances in the extracellular fluid.

hilum = hil/o

The Nephron

The nephrons filter all of the blood in the body approximately every 5 minutes. The **renal afferent arteries** transport unfiltered blood to the kidneys. Once in the kidneys, the blood travels through small arteries called **arterioles** (ar TEER ree ohls) and finally into tiny balls of renal capillaries called **glomeruli** (gloh MER yoo lye) (*sing.* glomerulus). These glomeruli cluster at the entrance to each nephron. It is here that the process of filtering the blood to form urine begins.

The nephron consists of four parts: (1) the **renal corpuscle** (KORE pus sul), which is composed of the glomerulus and its surrounding Bowman capsule; (2) a **proximal convoluted tubule;** (3) the **nephronic loop,** also known as the *loop of Henle;* and (4) the **distal convoluted tubule.** As blood flows through the capillaries, water, electrolytes, glucose, and nitrogenous wastes are passed through the glomerular membrane and collected. The most common electrolytes are sodium (Na), chloride (Cl), and potassium (K). Blood cells and

artery = arteri/o

glomerulus = glomerul/o

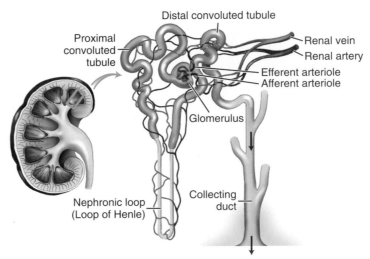

Fig. 6-4 The nephron.

urine = ur/o, urin/o

proteins are too large to pass through the glomerular membrane. Selective filtration and reabsorption continue along the renal tubules, with the end result of **urine** concentration and subsequent dilution occurring in the renal medulla. From there, the urine flows to the calyces and exits the kidney, flowing through the ureter into the bladder, where it is stored until it can be expelled from the body through the urethra.

EXERCISE 1: The Urinary System

Match the combining form with its term.

_____ 1. opening of the urethra

_____ 2. tubes connecting kidneys and bladder

_____ 3. tube conducting urine out of the bladder

_____ 4. same as ren/o

_____ 5. sac that stores urine

_____ 6. area between ureters coming in and urethra going out in the sac that stores urine

_____ 7. urine, urinary system

_____ 8. renal pelvis

_____ 9. outer portion of the kidney

_____ 10. inner portion of the kidney

_____ 11. artery

_____ 12. renal calyx

_____ 13. location where ureter and renal vein leave kidney and renal artery enters

A. nephr/o
B. ur/o, urin/o
C. meat/o
D. urethr/o
E. cyst/o, vesic/o
F. ureter/o
G. trigon/o
H. medull/o
I. calic/o, cali/o, calyc/o
J. cortic/o
K. hil/o
L. pyel/o
M. arteri/o

Decode the terms.

14. transurethral _____

15. paranephric _____

16. retroperitoneal _____

17. suprarenal _____

18. perivesical _____

Combining and Adjective Forms for the Anatomy of the Urinary System

Meaning	Combining Form	Adjective Form
artery	arteri/o	arterial
bladder	cyst/o, vesic/o	cystic, vesical
calyx	calic/o, cali/o, calyc/o	caliceal, calyceal
cell	cellul/o	cellular
cortex	cortic/o	cortical
glomerulus	glomerul/o	glomerular
hilum	hil/o	hilar
kidney	nephr/o, ren/o	nephric, renal
medulla	medull/o	medullary
parenchyma	parenchym/o	parenchymal
peritoneum	peritone/o	peritoneal
renal pelvis	pyel/o	
stroma	strom/o	stromal
trigone	trigon/o	trigonal
ureter	ureter/o	ureteral
urethra	urethr/o	urethral
urinary meatus	meat/o	meatal
urine, urinary system	urin/o, ur/o	urinary

Prefixes for the Anatomy of the Urinary System

Prefix	Meaning
extra-	outside
en-	in
par-	beside, near
retro-	backward

Suffixes for the Anatomy of the Urinary System

Suffix	Meaning
-al, -ar, -ic	pertaining to
-ation, -ion	process of

 *You can review the anatomy of the urinary system by clicking on **Body Spectrum Electronic Anatomy Coloring Book → Urinary Tract.** Click on **Hear It, Spell It** to practice spelling the anatomy and physiology terms you have learned in this chapter.*

EXERCISE 2: The Urinary System

Label the images using the terms provided.

urethra
ureter
kidney
bladder

renal cortex
renal calyx
hilum
ureter
renal pelvis
renal medulla

 *Click on **Label It** to practice labeling the kidney and nephron.*

PATHOLOGY

Terms Related to Urinary Signs

Term	Word Origin	Definition
abscess, urinary AB ses		Cavity containing pus and surrounded by inflamed tissue in the urinary system.
albuminuria al byoo mih NOOR ee ah	*albumin/o* protein *-uria* urinary condition	Albumin (a protein) in the urine. Also called **proteinuria** (pro teen NOOR ee ah).

Terms Related to Urinary Signs—cont'd

Term	Word Origin	Definition
azotemia a zoh TEE mee ah	*azot/o* nitrogen *-emia* blood condition	Condition of excessive urea in the blood indicating nonfunctioning kidneys; also called **uremia.**
azoturia a zoh TOOR ee ah	*azot/o* nitrogen *-uria* urinary condition	Excessive nitrogenous compounds, including urea, in the urine.
bacteriuria back tur ee YOOR ee ah	*bacteri/o* bacteria *-uria* urinary condition	Bacteria in the urine.
edema eh DEE mah		Accumulation of fluid in the tissues; can result from kidney failure.
glycosuria gly kohs YOOR ee ah	*glycos/o* sugar, glucose *-uria* urinary condition	Sugar in the urine.
hematuria hee mah TOOR ee ah	*hemat/o* blood *-uria* urinary condition	Blood in the urine.
hypertension hye pur TEN shun	*hyper-* excessive *tens/o* stretching *-ion* process of	Condition of high blood pressure.
pyuria pye YOOR ee ah	*py/o* pus *-uria* urinary condition	Pus in the urine.

Terms Related to Urinary Symptoms

Term	Word Origin	Definition
anuria a NOOR ee ah	*an-* without *-uria* urinary condition	Condition of no urine.
diuresis dye yoor EE sis	*di-* through, complete *ur/o* urine *-esis* state of	Condition of increased formation and excretion of urine, of large volumes of urine. Caffeine and alcohol are **diuretics** (dye yoor RET icks)—that is, they increase the amount of urine produced.
dysuria dis YOOR ee ah	*dys-* painful, abnormal *-uria* urinary condition	Condition of painful urination.
enuresis en yoor EE sis	*en-* in *ur/o* urine *-esis* state of	Also commonly known as "bed-wetting," enuresis can be nocturnal (at night) or diurnal (during the day).
incontinence, urinary in KON tih nense		Inability to hold urine.
nocturia nock TOOR ee ah	*noct/i* night *-uria* urinary condition	Condition of excessive urination at night.
oliguria ah lig GYOOR ee ah	*olig/o* scanty, few *-uria* urinary condition	Condition of scanty urination.
polydipsia pah lee DIP see ah	*poly-* excessive, frequent *-dipsia* condition of thirst	Condition of excessive thirst (usually accompanied by polyuria).
polyuria pah lee YOOR ee ah	*poly-* excessive, frequent *-uria* urinary condition	Condition of excessive urination.
retention, urinary		Inability to release urine.
urgency		Intense sensation of the need to urinate immediately.

EXERCISE 3: Urinary Signs and Symptoms

Fill in the blank.

1. Urinary _____ is the inability to release urine.

2. If a patient complains of an accumulation of fluid around her ankles, she may be exhibiting _____.

3. A patient with a renal _____ has a cavity containing pus and surrounded by inflamed tissue in the kidneys.

4. A sign of kidney failure may be excessive urea in the blood, called _____.

5. A concerned parent calls in to discuss her 4-year-old son's inability to remain dry during the night. This bed-wetting may be diagnosed as _____.

6. Caffeine and alcohol are substances that cause an increase in the volume of fluids excreted from the body, causing _____.

7. A feeling of a need to urinate immediately is called _____.

8. The elderly gentleman was seen by his physician because he was unable to control his urination. He was suffering from urinary _____.

Build the terms.

9. urinary condition of pus _____

10. condition of excessive thirst _____

11. condition of painful urination _____

Decode the terms.

12. glycosuria _____

13. hematuria _____

14. anuria _____

⊗ Be Careful!

Py/o *means pus, and* **pyel/o** *means renal pelvis. A dilation of the renal pelvis caused by an accumulation of pus would be pyopyelectasis.*

Terms Related to Urinary System Disorders, Stones, and Diabetes

Term	Word Origin	Definition
diabetes insipidus (DI) dye ah BEE teez in SIP ih dus		Deficiency of antidiuretic hormone (ADH), which causes the patient to excrete large quantities of urine **(polyuria)** and exhibit excessive thirst **(polydipsia)**.

Terms Related to Urinary System Disorders, Stones, and Diabetes—cont'd

Term	Word Origin	Definition
diabetes mellitus (DM) dye ah BEE teez meh LYE tus		A group of metabolic disorders characterized by high glucose levels that result from inadequate amounts of insulin, resistance to insulin, or a combination of both (see Chapter 14).
nephrolithiasis neff roh lih THIGH uh sis	*nephr/o* kidney *lith/o* stone *-iasis* condition, presence of	Stones in the kidney.
polycystic kidney disease (PKD) pah lee SIS tick	*poly-* excessive, many *cyst/o* sac *-ic* pertaining to	Inherited disorder characterized by an enlargement of the kidneys caused by many renal cysts bilaterally that reduce functioning of renal tissue (Fig. 6-5).
renal colic REE null KAH lick	*ren/o* kidney *-al* pertaining to	Severe pain associated with kidney stones lodged in the ureter. The term "colic" means pain.
urinary tract infection (UTI)	*urin/o* urine, urinary system	Infection anywhere in the urinary system, caused most commonly by bacteria, but also by parasites, yeast, and protozoa (*sing.* protozoon). Most frequently occurring disorder in the urinary system.
urolithiasis yoo roo lih THIGH uh sis	*ur/o* urine, urinary system *lith/o* stone *-iasis* condition, presence of	Stones anywhere in the urinary tract, but usually in the renal pelvis or urinary bladder. Usually formed in patients with an excess of the mineral calcium. Also called **urinary calculi** (KAL kyoo lye) (Fig. 6-6).

Staghorn calculus

Renal stone

Ureteral stones

Bladder stones

Fig. 6-5 Comparison of a polycystic kidney *(right)* with a normal kidney *(left)*.

Fig. 6-6 A, Sonogram of stones in the renal pelvis. **B,** Locations of ureteral calculi.

EXERCISE 4: Urinary Disorders, Stones, and Diabetes

Match the disorders with their definitions.

_____ 1. inherited congenital disorders of the kidneys

_____ 2. pain caused by a stone lodged in the ureter

_____ 3. disease caused by deficiency of insulin

_____ 4. infection anywhere in the urinary system

_____ 5. deficiency of antidiuretic hormone

_____ 6. stones in the urinary tract

_____ 7. excessive thirst

A. urolithiasis
B. polydipsia
C. polycystic kidney disease (PKD)
D. diabetes mellitus (DM)
E. urinary tract infection (UTI)
F. renal colic
G. diabetes insipidus (DI)

Build terms for the following conditions.

8. condition of stones in the kidney _____

9. condition of stones in the ureter _____

10. condition of stones in the bladder _____

11. condition of stones in the urethra _____

Case Study   Victor Molina

Victor Molina comes to his physician with complaints of blood in his urine, pain in his abdomen, and the need to get up several times each night to urinate. Victor is afraid that he has PKD because both his father and uncle died from this disorder. His doctor tells him that PKD is a hereditary condition but that she doesn't want to assume anything until testing and imaging are performed. She sends a sample of Victor's urine for urinalysis (UA) and orders a computed tomography (CT) scan and sonogram of his kidneys.

1. PKD stands for _____.

2. The suffix -*cystic* means _____.

3. What is the term that means blood in the urine?
   _____

4. What is the term that means getting up frequently at night to urinate? _____

Terms Related to Kidney Disorders

Term	Word Origin	Definition
glomerulonephritis (GN) gloh MUR yoo loh neh FRY tis	glomerul/o glomerulus nephr/o kidney -itis inflammation	Inflammation of the glomeruli of the kidney characterized by proteinuria, hematuria, decreased urine production, and edema.
hydronephrosis hye droh neh FROH sis	hydr/o water nephr/o kidney -osis abnormal condition	Dilation of the renal pelvis and calices of one or both kidneys resulting from obstruction of the flow of urine.
nephritis neh FRY tis	nephr/o kidney -itis inflammation	Inflammation of the kidney; a general term that does not specify the location of the inflammation or its cause.
nephropathy neh FROP ah thee	nephr/o kidney -pathy disease process	Disease of the kidneys; a general term that does not specify a disorder.
nephroptosis neh frop TOH sis	nephr/o kidney -ptosis drooping, prolapse	Prolapse or sagging of the kidney.
nephrosclerosis neh froh sklih ROH sis	nephr/o kidney -sclerosis a hardening	Hardening of the arteries of the kidneys. Also known as **renal sclerosis.**
nephrotic syndrome neh FRAH tick	nephr/o kidney -tic pertaining to	Abnormal group of symptoms in the kidney characterized by proteinuria, hypoalbuminemia, and edema; may occur in glomerular disease and as a complication of many systemic diseases (e.g., DM). Also called **nephrosis** (neh FROH sis).
pyelonephritis pye uh loh neh FRY tis	pyel/o renal pelvis nephr/o kidney -itis inflammation	Infection of the renal pelvis and parenchyma of the kidney, usually the result of lower UTI.
renal failure	ren/o kidney -al pertaining to	Inability of the kidneys to excrete waste, concentrate urine, and conserve electrolytes. May be acute or chronic.
acute renal failure (ARF)		Sudden inability of the kidneys to excrete wastes, resulting from hemorrhage, trauma, burns, toxic injury to the kidney, pyelonephritis or GN, or lower urinary tract obstruction. Characterized by oliguria and rapid azotemia.
chronic kidney disease (CKD) (formerly chronic renal failure)		CKD is measured in stages of increasing severity, from 1 (mild damage with a normal glomerular filtration rate [GFR]) to 5 (complete kidney failure requiring either dialysis or a renal transplant). Stage 5 is also called **end-stage renal disease (ESRD).**
renal hypertension	ren/o kidney -al pertaining to hyper- excessive tens/o stretching -ion process of	High blood pressure secondary to kidney disease.

Terms Related to Bladder, Ureter, and Urethra Disorders

Term	Word Origin	Definition
cystitis sis TYE tis	*cyst/o* urinary bladder *-itis* inflammation	Inflammation of the urinary bladder. **Trigonitis** is inflammation of the trigone of the bladder.
cystocele SIS toh seel	*cyst/o* urinary bladder *-cele* herniation	Herniation of the urinary bladder (Fig. 6-7).
ureterocele yoo REE tur oh seel	*ureter/o* urethra *-cele* herniation	Prolapse of the terminal end of the ureter into the bladder.
urethral stenosis yoo REE thruhl sten NOH sis	*urethr/o* urethra *-al* pertaining to *stenosis* a narrowing	Narrowing of the urethra. Also called a **urethral stricture.**
urethritis yoo ree THRY tis	*urethr/o* urethra *-itis* inflammation	Inflammation of the urethra.
vesicoureteral reflux ves ih koh yoo REE tur ul REE flucks	*vesic/o* urinary bladder *ureter/o* ureter *-al* pertaining to *re-* back *-flux* flow	Abnormal backflow of urine from the bladder to the ureter. May be the result of an obstruction, an infection, or a congenital defect (Fig. 6-8).

Fig. 6-7 Cystocele. The urinary bladder is displaced downward *(arrow)*, which causes bulging of the anterior vaginal wall.

Fig. 6-8 Serial voiding cystourethrograms in an infant girl with vesicoureteral reflux *(arrowheads).*

EXERCISE 5: Kidney, Ureter, Bladder, and Urethral Disorders

Match the kidney disorders with their definitions.

_____ 1. inability of the kidneys to excrete wastes

_____ 2. hardening of the arteries of the kidneys

_____ 3. prolapse of the kidney

_____ 4. inflammation of the renal parenchyma and the renal pelvis

_____ 5. disease of the kidney

_____ 6. inflammation of the kidney

_____ 7. proteinuria, hypoalbuminemia, and edema characterize this syndrome

_____ 8. inflammation of the capillaries within the renal corpuscles

_____ 9. inflammation of the tube leading from the bladder to the outside of the body

_____ 10. inflammation of the bladder

_____ 11. herniation of the tube from the kidney to the bladder

_____ 12. backward flow of urine from the bladder toward the kidney

A. glomerulonephritis (GN)
B. cystitis
C. nephritis
D. nephroptosis

E. vesicoureteral reflux
F. urethritis
G. pyelonephritis
H. nephrotic syndrome

I. nephrosclerosis
J. nephropathy
K. ureterocele
L. renal failure

Decode the terms.

13. hydronephrosis _____

14. cystocele _____

15. nephrolithiasis _____

16. renal sclerosis _____

Case Study Paulina Abernathy

Paulina Abernathy is a 41-year-old event planner who has been experiencing scanty urine and generalized swelling. UA shows that she has proteinuria and hypoalbuminemia (low protein in the blood). Testing shows increased blood urea nitrogen (BUN), and a creatinine clearance test shows abnormal findings. She is diagnosed with nephrotic syndrome.

1. What is the medical term for scanty urination? _____

2. What is the term for generalized swelling? _____ _____

3. Another term for proteinuria is _____ _____.

4. Another term for nephrotic syndrome is _____ _____.

Terms Related to Benign Neoplasms

Term	Word Origin	Definition
renal adenoma REE nuhl add ih NOH mah	*ren/o* kidney *-al* pertaining to *aden/o* gland *-oma* tumor, mass	Small, slow-growing glandular noncancerous tumor of the kidney, usually found at autopsy.
renal oncocytoma REE null on koh sye TOH mah	*onc/o* tumor *cyt/o* cell *-oma* tumor, mass	The most common benign solid renal tumor. An adenoma composed of oncocytes (abnormal epithelial cells) that develops in the nephron of the kidney.
transitional cell papilloma pap ih LOH mah	*papill/o* nipple *-oma* tumor, mass	Also referred to as **bladder papilloma.** Although this type of tumor is benign when found, recurrences are occasionally malignant.

Terms Related to Malignant Neoplasms

Term	Word Origin	Definition
nephroblastoma nef roh blass TOH mah	*nephr/o* kidney *blast/o* embryonic *-oma* tumor, mass	Also called **Wilms tumor,** these tumors develop from kidney cells that did not develop fully before a child's birth. These cancerous tumors of the kidney occur mainly in children (Fig. 6-9).
renal cell carcinoma REE nul sell kar sih NOH mah	*ren/o* kidney *-al* pertaining to *carcinoma* cancerous tumor of epithelial origin	Also referred to as **hypernephroma** or **adenocarcinoma of the kidney,** this is one of the most common cancers. Although the cause is unknown, risk factors include smoking and obesity.
transitional cell carcinoma (TCC) of the bladder tran SIH shuh null kar sih NOH mah	*carcinoma* cancerous tumor of epithelial origin	These malignant tumors account for approximately 90% of all bladder cancers and arise from the cells lining the bladder (Fig. 6-10). Also called **urothelial cell carcinoma.**

Fig. 6-9 Wilms tumor of the kidney.

Fig. 6-10 Transitional cell carcinoma (TCC) of the bladder.

EXERCISE 6: Neoplasms

Match the neoplasms with their definitions.

_____ 1. nephroblastoma

_____ 2. renal adenoma

_____ 3. renal cell carcinoma

_____ 4. transitional cell carcinoma (TCC) of the bladder

_____ 5. renal oncocytoma

_____ 6. transitional cell papilloma

A. most common benign solid renal tumor
B. malignant tumor arising from cells lining the bladder
C. small, slow-growing benign tumor of the kidney
D. also known as bladder papilloma
E. also called Wilms tumor
F. also called hypernephroma or adenocarcinoma of the kidney

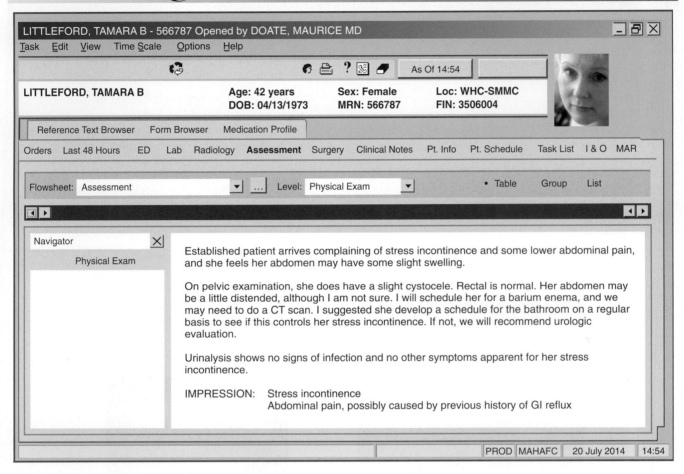

Medical Record Tamara Littleford

LITTLEFORD, TAMARA B - 566787 Opened by DOATE, MAURICE MD

Task Edit View Time Scale Options Help

As Of 14:54

| LITTLEFORD, TAMARA B | Age: 42 years | Sex: Female | Loc: WHC-SMMC |
| | DOB: 04/13/1973 | MRN: 566787 | FIN: 3506004 |

Reference Text Browser   Form Browser   Medication Profile

Orders Last 48 Hours ED Lab Radiology **Assessment** Surgery Clinical Notes Pt. Info Pt. Schedule Task List I & O MAR

Flowsheet: Assessment   Level: Physical Exam   • Table   Group   List

Navigator

Physical Exam

Established patient arrives complaining of stress incontinence and some lower abdominal pain, and she feels her abdomen may have some slight swelling.

On pelvic examination, she does have a slight cystocele. Rectal is normal. Her abdomen may be a little distended, although I am not sure. I will schedule her for a barium enema, and we may need to do a CT scan. I suggested she develop a schedule for the bathroom on a regular basis to see if this controls her stress incontinence. If not, we will recommend urologic evaluation.

Urinalysis shows no signs of infection and no other symptoms apparent for her stress incontinence.

IMPRESSION: Stress incontinence
Abdominal pain, possibly caused by previous history of GI reflux

PROD MAHAFC 20 July 2014 14:54

EXERCISE 7: Progress Note

Using the preceding progress report, answer the following questions.

1. Aside from pain and possibly some swelling, what is this patient's main complaint?

    _____

2. What type of herniation does she exhibit? _____

3. What imaging tests are the doctors considering? _____

 *Click on **Hear It, Spell It** to practice spelling the pathology terms that you have learned in this chapter. To review the pathology terms that you have learned in this chapter, play **Medical Millionaire.***

DIAGNOSTIC PROCEDURES

Urinalysis

Urinalysis (UA) is the physical, chemical, and/or microscopic examination of urine. The following table gives examples of the constituents examined and of normal and abnormal findings with their possible interpretations.

Urinalysis

Physical Examination

Appearance (Fig. 6-11)
Normal finding: Clear
Abnormal finding with interpretation: Cloudiness may indicate a UTI.

Color (Fig. 6-12)
Normal finding: Straw-colored or light amber
Abnormal findings with interpretations: Lighter color may indicate DI or overhydration. Darker colors may indicate concentrated urine caused by dehydration, drugs, or liver disease.

Quantity
Normal finding: Approximately 1½ L per day
Abnormal findings with interpretations: Profusion may indicate DI or a variety of other conditions precipitating diuresis. Smaller than normal amounts may be a result of dehydration, blockages, or strictures.

Specific gravity (SG): Measures the ability of the kidneys to regulate the concentration of urine
Normal finding: A reading of 1.015 to 1.025, which is slightly denser than the weight of water
Abnormal findings with interpretations: Diabetes or kidney damage may be the cause of a low SG.

Fig. 6-11 Appearance of urine.

Fig. 6-12 Color of urine.

Continued

Urinalysis—cont'd

Chemical Examination

Bilirubin
Normal finding: Not present
Abnormal finding with interpretation: Presence may indicate liver disease or biliary obstruction.

Blood
Normal finding: Not present
Abnormal findings with interpretations: Red blood cells may indicate an inflammation or trauma in the urinary tract. White blood cells may indicate a UTI.

Creatinine
Normal finding: 1 to 2.5 mg/24 hours
Abnormal findings with interpretations: An increase may indicate infection. A decrease may indicate kidney disease.

Glucose
Normal finding: Not present
Abnormal finding with interpretation: Presence may indicate DM.

Ketones
Normal finding: Not present
Abnormal finding with interpretation: DM or starvation may be the cause.

pH
Normal finding: 5.0 to 7.0; slightly acidic
Abnormal findings with interpretations: pH increases in alkalosis, decreases in high-protein diets.

Protein
Normal finding: Not present
Abnormal findings with interpretations: Increased amounts present in kidney disease; albumin present when glomeruli are damaged.

Microscopic Examination

Bacteria
Normal finding: Not present
Abnormal finding with interpretation: UTI

Pus
Normal finding: Not present
Abnormal finding with interpretation: Pyelonephritis

⊗ Be Careful!

Creatine *is a substance that is synthesized by the body and used to store energy.*
Creatinine *(a substance produced from creatine) is a waste product of muscle metabolism that is excreted by the kidneys.*

Terms Related to Laboratory Tests

Term	Word Origins	Definitions
blood urea nitrogen (BUN) YOOR ee ah		Blood test that measures the amount of nitrogenous waste in the circulatory system; an increased level is an indicator of kidney dysfunction.
creatinine clearance test kree AT ih nin		Test of kidney function that measures the rate at which nitrogenous waste is removed from the blood by comparing its concentration in the blood and urine over a 24-hour period.
glomerular filtration rate (GFR) gloh MARE yoo lure		The amount of blood that is filtered by the glomeruli of the kidneys. This rate is decreased when the kidneys are dysfunctional.

Terms Related to Imaging

Term	Word Origin	Definition
computed tomography (CT) scan toh MAH gruh fee	*tom/o* section, cutting *-graphy* process of recording	Computerized image that shows a "slice" of the body (Fig. 6-13).
cystourethroscopy sis toh yoor ee THRAH skup ee	*cyst/o* bladder *urethr/o* urethra *-scopy* process of viewing	Visual examination of the bladder and urethra, often with a biopsy of the ureter.
intravenous urography (IVU) in truh VEE nus yoo RAH gruh fee	*intra-* within *ven/o* vein *-ous* pertaining to *ur/o* urine, urinary system *-graphy* process of recording	Radiographic imaging of the kidneys, ureters, and bladder done with a contrast medium (Fig. 6-14). Also called **intravenous pyelography (IVP)**.
kidney, ureter, and bladder (KUB)		Radiographic imaging of the kidney, ureters, and bladder without a contrast medium.
nephrotomography neh froh toh MAH gruh fee	*nephr/o* kidney *tom/o* section *-graphy* process of recording	Sectional radiographic exam of the kidneys.
voiding cystourethrography (VCUG) VOY ding sis toh yoor ee THRAH gruh fee	*cyst/o* bladder *urethr/o* urethra *-graphy* process of recording	Radiographic imaging of the urinary bladder and urethra done with a contrast medium while patient is urinating (Fig. 6-15).

Fig. 6-13 Three-dimensional computed tomography (CT) image of urinary system in relation to bony structures.

Pelvis of kidney

Fig. 6-14 Intravenous urogram (IVU).

Fig. 6-15 Female voiding cystourethrogram (VCUG).

Terms Related to Other Diagnostic Procedures

Term	Word Origin	Definition
biopsy BYE op see	*bi/o* life, living *-opsy* process of viewing	Taking a piece of tissue for microscopic study. A **closed biopsy** is done by an endoscopy or aspiration (by suction through a fine needle). An **open biopsy** is done through an incision.
cystoscopy sis TOSS koh pee	*cyst/o* bladder *-scopy* process of viewing	Visual examination of the urinary bladder using a cystoscope (Fig. 6-16).

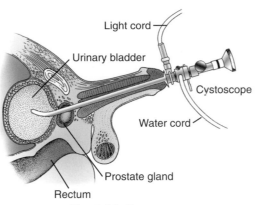

Light cord

Urinary bladder

Cystoscope

Water cord

Prostate gland

Rectum

Fig. 6-16 Cystoscopy.

Terms Related to Instruments

Term	Word Origin	Definition
catheter KATH uh tur		Hollow, flexible tube that can be inserted into a vessel, organ, or cavity of the body to withdraw or instill fluid, monitor types of various information, and visualize a vessel or cavity. Catheters can be inserted through the urethra into the bladder to drain urine (Fig. 6-17). An indwelling catheter is one that remains in the bladder; a straight catheter is removed when urine has been drained.
cystoscope SIS toh skohp	*cyst/o* urinary bladder *-scope* instrument to view	Instrument for visual examination of the inside of the bladder. (See Fig. 6-16 for a drawing of a cystoscope.)
laparoscope LAP ur oh skohp	*lapar/o* abdomen *-scope* instrument to view	Type of endoscope consisting of an illuminated tube with an optical system, inserted through the abdominal wall for examining the peritoneal cavity.
lithotripter lith oh TRIP tur	*lith/o* stone *-tripter* machine to crush	A machine that is used to crush stones, especially in extracorporeal shock wave lithotripsy (ESWL) (see Fig. 6-19).
lithotrite LITH oh tryte	*lith/o* stone *-trite* instrument to crush	Instrument used to crush a calculus in the urinary bladder; fragments may then be expelled or washed out.
nephroscope NEFF roh skohp	*nephr/o* kidney *-scope* instrument to view	Fiberoptic instrument used specifically for the disintegration and removal of renal calculi; an ultrasonic probe emitting high-frequency sound waves breaks up the calculi, which are removed by suction through the scope.
stent stehnt		Tubular device for supporting hollow structures during surgical anastomosis or for holding arteries open after angioplasty.
urinometer yoor ih NOM meh tur	*urin/o* urine *-meter* instrument to measure	Type of hydrometer used to measure the SG of a urine sample. Also known as an **urometer** (Fig. 6-18).

Fig. 6-17 *Top,* Indwelling catheter kit. *Bottom,* Straight catheter.

Fig. 6-18 Urinometer.

⊘ EXERCISE 8: Diagnostic Procedures

Match the diagnostic tests with their definitions.

_____ 1. blood urea nitrogen (BUN)

_____ 2. glomerular filtration rate (GFR)

_____ 3. creatinine clearance test

_____ 4. nephrotomography

_____ 5. cystoscopy

_____ 6. biopsy

_____ 7. intravenous urography (IVU)

_____ 8. voiding cystourethrography (VCUG)

A. radiographic imaging of bladder and urethra with a contrast medium while patient is urinating
B. radiographic imaging of kidneys, ureters, and bladder done with a contrast medium
C. taking a piece of tissue for microscopic study
D. visual examination of the bladder
E. test comparing the concentration of nitrogenous waste in blood and urine over a 24-hour period
F. lab test done to measure nitrogenous waste
G. test performed to measure the amount of blood filtered by the glomeruli
H. sectional radiographic examination of the kidneys

Build the terms.

9. an instrument to crush stones _____

10. an instrument to view the kidney _____

11. an instrument used to measure (the specific gravity [SG] of) urine _____

Case Study Maria Alonsa Cortez

Maria Alonsa Cortez is a 33-year-old with a history of recurring UTIs. She is being seen today for lower abdominal pain and oliguria. An IVU and cystoscopy reveal vesicoureteral reflux and urethral stenosis. Urethroplasty is indicated for correction of the stenosis.

1. What is a synonym for urethral stenosis? _____ _____

2. What does UTI stand for? _____ _____

3. Vesicoureteral reflux is the backflow of urine from the _____ to the ureters.

4. The tube that conducts urine out of the bladder is the _____.

5. An endoscopic examination of the bladder is called _____.

Medical Record — *Karen McLoud*

McCLOUD, KAREN K - 616784 Opened by DOATE, MAURICE MD

Task   Edit   View   Time Scale   Options   Help

McCLOUD, KAREN K   Age: 56 years   Sex: Female   Loc: WHC-SMMC
                       DOB: 03/14/1959   MRN: 616784   FIN: 3506004

Reference Text Browser | Form Browser | Medicat on Profile

Orders | Last 48 Hours | **ED** | Lab | Radiology | Assessment | Surgery | Clinical Notes | Pt. nfo | Pt. Schedule | Task List | I & O | MAR

Flowsheet: ED   Level: ED report   ⊙ Table ○ Gro_p ○ List

Navigator

✓ ED report

Patient is a 56-year-old who had hysterectomy performed approximately 1 week ago. She called our office this morning complaining of fever, nausea, and vomiting over the past 24 hours.

Upon arrival, the patient relates a 24-hour history of nausea, vomiting, and abdominal tenderness. Of note, the patient has an indwelling catheter, which was inserted postoperatively because of her inability to void. She was to return to the office postoperatively on the third postop day for possible removal of the catheter.

Urine sample taken from the catheter shows red and white blood cells. Urine culture is performed, and the patient is given antibiotics.

ASSESSMENT: Bladder infection caused by indwelling catheter

PROD | MAHAFC | 17 July 2015 | 15:22

EXERCISE 9: Emergency Department Report

Using the preceding emergency department report, answer the following questions.

1. What is an indwelling catheter? _____

2. Which prefix tells you that the catheter was inserted after surgery? _____

3. What types of tests were done to test for a bladder infection? _____

THERAPEUTIC INTERVENTIONS

Surgical procedures on the urinary system may be done through an open incision or laparoscopically.

Terms Related to Therapeutic Interventions

Term	Word Origin	Definition
ileal conduit ILL ee ul KON doo it	*ile/o* ileum *-al* pertaining to	Channel, pipe, or tube that guides urine from the ureters to the ileum in the digestive system to be excreted through the large intestine when the bladder is no longer available for storing the urine and releases it through the urethra. Also known as an **ureteroileostomy** (yoo ree tur oh ill ee AH stuh mee).
lithotripsy LITH oh trip see	*lith/o* stone *-tripsy* process of crushing	Process of crushing stones either to prevent or clear an obstruction in the urinary system; crushing may be done manually, by high-energy shock waves, or by pulsed dye laser. In each case, the fragments may be expelled naturally or washed out (Fig. 6-19). Use of shock waves is termed **extracorporeal shock wave lithotripsy (ESWL).**
meatotomy mee ah TOT uh mee	*meat/o* meatus, opening *-tomy* incision	An incision of the urinary meatus.
nephrectomy neh FRECK tuh mee	*nephr/o* kidney *-ectomy* removal	Resection of the kidney.
nephrolithotomy neh froh lith AH tuh mee	*nephr/o* kidney *-lithotomy* removal of a stone	Incision of the kidney for removal of a kidney stone.
nephropexy neh froh peck see	*nephr/o* kidney *-pexy* suspension	Suspension or fixation of the kidney.
nephrostolithotomy neh froh stoh lith AH tuh mee	*nephr/o* kidney *stom/o* opening *-lithotomy* removal of a stone	Removal of a stone from the kidney through a preexisting nephrostomy.
nephrostomy neh FRAH stuh mee	*nephr/o* kidney *-stomy* new opening	Opening made in the kidney so that a catheter can be inserted.
nephrotomy neh FRAH tuh mee	*nephr/o* kidney *-tomy* incision	Incision of the kidney.
transurethral procedure trans yoo REE thrul	*trans-* through *urethr/o* urethra *-al* pertaining to	Any procedure conducted through the urethra.
urethrolysis yoo ree THRAWL ih sis	*urethr/o* urethra *-lysis* separation, breakdown	Destruction of adhesions of the urethra.
vesicotomy vess ih KAH tuh mee	*vesic/o* bladder *-tomy* incision	Incision of the urinary bladder.

Fragments passed
through ureter

Kidney stone
being shattered

Focused shock wave

Fig. 6-19 Lithotripsy performed with a lithotripter.

Be Careful!

Do not confuse **ilium**, which is a pelvic bone, with **ileum**, which is a part of the small intestine.

Terms Related to Kidney Failure Treatment

Term	Word Origin	Definition
renal dialysis dye AL ih sis	*ren/o* kidney *-al* pertaining to *dia-* through, complete *-lysis* separation, breakdown	Process of diffusing blood across a semipermeable membrane to remove substances that a healthy kidney would eliminate, including poisons, drugs, urea, uric acid, and creatinine.
peritoneal dialysis pair eh tuh NEE ul dye AL ih sis	*peritone/o* peritoneum *-al* pertaining to *dia-* through, complete *-lysis* separation, breakdown	Type of renal dialysis in which the peritoneum is used as the semipermeable membrane to cleanse the blood. In **continuous ambulatory peritoneal dialysis (CAPD)** and **continuous cycling peritoneal dialysis (CCPD)** (Fig. 6-20), an indwelling catheter in the abdomen permits dialysis fluid to drain in and out of the peritoneal cavity.
hemodialysis (HD) hee moh dye AL ih sis	*hem/o* blood *dia-* through, complete *-lysis* separation, breakdown	Type of renal dialysis that cleanses the blood by shunting it from the body through a machine for diffusion and ultrafiltration and then returning it to the patient's circulation (Fig. 6-21).
renal transplant	*ren/o* kidney *-al* pertaining to *trans-* across	Surgical transfer of a complete kidney from a donor to a recipient (Fig. 6-22). Also called a **kidney transplant**.

Dialysate

Peritoneum

Abdominal
cavity

Catheter

Drainage bag

Fig. 6-20 Continuous ambulatory peritoneal dialysis (CAPD).

Pressure monitor

Clot and air bubble traps

Dialysate outflow

Dialyzer (artificial kidney)

Dialysate inflow

Blood pump

Arterial blood

Venous blood

A

B

Fig. 6-21 A, Hemodialysis (HD) circuit. **B,** HD machine.

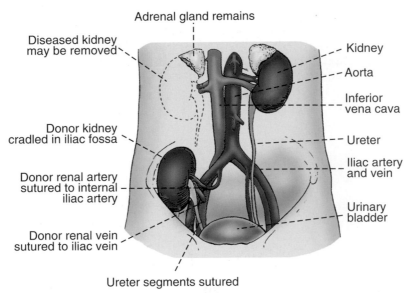

Adrenal gland remains

Diseased kidney may be removed

Kidney

Aorta

Inferior vena cava

Donor kidney cradled in iliac fossa

Ureter

Donor renal artery sutured to internal iliac artery

Iliac artery and vein

Donor renal vein sutured to iliac vein

Urinary bladder

Ureter segments sutured

Fig. 6-22 Kidney transplant.

⊘ EXERCISE 10:   Therapeutic Interventions

Match the therapeutic intervention terms with their definitions.

_____ 1. removal of a kidney

_____ 2. incision of a kidney

_____ 3. removal of a renal calculus

_____ 4. fixation of a kidney

_____ 5. new opening of a kidney

_____ 6. removal of a stone from the kidney through a preexisting opening

A. nephrostolithotomy
B. nephrolithotomy
C. nephrectomy
D. nephrostomy
E. nephrotomy
F. nephropexy

Build the terms.

7. destruction of adhesions of the urethra _____

8. process of crushing stones _____

9. incision of the urinary bladder _____

ⓔ   Click on **Hear It, Spell It** to practice spelling the diagnostic and therapeutic terms you have learned in this chapter.

PHARMACOLOGY

urinary pH modifiers: Increase (acidifiers) or decrease (alkalinizers) the pH of the urine to prevent kidney stones, treat acidosis, or promote excretion of some drugs and toxins. Examples of acidifiers include methionine and ammonium chloride, but are more commonly used in animals. Examples of alkalinizers include sodium bicarbonate (Neut) and potassium citrate (Urocit-K).

anticholinergics: Help control urinary incontinence by delaying the urge to void, increasing the bladder capacity, and relaxing the bladder muscles. Examples include tolterodine (Detrol), darifenacin (Enablex), and oxybutynin (Ditropan).

antidiuretics: Suppress urine formation. Examples include vasopressin (also known as *antidiuretic hormone, ADH*) and desmopressin (DDAVP).

antiinfectives: Fight infection in the urinary system, such as antibiotics, antiseptics, or antifungals. Nitrofurantoin (Macrobid), sulfamethoxazole/trimethoprim (Septra, Bactrim), and levofloxacin (Levaquin) are common examples of antiinfectives used for conditions of the urinary tract.

antispasmodics: Anticholinergic drugs that relax the bladder for the treatment of incontinence. Examples include flavoxate (Urispas) and dicyclomine (Bentyl).

diuretics: Increase the formation of urine by promoting excretion of water and sodium. These drugs are often used to treat high blood pressure, congestive heart failure, and peripheral edema. Examples include hydrochlorothiazide (HydroDIURIL, also found in many combinations), furosemide (Lasix), and triamterene (Dyrenium, also found in many combinations).

anti- = against

⟳ EXERCISE 11: Pharmacology

Match the pharmacology terms with their definitions.

_____ 1. diuretic

_____ 2. antiinfective

_____ 3. alkalinizer

_____ 4. anticholinergic

_____ 5. acidifier

_____ 6. antidiuretic

A. increases the pH of urine
B. suppresses urine formation
C. decreases the pH of urine
D. increases formation of urine
E. antibiotics, antifungals, antiseptics
F. helps control urinary incontinence

Case Study Henry Walker

Henry Walker is a 66-year-old retired professor who has had CKD due to DM. His initial testing showed abnormal GFR and proteinuria. Over a 5-year period he progressed from stage 1 CKD to stage 5 CKD. He has been on HD for 1 year and has been on a waiting list to receive a new kidney.

1. GFR stands for _____ _____.

2. CKD stands for _____ _____.

3. CKD is also known as _____ _____.

4. The type of renal dialysis that cleanses the blood by shunting it from the body through a machine for diffusion and filtration is called _____ _____.

5. If a donor kidney is found for Henry, he will undergo a _____.

Abbreviations

Abbreviation	Definition	Abbreviation	Definition
ADH	antidiuretic hormone	GFR	glomerular filtration rate
ARF	acute renal failure	GN	glomerulonephritis
BUN	blood urea nitrogen	HD	hemodialysis
CAPD	continuous ambulatory peritoneal dialysis	IVU	intravenous urography
		KUB	kidney, ureter, and bladder
CCPD	continuous cycling peritoneal dialysis	pH	acidity/alkalinity
		PKD	polycystic kidney disease
CKD	chronic kidney disease	SG	specific gravity
CT	computed tomography	TCC	transitional cell carcinoma
DI	diabetes insipidus	UA	urinalysis
DM	diabetes mellitus	UTI	urinary tract infection
ESRD	end-stage renal disease	VCUG	voiding cystourethrography
ESWL	extracorporeal shock wave lithotripsy		

EXERCISE 12: Abbreviations

Write the meanings of the abbreviations.

1. The patient with DM had produced 3.0 liters of urine in the last 24 hours.

2. The patient with CKD was treated with HD.

3. Ellen's UA noted a low SG. The diagnosis was DI.

4. Antonia was treated for a UTI.

5. A VCUG helped to confirm the patient's diagnosis of hydronephrosis.

Chapter Review

Match the word parts to their definitions.

Word Part Definitions

Suffix		Definition
-cele	1. _____	removal of a stone
-dipsia	2. _____	herniation
-esis	3. _____	separation, breakdown
-lithotomy	4. _____	machine to crush
-lysis	5. _____	condition of thirst
-pexy	6. _____	process of viewing
-ptosis	7. _____	suspension
-scopy	8. _____	drooping, prolapse
-tripter	9. _____	urinary condition
-uria	10. _____	state of

Combining Form		Definition
azot/o	11. _____	sugar, glucose
albumin/o	12. _____	urinary bladder
calic/o	13. _____	ureter
cortic/o	14. _____	potassium
cyst/o	15. _____	night
glomerul/o	16. _____	trigone
glycos/o	17. _____	sodium
hil/o	18. _____	urine, urinary system
lith/o	19. _____	stone
meat/o	20. _____	urinary meatus
natr/o	21. _____	kidney
nephr/o	22. _____	scanty, few
noct/i	23. _____	glomerulus
olig/o	24. _____	kidney
pyel/o	25. _____	calyx
ren/o	26. _____	renal pelvis
trigon/o	27. _____	urethra
ureter/o	28. _____	urinary bladder
urethr/o	29. _____	protein
ur/o	30. _____	nitrogen
vesic/o	31. _____	cortex

Word Shop

Prefixes	Combining Forms	Suffixes
a–	azot/o	-al
an–	cyst/o	-cele
dys–	glomerul/o	-dipsia
per–	glycos/o	-emia
peri–	hemat/o	-graphy
poly–	lith/o	-iasis
pre–	nephr/o	-itis
	pyel/o	-lysis
	py/o	-oma
	tom/o	-scope
	ureter/o	-scopy
	urethr/o	-tomy
	ur/o	-tripsy
	vesicul/o	-uria

Build the following terms by combining the preceding word parts. Some word parts may be used more than once. Some may not be used at all. The number in parenthesis is the number of word parts needed to build the term.

Definition	Term
1. pertaining to surrounding the bladder (3)	_____
2. process of recording a section of kidney (3)	_____
3. instrument to visually examine the kidney (2)	_____
4. herniation of a ureter (2)	_____
5. condition of painful/difficult urination (2)	_____
6. condition of blood in the urine (2)	_____
7. inflammation of the glomerulus in the kidney (3)	_____
8. condition of stones in the urinary tract (3)	_____
9. condition of no urination (2)	_____
10. process of crushing stones (2)	_____
11. condition of urea in the blood (2)	_____
12. freeing from adhesions in the urethra (2)	_____
13. condition of excessive urination (2)	_____
14. inflammation of the renal pelvis of the kidney (3)	_____
15. condition of excessive thirst (2)	_____

Sort the terms below into the correct categories.

Term Sorting

Anatomy and Physiology	Pathology	Diagnostic Procedures	Therapeutic Interventions

albuminuria	HD	nephropexy	urea
BUN	hilum	nephroptosis	urethra
CAPD	IVU	nephrostomy	urethral stenosis
cortex	KUB	nephrotomography	ureterolysis
cystoscopy	lithotripsy	pyuria	UA
cystourethroscopy	medulla	renal adenoma	urinary meatus
DM	meatotomy	renal colic	urinometer
enuresis	micturition	renal dialysis	UTI
GFR	nephritis	renal medulla	VCUG
glomeruli	nephrolithotomy	trigone	vesicotomy

Replace the highlighted words with the correct terms.

Translations

1. Emily was admitted with **accumulation of fluid in the tissues** and **condition of high blood pressure.**

2. Dr. Garcia ordered a **blood test that measures the amount of nitrogenous waste** and a **test of kidney function that measures the rate at which nitrogenous waste is removed from the blood.**

3. Moumoud was admitted for **severe pain associated with kidney stones lodged in the ureter** and **stones anywhere in the urinary tract.**

4. Mr. Samuels was treated for his **stones in the kidney** with **process of crushing stones to prevent or clear an obstruction in the urinary system.**

5. Once **an infection anywhere in the urinary system** was ruled out, Rebecca was evaluated for ongoing **bed-wetting.**

6. A/an **instrument for visual examination of the inside of the bladder** was used to locate the site of a **herniation of the urinary bladder.**

7. Mr. Alton's acute renal failure was diagnosed after examination findings that included **condition of scanty urination** and **condition of excessive urea in the blood.**

8. The patient's **prolapse or sagging of the kidney** was surgically corrected with a suspension or **fixation of the kidney.**

9. A **sectional radiographic exam of the kidneys** was performed to diagnose Mr. Woo's **adenoma composed of oncocytes.**

10. Mary's DM was diagnosed after she presented with **condition of excessive urination** and **condition of excessive thirst.**

11. Kevin Allen was afraid he had **a group of metabolic disorders characterized by high glucose levels** but was instead diagnosed with **deficiency of ADH.**

12. The patient showed symptoms of **infection of the renal pelvis and parenchyma of the kidney.**

13. Dr. Simons told Marqueta that she had **high blood pressure secondary to kidney disease** due to **inability of the kidneys to excrete wastes.**

14. After several years of **process of diffusing blood across a semipermeable membrane,** Johnna underwent **a surgical transfer of a complete kidney from a donor.**

Medical Record *Brian Coulter*

COULTER, BRIAN S - 724001 Opened by RAMIREZ, GINA, SURGEON

Task   Edit   View   Time Scale   Options   Help

As Of 07:37

| COULTER, BRIAN S | Age: 60 years | Sex: Male | Loc: WHC-SMMC |
| | DOB: 11/11/1955 | MRN: 724001 | FIN: 3506004 |

Reference Text Browser   Form Browser   Medication Profile

Orders | Last 48 Hours | ED | Lab | Radiology | Assessment | Surgery | **Clinical Notes** | Pt. Info | Pt. Schedule | Task List | I & O | MAR

Flowsheet: Clinical Notes   ...   Level: Progress Note   ⊙ Table ○ Group ○ List

Navigator

✓ Operative Report

Description: Nephrolithiasis status post lithotripsy. Stent was placed in the left ureter, urinary incontinence, recent sepsis.

SUBJECTIVE: The patient returns today for a follow up. He was recently in the hospital and was found to be septic from nephrolithiasis. This was all treated. He did require a stent in the left ureter. He had a calculus, which was treated with lithotripsy. He is now back for follow up.

ALLERGIES: Sulfa.

CURRENT MEDICATIONS: Levaquin, Prinivil 20 mg a day, Bumex 0.5 mg a day, Levsinex 0.375 mg a day, cimetidine 400 mg a day, potassium chloride 8 mEq a day, and atenolol 25 mg a day.

REVIEW OF SYSTEMS: He says he is voiding okay. He denies fever, chills, or sweats.

OBJECTIVE:
Vital Signs: Blood pressure 120/70   Temp: 99.3°   Pulse: 87
Neck: Supple.
Lungs: Clear.
Heart: Regular rate and rhythm.
Abdomen: Soft.
Extremities: No edema.

IMPRESSION:
1. Hypertension controlled.
2. Nephrolithiasis status post lithotripsy and stent placed in the left ureter
3. Urinary incontinence.
4. Recent sepsis.

PLAN:
1. Instructions given to call for followup appt regarding his stent.
2. See me back here in two months.
3. No changes made to his medications.

PROD | MAHAFC | 11 Nov 2015 | 07:37

OPERATIVE REPORT

Answer the questions using the preceding operative report.

1. What is a left ureteral calculus? _____

2. What term describes the sudden onset of symptoms? _____

3. Did the ureteral calculus cause an obstruction? _____

    How do you know?

4. What were all the instruments and/or procedures that were used to visualize the problem?

    _____

5. What term indicates that no further injury was caused by the surgery?

    _____

7

Male Reproductive System

OBJECTIVES

- Recognize and use terms related to the anatomy and physiology of the male reproductive system.
- Recognize and use terms related to the pathology of the male reproductive system.

- Recognize and use terms related to the diagnostic procedures for the male reproductive system.
- Recognize and use terms related to the therapeutic interventions for the male reproductive system.

For more interactive learning, go to the Shiland Evolve website, and click on:
- **Match the Word Parts** to review male reproductive word parts.
- **Word Shop** to practice word building.
- **Tournament of Terminology** to test your knowledge of male reproductive terms.
- **Term Sorting** to practice sorting male reproductive terms into categories.

*Click on **Chapter at a Glance** for a list of key word parts and terms for this chapter.*

FUNCTIONS OF THE MALE REPRODUCTIVE SYSTEM

The function of the male reproductive system is to reproduce. In the process of providing half of the genetic material (in the form of spermatozoa) necessary to form a new person—and then successfully storing, transporting, and delivering this material to fertilize the female counterpart, the ovum—the species survives.

SPECIALTIES/SPECIALISTS

Andrology is the study of the male reproductive system, especially in reference to fertility issues. **Urologists** treat male urinary and reproductive disorders.

ANATOMY AND PHYSIOLOGY

Both male and female anatomy can be divided into two parts: **parenchymal** (puh REN kih mul), or **primary tissue,** which produces sex cells for reproduction; and **stromal** (STROH mul), or **secondary tissue,** which includes all of the glands nerves, ducts, and other tissues that serve a supportive function in producing, maintaining, and transmitting these sex cells. Together these types of reproductive tissue, in either sex, are called **genitalia** (jen ih TAIL ee ah). The parenchymal organs that produce the sex cells in both sexes are called **gonads** (GOH nads). The sex cells themselves are called **gametes** (GAM eets).

In the male, the gonads are the **testes** (TESS teez) (*sing.* testis) or **testicles** (TESS tick kuls), paired organs that produce the gametes called **spermatozoa** (spur mat ah ZOH ah) (*sing.* spermatozoon). The testes are suspended in a sac called the **scrotum** (SKROH tum) (*pl.* scrota) outside the body's trunk (Fig. 7-1).

At **puberty** (PYOO bur tee), the stage of life in which males and females become functionally capable of sexual reproduction, the interstitial cells in the testicles begin to produce **testosterone** (tess TOSS tur rohn), a sex hormone responsible for the growth and development of male sex characteristics. The spermatozoa are formed in a series of tightly coiled tiny tubes in each testis called the **seminiferous tubules** (sem ih NIFF ur us TOO byools). The formation of sperm is called **spermatogenesis** (spur mat toh JEN ih sis). The serous membrane that surrounds the front and sides of the testicle is called the **tunica vaginalis testis** (TOON ih kah vaj ih NAL is TESS tis). From the seminiferous tubules, the formed spermatozoa travel to the **epididymis** (eh pih DID ih mis) (*pl.* epididymides), where they are stored.

When the seminal fluid is about to be ejected from the urethra **(ejaculation),** the spermatozoa travel through the left and right **vas deferens** (vas DEH fur ens), also called the **ductus deferens** (DUCK tus DEH fur ens), from the epididymides, around the bladder. The **spermatic cord** is an enclosed sheath that includes the vas deferens, along with arteries, veins, and nerves.

To survive and thrive, the sperm are nourished by fluid from a series of glands. The **seminal vesicles** (SEM ih nul VESS ih kuls), **Cowper** (or **bulbourethral** [bul boh yoo REE thrul]) **glands,** and the **prostate** (PROS tate) **gland** provide fluid either to nourish or to aid in motility and lubrication. The sperm and the fluid together make up a substance called **semen** (SEE men). The **ejaculatory duct** (ee JACK yoo lah tore ee) begins where the seminal vesicles join the vas deferens, and this "tube" joins the urethra. Once the sperm reach the **urethra,** they travel out through the shaft, or body, of the **penis** (PEE nuss), which is composed of three columns of highly vascular erectile tissue. There are two columns of **corpora cavernosa** (KORE poor ah kav ur NOH suh) and one of **corpus spongiosum** (KORE puss spun jee OH sum) that fill with blood through the dorsal veins during sexual arousal. During ejaculation, the sperm

andrology
 andr/o = male
 -logy = the study of

parenchymal
 par- = near
 en- = in
 chym/o = juice
 -al = pertaining to

stromal tissue = strom/o

gonad = gonad/o

testis, testicle = test/o, testicul/o, orchi/o, orchid/o, orch/o

spermatozoon = sperm/o, spermat/o

scrotum = scrot/o

testosterone
 test/o = testis
 ster/o = steroid
 -one = substance that forms

seminiferous
 semin/i = semen
 -ferous = pertaining to carrying

spermatogenesis
 spermat/o = spermatozoon
 -genesis = production

epididymis = epididym/o

vas deferens, ductus deferens = vas/o

seminal vesicle = vesicul/o

prostate = prostat/o

semen = semin/i

urethra = urethr/o

penis = pen/i, phall/o

Be Careful!

Don't confuse **vesic/o,** which means the urinary bladder, and **vesicul/o,** which means the seminal vesicle.

Be Careful!

Don't confuse **phall/o,** which means penis, and **phalang/o,** which is a bone in the finger or toe.

Be Careful!

Don't confuse **urethr/o,** which means urethra, and **ureter/o,** which means the ureter.

glans penis = balan/o

prepuce, foreskin = preputi/o, posth/o

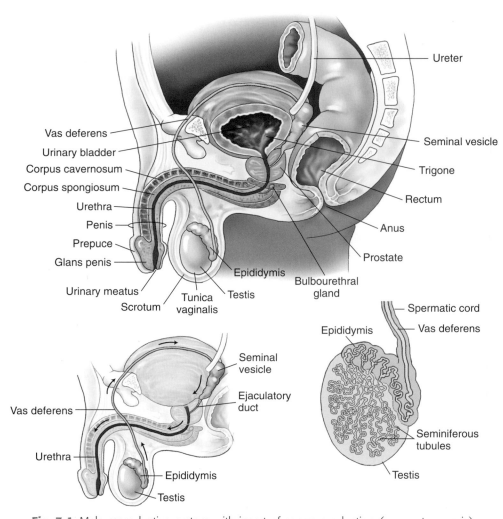

Fig. 7-1 Male reproductive system with insert of sperm production (spermatogenesis).

exit through the enlarged tip of the penis, the **glans penis.** At birth, the glans penis is surrounded by a fold of skin called the **prepuce** (PREE pyoos), or **foreskin.** The removal of this skin is termed **circumcision** (sur kum SIH zhun).

When ejaculation occurs during sexual intercourse (**coitus** [KOH ih tus] or **copulation** [kop yoo LAY shun]), the sperm then race toward the female sex cell, or ovum. If a specific sperm penetrates and unites with the ovum, **conception** takes place, and formation of an embryo begins.

EXERCISE 1: Anatomy of the Male Reproductive System

Match the word parts with their meanings.

_____ 1. penis

_____ 2. prostate

_____ 3. seminal vesicle

_____ 4. scrotum

_____ 5. prepuce

_____ 6. semen

_____ 7. urethra

_____ 8. glans penis

_____ 9. ductus deferens

_____ 10. spermatozoon

_____ 11. epididymis

_____ 12. testis

A. vesicul/o
B. preputi/o
C. orchid/o
D. phall/o
E. epididym/o
F. spermat/o

G. scrot/o
H. vas/o
I. semin/i
J. urethr/o
K. prostat/o
L. balan/o

Decode the terms.

13. unitesticular _____

14. preputial _____

15. vesicular _____

16. periprostatic _____

17. intrascrotal _____

 *You can review the anatomy of the male reproductive system by clicking on **Body Spectrum Electronic Anatomy Coloring Book** → **Reproductive** → **Male.** Click on **Hear It, Spell It** to practice spelling the anatomy and physiology terms you have learned in this chapter.*

 EXERCISE 2: Anatomy of the Male Reproductive System

Label the drawing using the terms provided.

prostate
scrotum
urethra
prepuce
seminal vesicle
testis
glans penis
vas deferens
penis
epididymis

 *Click on **Label It** to practice labeling the structures of the male reproductive system.*

Combining and Adjective Forms for the Anatomy of the Male Reproductive System

Meaning	Combining Form	Adjective Form
epididymis	epididym/o	epididymal
glans penis	balan/o	balanic
gonad	gonad/o	gonadal
juices	chym/o	chymous
male	andr/o	
penis	pen/i, phall/o	penile, phallic
prepuce, foreskin	preputi/o, posth/o	preputial
prostate	prostat/o	prostatic
scrotum	scrot/o	scrotal
semen	semin/i	seminal
seminal vesicle	vesicul/o	vesicular
spermatozoon	sperm/o, spermat/o	spermatic
steroid	ster/o	steroidal
stroma	strom/o	stromal
testis, testicle	test/o, testicul/o, orchid/o, orch/o	testicular
urethra	urethr/o	urethral
vas deferens, ductus deferens	vas/o	vasal, ductal

Prefixes for the Anatomy of the Male Reproductive System

Prefix	Meaning
en-	in
par-	near

Suffixes for the Anatomy of the Male Reproductive System

Suffix	Meaning
-al, -ous, -ar, -ile, -atic, -ic	pertaining to
-ferous	pertaining to carrying
-genesis	production
-logy	the study of
-one	substance that forms

PATHOLOGY

Terms Related to Congenital Disorders

Term	Word Origin	Definition
anorchism AN or kih zum	*an-* without *orch/o* testis *-ism* condition	Condition of being born without a testicle. May also be an acquired condition due to trauma or disease.
chordee KORE dee	*chord/o* cord	Congenital defect resulting in a downward (ventral) curvature of the penis due to a fibrous band (cord) of tissue along the corpus spongiosum. Often associated with hypospadias (Fig. 7-2).
cryptorchidism kript OR kid iz um	*crypt-* hidden *orchid/o* testis *-ism* condition	Condition in which the testicles fail to descend into the scrotum before birth. Also called **cryptorchism** (Fig. 7-3).
epispadias eh pee SPAY dee ahs	*epi-* above *-spadias* a rent or tear	Urethral opening on the dorsum (top) of the penis rather than on the tip. Also called **hyperspadias.**
hypospadias hye poh SPAY dee ahs	*hypo-* below *-spadias* a rent or tear	Urethral opening on the ventral surface (underside) of the penis instead of on the tip (Fig. 7-4). May be acquired as a result of the disease process.
phimosis fih MOH sis		Congenital condition of tightening of the prepuce around the glans penis so that the foreskin cannot be retracted.

Fig. 7-2 Chordee.

Fig. 7-3 Cryptorchidism in left testicle of a neonate.

Fig. 7-4 Hypospadias.

Terms Related to Other Male Reproductive Disorders

Term	Word Origin	Definition
aspermia a SPUR mee ah	*a-* without *sperm/o* sperm *-ia* condition	Condition in which no spermatozoa are present, nor any semen formed or ejaculated.
azoospermia a zoh uh SPUR mee ah	*a-* without *zo/o* animal *sperm/o* sperm *-ia* condition	Condition of no living sperm in the semen. This may be a desired condition, as when it follows a vasectomy.
balanitis bal en EYE tis	*balan/o* glans penis *-itis* inflammation	Inflammation of the glans penis.
benign prostatic hyperplasia (BPH) beh NYNE pros TAT ick hye pur PLAY zsa	*prostat/o* prostate *-ic* pertaining to *hyper-* excessive *-plasia* formation	Abnormal enlargement of the prostate gland surrounding the urethra, leading to difficulty with urination (Fig. 7-5). Also known as **benign prostatic hypertrophy.**
epididymitis ep ih did ih MYE tis	*epididym/o* epididymis *-itis* inflammation	Inflammation of the epididymis, usually as a result of an ascending infection through the genitourinary (GU) tract.
erectile dysfunction (ED)		Inability to achieve or sustain a penile erection for sexual intercourse. Also known as **impotence** (IM poh tense).
gynecomastia gye neh koh MASS tee ah	*gynec/o* female *mast/o* breast *-ia* condition	Enlargement of either unilateral or bilateral breast tissue in the male. The gynec/o is a reference to the appearance of the breast, not to a female (Fig. 7-6).
hydrocele HYE droh seel	*hydr/o* water, fluid *-cele* herniation, protrusion	Accumulation of fluid in the tunica vaginalis testis (Fig. 7-7).
oligospermia oh lih goh SPUR mee ah	*olig/o* scanty *sperm/o* sperm *-ia* condition	Condition of temporary or permanent deficiency of sperm in the seminal fluid; related to azoospermia.
orchitis or KYE tis	*orch/o* testis *-itis* inflammation	Inflammation of one or both of the testicles; may or may not be associated with the mumps virus. Also known as **testitis** (tess TYE tis).

Fig. 7-5 Benign prostatic hyperplasia (BPH).

Bladder

Compressed urethra

Seminal vesicle

Rectum

Enlarged median lobe of prostate gland

Fig. 7-6 Gynecomastia.

Terms Related to Other Male Reproductive Disorders—cont'd

Term	Word Origin	Definition
priapism PRY ah piz um		An abnormally prolonged erection.
prostatitis pros tah TYE tis	*prostat/o* prostate *-itis* inflammation	Inflammation of the prostate gland.
testicular torsion tes TICK kyoo lur	*testicul/o* testicle *-ar* pertaining to	Twisting of a testicle on its spermatic cord, usually caused by trauma. May lead to ischemia of the testicle.
varicocele VAIR ih koh seel	*varic/o* varices *-cele* herniation, protrusion	Abnormal dilation of the veins of the spermatic cord; can lead to infertility (Fig. 7-8).
vesiculitis veh sick yoo LYE tis	*vesicul/o* seminal vesicle *-itis* inflammation	Inflammation of a seminal vesicle, usually associated with prostatitis.

Fig. 7-7 Hydrocele.

Fig. 7-8 Varicocele.

EXERCISE 3: Male Reproductive Disorders

Match the male reproductive disorders with their definitions.

_____ 1. tightening of foreskin

_____ 2. opening of urethra on underside of penis

_____ 3. twisting of testicle on spermatic cord

_____ 4. inability to achieve or sustain a penile erection

_____ 5. accumulation of fluid in tunica vaginalis testis

_____ 6. opening of urethra on dorsum of penis

_____ 7. enlargement of breast tissue in a male

_____ 8. abnormal dilation of veins of the spermatic cord

A. hypospadias
B. varicocele
C. gynecomastia
D. epispadias
E. testicular torsion
F. erectile dysfunction (ED)
G. phimosis
H. hydrocele

Build the terms.

9.   inflammation of the glans penis _____

10. condition of no living sperm (in the semen) _____

11. inflammation of the prostate _____

12. excessive formation, pertaining to the prostate (two words) _____

Decode the terms.

13. orchitis _____

14. oligospermia _____

15. vesiculitis _____

Case Study Mario Polanco

Six-week-old Mario Polanco is seen by his pediatrician to evaluate the abnormal urethral opening on the dorsal side of his penis. The pediatrician advises the parents that a urethroplasty will be necessary to correct the location of the urethral opening. Mario does not exhibit chordee, which is often associated with hyperspadias.

1. The tube that conducts urine from the bladder through the penis is the _____.

2. Another term for hyperspadias is _____.

3. The prefix *epi-* means _____.

4. The dorsal side of the penis is the _____ of the penis.
   a. top
   b. bottom

5. An abnormal ventral curvature of the penis is called _____.

The pathogens that cause sexually transmitted infections (STIs) are various, but what they have in common is that all of them are most efficiently transmitted by sexual contact. The other terms for STI include venereal disease (VD) and sexually transmitted disease (STD).

Terms Related to Sexually Transmitted Infections

Term	Word Origin	Definition
gonorrhea gon uh REE ah	*gon/o* seed *-rrhea* flow, discharge	Disease caused by the gram-negative diplococcus *Neisseria gonorrhoeae* bacterium (Gc), which manifests itself as inflammation of the urethra, prostate, rectum, or pharynx. The cervix and fallopian tubes may also be involved in females, although they may appear to be **asymptomatic,** meaning without symptoms (Fig. 7-9)
herpes genitalis (herpes simplex virus-2, HSV-2) HER peez jen ih TAL is		Form of the herpesvirus transmitted through sexual contact, causing recurring painful vesicular eruptions (Fig. 7-10).
human papillomavirus (HPV) pap ih LOH mah		Virus that causes common warts of the hands and feet and lesions of the mucous membranes of the oral, anal, and genital cavities. A genital wart is referred to as a **condyloma** (kon dih LOH mah) (*pl.* condylomata).
nongonococcal urethritis (NGU) non gon uh KOCK ul yoor ih THRY tis	*urethr/o* urethra *-itis* inflammation	Inflammation of the urethra caused by *Chlamydia trachomatis, Mycoplasma genitalium,* or *Ureaplasma urealyticum.*
syphilis SIFF ill is		Multistage STI caused by the spirochete *Treponema pallidum* bacterium. A highly infectious **chancre** (SHAN kur), a painless, red pustule, appears in the first stage, usually on the genitals.

Fig. 7-9 Gonorrhea in a male patient.

Fig. 7-10 Genital herpes.

EXERCISE 4: Sexually Transmitted Infections

Fill in the blanks with one of the following terms.

condylomata, asymptomatic, human papillomavirus, chancres, herpes simplex virus-2, nongonococcal urethritis, syphilis, gonorrhea

1. HPV causes genital warts that are referred to as _____.

2. Which STI has multiple stages? _____

3. Inflammation of the urethra not caused by the gonorrhea bacterium is called _____.

4. An STI caused by gram-negative bacteria is called _____.

5. Syphilitic lesions that are painless ulcers are called _____.

6. When a patient has no symptoms, he is considered to be _____.

7. Genital warts are caused by the _____.

8. A viral infection that results in painful, recurring vesicular eruptions is called _____.

Terms Related to Benign Neoplasms		
Term	Word Origin	Definition
Leydig and Sertoli cell tumors LAY dig sur TOH lee		These testicular tumors arise from the stromal tissue of the testes that produce hormones. They are usually benign.

Terms Related to Malignant Neoplasms

Term	Word Origin	Definition
adenocarcinoma of the prostate ad eh noh kar sih NOH mah	*aden/o* gland *-carcinoma* cancer of epithelial origin	Prostate cancer is diagnosed in one of every six men. With early detection, however, this cancer is treatable (Fig. 7-11).
seminoma seh mih NOH mah	*semin/i* semen *-oma* tumor, mass	This malignancy is one type of germ cell tumor (GCT) that develops from the cells that form sperm (Fig. 7-12).
nonseminoma non seh mih NOH mah	*non-* not *semin/i* semen *-oma* tumor, mass	Nonseminoma is the second type of GCT. It accounts for the majority of testicular cancer cases and occurs in younger men, usually between the ages of 15 and 35.
teratoma, malignant tair uh TOH mah	*terat/o* deformity *-oma* tumor, mass	This tumor is a type of nonseminoma that is usually benign in children. Because these tumors are created from germ cells, they have half of the necessary genetic information to form an individual. A synonym is the term **dermoid cyst**.

Fig. 7-11 Adenocarcinoma of the prostate.

Fig. 7-12 Seminoma of the testicle.

EXERCISE 5: Neoplasms

Match the neoplasms with their definitions.

_____ 1. nonseminoma

_____ 2. teratoma

_____ 3. seminoma

_____ 4. adenocarcinoma of the prostate

_____ 5. Leydig and Sertoli cell tumors

A. benign tumors that arise from testicular stromal tissue
B. prostate cancer
C. majority of germ cell tumors (GCTs)
D. germ cell tumor (GCT) developing from cells that form sperm
E. synonym is dermoid cyst

Build the terms.

6. tumor of semen _____

7. glandular cancerous tumor of epithelial origin _____

 *Click on **Hear It, Spell It** to practice spelling the pathology terms you have learned. To review the pathology terms you've learned in this chapter, play **Medical Millionaire.***

Case Study   Roger Bradford

Roger Bradford is concerned about a painless red sore on his penis that appeared about 2 weeks ago. The physician's assistant (PA) examines the sore and notes no purulent discharge. He suspects that Roger has syphilis, although his history is negative for STIs.

1. If Roger indeed has syphilis, what is the painless red sore on his penis called? _____

2. What is the term that means "pus-filled?" _____ _____

3. STI stands for _____ _____.

4. Another abbreviation for STI is _____.

Age Matters

Pediatrics

Aside from the congenital disorders that a male child may be born with, very few male reproductive system disorders are specific to childhood. Seminoma, a cancer of the testicles, is one of the few cancers that afflicts youth. Fortunately, early detection makes this cancer almost 100% curable.

Geriatrics

Senior men have some very significant disorders. Disorders of the prostate gland are common and are usually accompanied by difficulty with urination because of the location of the prostate around the urethra. Usually benign, this also has a malignant form, and prostate cancer is the second greatest cause of cancer deaths. Erectile disorders, now treatable with a variety of different medications on the market, have also emerged as a significant "reason for visit" to the family physician.

DIAGNOSTIC PROCEDURES

Terms Related to Diagnostic Procedures

Term	Word Origin	Definition
digital rectal examination (DRE)	*digit/o* digit (finger or toe) *-al* pertaining to *rect/o* rectum *-al* pertaining to	Insertion of a gloved finger into the rectum to palpate the prostate (Fig. 7-13).
epididymovesiculography eh pih did ih moh veh sih kuh LAH grah fee	*epididym/o* epididymis *vesicul/o* seminal vesicle *-graphy* process of recording	Imaging of the epididymis and seminal vesicle using a contrast medium.
fluorescent treponemal antibody absorption (FTA-ABS) test floor ES unt trep uh NEE mul		Definitive test for diagnosing syphilis (Fig. 7-14).

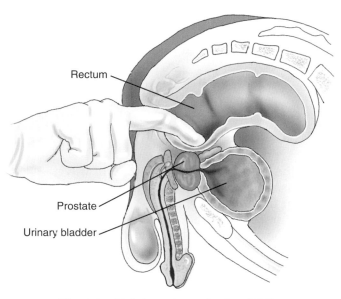

Fig. 7-13 Digital rectal examination (DRE).

Fig. 7-14 Fluorescent treponemal antibody absorption (FTA-ABS) test.

Terms Related to Diagnostic Procedures—cont'd

Term	Word Origin	Definition
Gram stain		A laboratory method of staining microorganisms as a means of identifying them as either gram-negative or gram-positive. Gonorrhea, gram-negative bacteria is diagnosed using Gram stain (Fig. 7-15).
plethysmography, penile pleth iz MAH grah fee	*plethysm/o* volume *-graphy* process of recording	The measurement of changes in volume of the penis.
prostate-specific antigen (PSA) AN tih jen		Blood test for prostatic hypertrophy. Very high levels may indicate prostate cancer. Above 2.6 ng/mL is considered elevated.
sonography, transrectal	*son/o* sound *-graphy* process of recording	Use of high-frequency sound waves to examine the prostate for abnormalities (Fig. 7-16).
sperm analysis		Count and analysis of the number and health of the spermatozoa as a test for male fertility. Also called **sperm count** or **semen analysis**.
testicular self-examination (TSE)	*testicul/o* testicle *-ar* pertaining to	Examination of the testicles by the patient.
Venereal Disease Research Laboratory (VDRL) test		Test used to screen for syphilis.

Fig. 7-15 Gram stain. **A,** Red blood cells (RBCs) and gram-positive cocci. **B,** RBCs with gram-negative bacilli.

Fig. 7-16 Transrectal ultrasound scan of the prostate, showing benign prostatic hyperplasia (BPH).

Be Careful!   *Don't confuse* **proct/o**, *which means rectum and anus, and* **prostat/o**, *which means prostate.*

⟳ EXERCISE 6: Diagnostic Procedures

Match the diagnostic procedures with their definitions.

_____ 1. digital rectal examination (DRE)

_____ 2. fluorescent treponemal antibody absorption (FTA-ABS) test

_____ 3. Gram stain

_____ 4. prostate-specific antigen (PSA)

_____ 5. sperm analysis

_____ 6. sonography

_____ 7. Venereal Disease Research Laboratory (VDRL) test

A. imaging with high-frequency sound waves
B. test used to screen for syphilis
C. test of male fertility
D. blood test for prostatic hypertrophy
E. insertion of a gloved finger to palpate the prostate
F. definitive test for diagnosing syphilis
G. test used to diagnose gonorrhea

Decode the terms.

8. plethysmography _____

9. epididymovesiculography _____

Case Study Daniel Grey

Fifty-year-old Daniel Grey has had difficulty urinating with only a small amount of urine coming out at a time. The urologist performs a DRE and notes that Daniel's prostate is enlarged. He orders a PSA test and a biopsy. Daniel isn't happy to hear about the biopsy. He says that he had had a biopsy 6 months earlier, but that it was normal. The urologist assures Daniel that the biopsy is very important to diagnose whether he has prostate cancer or BPH.

1. BPH stands for _____ _____.

2. What is enlarged in BPH? _____ _____

3. PSA stands for _____ _____.

4. DRE stands for _____ _____.

THERAPEUTIC INTERVENTIONS

Terms Related to Therapeutic Interventions

Term	Word Origin	Definition
ablation ah BLAY shun		Removal of tissue by surgery, chemical destruction, cryoprobe, electrocautery, or radiofrequency energy.
castration kas TRAY shun		Removal of both gonads in the male or the female.
circumcision sur kum SIH zhun	*circum-* around *-cision* process of cutting	Surgical procedure in which the prepuce of the penis (or that of the clitoris of the female) is excised.
hydrocelectomy hye droh sell ECK tuh mee	*hydr/o* water, fluid *-cele* herniation, protrusion *-ectomy* removal, excision	Removal of a hydrocele.
orchidectomy or kih DECK tuh mee	*orchid/o* testis *-ectomy* removal	Removal of one or both testicles.
orchiopexy or kee oh PECK see	*orchi/o* testis *-pexy* fixation, suspension	Surgical procedure to mobilize an undescended testicle, attaching it to the scrotum.
prostatectomy pros tuh TECK tuh mee	*prostat/o* prostate *-ectomy* removal	Removal of the prostate gland. If termed a **radical prostatectomy,** the seminal vesicles and area of vas ampullae of the vas deferens are also removed.
transurethral resection of the prostate (TUR, TURP) trans yoo REE thrul	*trans-* through *urethr/o* urethra *-al* pertaining to	Removal of the prostate in sections through a urethral approach (Fig. 7-17). This procedure is the most common type of prostatectomy.
transurethral incision of the prostate (TUIP) trans yoo REE thruhl	*trans-* through *urethr/o* urethra *-al* pertaining to	Form of prostate surgery involving tiny incisions of the prostate. The prostate is not removed.
sterilization		Process of rendering a male or female unable to conceive a child while retaining gonads.
vasectomy vas SECK tuh mee	*vas/o* vas deferens *-ectomy* removal	Incision, ligation, and cauterization of both of the vas deferens for the purpose of male sterilization.
vasovasostomy vas zoh vuh SOS tuh mee	*vas/o* vas deferens *-stomy* new opening	Anastomosis of the ends of the vas deferens as a means of reconnecting them to reverse the sterilization procedure.

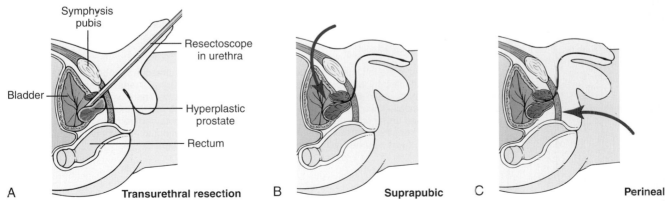

Fig. 7-17 A, Transurethral resection of the prostate (TURP). The approach may be **(A)** through the urethra (transurethral), **(B)** above the pubic bone (suprapubic), or **(C)** through the perineum (perineal).

EXERCISE 7: Therapeutic Interventions

Match the therapeutic interventions with their definitions.

_____ 1. removal of both gonads   _____ 5. fixation of a testicle   A. orchidectomy
                                                                                  B. ablation
_____ 2. destruction of tissue   _____ 6. rendering barren   C. circumcision
                                                                                  D. sterilization
_____ 3. removal of prepuce   _____ 7. ligation of ductus deferens   E. vasectomy
                                                                                  F. castration
_____ 4. removal of testicle   G. orchiopexy

Decode the terms.

8. vasovasotomy _____

9. transurethral _____

10. prostatectomy _____

Medical Record **Tyson Bernard**

BERNARD, TYSON Q. - 732723 Opened by PEREZ, RAECHAL, MD

Task   Edit   View   Time Scale   Options   Help

As Of 11:04

| BERNARD, TYSON Q. | Age: 64 years | Sex: Male | Loc: WHC-SMMC |
| | DOB: 05/05/1951 | MRN: 732723 | FIN: 3506004 |

Reference Text Browser | Form Browser | Medication Profile

Orders | Last 48 Hours | ED | Lab | Radiology | Assessments | **Surgery** | Clinical Notes | Pt. Info | Pt. Schedule | Task List | I & O | MAR

Flowsheet: Surgery   Level: Operative Report   ⦿ Table ○ Group ○ List

Navigator
✔ Operative Report

Preoperative diagnosis: Elevated prostate-specific antigen

Surgical procedure: Transrectal ultrasound of prostate

A 64-year-old male with PSA of 21.8. He had normal biopsy results 6 months ago. The PSA continues to rise incrementally and the patient comes in now for repeat prostate ultrasound with biopsy.

Patient was placed in the left lateral decubitus position. A lubricated ultrasound probe passed per rectum without difficulty. Multiple images of the prostate were obtained, transverse and sagittal axes. Seminal vesicles were nondilated. Prostate capsule intact. There were prostatic calcifications especially toward the base of the gland. At this point, the needle biopsy device was positioned, and under ultrasound guidance, five biopsies were obtained from the right side and five biopsies from the left. Prostate volume measured 71 mL. Patient tolerated the procedure well and was returned to the recovery room in good condition.

PROD | MAHAFC | 03 April 2015 | 11:04

⊘ EXERCISE 8: Operative Report

Using the operative report on p. 260, answer the following questions.

1. What was the route of the approach for the ultrasound? _____

2. What is the significance of an elevated PSA? _____

3. The report says that the "seminal vesicles were nondilated." What is the function of the seminal

   vesicles? _____

PHARMACOLOGY

alpha-adrenergic inhibitors: Block alpha-1 adrenergic receptors to relax smooth muscle in prostate to improve urinary flow. Examples include tamsulosin (Flomax) and terazosin (Hytrin).

androgen antagonists: Block receptors or inhibit synthesis of androgen hormones. Finasteride (Proscar) and dutasteride (Avodart) block the conversion of testosterone to the more potent hormone 5-alpha-dihydrotestosterone (DHT) to suppress growth of and even shrink the enlarged prostate. Saw palmetto (Serenoa repens) is an alternative medicine that has been shown to be effective in treating sumptoms of BPH.

antibiotics: Treat bacterial infection. Penicillin G, tetracycline, and doxycycline all can be used to treat syphilis.

anti-impotence agents: Used to alleviate ED. Sildenafil (Viagra) and tadalafil (Cialis) are examples of oral agents. Alprostadil (Caverject) is injected directly into the corpus cavernosum of the penis.

antivirals: Treat viral infections. Acyclovir (Zovirax) is used to treat genital herpes virus.

andr/o = male

anti- = against

⊘ EXERCISE 9: Pharmacology

Match the pharmacology terms with their definitions.

_____ 1. class of drug used to treat bacterial infection

_____ 2. class of drug used to treat viral infections

_____ 3. class of drug used to treat erectile dysfunction (ED)

_____ 4. an example of a drug used to treat benign prostatic hyperplasia (BPH)

_____ 5. class of drug used to improve urine flow in patients with BPH

A. antivirals
B. anti-impotence agents
C. alpha-adrenergic inhibitors
D. antibiotics
E. finasteride

Case Study   Vithy Gupta

Vithy Gupta, a 9-month-old male, is diagnosed with an undescended testicle. The pediatrician explains to Vithy's parents that if the testicle does not descend on its own, orchiopexy will be needed to place the testicle in its normal position.

1. The term for a condition of an undescended testicle is _____.

2. The prefix *crypt-* means _____.

3. The term meaning to fix a testicle in place is _____.

4. The suffix *-pexy* means _____.

5. List all the combining forms that mean testicle. _____ _____.

Click on **Hear It, Spell It** to practice spelling the diagnostic and therapeutic terms you have learned in this chapter.

Abbreviations

Abbreviation	Definition
BPH	benign prostatic hyperplasia/hypertrophy
Bx	biopsy
DRE	digital rectal exam
FTA-ABS	fluorescent treponemal antibody (test)
Gc	gonococcus
GCT	germ cell tumor
GU	genitourinary
HPV	human papillomavirus
HSV-2	herpes simplex virus-2, herpes genitalis

Abbreviation	Definition
NGU	nongonococcal urethritis
PSA	prostate-specific antigen
STI	sexually transmitted infection
TSE	testicular self-examination
TUIP	transurethral incision of the prostate
TUR	transurethral resection (of the prostate)
TURP	transurethral resection of the prostate
VD	venereal disease
VDRL	Venereal Disease Research Laboratory (test for syphilis)

EXERCISE 10: Abbreviations

1. The patient had a TURP to relieve his _____ (answer with another abbreviation).

2. Someone who has a Gc infection has a/an _____ (answer with another abbreviation).

3. A patient tested with VDRL may be suspected of having _____.

4. What is a DRE, and what is it used for? _____

5. If condylomata are present, the patient may have _____.

6. What is the GU system? _____

⊗ **Be Careful!**   Don't confuse the gastrointestinal (**GI**) system with the genitourinary (**GU**) system.

Chapter Review

Match the word parts to their definitions.

Word Part Definitions

Prefix/Suffix		Definition
a-	1. _____	below
-cele	2. _____	excessive
circum-	3. _____	tumor, mass
-cision	4. _____	through
crypt-	5. _____	inflammation
-ectomy	6. _____	around
-genesis	7. _____	process of recording
-graphy	8. _____	herniation, protrusion
hyper-	9. _____	without
hypo-	10. _____	hidden
-itis	11. _____	removal
-oma	12. _____	production
-plasia	13. _____	process of cutting
-spadias	14. _____	a rent or tear
trans-	15. _____	formation

Combining Form		Definition
andr/o	16. _____	male
balan/o	17. _____	semen
epididym/o	18. _____	glans penis
hydr/o	19. _____	spermatozoon
olig/o	20. _____	epididymis
orchid/o	21. _____	testis
pen/i	22. _____	foreskin
phall/o	23. _____	seminal vesicle
plethysm/o	24. _____	penis
preputi/o	25. _____	scrotum
prostat/o	26. _____	vas deferens
scrot/o	27. _____	scanty
semin/i	28. _____	prostate
sperm/o	29. _____	volume
vas/o	30. _____	water, fluid
vesicul/o	31. _____	animal
zo/o	32. _____	penis

Word Shop

Prefixes	Combining Forms	Suffixes
a	andr/o	-cision
aan	balan/o	-ectomy
circum	epididym/o	-genesis
crypt	olig/o	-ia
dys	orchid/o	-ism
e	orchi/o	-itis
post	orch/o	-logy
pre	prostat/o	-pexy
syn-	spermat/o	-plasty
	sperm/o	-stomy
	vas/o	-tomy
	vesicul/o	
	zo/o	

Build the following terms by combining the preceding word parts. Some word parts may be used more than once. Some won't be used at all. The number in parenthesis is the number of word parts needed to build the terms.

Definition	Term
1. condition of scanty sperm (3)	_____
2. inflammation of a seminal vesicle (2)	_____
3. fixation of a testicle (2)	_____
4. surgical repair of the glans penis (2)	_____
5. removal of the prostate (2)	_____
6. inflammation of the glans penis (2)	_____
7. the study of the male reproductive system (2)	_____
8. production of sperm (2)	_____
9. condition of no animals (life) in the sperm (4)	_____
10. process of cutting around (2)	_____
11. condition of a "hidden" testicle (3)	_____
12. inflammation of the vessels that store sperm (2)	_____
13. removal of the epididymis (2)	_____
14. condition of no testicle (3)	_____
15. removal of a testicle (2)	_____

Sort the terms below into the correct categories.

Term Sorting

Anatomy and Physiology	Pathology	Diagnostic Procedures	Therapeutic Interventions

ablation	epididymovesiculography	orchiopexy	spermatogenesis
anorchism	FTA-ABS	phimosis	sterilization
BPH	gametes	plethysmography	TSE
castration	genitalia	prepuce	TUIP
circumcision	glans penis	prostatectomy	TURP
corpora cavernosa	gonorrhea	PSA	tunica vaginalis
ductus deferens	Gram stain	semen	vasectomy
ED	hydrocele	seminoma	VDRL
epididymis	oligospermia	sonography	
epididymitis	orchidectomy	sperm analysis	

Replace the highlighted words with the correct term.

Translations

1. A **count and analysis of the number and health of spermatozoa** revealed a **condition of temporary or permanent deficiency of sperm in the seminal fluid** that caused the couple's infertility.

2. Mr. Steinman's **abnormal enlargement of the prostate gland** was treated with a **form of prostate surgery involving tiny incision of the prostate.**

3. Sam's painful testicular swelling was diagnosed as **an inflammation of the epididymis.**

4. The physician suggested a **surgical procedure in which the prepuce of the penis is excised** to treat the patient's **congenital condition of tightening of the prepuce around the glans penis.**

5. Dr. Adams explained that **the painless, red, highly infectious pustule** was the first stage of **a multistage STI** caused by the spirochete *Treponema pallidum* bacterium.

6. The physician ordered **a laboratory method of staining microorganisms as a means of identifying them as gram-negative or gram-positive** to diagnose the patient's disease caused by the gram-negative diplococcus *Neisseria gonorrhoeae* bacterium.

7. When Ken remarried, he decided to have his **incision, ligation, and cauterization of both of the vas deferens** reversed and was scheduled for a/an **anatomosis of the ends of the vas deferens as a means of reconnecting them.**

8. Hunter underwent a **removal of one or both testicles** to treat his **condition in which the testicles fail to descend into the scrotum before birth.**

9. As part of a work-up for **the inability to achieve or sustain a penile erection for sexual intercourse,** the patient underwent **the measurement of changes in volume of organs or body parts.**

10. The patient was treated for the **genital warts** that accompanied his **form of the herpesvirus transmitted through sexual contact, causing painful eruptions.**

11. Harold was diagnosed with a/an **germ cell tumor that develops from the cells that form sperm.**

12. **The healthcare specialist who treats male urinary and reproductive disorders** treated Mr. Mason's **abnormal dilation of the veins of the spermatic cord.**

13. Tanner was embarrassed about his **enlargement of breast tissue in the male.**

14. Robert's **condition of no living sperm in the semen,** following a vasectomy was the result of **the process of rendering a male unable to to conceive a child while retaining gonads.**

Medical Record Sam Trudell

TRUDELL, SAMUEL H. - 453768 Opened by JAMES, ZACHARY MD

Task Edit View Time Scale Options Help

TRUDELL, SAMUEL H.

Age: 67 years — Sex: Male — Loc: WHC-SMMC
DOB: 10/17/1947 — MRN: 453768 — FIN: 3506004

Reference Text Browser | Form Browser | Medication Profile

Orders | Last 48 Hours | ED | Lab | Radiology | Assessments | **Surgery** | Clinical Notes | Pt. Info | Pt. Schedule | Task List | I & O | MAR

Flowsheet: Surgery — Level: Operative Report — ○ Table ○ Group ○ List

Navigator
✔ Operative Report

Preoperative Diagnosis: BPH, urinary retention
Postoperative Diagnosis: BPH, urinary retention
   History of Present Illness: Patient is a 67-year-old African American male with past medical history of hiatal hernia with gastritis, BPH, and UTI with a history of urinary retention. Patient denies dysuria, incontinence, hematuria, urgency, and urinary frequency. Urinary retention has been managed with a Foley catheter after a bout of UTI on past admission.
   Operation: TURP
   Anesthesia: Spinal
   Procedure: The patient was brought to the operating room, was properly identified, and, following adequate administration of spinal anesthetic, was placed in the dorsal lithotomy position, and the genitalia prepared with Betadine and draped in the sterile manner.
   A #26 French scope was used to inspect the urethra and bladder. Bilobar hypertrophy of the prostate was easily identified.
   A transurethral resection of the prostate was carried out in the usual fashion. Chips of prostatic tissue were evacuated from the bladder with a Toomey syringe. Hemostasis was achieved with a Bovie. On final inspection, the urethra was free of obstruction, and both the external sphincter and the ureteral orifices were intact. A Foley catheter was attached for drainage, and the patient was sent to the recovery room in satisfactory condition.

PROD | MAHAFC | 01 August 2015 | 16:24

OPERATIVE REPORT

Answer the questions using the preceding operative report.

1. The patient's past medical history included BPH. Describe this condition.

2. Define what the patient does *not* complain of:

   A. dysuria _____

   B. incontinence _____

   C. urgency _____

   D. urinary frequency _____

   E. hematuria _____

3. How many lobes of the prostate were enlarged?

4. What does the abbreviation TURP mean?

5. If this patient had had periprostatic lesions, where would they have been?

8

Female Reproductive System and Pregnancy

CHAPTER OUTLINE

Functions of the Female
  Reproductive System
Specialists/Specialties
Anatomy and Physiology
Pregnancy and Delivery
Pathology
  Case Study: Magda Petersen
  Case Study: Antoinette Song
  Medical Record: Olivia Carter

Diagnostic Procedures
  Case Study: Marina Santiago
Therapeutic Interventions
  Case Study: Phoebe Gilliam
  Case Study: Elizabeth Dardenne
  Medical Record: Hortencia Garcia

Pharmacology
  Case Study: Sharifa Kha
Chapter Review
  Medical Record: Suzanne Goldstein

OBJECTIVES

- Recognize and use terms related to the anatomy and physiology of the female reproductive system and pregnancy.
- Recognize and use terms related to the pathology of the female reproductive system and pregnancy.

- Recognize and use terms related to the diagnostic procedures for the female reproductive system and pregnancy.
- Recognize and use terms related to the therapeutic interventions for the female reproductive system and pregnancy.

For interactive learning, go to the Evolve website and click on:
- **Match the Word Parts** to review female reproductive and pregnancy word parts.
- **Word Shop** to practice word building.
- **Tournament of Terminology** to test your knowledge of female reproductive and pregnancy terms.
- **Term Sorting** to practice sorting female reproductive and pregnancy terms into categories.

*Click on **Chapter at a Glance** for a list of key word parts and terms for this chapter.*

FUNCTIONS OF THE FEMALE REPRODUCTIVE SYSTEM

The role of the female reproductive system is to keep one's genetic material in the world's gene pool. Through sexual reproduction, the 23 pairs of chromosomes of the **female** must join with 23 pairs of chromosomes from a male to create new life. To do this, the system must produce the hormones necessary to provide a hospitable environment for the **ovum** (OH vum) (*pl.* **ova**), the female gamete, to connect with the spermatozoon, the male gamete, for fertilization to occur. Once an egg is fertilized, it is nurtured throughout its growth process until the delivery of the neonate (newborn).

female = gynec/o

ovum = o/o, ov/o, ov/i, ovul/o

SPECIALTIES/SPECIALISTS

Obstetricians are medical doctors who treat women during pregnancy, deliver infants, and follow women through the postpartum period. Many obstetricians are also trained as **gynecologists,** medical doctors who monitor health and treat diseases of the female reproductive system. The medical specialties for these fields are called **obstetrics** and **gynecology,** respectively.

    Midwives are healthcare providers, usually nurses, who assist women through labor and delivery.

    Doulas care for a pregnant mother through labor and delivery and/or after delivery provide care for the mother and baby.

gynecologist
  gynec/o = female
  -logist = one who specializes in the study of

 Be Careful!

The term **germ** *comes from the Latin word for sprout or fetus, here referring to its reproductive nature; however, it can also mean a type of microorganism that can cause disease.*

ANATOMY AND PHYSIOLOGY

Internal Anatomy

Because the primary function of the female reproductive system is to create new life through the successful fertilization of an ovum, discussion of this system begins with this very important germ cell.

Ova and Ovaries

From **menarche** (meh NAR kee), the first menstrual period, to **menopause** (MEN oh poz), the cessation of menstruation, mature ova are produced by the female gonads, the **ovaries** (OH vuh reez) (Fig. 8-1). The ovaries are small, almond-shaped, paired organs located on either side of the uterus in the female pelvic cavity. They are attached to the uterus by the ovarian ligaments and lie close to the opening of the **fallopian** (fuh LOH pee un) **tubes,** the ducts that

menarche
  men/o = menstruation
  -arche = beginning

menopause
  men/o = menstruation
  -pause = stop, cease

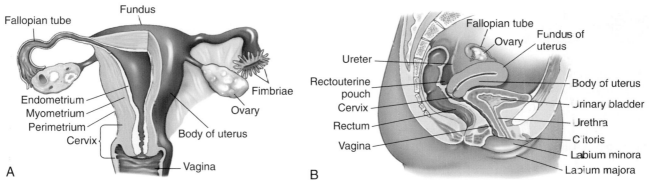

Fig. 8-1 Female reproductive organs. **A,** Frontal view. **B,** Sagittal view.

menstruation = men/o, menstru/o

ovary = oophor/o, ovari/o

uterus = hyster/o, metri/o, metr/o, uter/o

fallopian tube = salping/o, -salpinx

ovulation
   ovul/o = egg
   -ation = process of

Be Careful!

Do not confuse
ureter/o, *which means the ureter, with* **uter/o,** *which means uterus.*

perimetrium = perimetri/o

myometrium = myometri/o

endometrium = endometri/o

fundus = fund/o

cervix = cervic/o

rectouterine pouch = culd/o

Be Careful!

Don't confuse **culd/o,** *which means the rectouterine pouch, with* **colp/o,** *which means vagina.*

vagina = colp/o, vagin/o

convey the ova from the ovaries to the uterus. Fallopian tubes are also called **oviducts** or **uterine tubes.** Approximately every 28 days, in response to hormonal stimulation, the ovaries alternate releasing one ovum. This egg matures in one of the **follicles** (FALL ih kuls), which are tiny secretory sacs within an ovary. The **pituitary** (pih TOO ih tair ee) **gland,** an endocrine gland located in the cranial cavity, secretes two hormones that influence the activity of the ovaries. **Follicle-stimulating hormone (FSH)** causes the ovarian follicles to begin to mature and secrete estrogen. Because of the increase of estrogen in the bloodstream, **luteinizing** (LOO tin eye zing) **hormone (LH)** is released by the anterior lobe of the pituitary gland. LH then stimulates the follicle to mature and release its ovum **(ovulation)** and aids in the development of the **corpus luteum** (KORE pus LOO tee um). The corpus luteum is then responsible for secreting **estrogen** (ES troh jen) and **progesterone** (proh JES teh roan), hormones responsible for female secondary sex characteristics and the cyclical maintenance of the uterus for pregnancy.

If two eggs are released and fertilized, the resulting twins will be termed **fraternal,** because they will be no more or less alike in appearance than brothers (or sisters) occurring in sequential pregnancies. If, however, one of the fertilized eggs divides and forms two infants, these are **identical** twins, who share the same appearance and genetic material.

Fallopian Tubes
Once the mature ovum has been released, it is drawn into the **fimbriae** (FIM bree ee) (*sing.* fimbria), the feathery ends of the fallopian tube (see Fig. 8-1). These tubes, about the width of a pencil, and about as long (10 to 12 cm), transport the ovum to the uterus. The fallopian tubes (also called *oviducts* or *uterine tubes*) and the ovaries make up what is called the **uterine adnexa** (YOO tuh rin add NECKS ah), or accessory organs of the uterus.

Uterus
Once the ovum has traversed the fallopian tube, it is secreted into the uterus, or womb, a pear-shaped organ that is designed to nurture a developing embryo/fetus (see Fig. 8-1). The uterus is composed of three layers: the outer layer, called the **perimetrium** (pair ih MEE tree um), or serosa; the **myometrium** (mye oh MEE tree um), or muscle layer; and the **endometrium** (en doh MEE tree um), the lining of the uterus. As a whole, it can be divided into several areas. The body or **corpus** (which means *body* in Latin) is the large central area; the **fundus** (FUN dus) is the raised area at the top of the uterus between the outlets for the fallopian tubes; and the **cervix** (SUR vicks) **(Cx)** is the narrowed lower area, often referred to as the neck of the uterus. The opening of the cervix is called the **cervical os.**

Rectouterine Pouch
An area associated with the female reproductive system that does not play a direct role in its function, the **rectouterine pouch** (reck toh YOO tur in), is also called **Douglas' cul-de-sac,** a space in the pelvic cavity between the uterus and the rectum.

Vagina
If the ovum does not become fertilized by a spermatozoon, the corpus luteum stops producing estrogen and progesterone, and the lining of the uterus is shed through the muscular, tubelike **vagina** by the process of **menstruation (menses).** The vagina extends from the uterine cervix to the vulva (the external genitalia).

EXERCISE 1: Combining Forms for Internal Female Genitalia

Match the following. There may be more than one answer per question. Answers may be used more than once.

_____ 1. culd/o   _____ 5. colp/o   _____ 9. ovari/o

_____ 2. oophor/o   _____ 6. ov/o   _____ 10. uter/o

_____ 3. metr/o   _____ 7. salping/o   _____ 11. vagin/o

_____ 4. hyster/o   _____ 8. cervic/o   _____ 12. men/o

A. uterus
B. vagina
C. fallopian tube
D. cervix
E. rectouterine pouch
F. ovary
G. female germ cell
H. menstruation, menses

Decode the terms.

13. supracervical _____

14. intrauterine _____

15. premenstrual _____

16. transvaginal _____

 EXERCISE 2: Internal Female Anatomy

Label the drawing below using the terms provided.

ovary
fallopian tube
cervix
endometrium
myometrium
fimbriae
perimetrium
vagina

Label the drawing below using the terms provided.

vagina
rectouterine pouch
rectum
cervix
ovary
urinary bladder
ureter
urethra
fallopian tube

vulva = vulv/o, episi/o

hymen = hymen/o

labia = labi/o

clitoris = clitorid/o

perineum = perine/o

Bartholin gland = bartholin/o

breast = mamm/o, mast/o

milk = lact/o, galact/o

nipple = papill/o, thel/e

External Genitalia

The external female genitalia collectively are called the **vulva** (VUL vah) (Fig. 8-2). The vulva consists of the vaginal opening, or **orifice** (ORE ih fis); the membrane covering the opening, or **hymen** (HYE men); the two folds of skin surrounding the opening, or **labia majora** (LAY bee ah muh JOR ah) (the larger folds) and **labia minora** (LAY bee ah min NOR uh) (the smaller folds); the **clitoris** (KLIT uh ris), which is sensitive, erectile tissue; and the **perineum** (pair ih NEE um), the area between the opening of the vagina and the anus. The paired glands in the vulva that secrete a mucous lubricant for the vagina are the **Bartholin** (BAR toh lin) **glands.** The **mons pubis** (mons PYOO bis) is a fatty cushion of tissue over the pubic bone.

The Breast

The **breasts,** or mammary glands, function to secrete milk. The breast tissue is composed of glandular **milk**-producing, fatty, and fibrous tissue. The **nipple** of the breast is the **mammary papilla** (MAM uh ree puh PILL ah) (*pl.* **papillae**), and the darker colored skin surrounding the nipple is the **areola** (ah REE oh lah) (*pl.* **areolae**) (Fig. 8-3).

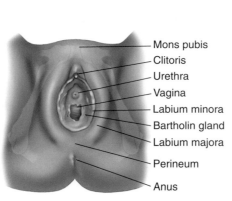

Fig. 8-2 Female external genitalia.

Fig. 8-3 Breast quadrants.

EXERCISE 3: External Female Genitalia and the Breast

Match the following combining forms with their meanings. There may be more than one answer.

_____ 1. vulva   _____ 6. breast   A. galact/o   H. perine/o
                                                  B. episi/o   I. lact/o
_____ 2. nipple   _____ 7. perineum   C. bartholin/o   J. vulv/o
                                                  D. papill/o   K. mast/o
_____ 3. hymen   _____ 8. Bartholin glands E. mamm/o   L. labi/o
                                                  F. thel/e   M. clitorid/o
_____ 4. milk   _____ 9. clitoris   G. hymen/o

_____ 5. labia

Decode the terms.

10. interlabial _____

11. intramammary _____

 *You can review the anatomy of the female reproductive system by clicking on **Body Spectrum Electronic Anatomy Coloring Book → Reproductive → Female.***

PREGNANCY AND DELIVERY

Pregnancy begins with the fertilization of an ovum by a spermatozoon, often in the fallopian tube, as the ovum travels toward the uterus (Fig. 8-4). Conception is usually the result of sexual intercourse (also termed *copulation* or *coitus*). However, other methods of conception are possible if the couple has difficulty conceiving. These methods are discussed in the section on therapeutic interventions and may include artificial insemination (AI) and in vitro fertilization (IVF).

pregnancy = gravid/o, -gravida, -cyesis

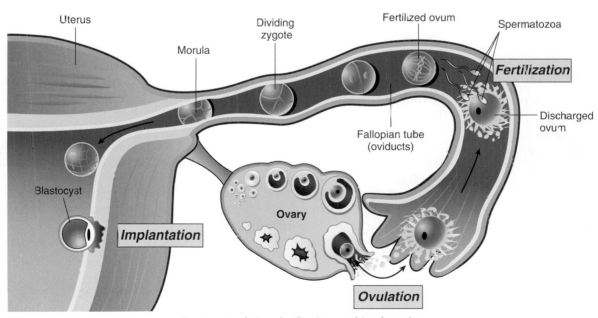

Fig. 8-4 Ovulation, fertilization, and implantation.

Fig. 8-5 The developing embryo.

The fertilized egg, or **zygote** (ZYE gote), divides as it moves through the fallopian tube to the uterus, where it becomes implanted. In the first few days after fertilization, when the zygote has become a solid ball of cells from repeated divisions, it is called a **morula**. As it continues to develop, it moves from the fallopian tube into the uterus and implants into the uterine wall. At this point it is called a **blastocyst**.

During implantation, the zygote functions as an endocrine gland by secreting **human chorionic gonadotropin (hCG)** (kore ee AH nick goh nad doh TROH pin). The function of the hormone is to prevent the corpus luteum from deteriorating, which allows the continued production of estrogen and progesterone to support the pregnancy and prevent menstruation. From the third to the eighth week of life, the organism is called an **embryo** (EM bree oh). From the ninth through the thirty-eighth week of life (a normal length for **gestation** [jes TAY shun], or pregnancy), it is called a **fetus** (FEE tus).

At the same time that the embryo is developing, extraembryonic membranes are forming to sustain the pregnancy: Two of these, the **amnion** (AM nee on) and the **chorion** (KORE ee on), form the inner and outer sacs that contain the embryo (Fig. 8-5). The fluid that forms inside the amnion is the **amniotic** (am nee AH tick) **fluid.** It functions to cushion the embryo, protect it against temperature changes, and allow it to move. The **placenta** (plah SEN tah) is a highly vascular structure that acts as a physical communication between the mother and the embryo. The **umbilical** (um BILL ih kul) **cord** is the tissue that connects the embryo to the placenta (and hence to the mother). When the baby is delivered, the umbilical cord is cut, and the baby is then dependent on his/her own body for all physiologic processes. The remaining "scar" is the **umbilicus** (um BILL il kus), or navel. The delivery of an infant is termed **parturition** (par tur RIH shun).

A woman who is pregnant for the first time is a **primigravida**. If she has two or more pregnancies, she is referred to as a **multigravida**. If she has never been pregnant, she is a **nulligravida.**

A woman who has delivered her first baby is referred to as a **primipara**. If she delivers more than one baby, she is a **multipara**. A woman who has never delivered a child is referred to as a **nullipara.**

The abbreviation GPA is used in obstetric notation to indicate the *number of pregnancies* (G for gravida), *the number of deliveries* of a live or stillborn infant at more than 20 weeks of gestation (P for para), and *the number of miscarriages/abortions* that occur before 20 weeks of gestation (A for abortion). A woman described as G4P3A1 has had 4 pregnancies, 3 deliveries, and 1 abortion.

---

fetus = fet/o

amnion = amni/o, amnion/o, -amnios

chorion = chori/o, chorion/o

placenta = placent/o

umbilicus = omphal/o, umbilic/o

parturition = part/o, -para, -partum, -tocia

birth, born = nat/o

primigravida
 primi- = first
 -gravida = pregnancy

multigravida
 multi- = many
 -gravida = pregnancy

nulligravida
 nulli- = none
 -gravida = pregnancy

The terms **antenatal** and **prenatal** both mean "pertaining to before birth," and **postnatal** means "pertaining to after birth." **Antepartum** means "before delivery," and **postpartum** means "after delivery." The **puerperium** (pyoo ur PER ee um) is the approximate 6-week time period after childbirth.

Babies born before 37 weeks are referred to as *premature infants*. Those weighing less than 2500 g (5 lbs, 8 oz) are referred to as *low–birth-weight infants*.

Time periods are important when using the terminology of pregnancy. A normal pregnancy is approximately 38 to 40 weeks. Each pregnancy is divided into three equal **trimesters** of 3 months each. The first trimester is week 1 to 12, the second trimester is week 13 to 28, and the third trimester is week 29 to the day of delivery. The **estimated date of delivery (EDD)** of the infant can be calculated using a formula, Naegli's rule, that uses the first day of a woman's **last menstrual period (LMP)**, subtracts 3 months and adds 7 days to come up with a "due" date.

primipara	
primi- = first	
-para = delivery	
multipara	
multi- = many	
-para = delivery	
nullipara	
nulli- = none	
-para = delivery	
puerper/o = childbirth	

 EXERCISE 4: Pregnancy

Match the word parts with their correct meanings. There may be more than one answer.

_____ 1. pregnancy

_____ 2. navel

_____ 3. labor, delivery

_____ 4. organ of communication between mother and baby

_____ 5. inner sac that encircles the embryo

_____ 6. outer sac that encircles the embryo

_____ 7. fetus

_____ 8. birth

A. -tocia
B. omphal/o
C. gravid/o
D. amni/o
E. umbilic/o
F. chori/o
G. nat/o
H. -para
I. -cyesis
J. chorion/o
K. -gravida
L. fet/o
M. placent/o

Decode the terms.

9. antenatal _____

10. periumbilical _____

 EXERCISE 5: Pregnancy

Label the drawing using the terms provided.

embryo
umbilical cord
chorion
placenta
yolk sac
amnion
amniotic fluid
chorionic villi

*Choose **Hear It, Spell It** to practice spelling the anatomy and physiology terms you have learned in this chapter.*

The following word part tables can be used as a reference and a review of the anatomy and physiology word parts you have learned for the female reproductive system.

Combining and Adjective Forms for the Anatomy and Physiology of the Female Reproductive System

Meaning	Combining Form	Adjective Form
amnion	amni/o, amnion/o	amniotic
Bartholin gland	bartholin/o	
birth, born	nat/o	natal
breast	mamm/o, mast/o	mammary
cervix	cervic/o	cervical
chorion	chori/o, chorion/o	chorionic
clitoris	clitorid/o	
endometrium	endometri/o	endometrial
fallopian tube	salping/o, fallopi/o	salpingeal, fallopian
female	gynec/o	
fetus	fet/o	fetal
fundus	fund/o	fundal
hymen	hymen/o	hymenal
labia	labi/o	labial
menstruation, menses	men/o	menstrual
milk	lact/o, galact/o	lactic, galactic
myometrium	myometri/o	myometrial
nipple	papill/o, thel/e	papillary, thelial
ovary	oophor/o, ovari/o	ovarian
ovum, egg	ov/o, ov/i, ovul/o, o/o	
parturition, delivery	part/o	
perimetrium	perimetri/o	perimetrial
perineum	perine/o	perineal
placenta	placent/o	placental
pregnancy	gravid/o	
puerperium	puerper/o	
rectouterine pouch	culd/o	
umbilicus, navel	omphal/o, umbilic/o	umbilical, omphalic
uterus	hyster/o, metri/o, metr/o, uter/o	uterine
vagina	colp/o, vagin/o	vaginal
vulva	vulv/o, episi/o	vulvar

Prefixes for the Anatomy and Physiology of the Female Reproductive System

Prefix	Meaning
endo-	within
multi-	many
neo-	new
nulli-	none
peri-	surrounding
primi-	first

Suffixes for the Anatomy and Physiology of the Female Reproductive System

Suffix	Meaning
-arche	beginning
-ation	process of
-gravida, -cyesis	pregnancy, gestation
-ic, -al, -ine	pertaining to
-ician, -logist	one who specializes in the study of
-para, -partum, -tocia	delivery, parturition
-pause	stop, cease
-salpinx	fallopian tube
-um	structure

 *Click on **Label It** to practice labeling the female reproductive system.*

PATHOLOGY

Terms Related to Disorders of the Ovaries

Term	Word Origin	Definition
anovulation an ah vyoo LAY shun	*an-* without *ovul/o* ovum *-ation* process of	Failure of the ovary to release an ovum.
oophoritis oh off oh RYE tis	*oophor/o* ovary *-itis* inflammation	Inflammation of an ovary.
polycystic ovary syndrome (PCOS) pall ee SIS tick	*poly-* many *cyst/o* sac, cyst *-ic* pertaining to	Bilateral presence of numerous cysts, caused by a hormonal abnormality leading to the secretion of androgens. Can cause acne, facial hair, and infertility.

Terms Related to Disorders of the Fallopian Tubes

Term	Word Origin	Definition
adhesions, fallopian tubes add HEE zhuns		Scar tissue that binds surfaces together; a sequela of **pelvic inflammatory disease (PID)**, in which (as a result of the inflammation) the tubes heal closed, causing infertility.
hematosalpinx hee mah toh SAL pinks	*hemat/o* blood *-salpinx* fallopian tube	Condition of blood in a fallopian tube; usually caused by a tubal pregnancy.
hydrosalpinx hye droh SAL pinks	*hydr/o* fluid, water *-salpinx* fallopian tube	Condition of fluid in a fallopian tube.
pyosalpinx pye oh SAL pinks	*py/o* pus *-salpinx* fallopian tube	Condition of pus in a fallopian tube.
salpingitis sal pin JYE tis	*salping/o* fallopian tube *-itis* inflammation	Inflammation of a fallopian tube.

EXERCISE 6: Ovarian and Fallopian Tube Disorders

Fill in the blanks with the terms provided.

polycystic ovary syndrome, adhesions, hematosalpinx, salpingitis, hydrosalpinx, pyosalpinx

1. condition of pus in the fallopian tubes _____

2. scar tissue that binds surfaces together _____

3. inflammation of the fallopian tubes _____

4. condition of fluid in the fallopian tubes _____

5. condition of multiple cysts on both ovaries leading to acne, facial hair, and infertility

_____

Decode the terms.

6. oophoritis _____

7. anovulation _____

8. hematosalpinx _____

Case Study   Magda Petersen

Magda Petersen is visiting her obstetrician to discuss her inability to become pregnant. She had salpingitis as a teenager. Tests show a bilateral occlusion of both oviducts. Magda is scheduled for salpingolysis.

1. What is the combining form that means fallopian tube? _____

2. Which term means "an inflammation of the fallopian tubes?" _____

3. Obstetricians are medical doctors who treat women during _____.

4. What is another term that means fallopian tube? _____

Terms Related to Disorders of the Uterus

Term	Word Origin	Definition
endometritis en doh mee TRY tis	*endometri/o* endometrium *-itis* inflammation	Inflammation of the inner layer of the uterus, the endometrium.
endometriosis en doh mee tree OH sis	*endometri/o* endometrium *-osis* abnormal condition	Condition in which the tissue that makes up the lining of the uterus, the endometrium, is found ectopically (outside the uterus); causes are unknown (Fig. 8-6).
hysteroptosis hiss tur op TOH sis	*hyster/o* uterus *-ptosis* drooping, sagging	Falling or sliding of the uterus from its normal location in the body. Also called **uterine prolapse** (Fig. 8-7).
retroflexion of uterus reh troh FLECK shun	*retro-* backward *flex/o* bend *-ion* process	Condition in which the body of the uterus is bent backward, forming an angle with the cervix.

Fig. 8-6 *Black spots* indicate common sites of endometriosis.

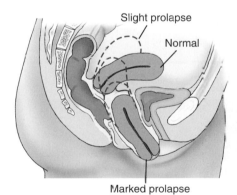

Slight prolapse

Normal

Marked prolapse

Fig. 8-7 Prolapse of uterus.

Terms Related to Disorders of the Cervix

Term	Word Origin	Definition
cervicitis sur vih SYE tis	*cervic/o* cervix *-itis* inflammation	Inflammation of the cervix.
leukorrhea loo kuh REE ah	*leuk/o* white *-rrhea* discharge, flow	Whitish discharge usually resulting from an inflammation of the cervix.

EXERCISE 7: Disorders of the Uterus and Cervix

Fill in the blanks with the terms provided.

leukorrhea, endometriosis, retroflexion of uterus

1. white cervical discharge _____

2. uterus bent toward spine _____

3. condition of ectopic endometrial tissue _____

Decode the terms.

4. endometritis _____

5. hysteroptosis _____

6. cervicitis _____

Terms Related to Disorders of the Vagina and Vulva

Term	Word Origin	Definition
vaginal prolapse PRO laps	*pro-* forward *-lapse* fall	Downward displacement of the vagina. Also called **colpoptosis** (kohl pop TOH sis).
vaginitis vaj ih NYE tis	*vagin/o* vagina *-itis* inflammation	Inflammation of the vagina.
vulvitis vul VYE tis	*vulv/o* vulva *-itis* inflammation	Inflammation of the external female genitalia.
vulvodynia vul voh DIN ee ah	*vulv/o* vulva *-dynia* pain	Idiopathic syndrome of nonspecific complaints of pain of the vulva.
vulvovaginitis vul voh vaj ih NYE tis	*vulv/o* vulva *vagin/o* vagina *-itis* inflammation	Inflammation of the vulva and the vagina.

Terms Related to Disorders of the Breast

Term	Word Origin	Definition
galactorrhea gah lack toh REE ah	*galact/o* milk *-rrhea* flow, discharge	An abnormal discharge of milk from the breasts.
mastitis mass TYE tis	*mast/o* breast *-itis* inflammation	Inflammation of the breast.
mastoptosis mass top TOH sis	*mast/o* breast *-ptosis* drooping, sagging	Downward displacement of the breasts.
thelitis thee LYE tis	*thel/e* nipple *-itis* inflammation	Inflammation of the nipples; also referred to as **acromastitis** (ack kroh mass TYE tis), meaning an inflammation of the extremities of the breast.

EXERCISE 8: Disorders of the Vagina, Vulva, and Breasts

Fill in the blanks with the terms provided.

vulvitis, thelitis, mastitis, vulvodynia, vaginal prolapse, vulvovaginitis

1. also known as colpoptosis _____

2. inflammation of the external female genitalia _____

3. pain of external female genitalia _____

4. also known as acromastitis _____

5. inflammation of the breast _____

6. inflammation of female external genitalia and vagina _____

Decode the terms.

7. galactorrhea _____

8. mastoptosis _____

9. vaginitis _____

Terms Related to Menstrual Disorders

Term	Word Origin	Definition
amenorrhea ah men uh REE ah	*a-* without *men/o* menses *-rrhea* discharge	Lack of menstrual flow. This is a normal, expected condition before puberty, after menopause, and during pregnancy.
dysfunctional uterine bleeding (DUB)		Abnormal uterine bleeding not caused by a tumor, inflammation, or pregnancy. **PMB** stands for **postmenopausal bleeding.**
dysmenorrhea diss men uh REE ah	*dys-* painful *men/o* menses *-rrhea* discharge	Painful menstrual flow, cramps.
menometrorrhagia men oh meh troh RAH zsa	*men/o* menses *metr/o* uterus *-rrhagia* bursting forth	Excessive menstrual flow and uterine bleeding other than that caused by menstruation.
menorrhagia men or RAH zsa	*men/o* menses *-rrhagia* bursting forth	Abnormally heavy menstrual flow or prolonged menstrual period. May be an indication of fibroids.
metrorrhagia meh troh RAH zsa	*metr/o* uterus *-rrhagia* bursting forth	Uterine bleeding other than that caused by menstruation. May be caused by uterine lesions.
oligomenorrhea oh lig oh men oh REE ah	*olig/o* scanty, few *men/o* menses *-rrhea* discharge	Abnormally light or infrequent menstrual flow; *menorrhea* refers to the normal discharge of blood and tissue from the uterus.
polymenorrhea pol ee men or REE ah	*poly-* many *men/o* menses *-rrhea* discharge	Abnormally frequent menstrual flow.

Continued

Terms Related to Menstrual Disorders—cont'd		
Term	Word Origin	Definition
premenstrual dysphoric disorder (PMDD)	*pre-* before *menstru/o* menses *-al* pertaining to *dys-* abnormal *phor/o* carry, bear *-ic* pertaining to	Mood disorder that includes depression, irritability, fatigue, changes in appetite or sleep, and difficulty in concentrating; occurs 1 to 2 weeks before the onset of the menstrual flow.
premenstrual syndrome (PMS)	*pre-* before *menstru/o* menses *-al* pertaining to *syn-* together *-drome* run	Poorly understood group of symptoms that occur in some women on a cyclical basis: Breast pain, irritability, fluid retention, headache, and lack of coordination are some of the symptoms.

EXERCISE 9: Menstrual Disorders

Fill in the blanks with the terms provided.

premenstrual syndrome, menometrorrhagia, dysfunctional uterine bleeding, menorrhagia, premenstrual dysphoric disorder

1. What is the term for an excessively heavy menstrual period? _____

2. What is the term for bleeding from the uterus that is not a result of menstruation?

   _____

3. What is the term for the group of symptoms that occurs on a cyclical basis that include irritability, retention of fluid, and lack of coordination? _____

4. What is the term for excessive menstrual and dysfunctional bleeding? _____

5. What mood disorder occurs before menstruation and includes depression, appetite loss, and sleep disorders? _____

6. What is the term for uterine bleeding not caused by a tumor, inflammation, or pregnancy?

   _____

Decode the terms.

7. dysmenorrhea _____

8. amenorrhea _____

9. polymenorrhea _____

10. oligomenorrhea _____

Case Study — Antoinette Song

Antoinette Song, who is 33 years old, has pain in her lower left quadrant that she thinks is related to her menstrual cycle. She reports that her cycles are irregular and very, very light. She says that not having a menstrual cycle was "not a problem for her" in her twenties, but now that she is thinking of having a family, she wants to be healthy. Previous history includes vaginitis and cystitis.

Her gynecologist suspects a possible ovarian cyst and tells Antoinette that she wants her to have sonography of her ovaries.

1. What is the term for a light or scanty menstrual flow? _____

2. What is the term for the absence of a menstrual flow? _____

3. Vaginitis is a/an _____ of the vagina.

4. Cystitis is inflammation of the _____.

5. What is the term that means painful menstrual cramps? _____

Infertility

Couples who are infertile are unable to produce offspring. The causes of infertility in the female may be endometriosis, ovulation problems, poor egg quality, polycystic ovarian syndrome, or female tube blockages. In the male, the problem may be lack of sperm production or viability, or male tube blockages. His partner may even be allergic to his sperm. Treatments are dependent on the variety of causal factors and are discussed in the Therapeutic Interventions and Pharmacology sections.

Terms Related to Pregnancy Disorders

Term	Word Origin	Definition
abruptio placentae ah BRUP she oh plah SEN tee		Premature separation of the placenta from the uterine wall; may result in a severe hemorrhage that can threaten both infant and maternal lives. Also called **ablatio** (ah BLAY she oh) **placentae** (Fig. 8-8).
agalactia a gah LACK tee ah	**a-** without **galact/o** milk **-ia** condition	Condition of mother's inability to produce milk.
cephalopelvic disproportion seh fah loh PELL vick	**cephal/o** head **pelv/i** pelvis **-ic** pertaining to	Condition in which the infant's head is larger than the pelvic outlet it must pass through, thereby inhibiting normal labor and birth. It is one of the indications for a cesarean section (C-section, CS).
eclampsia eh KLAMP see ah		Extremely serious form of hypertension secondary to pregnancy. Patients are at risk for coma, convulsions, and death.
ectopic pregnancy eck TAH pick	**ec-** out **top/o** place **-ic** pertaining to	Implantation of the embryo in any location but the uterus (Fig. 8-9).
erythroblastosis fetalis eh RITH roh blas toh sis feh TAL is	**erythr/o** red (blood cell) **blast/o** immature **-osis** abnormal condition	Condition in which the mother is Rhesus factor (Rh) negative and her fetus is Rh positive, causing the mother to form antibodies to the Rh-positive factor. Subsequent Rh-positive pregnancies will be in jeopardy because the mother's anti-Rh antibodies will cross the placenta and destroy fetal blood cells (Fig. 8-10).

Continued

Terms Related to Pregnancy Disorders—cont'd

Term	Word Origin	Definition
miscarriage/abortion		Termination of a pregnancy before the fetus is viable. If spontaneous, it may be termed a **miscarriage** or a **spontaneous abortion**. If induced, it can be referred to as a **therapeutic abortion**.
oligohydramnios oh lih goh hye DRAM nee ohs	*olig/o* scanty *hydr/o* water, fluid *-amnios* amnion	Condition of low or missing amniotic fluid.
placenta previa plah SEN tah PREE vee ah	*previa* in front of	Placenta that is malpositioned in the uterus so that it covers the opening of the cervix.
polyhydramnios pah lee hye DRAM nee ohs	*poly-* excessive *hydr/o* water, fluid *-amnios* amnion	Condition of excessive amniotic fluid.
preeclampsia pree eh KLAMP see ah	*pre-* before	Abnormal condition of pregnancy with unknown cause, marked by hypertension, edema, and proteinuria. Formerly called **toxemia of pregnancy.**

Fig. 8-8 Abruptio placentae.

Fig. 8-9 Sites of ectopic pregnancy.

Fig. 8-10 Diagram illustrating the concept of Rhesus factor (Rh) sensitization.

Terms Related to Neonatal Disorders

Term	Word Origin	Definition
meconium staining meh KOH nee um		Refers to fetal defecation while in utero and indicates fetal distress. Meconium is the first feces of the newborn.
nuchal cord NOO kul	*nuch/o* neck *-al* pertaining to	Abnormal but common occurrence of the umbilical cord wrapped around the neck of the neonate.

EXERCISE 10: Disorders of Pregnancy and the Newborn

Fill in the blanks with the terms provided.

ectopic pregnancy, nuchal cord, abortion, eclampsia, placenta previa, meconium, erythroblastosis fetalis, preeclampsia, abruptio placentae, cephalopelvic disproportion

1. What are the first feces of the newborn called? _____

2. What is the term for the cord wrapped around the neck of the neonate?

3. What is the term for a placenta that separates prematurely from the wall of the uterus?

4. What is the term for a baby's head being larger than the pelvic outlet?

5. What is the term for a pregnancy that takes place anywhere but in the uterus?

6. What is the term for the termination of a pregnancy, intentionally or not, before the fetus is viable?

7. What is the term for a complication of pregnancy characterized by protein in the mother's urine, hypertension, and swelling? _____

8. What is the term for a placenta that is attached to the opening of the cervix?

9. What is the term for a severe form of toxemia that may result in convulsions, coma, and death?

10. Incompatibility between Rh factors of mother and baby that leads to destruction of red blood cells in the fetus is called _____.

Build the terms.

11.   condition of no milk _____

12.   excessive amniotic fluid _____

13.   scanty amniotic fluid _____

Terms Related to Benign Neoplasms

Term	Word Origin	Definition
cervical intraepithelial neoplasia (CIN) SUR vih kull intruh ehp ih THEE lee ahl nee oh PLAY zha	*cervic/o* cervix *-al* pertaining to *neo-* new *-plasia* formation, development	Also termed "cervical dysplasia," this abnormal cell growth may or may not develop into cancer. It is reported in grades I, II, and III, with I being the mildest and III the most severe.
endometrial hyperplasia en doh MEE tree uhl hye pur PLAY zha	*endometri/o* endometrium *-al* pertaining to *hyper-* excessive *-plasia* formation, development	An excessive development of cells in the lining of the uterus; this condition is benign but can become malignant.
fibroadenoma of the breast fye broh add eh NOH mah	*fibr/o* fiber *aden/o* gland *-oma* tumor, mass	Noncancerous breast tumors composed of fibrous and glandular tissue (Fig. 8-11).
fibrocystic changes of the breast	*fibr/o* fiber *cyst/o* sac, cyst *-ic* pertaining to	Formerly called "fibrocystic disease," this benign condition affects the glandular and stromal tissue. The changes may take a variety of forms with typical symptoms of cysts, lumpiness, and/or pain.
leiomyoma of the uterus lye oh mye OH mah	*leiomy/o* smooth muscle *-oma* tumor, mass	Also termed **fibroids,** these smooth muscle tumors of the uterus are usually nonpainful growths, which may be removed surgically (Fig. 8-12).

Fig. 8-11 Fibroadenoma in the right *(R)* breast.

Fig. 8-12 Leiomyoma of the uterus.

Terms Related to Benign Neoplasms—cont'd

Term	Word Origin	Definition
mature teratoma of the ovary tare ih TOH mah	*terat/o* deformity *-oma* tumor, mass	Also termed "dermoid cysts," these usually noncancerous ovarian growths arise from germ cells.
ovarian cyst	*ovari/o* ovary *-an* pertaining to	Benign, fluid-filled sac. Can be either a follicular cyst, which occurs when a follicle does not rupture at ovulation, or a cyst of the corpus luteum, which is caused when it does not continue its transformation (Fig. 8-13).

 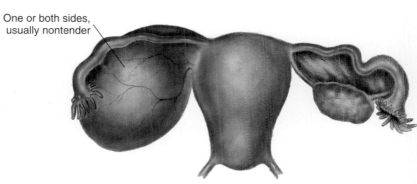

One or both sides, usually nontender

Fig. 8-13 Ovarian cyst.

Terms Related to Malignant Neoplasms

Term	Word Origin	Definition
choriocarcinoma kore ee oh kar sih NOH mah	*chori/o* chorion *-carcinoma* cancer of epithelial origin	A malignant tumor arising from the chorionic membrane surrounding the fetus.
endometrial adenocarcinoma en doh MEE tree uhl add eh noh kar sih NOH mah	*endometri/o* endometrium *-al* pertaining to *aden/o* gland *-carcinoma* cancer of epithelial origin	By far the most common cancer of the uterus, this type develops from the cells that line the uterus.
epithelial ovarian cancer (EOC) epp ih THEE lee uhl	*epitheli/o* epithelium *-al* pertaining to *ovari/o* ovary *-an* pertaining to	An inherited mutation of the *BRCA1* or *BRCA2* gene is linked to the risk of this malignancy and breast cancer.
infiltrating ductal carcinoma (IDC)	*duct/o* carry *-al* pertaining to *-carcinoma* cancer of epithelial origin	The most common type of breast cancer, IDC arises from the cells that line the milk ducts.
leiomyosarcoma lye oh mye oh sar KOH mah	*leiomy/o* smooth muscle *-sarcoma* cancerous tumor of connective tissue	A rare type of cancer of the smooth muscle of the uterus.

Continued

Terms Related to Malignant Neoplasms—cont'd

Term	Word Origin	Definition
lobular carcinoma LAH byoo lure kar sih NOH mah	*lobul/o* small lobe *-ar* pertaining to *-carcinoma* cancer of epithelial origin	About 15% of breast cancers are lobular carcinomas. These tumors begin in the glandular tissue of the breast at the ends of the milk ducts (Fig. 8-14).
Paget disease of the breast PAJ ett		A rare form of cancer, this malignancy of the nipple can occur in men and women.
squamous cell carcinoma of the cervix SKWAY muss	*squam/o* scaly *-ous* pertaining to *-carcinoma* cancer of epithelial origin	The most common type of cervical cancer. Thought to be caused by the human papilloma virus (HPV), it is also one of the most curable cancers if detected in its early stage.

Fig. 8-14 Magnetic resonance imaging (MRI) breast image using contrast and demonstrating lobular carcinoma in the left breast *(arrow).*

EXERCISE 11: Neoplasms

Match the benign neoplasms with their definitions.

_____ 1. ovarian cyst

_____ 2. endometrial hyperplasia

_____ 3. cervical intraepithelial neoplasia (CIN)

_____ 4. fibroadenoma of breast

_____ 5. mature teratoma of ovary

_____ 6. fibrocystic changes of breast

_____ 7. leiomyoma of uterus

A. fibroid
B. dermoid cyst
C. benign breast tumors of fibrous and glandular tissue
D. cervical dysplasia
E. benign, fluid-filled sac
F. excessive cell development in lining of uterus
G. benign breast condition with symptoms of cysts, lumpiness, and/or pain

Match the malignant neoplasms with their definitions.

_____ 8. endometrial adenocarcinoma

_____ 9. lobular carcinoma

_____ 10. Paget disease of the breast

_____ 11. infiltrating ductal carcinoma (IDC)

_____ 12. epithelial ovarian cancer (EOC)

_____ 13. squamous cell carcinoma of the cervix

_____ 14. leiomyosarcoma of the uterus

A. most common cancer of the uterus
B. rare smooth muscle tumor of uterus
C. breast cancer arising from ends of milk ducts
D. most common type of cervical cancer
E. inherited mutation linked to this form of ovarian cancer
F. most common type of breast cancer arising from cells that line milk ducts
G. malignancy of nipple

Medical Record Olivia Carter

CARTER, OLIVIA M. - 599333 Opened by MACHAR A, LOUIS MD

Task   Edit   View   Time Scale   Options   Help

As Of 13:02

CARTER, OLIVIA M.	Age: 19 years	Sex: Female	Loc: WHC-SMMC
	DOB: 05/27/1996	MRN: 599333	FIN: 3506004

Reference Text Browser | Form Browser | Medication Profile

Orders | Last 48 Hours | ED | Lab | Radiology | **Assessments** | Surgery | Clinical Notes | Pt. Info | Pt. Schedule | Task List | I & O | MAR

Flowsheet: Assessments   Level: Progress Note   ● Table ○ Group ○ List

Navigator

✓ Progress Note

This 19-year-old female states that her last menstrual period ended approximately 2 weeks ago. She reports she had heavy vaginal bleeding with passage of clots and crampy lower abdominal pain, and she felt weak. She is on OCPs.

　Gravida 1 para 1, history of normal vaginal delivery approximately 1 year ago. History of PID before pregnancy and recurrent dysmenorrhea.

　There is a minimum amount of blood in the vaginal vault. No tissue noted. Cervix is normal in appearance. The os is closed. The fundus of the uterus is not well appreciated. Serum pregnancy test was negative. WBC was 11,300 with normal Hgb and Hct.

　Vaginal bleeding, possibly involving past pelvic inflammatory disease.

PROD | MAHAFC | 25 May 2015 | 13:02

EXERCISE 12: Progress Note

Using the preceding progress note, answer the following questions.

1. What does gravida 1 para 1 mean? _____

2. What is the meaning of the abbreviation for the disorder she had before pregnancy?

    _____

3. How do you know that she experienced painful menstrual periods? _____

4. What type of pregnancy test is a "serum pregnancy test?"

    _____

 Click on **Hear It, Spell It** to practice spelling the pathology terms that you have learned in this chapter. To review the pathology terms in this chapter, play **Medical Millionaire.**

 Age Matters

Pediatrics

A review of the most recent national statistics for all diagnoses for hospital inpatients for newborns and children under the age of 17 revealed some surprises. For neonates (28 days old and younger), diagnoses that included complications of delivery were common. Meconium staining and cord entanglement were high on the list. However, for fertile females between the ages of 1 and 17, the delivery of a single liveborn is second only to hypovolemia for all diagnoses. (Pneumonia and asthma follow close behind.) Still within the top 50 diagnoses are a large number of complications of delivery.

Geriatrics

Later in life, senior women are seen most often for neoplasms of the breast, uterus, cervix, and ovaries. Breast cancer alone will be diagnosed in one in eight women in their lifetime in this country.

DIAGNOSTIC PROCEDURES

Terms Related to Imaging

Term	Word Origin	Definition
cervicography sur vih KAH gruh fee	cervic/o cervix -graphy process of recording	Photographic procedure in which a specially designed 35-mm camera is used to image the entire cervix to produce a slide called a **cervigram.** It is used to detect early CIN or invasive cervical cancer. Can be combined with **colposcopy** or can be done independently.
hysterosalpingography (HSG) his tur oh sal pin GAH gruh fee	hyster/o uterus salping/o fallopian tube -graphy process of recording	X-ray procedure in which contrast medium is used to image the uterus and fallopian tubes (Fig. 8-15).

Terms Related to Imaging—cont'd

Term	Word Origin	Definition
mammography mam MOG gruh fee	*mamm/o* breast *-graphy* process of recording	Imaging technique for the early detection of breast cancer. The record produced is called a **mammogram** (see Fig. 8-11).
pelvimetry pell VIH meh tree	*pelv/i* pelvis *-metry* process of measurement	Measurement of the birth canal. Types of pelvimetry include clinical and x-ray, although x-ray pelvimetry is not commonly done.
sonography	*son/o* sound *-graphy* process of recording	Use of high-frequency sound waves to image the pelvic area **(pelvic sonography)** and the uterus **(sonohysterography)**. **Transvaginal sonography** of the pelvic cavity is obtained through the use of a probe introduced into the vagina (Fig. 8-16).

Fig. 8-15 A, Hysterosalpingography (HSG). **B,** Resulting hysterosalpingogram demonstrating coronal image of a dilated fallopian tube. When swollen with fluid, the tube bends and curls.

Fig. 8-16 A, Transvaginal sonography. **B,** Transvaginal sagittal view of the uterus. **C,** Uterus with fibroids *(right)* and fetus *(left)*.

⊗ **Be Careful!**   *Don't confuse the suffix* **-metry,** *which means the process of measurement, with* **metr/o,** *the combining form for the uterus.*

Terms Related to Endoscopies

Term	Word Origin	Definition
colposcopy kohl PAH skuh pee	*colp/o* vagina *-scopy* process of viewing	Endoscopic procedure used for a cervical/vaginal biopsy. The instrument used is called a **colposcope** (Fig. 8-17).
culdoscopy kull DAH skuh pee	*culd/o* cul-de-sac *-scopy* process of viewing	Endoscopic procedure used for biopsy of Douglas' cul-de-sac. The instrument used is called a **culdoscope**.
hysteroscopy hiss tuh RAH skuh pee	*hyster/o* uterus *-scopy* process of viewing	Endoscopic procedure used for a myomectomy (fibroid removal) or polypectomy (polyp removal). The instrument used is called a **hysteroscope**.
laparoscopy lap uh RAH skuh pee	*lapar/o* abdomen *-scopy* process of viewing	Endoscopic procedure for removing lesions (lysis) or performing a hysterectomy or an ovarian biopsy. The instrument used is called a **laparoscope**.

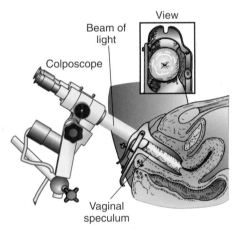

View

Beam of light

Colposcope

Vaginal speculum

Fig. 8-17 Colposcopy.

Terms Related to Laboratory Tests

Term	Word Origin	Definition
culdocentesis kull doh sen TEE sis	*culd/o* cul-de-sac *-centesis* surgical puncture	Removal of fluid and cells from the rectouterine pouch to detect dysplasia.
hormone levels		Laboratory measurements of the presence and extent of specific hormones in specimens of blood, urine, or body tissues. Information is useful in evaluating a range of conditions from pregnancy to menopause.
Papanicolaou (Pap) smear		Exfoliative cytology procedure useful for the detection of vaginal and cervical cancer (Fig. 8-18).

A   Swab   Cervix

Fig. 8-18 A, Obtaining a Pap smear. **B,** Malignant cells have enlarged hyperchromatic nuclei in contrast to the small nuclei of normal cells.

 EXERCISE 13: Female Reproductive Imaging Techniques, Endoscopies, and Laboratory Tests

Fill in the blanks with the terms provided.

cervicography, pelvimetry, hysterosalpingography, sonohysterography, hysteroscopy, laparoscopy, hormone levels, Pap smear

1. process of imaging the uterus and fallopian tubes _____

2. measurement of the birth canal _____

3. photographic recording of the cervix _____

4. endoscopic procedure for fibroid/polyp removal _____

5. high-frequency sound waves used to image the uterus _____

6. endoscopic procedure for removing lesions _____

7. lab test to detect a range of conditions from pregnancy to menopause _____

8. removal of cells from the cervix to detect abnormal cells _____

Decode the terms.

9. culdocentesis _____

10. mammography _____

11. culdoscopy _____

12. colposcopy _____

Case Study   *Marina Santiago*

Marina Santiago is a 35-year-old woman who is visiting her gynecologist with complaints of painful menses with heavy flow. Both have become increasingly worse during the past 6 months. Pelvic examination reveals a tender and enlarged uterus. After several diagnostic tests, this was confirmed along with the fact that she also had fragments of the uterine lining attached to the fallopian tubes and the ovaries.

1. Based on Marina's complaints and findings from the pelvic and diagnostic examination, her probable diagnosis would be _____.

2. A number of causes are believed to be responsible for this condition, including the backward flow during _____ of fragments of endometrium.

3. _____ means an abnormally heavy menstrual flow.

4. In severe cases, if her condition does not respond to drug therapy, a woman with this disorder may be advised to consider surgical removal of the uterus, a procedure known as a _____.

5. The condition is definitively diagnosed by means of hysterosalpingography, the process of recording of the _____ and _____.

Signs and Symptoms of Pregnancy

Presumptive	Probable	Positive
Amenorrhea	Goodell sign (softening of cervix)	Fetal heart tone (FHTs) heard
Chloasma (hyperpigmentation of face, "mask of pregnancy")	Hegar sign (softening of lower segment of uterus)	Fetal movement felt by examiner
Nausea and vomiting (N&V)	Ballottement of fetus (palpation to detect floating object)	Fetus observed on ultrasound
Fatigue	Positive pregnancy test	
Quickening	Chadwick sign (vaginal hyperemia)	

Terms Related to Prenatal Diagnosis

Term	Word Origin	Definition
alpha fetoprotein (AFP) test al fah fee toh PROH teen		Maternal serum (blood) AFP test performed between 14 and 19 weeks of gestation; may indicate a variety of conditions, such as neural tube defects (spina bifida is the most common finding) and multiple gestation.
amniocentesis am nee oh sen TEE sis	*amni/o* amnion *-centesis* surgical puncture	Removal and analysis of a sample of the amniotic fluid with the use of a guided needle through the abdomen of the mother into the amniotic sac to diagnose fetal abnormalities (Fig. 8-19).
chorionic villus sampling (CVS) kore ee AH nick VILL us	*chorion/o* chorion *-ic* pertaining to	Removal of a small piece of the chorionic villi that develop on the surface of the chorion, either transvaginally or through a small incision in the abdomen, to test for chromosomal abnormalities (Fig. 8-20).
contraction stress test (CST)		Test to predict fetal outcome and risk of intrauterine asphyxia by measuring fetal heart rate throughout a minimum of three contractions within a 10-minute period. Also called a **stress test** or **oxytocin challenge test.**
nonstress test (NST)		The fetus is monitored for a normal, expected acceleration of the fetal heart rate. A reactive NST should be followed by a CST and possible ultrasound studies.
pregnancy test		Test available in two forms: a standard over-the-counter (OTC) pregnancy test, which examines urine for the presence of hCG; and a serum (blood) pregnancy test performed in a physician's office or laboratory to get a quantitative hCG. A "triple-screen" is a blood test for hCG, AFP, and unconjugated estradiol (uE3).

Fig. 8-19 Amniocentesis.

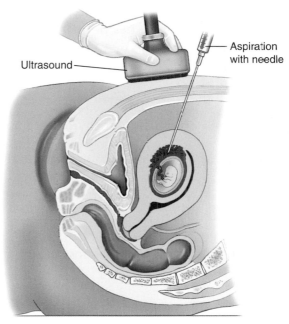

Fig. 8-20 Chorionic villus sampling (CVS).

Terms Related to Postnatal Diagnosis

Term	Word Origin	Definition
Apgar score		Rates the physical health of the infant with a set of criteria 1 minute and 5 minutes after birth.
congenital hypothyroidism test kon JEN ih tuhl hye poh THIGH royd iz um	*hypo-* below *thyroid/o* thyroid *-ism* condition	Test for deficient thyroid hormones. Undiscovered and untreated, this condition can lead to retarded growth and brain development. If caught at birth, oral doses of the missing thyroid hormone will allow normal development.
phenylketonuria (PKU) test fee null kee tone YOOR ee ah		Test for deficiency of enzyme phenylalanine hydroxylase, which is responsible for converting phenylalanine, found in certain foods, into tyrosine. Failure to treat this condition will lead to brain damage and mental retardation.

EXERCISE 14: Prenatal and Postnatal Diagnosis

Fill in the blanks with the terms provided.

alpha fetoprotein, human chorionic gonadotropin, Apgar score, nonstress test, chorionic villus sampling, contraction stress test, congenital hypothyroidism

1. What hormone does a pregnancy test look for? _____

2. What is the name of the test done 1 and 5 minutes after birth that scores the physical health of the

    neonate? _____

3. What is a measurement of fetal heart rate through contractions? _____

4. What test determines fetal health by measuring the heart rate? _____

5. What test of maternal blood between 14 and 19 weeks indicates neural tube defects and/or multiple

    gestation? _____

6. What is a condition of deficient thyroid hormones that is present at birth? _____

7. What test of a sample from the outer covering of the fetus determines chromosomal abnormalities?

    _____

Build the term.

8. removal of amniotic fluid for diagnostic testing _____

THERAPEUTIC INTERVENTIONS

Terms Related to Non-Pregnancy Procedures

Term	Word Origin	Definition
cervicectomy sur vih SECK tuh mee	*cervic/o* cervix *-ectomy* removal	Resection (removal) of the uterine cervix.
clitoridectomy klit er oh DECK toh mee	*clitorid/o* clitoris *-ectomy* removal	Removal of the clitoris. Referred to as "female circumcision" in some cultures.
colpopexy KOHL poh peck see	*colp/o* vagina *-pexy* fixation, suspension	Fixation of the vagina to an adjacent structure to hold it in place.
colpoplasty KOHL poh plas tee	*colp/o* vagina *-plasty* surgical repair	Surgical repair of the vagina.
culdoplasty KULL doh plas tee	*culd/o* cul-de-sac *-plasty* surgical repair	Surgical repair of the cul-de-sac.
dilation and curettage (D&C) dye LAY shun kyoor ih TAHZH		Procedure involving widening (dilation) of the cervix until a curette, a sharp scraping tool, can be inserted to remove the lining of the uterus (curettage). Used to treat and diagnose conditions, such as heavy menstrual bleeding, or to empty the uterus of the products of conception.
hymenotomy hye meh NAH tuh mee	*hymen/o* hymen *-tomy* incision	Incision of the hymen to enlarge the vaginal opening.
hysterectomy hiss tur RECK tuh mee	*hyster/o* uterus *-ectomy* removal	Resection (removal) of the uterus; may be partial, pan- (all), or include other organs as well (e.g., total abdominal hysterectomy with a bilateral salpingo-oophorectomy [TAH-BSO]). The surgical approach is usually stated—whether it is laparoscopic, vaginal, or abdominal.
hysteropexy HISS tur oh peck see	*hyster/o* uterus *-pexy* fixation, suspension	Suspension and fixation of a prolapsed uterus.
loop electrocautery excision procedure (LEEP) ee leck troh KAH tur ee	*electr/o* electricity *cauter/i* burning *-y* process of	A procedure done to remove abnormal cells in cervical dysplasia.
lumpectomy lum PECK tuh mee	*-ectomy* removal	Removal of a tumor from the breast.
mammoplasty MAM oh plas tee	*mamm/o* breast *-plasty* surgical repair	Surgical or cosmetic repair of the breast. Options may include augmentation, to increase the size of the breasts, or reduction, to reduce the size of the breasts.
mastectomy mass TECK tuh mee	*mast/o* breast *-ectomy* removal	Removal of the breast; may be unilateral or bilateral.
mastopexy MASS toh peck see	*mast/o* breast *-pexy* fixation, suspension	Reconstructive procedure to lift and fixate the breasts.

Continued

Terms Related to Non-Pregnancy Procedures—cont'd

Term	Word Origin	Definition
oophorectomy oo ah fore ECK tuh mee	*oophor/o* ovary *-ectomy* removal	Resection of an ovary; may be unilateral or bilateral.
oophorocystectomy oo off oh roh sis TECK tuh mee	*oophor/o* ovary *cyst/o* sac, cyst *-ectomy* removal	Removal of an ovarian cyst (Fig. 8-21).
pelvic exenteration eck sen tuh RAY shun		Removal of the contents of the pelvic cavity. Pelvic exenteration is usually done in response to widespread cancer to remove the uterus, fallopian tubes, ovaries, bladder, vagina, rectum, and lymph nodes (Fig. 8-22).
salpingectomy sal pin JECK tuh mee	*salping/o* fallopian tube *-ectomy* removal	Resection of a fallopian tube; may be unilateral or bilateral.
salpingolysis sal ping GALL ih sis	*salping/o* fallopian tube *-lysis* freeing from adhesions; destruction	Removal of the adhesions in a fallopian tube to reestablish patency with the goal of fertility.
theleplasty THEE leh plas tee	*thel/e* nipple *-plasty* surgical repair	Surgical and/or cosmetic repair of the nipple.
uterine artery embolization (UAE) em boh lye ZAY shun		Injection of particles to block a uterine artery supplying blood to a fibroid with resultant death of fibroid tissue.

Fig. 8-21 Oophorocystectomy.

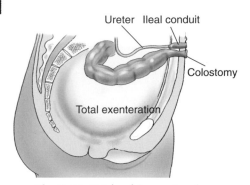

Ureter   Ileal conduit

Colostomy

Total exenteration

Fig. 8-22 Total pelvic exenteration.

EXERCISE 15: Therapeutic Interventions Not Related to Pregnancy

Fill in the blanks with the terms provided.

lumpectomy, dilation and curettage, salpingolysis, colpoplasty, hysteropexy, pelvic exenteration, uterine artery embolization, mastopexy, bilateral oophorectomy, TAH-BSO

1. What surgical procedure suspends the uterus? _____

2. What surgical procedure removes adhesions from the fallopian tubes? _____

3. What surgical procedure resects both ovaries? _____

4. What surgical procedure resects the entire uterus, fallopian tubes, and ovaries through an incision in the abdomen? _____

5. What is removal of a tumor from the breast called? _____

6. What is the term for the removal of the contents of the pelvic cavity? _____

7. What procedure treats fibroids without surgically removing them? _____

8. What is the term for a procedure that widens the cervix to remove the lining of the uterus?

   _____

9. What is surgical repair of the vagina called? _____

10. What is the term for the lifting and fixation of sagging breasts? _____

Decode the terms.

11. clitoridectomy _____

12. culdoplasty _____

13. hymenotomy _____

Build the terms.

14. removal of an ovarian cyst _____

15. surgical repair of the nipple _____

Case Study *Phoebe Gilliam*

Phoebe Gilliam was admitted to the hospital with pelvic pain and vaginal bleeding. A pregnancy test was positive but the sonogram was negative. A left ruptured ectopic pregnancy is diagnosed. A left salpingectomy was performed and Phoebe recovered without complications.

1. What is the term that means uterine bleeding other than that caused by menstruation? _____ _____

2. What hormone does a pregnancy test measure? _____

3. How does sonography produce images?
   a. sound waves
   b. x-rays
   c. magnets

4. A pregnancy that occurs anywhere except the uterus is called a/an _____ pregnancy.

5. A salpingectomy is a removal of a _____ _____.

Terms Related to Pregnancy and Delivery Procedures

Term	Word Origin	Definition
cephalic version seh FAL ick	*cephal/o* head *-ic* pertaining to version process of turning	Process of turning the fetus so that the head is at the cervical outlet for a vaginal delivery. **Cephalic presentation** means a fetus is in a head-down position.
cerclage sur KLAHZH		Suturing the cervix closed to prevent a spontaneous abortion in a woman with an incompetent cervix. The suture is removed when the pregnancy is at full term to allow the delivery to proceed normally (Fig. 8-23).
cesarean section (C-section, CS) seh SARE ree un		Delivery of an infant through a surgical abdominal incision (Fig. 8-24).
episiotomy eh pee zee AH tuh mee	*episi/o* vulva *-tomy* incision	Incision to widen the vaginal orifice to prevent tearing of the tissue of the vulva during delivery (Fig. 8-25).
oxytocia ock see TOH sha	*oxy-* rapid *-tocia* labor, delivery	Rapid birth. **Dystocia** is a difficult labor. **Eutocia** is a normal, "good" delivery.
vaginal birth after cesarean section (VBAC) VAJ ih nul	*vagin/o* vagina *-al* pertaining to	Delivery of subsequent babies vaginally after a C-section. In the past, women were told "once a C-section, always a C-section." Currently, this is being changed by recent developments in technique.
vaginal delivery	*vagin/o* vagina *-al* pertaining to	Usually cephalic presentation (head first) through the vagina. Feet or buttock presentation is a **breech** delivery.

Fig. 8-23 A, Cerclage correction of premature dilation of the cervix. **B,** Cross-sectional view of closed cervix.

Fig. 8-24 Cesarean birth.

Mediolateral

Median
(or midline)

Fig. 8-25 Types of episiotomies.

Terms Related to Infertility Procedures

Term	Word Origin	Definition
artificial insemination (AI)	*in-* in *semin/i* semen *-ation* process of	Introduction of semen into the vagina by mechanical or instrumental means.
gamete intrafallopian transfer (GIFT) GAM eet in trah fah LOH pee un	*intra-* within *fallopi/o* fallopian tube *-an* pertaining to	Laboratory mixing and injection of the ova and sperm into the fallopian tubes so that fertilization occurs naturally within the body.
intracytoplasmic sperm injection (ICSI) in trah sye toh PLAZ mick	*intra-* within *cyt/o* cell *plasm/o* formation *-ic* pertaining to	Injection of one sperm into the ovum and subsequent transplantation of the resulting zygote into the uterus (Fig. 8-26).
in vitro fertilization (IVF) in VEE troh	*in* in *vitro* life	Procedure that allows the mother's ova to be fertilized outside the body and then implanted in the uterus of the biologic mother or a surrogate to carry to term.
salpingosalpingostomy sal pin goh sal pin GOS tuh mee	*salping/o* fallopian tube *salping/o* fallopian tube *-stomy* new opening	The rejoining of previously cut fallopian tubes to reestablish patency. A reversal of a tubal ligation.
zygote intrafallopian transfer (ZIFT) ZYE gote in trah fuh LOH pee un	*intra-* within *fallopi/o* fallopian tube *-an* pertaining to	Mixing of the ova and sperm in the laboratory with fertilization confirmed before the zygotes are returned to the fallopian tubes.

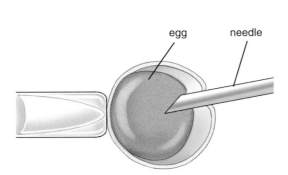

Fig. 8-26 Intracytoplasmic sperm injection (ICSI).

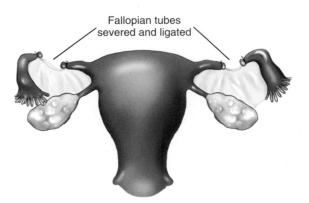

Fig. 8-27 Tubal ligation.

Terms Related to Sterilization

Term	Word Origin	Definition
sterilization		Surgical procedure rendering a person unable to produce children; for women, may involve hysterectomy, bilateral oophorectomy, or tubal ligation.
tubal ligation TOO bul lye GAY shun	*tub/o* tube *-al* pertaining to *ligat/o* tying *-ion* process of	Sterilization procedure in which the fallopian tubes are cut, ligated (tied), and cauterized to prevent released ova from being fertilized by spermatozoa (Fig. 8-27).

EXERCISE 16: Interventions Related to Procreation and Contraception

Fill in the blanks with the terms provided.

C-section, VBAC, tubal ligation, cerclage, cephalic version, sterilization, eutocia

1. The fallopian tubes are cut, tied, and cauterized in which procedure? _____

2. A patient who has a baby vaginally after having a C-section may have what abbreviation on

   her chart? _____

3. What is the term for a normal, good delivery? _____

4. What is the procedure to turn the infant if its head is not down? _____

5. What is the term for a delivery via an incision? _____

6. A bilateral oophorectomy would effectively cause _____.

7. A procedure to keep an incompetent cervix closed until the due date is called _____.

Match the abbreviations with the type of fertilization technique.

_____ 8. IVF

_____ 9. ZIFT

_____ 10. AI

_____ 11. GIFT

_____ 12. ICSI

A. ova fertilized outside of the body, then implanted in the uterus of biologic mother or surrogate
B. semen introduced in vagina by means other than sexual intercourse
C. ova and sperm mixed outside of the body; confirmed zygotes are implanted in fallopian tubes
D. ova and sperm injected in oviducts; fertilization occurs within the body
E. ovum injected with one sperm; confirmed zygote is implanted in uterus

Decode the terms.

13. episiotomy _____

14. oxytocia _____

15. salpingosalpingostomy _____

Case Study Elizabeth Dardenne

Elizabeth Dardenne is a preeclamptic, multigravida 35-year-old who is in the early stages of labor. Because the baby is not in the cephalic position, the obstetrician has to perform cephalic version. If the baby does not turn, a C-section will probably need to be performed.

1. Elizabeth has had 0, 1, or multiple pregnancies? _____

2. The main symptom of preeclampsia is _____ _____.

3. Cephalic version is the _____ of a baby so that the head is pointing down toward the vagina.

4. What does C-section stand for? _____

Within the medical record screen:

Medical Record Hortencia Garcia

GARCIA, HORTENCIA T. - 538437 Opened by Chung, Patrick MD

Task   Edit   View   Time Scale   Options   Help

GARCIA, HORTENCIA T.   Age: 27 years   Sex: Female   Loc: WHC-SMMC
                              DOB: 04/04/1985   MRN: 538437   FIN: 3506004

Reference Text Browser | Form Browser | Medication Profile

Orders | Last 48 Hours | ED | Lab | Radiology | Assessments | **Surgery** | Clinical Notes | Pt. Info | Pt. Schedule | Task List | I & O | MAR

Flowsheet: Surgery   Level: Operative Report   ● Table   ○ Group   ○ List

Navigator
✓   Operative Report

Diagnosis: Desired sterilization, multiparity
Surgery: Laparoscopic tubal ligation

This 27-year-old multigravida female desired tubal sterilization. The patient was taken to the operating room, where, under adequate general anesthetic, the abdomen and perineum were prepped and draped in a sterile fashion. The bladder was drained. An infraumbilical incision was made, and the Veress needle was used for institution of pneumoperitoneum. A 10-mm and a 5-mm port were placed. Both tubes were electrocoagulated and divided under direct vision. After hemostasis was ensured, the wounds were closed with 2-0 Vicryl and 4-0 Vicryl subcuticular. Skin incisions were infiltrated with Marcaine. The patient went to the recovery room in stable condition.

PROD | MAHAFC | 13 July 2012 | 11:27

EXERCISE 17: Operative Report

Using the preceding operative report, answer the following questions.

1. What does this diagnosis mean, "Desired sterilization, multiparity?" (Define sterilization and multiparity.) _____

2. The patient is also described as being "multigravida." What is the difference between multiparous and multigravida? _____

3. What approach is used for the procedure? _____

4. What does the term "ligation" mean? _____

5. Where was the incision made? _____

*Click on **Hear It, Spell It** to practice spelling the diagnostic and therapeutic terms that you have learned in this chapter.*

PHARMACOLOGY

Contraceptive Management

abortifacient (ah bore tih FAY shee ent): Medication that terminates pregnancy. Mifepristone (Mifeprex) and dinoprostone (Prostin E2) may be used as abortifacients.

abstinence: Total avoidance of sexual intercourse as a contraceptive option.

barrier methods: See *diaphragm* and *cervical cap.*

birth control patch: Timed-release contraceptive worn on the skin that delivers hormones transdermally.

cervical cap: Small rubber cup that fits over the cervix to prevent sperm from entering.

contraceptive sponge: Intravaginal barrier with a spermicidal additive.

diaphragm: Soft, rubber hemisphere that fits over the cervix, which can be lined with a spermicidal lubricant prior to insertion.

emergency contraception pill (ECP): Medication that can prevent pregnancy after unprotected vaginal intercourse; does not affect existing pregnancies or cause abortions. Plan B is a popular brand-name available ECP that is now available OTC behind the counter. Commonly called the "day-after pill."

female condom: Soft, flexible sheath that fits within the vagina and prevents sperm from entering the vagina.

hormone implant: Timed-release medication placed under the skin of the upper arm, providing long-term protection. The Norplant system is an example.

hormone injection: Contraceptive hormones (such as medroxyprogesterone [Depo-Provera]) that may be given every few months to provide reliable pregnancy prevention.

intrauterine device (IUD): Small, flexible device inserted into the uterus that prevents implantation of a zygote (Fig. 8-28).

male condom: Soft, flexible sheath that covers the penis and prevents sperm from entering the vagina. If may also be coated with a spermicide.

oral contraceptive pill (OCP) or **birth control pill (BCP):** Pill containing estrogen and/or progesterone that is taken daily to fool the body into thinking it is pregnant so that ovulation is suppressed.

procreative and contraceptive management: Term for a variety of medications and techniques that describe the options available for women's reproductive health.

intrauterine
intra- = within
uter/o = uterus

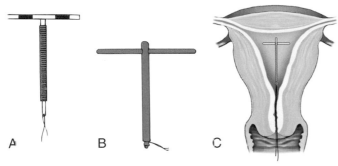

Fig. 8-28 Intrauterine devices (IUDs). **A,** Copper T380A. **B,** Progesterone T. **C,** Levonorgestrel-releasing IUD in place in the uterus.

spermicide
sperm/o = sperm
-cide = to kill

rhythm method: A natural family planning method that involves charting the menstrual cycle to recognize fertile and infertile periods.

spermicides: Foam or gel applied as directed prior to intercourse to kill sperm.

vaginal ring: Flexible ring containing contraceptive hormones inserted into the vagina to prevent pregnancy.

 EXERCISE 18: Contraceptive Options

Fill in the blanks with the terms provided.

abstinence, rhythm method, abortifacient, OCP, spermicides, IUDs, condoms, ECP, barrier methods

1. A contraceptive oral medication that works by suppressing ovulation is _____.

2. Diaphragms and cervical caps are examples of what type of contraceptive method? _____

   _____

3. Soft, flexible sheaths that prevent sperm from entering the vagina are called _____

   _____.

4. Small flexible devices that fit within the uterus are called _____

   _____.

5. A medication intended to terminate a pregnancy is a/an _____.

6. A natural family planning method that has participants chart the woman's menstrual cycle

   to determine fertile and infertile periods is _____.

7. The only 100% effective contraceptive method is _____.

8. Foams and gels that kill sperm are called _____.

9. An emergency contraceptive measure that prevents pregnancy but does not affect an existing

   pregnancy is called a/an _____.

Fertility Drugs

All of the following fertility drugs support or trigger ovulation and may be referred to as *ovulation stimulants:*

bromocriptine (Parlodel): Oral medication typically used with IVF to reduce prolactin levels (which suppresses ovulation).

clomiphene (Clomid, Serophene): Oral medication that stimulates the pituitary gland to produce the hormones that trigger ovulation.

gonadotropin-releasing hormone (GRH) agonist (leuprolide; Lupron): Agent injected or inhaled nasally to prevent premature release of eggs.

human chorionic gonadotropin (hCG) (Novarel): Hormone given intramuscularly to trigger ovulation and typically given with another hormone that will stimulate the release of developed eggs.

human menopausal gonadotropin (hMGs) (menotropins; Repronex): Dual gonadotropins that both stimulate the production of egg follicles and cause the eggs to be released once they are developed. These are given by intramuscular or subcutaneous injection.

lutropin alfa (Luveris): A gonadotropin that stimulates the production of egg follicles.

urofollitropin (Bravelle): Hormone given subcutaneously that mimics FSH to directly stimulate the ovaries to produce egg follicles.

Drugs to Manage Delivery

oxytocic: Medication given to induce labor by mimicking the body's natural release of the oxytocin hormone or to manage postpartum uterine hemorrhage. Oxytocin (Pitocin) is the most commonly used agent to induce labor. Other available oxytocic agents are methylergonovine (Methergine) and ergonovine.

tocolytic: Medication given to slow down or stop preterm labor by inhibiting uterine contractions. Various drugs such as magnesium sulfate, terbutaline (Brethine), nifedipine (Procardia), or indomethacin (Indocin) may be used for this purpose.

Be Careful!

Do not confuse **oxytocin**, a labor-inducing drug, with **oxytocia**, which means rapid birth.

Hormone Replacements

hormone replacement therapy (HRT) and **estrogen replacement therapy (ERT):** The healthcare replacement of estrogen alone (ERT) or with progesterone (HRT) perimenopausally in several forms (tablet, transdermal patch, injection, or vaginal suppository) to relieve symptoms of menopause and protect against osteoporosis.

phytoestrogens: An alternative source of estrogen replacement that occurs through the ingestion of certain plants like soy beans. Phytoestrogens act similarly to human estrogens in the body.

 EXERCISE 19: Fertility, Delivery, and Hormone Replacement Drugs

Circle the correct answer in parentheses.

1. Bromocriptine, clomiphene, and hMG all are used to *(increase, decrease)* fertility.

2. Use of drugs to replace hormones that are missing as a result of menopause is called *(hormone replacement therapy, contraceptive management).*

3. A natural source of estrogen is in *(carbohydrates, soy beans).*

4. Oxytocin is used to *(inhibit, induce)* labor.

5. Medications given to slow down or stop labor are called *(tocolytics, phytoestrogens).*

Case Study Sharifa Khan

Sharifa Khan, a 27-year-old G1P0A0, presents for a D&C. She has had a 3-year history of menometrorrhagia due to fibroids. Hysteroscopy reveals a large endometrial fibroid. It is removed by UAE.

1. G1P0A0 means _____ _____.

2. Heavy menstrual bleeding and bleeding between periods is called _____.

3. The term that means pertaining to the lining of the uterus is _____.

4. Hysteroscopy is a viewing of the _____.

5. UAE stands for _____.

Abbreviations

Abbreviation	Definition
AFP	alpha fetoprotein (test)
AI	artificial insemination
BCP	birth control pill
CIN	cervical intraepithelial neoplasia
CS	cesarean section, C-section
CST	contraction stress test
CVS	chorionic villus sampling
Cx	cervix
D&C	dilation and curettage
DUB	dysfunctional uterine bleeding
ECP	emergency contraceptive pill
EDD	estimated delivery date
EOC	epithelial ovarian cancer
ERT	estrogen replacement therapy
FHR	fetal heart rate
FSH	follicle-stimulating hormone
GIFT	gamete intrafallopian transfer
GPA	gravida, para, abortion
hCG	human chorionic gonadotropin
hMG	human menopausal gonadotropin
HRT	hormone replacement therapy
HSG	hysterosalpingography
ICSI	intracytoplasmic sperm injection

Abbreviation	Definition
IDC	infiltrating ductal carcinoma
IUD	intrauterine device
IVF	in vitro fertilization
LEEP	loop electrocautery excision procedure
LH	luteinizing hormone
LMP	last menstrual period
NST	nonstress test
OB	obstetrics
OCP	oral contraceptive pill
PCOS	polycystic ovary syndrome
PID	pelvic inflammatory disease
PKU	phenylketonuria
PMB	postmenopausal bleeding
PMDD	premenstrual dysphoric disorder
PMS	premenstrual syndrome
Rh	Rhesus factor
TAH-BSO	total abdominal hysterectomy with a bilateral salpingo-oophorectomy
UAE	uterine artery embolization
VBAC	vaginal birth after cesarean section
ZIFT	zygote intrafallopian transfer

EXERCISE 20: Abbreviations

Matching.

_____ 1. baby is due

_____ 2. pregnancy hormone

_____ 3. multiple cysts on ovaries

_____ 4. birth control medication

_____ 5. bleeding after menopause

_____ 6. removal of uterine lining

_____ 7. test for cervical/vaginal cancer

_____ 8. removal of uterus, oviducts, and ovaries

A. TAH-BSO
B. OCP
C. Pap smear
D. hCG
E. D&C
F. PCOS
G. PMB
H. EDD

Chapter Review

Match the word parts to their definitions.

Word Parts

Prefix/Suffix

Prefix/Suffix
-gravida
multi-
neo-
nulli-
-para
primi-
-ptosis
-rrhea
-salpinx
-tocia

Definition

1. _____ new
2. _____ first
3. _____ pregnancy
4. _____ delivery
5. _____ fallopian tube
6. _____ many
7. _____ none
8. _____ dropping, sagging
9. _____ discharge, flow
10. _____ condition of labor, delivery

Combining Form

Combining Form
amni/o
cervic/o
chori/o
colp/o
culd/o
episi/o
gravid/o
gynec/o
hyster/o
lact/o
mamm/o
mast/o
men/o
metr/o
nat/o
o/o
olig/o
oophor/o
papill/o
part/o
salping/o
thel/e

Definition

11. _____ cervix
12. _____ pregnancy
13. _____ milk
14. _____ breast
15. _____ birth
16. _____ nipple
17. _____ breast
18. _____ amnion
19. _____ nipple
20. _____ female
21. _____ ovum, egg
22. _____ scanty, few
23. _____ uterus
24. _____ menstruation
25. _____ delivery
26. _____ chorion
27. _____ vagina
28. _____ uterus
29. _____ recto urine pouch
30. _____ fallopian tube
31. _____ ovary
32. _____ vulva

Word Shop

Prefixes	Combining Forms	Suffixes
a	colp/o	-ectomy
an	episi/o	-graphy
dys	galact/o	-gravida
eu	gynec/o	-ia
multi	hyster/o	-lysis
nulli	mamm/o	-para
poly	mast/o	-partum
post	men/o	-pexy
pre-	metr/o	-plasty
	oophor/o	-rrhea
	py/o	-salpinx
	salping/o	-tocia
	thel/e	-tomy

Build the following terms by combining the preceding word parts. Some word parts may be used more than once. Some may not be used at all. The number in parentheses indicates how many word parts are needed to build the term.

Definition	Term
1. no menstrual flow (3)	_____
2. process of recording the uterus and fallopian tube (3)	_____
3. frequent menstrual flow (3)	_____
4. no pregnancies (2)	_____
5. after delivery (2)	_____
6. many (more than one) deliveries (2)	_____
7. painful menstrual flow (3)	_____
8. removal of the uterus (2)	_____
9. freeing from adhesions in a fallopian tube (2)	_____
10. fixation of the breast (2)	_____
11. pus in a fallopian tube (2)	_____
12. condition of no milk (3)	_____
13. incision of the perineum (2)	_____
14. process of healthy, normal delivery, labor (2)	_____
15. surgical repair of the nipple (2)	_____

Sort the terms below into the correct categories.

Term Sorting

Anatomy and Physiology	Pathology	Diagnostic Procedures	Therapeutic Interventions

AFP	CST	hysteroptosis	Pap smear
amniocentesis	culdocentesis	LEEP	parturition
anovulation	CVS	leiomyoma	pelvimetry
Apgar	D&C	tubal ligation	PKU
areola	eclampsia	vulvodynia	polyhydramnios
cerclage	endometrium	mastopexy	progesterone
cervicectomy	fimbriae	menopause	puerperium
cervix	gestation	menorrhagia	pyosalpinx
colpopexy	hCG	oophorectomy	salpingolysis
colposcopy	hematosalpinx	oophoritis	theleplasty

Replace the highlighted words with the correct terms.

Translations

1. Ms. Costello made an appointment with her **medical doctor who monitors health and treat diseases of the female reproductive system** to discuss her **painful menstrual flow.**

2. Anna Walker's **medical doctor who treats women during pregnancy, delivery, and during the postpartum period** scheduled her for a **removal and analysis of a sample of amniotic fluid.**

3. The **newborn** was born with a/an **umbilical cord around his neck.**

4. Maria Olmos had a **white discharge** that was a symptom of **inflammation of the cervix.**

5. Ms. Robinson was treated for **closure of the uterine tubes** with **destruction of adhesions within the fallopian tubes.**

6. After her third **implantation of the embryo in any location but the uterus**, the patient requested a **sterilization procedure in which the fallopian tubes are cut, ligated, and cauterized.**

7. The 42-year-old **woman who is pregnant for the first time** was sent for a **stimulation of the fetus to monitor for a normal, expected acceleration of the fetal heart rate.**

8. Ms. Graf had a **removal of the breast** to treat her **breast cancer that arises from the cells that line the milk ducts.**

9. Because of an abnormal **exfoliative cytology procedure used for the detection of vaginal and cervical cancer,** the patient was scheduled for a/an **endoscopic procedure used for a cervical/vaginal biopsy.**

10. After delivering a baby two weeks ago, the patient was seen to treat **inflammation of the breast** and **inflammation of the nipples.**

11. The doctor ordered a/an **x-ray procedure in which contrast medium is used to image the uterus and fallopian tubes** to image the patient's **inflammation of the fallopian tubes.**

12. Janice had a **resection of the uterus** to treat her **rare cancer of the smooth muscle of the uterus.**

13. Maria experienced **rapid birth,** and her obstetrician did not have time to do an **incision to widen the vaginal orifice.**

14. Because of a/an **condition in which the infant's head is larger than the mother's pelvic outlet,** Suzanne had to have a **delivery of an infant through a surgical abdominal incision.**

Medical Record Suzanne Goldstein

BARFIELD, SUZANNE W. - 600001 Opened by MACHARIA, LOUIS, MD

Task   Edit   View   Time Scale   Options   Help

As Of 06:29

GOLDSTEIN, SUZANNE W.   Age: 36 years   Sex: Female   Loc: WHC-SMMC
                                DOB: 03/09/1979   MRN: 600001   FIN: 3506004

Reference Text Browser | Form Browser | Medication Profile

Orders | Last 48 Hours | ED | Lab | Radiology | Assessments | **Surgery** | Clinical Notes | Pt. Info | Pt. Schedule | Task List | I & O | MAR

Flowsheet: Surgery   ...   Level: Operative Report   ⊙ Table   ○ Group   ○ List

Navigator

✔ Operative Report

Preoperative Diagnosis: Pregnancy at 34 weeks, poor nonstress test, oligohydramnios, preeclampsia
Postoperative Diagnosis: Pregnancy at 34 weeks, poor nonstress test, oligohydramnios, preeclampsia
Procedure: Low transverse cervical cesarean section
Estimated Blood Loss: 300 ml
Anesthesia: Epidural anesthesia
Description of Procedure: Routine preparation and draping of the abdomen. Abdominal cavity was opened
with a Pfannenstiel skin incision. Bladder flap of peritoneum was incised and bluntly stripped downward
over the lower uterine segment.
    A transverse incision was made in the lower uterine segment, and a normal, viable female neonate weighing
6 lb 1 oz was delivered with meconium-stained amniotic fluid. Her Apgars were 5/9. Cord blood was obtained.
Placenta was removed complete with membranes.
    Edge of uterine incision was then closed with two layers of a continuous #1 chromic catgut, with the second
layer placed in a running type of Lembert suture. All bleeding was controlled. Bladder flap of peritoneum was
replaced.
    Sponge and pack counts were correct before and after the abdomen was closed. Routine closure of the
abdomen. Staples were used for the skin.
    Immediate postoperative condition of mother and baby was good. Amniotic fluid was noted to be meconium
stained.

PROD | MAHAFC | 09 Aug 2015 | 06:29

OPERATIVE REPORT

Answer the questions using the preceding operative report.

1. An infant born at 34 weeks of gestation would be considered what type of infant?

    _____

2. What is meconium? _____

3. What is a nuchal cord? _____

4. What does an Apgar score measure? _____

5. The NST probably was done because there was concern about _____

    _____.

9 Blood, Lymphatic, and Immune Systems

OBJECTIVES

- Recognize and use terms related to the anatomy and physiology of the blood, lymphatic, and immune systems.
- Recognize and use terms related to the pathology of the blood, lymphatic, and immune systems.
- Recognize and use terms related to the diagnostic procedures for the blood, lymphatic, and immune systems.
- Recognize and use terms related to the therapeutic interventions for the blood, lymphatic, and immune systems.

For interactive learning, go to the Shiland Evolve website, and click on:
- **Match the Word Parts** to review blood, lymph, and immune word parts.
- **Word Shop** to practice word building.
- **Tournament of Terminology** to test your knowledge of blood, lymph, and immune terms.
- **Term Sorting** to practice sorting blood, lymph, and immune terms into categories.

*Click on **Chapter at a Glance** for a printable list of key word parts and terms for this chapter.*

FUNCTIONS OF THE BLOOD, LYMPHATIC, AND IMMUNE SYSTEMS

Homeostasis (hoh mee oh STAY sis), or a "steady state," is a continual balancing act of the body systems to provide an internal environment that is compatible with life. The two liquid tissues of the body, the **blood** and **lymph** (limf), have separate but interrelated functions in maintaining this balance. They work with the **immune** (ih MYOON) system to protect the body against **pathogens** (PATH oh jenz) that could threaten the organism's viability. The **blood** is responsible for the following:

- Transportation of gases (oxygen [O_2] and carbon dioxide [CO_2]), chemical substances (hormones, nutrients, and salts), and cells that defend the body.
- Regulation of the body's fluid and electrolyte balance, acid-base balance, and body temperature.
- Protection of the body from infection.
- Protection of the body from loss of blood by the action of clotting.

The **lymphatic system** is responsible for the following:

- Cleansing the cellular environment.
- Returning proteins and tissue fluids to the blood (drainage).
- Providing a pathway for the absorption of fats and fat-soluble vitamins into the bloodstream.
- Defending the body against disease.

The **immune system** is responsible for the following:

- Defending the body against disease via the immune response.

Fig. 9-1 is a Venn diagram of the interrelationship among the three systems with the shared goals of homeostasis and protection at the intersection of the three circles.

homeostasis
home/o = same
-stasis = controlling, stopping

blood = hem/o, hemat/o

lymph = lymph/o, lymphat/o

pathogen
path/o = disease
-gen = producing

Fig. 9-1 Diagram of interrelationships among the hematic, lymphatic, and immune systems.

SPECIALISTS/SPECIALTIES

The study, diagnosis, and treatment of diseases of blood and blood-forming organs is called **hematology.** The specialist in this field is called a **hematologist.**

Immunology is the study of the body's response to foreign substances. The specialist in this field is called an **immunologist.**

hematologist
hemat/o = blood
-logist = one who studies

immunology
immun/o = safety, protection
-logy = study of

ANATOMY AND PHYSIOLOGY

The hematic (hem AT ick) and lymphatic (lim FAT ick) systems flow through separate yet interconnected and interdependent channels. Both are systems composed of vessels and the liquids that flow through them. The immune system, a very complex set of levels of protection for the body, includes blood and lymph cells.

Fig. 9-2 shows the relationship of the lymphatic vessels to the circulatory system. Note the close relationship between the distribution of the lymphatic vessels and the venous blood vessels. Tissue fluid is drained by the lymphatic capillaries and is transported by a series of larger lymphatic vessels toward the heart.

Circulation to lungs

Lymph capillaries

Pulmonary capillary network

Venule

Blood capillaries

Lymphatic capillaries

Arteriole

Lymph node

Lymphatic vessel

Tissue cell

Tissue space (interstitium)

Circulation to lower body

Fig. 9-2 Relationship of the lymphatic vessels to the circulatory system.

The clearest path to understanding the interconnected roles of these three systems is to look at the hematic system first.

Hematic System

The hematic system is composed of blood and the vessels that carry the blood throughout the body. The process of blood formation is called **hematopoiesis** (hee mah toh poy EE sis). All blood cells originate from a single type of cell called a **stem cell.** Because blood can be an extremely important part of the diagnostic process, students need to understand its normal composition. Blood is composed of a solid portion that consists of formed elements, or **cells,** and a liquid portion called **plasma** (PLAZ muh). Blood cells make up 45% of the total blood volume, and plasma makes up the other 55% (Fig. 9-3).

(Whole) Blood = Blood Cells (45%) + Plasma (55%)

The solid portion of blood is composed of three different types of cells:

1. **Erythrocytes** (eh RITH roh sites), also called **red blood cells (RBCs).**
2. **Leukocytes** (LOO koh sites), also called **white blood cells (WBCs).**
3. **Thrombocytes** (THROM boh sites), also called *clotting cells, cell fragments,* or **platelets** (PLATE lets).

hematopoiesis
  hemat/o = blood
  -poiesis = formation

erythrocyte
  erythr/o = red
  -cyte = cell

leukocyte
  leuk/o = white
  -cyte = cell

thrombocyte
  thromb/o = clotting, clot
  -cyte = cell

 Be Careful!   Hgb, HB, Hb, *and* HG *are all abbreviations for hemoglobin.* Hg *is the abbreviation for mercury.*

Fig. 9-3 Composition of blood.

Plasma 55%

Formed elements 45%

Platelets 250–400 thousand

Leukocytes 5–9 thousand

Erythrocytes 4.2–5 8 million

Fig. 9-4 Erythrocytes, or red blood cells (RBCs).

In a milliliter of blood, there are 4.2 to 5.8 million RBCs, 250,000 to 400,000 platelets, and 5000 to 9000 WBCs. These cells together account for approximately 8% of body volume. Converted to more familiar liquid measure, there are about 10.5 pt (5 L) of blood in a 150-lb (68-kg) person.

Components of Blood

Erythrocytes (Red Blood Cells)

The erythrocytes (which are normally present in the millions) have the important function of transporting O_2 and CO_2 throughout the body (Fig. 9-4). The vehicle for this transportation is a protein-iron pigment called **hemoglobin** (HEE moh gloh bin).

The formation of RBCs in the **red bone marrow,** the blood-producing cavities found in many bones, is stimulated by a hormone produced in the kidneys called **erythropoietin** (eh rith roh POY uh tin). RBCs have a life span of approximately 120 days, after which they decompose into **hemosiderin** (hee moh SID uh rin), an iron pigment resulting from **hemolysis** (heh MALL uh sis), and bilirubin. The iron is stored in the liver to be recycled into new RBCs, and the bile pigments are excreted via the liver.

Abnormal RBCs can be named by their **morphology** (more FALL uh jee), the study of shape or form. RBCs normally have a biconcave, disklike shape. (Although the center is depressed, there is not an actual hole.) Those that are shaped differently often have difficulty in carrying out their function.

For example, sickle cell anemia is a hereditary condition characterized by erythrocytes (RBCs) that are abnormally shaped. They resemble a crescent or sickle. Abnormal hemoglobin found inside these erythrocytes causes sickle-cell anemia.

Leukocytes (White Blood Cells)

Although there are fewer leukocytes (thousands, not millions), there are different types with different functions. In general, WBCs protect the body from invasion by pathogens. There are two main types of WBCs: granulocytes and agranulocytes.

hemoglobin
hem/o = blood
-globin = protein substance

bone marrow = myel/o

erythropoietin
erythr/o = red
-poietin = forming substance

hemosiderin
hem/o = blood
-siderin = iron substance

hemolysis
hem/o = blood
-lysis = breaking down

morphology
morph/o = shape
-logy = study of

granulocyte
granul/o = little grain
-cyte = cell

polymorphonucleocyte
poly- = many
morph/o = shape
nucle/o = nucleus
-cyte = cell

eosinophil
eosin/o = rosy-colored
-phil = attractio

neutrophil
neutr/o = neutral
-phil = attraction

phagocyte
phag/o = eat, swallow
-cyte = cell

basophil
bas/o = base
-phil = attraction

agranulocyte
a- = without
granul/o = little grain
-cyte = cell

monocyte
mono- = one
-cyte = cell

lymphocyte
lymph/o = lymph
-cyte = cell

Granulocytes (Polymorphonucleocytes)

Named for their appearance, **granulocytes** (GRAN yoo loh sites), also called **polymorphonucleocytes** (pah lee morf oh NOO klee oh sites) (PMNs, or polys), are WBCs that have small grains within the cytoplasm and multilobed nuclei. These names are used interchangeably.

There are three types of granulocytes, each with its own function. Each of them is named for the type of dye that it attracts.

1. **Eosinophils** (ee ah SIN oh fils) (eosinos) are cells that absorb an acidic dye, which causes them to appear reddish. An increase in eosinophils is a response to a need for their function in defending the body against allergens and parasites.
2. **Neutrophils** (NOO troh fils) (neuts) are cells that absorb neither an acidic nor a basic dye and consequently are a purplish color. They are also called **phagocytes** (FAG oh sites) because they specialize in **phagocytosis** (fag oh sye TOH sis) and generally combat bacteria in pyogenic infections. This means that these cells are drawn to the site of a pathogenic "invasion," where they consume the enemy and remove the debris resulting from the battle.
3. **Basophils** (BAY soh fils) are cells that absorb a basic (or alkaline) dye and stain a bluish color. Especially effective in combatting parasites, they release histamine (a substance that initiates an inflammatory response) and heparin (an **anticoagulant** [an tee koh AGG yoo lunt]), both of which are instrumental in healing damaged tissue.

Agranulocytes (Mononuclear Leukocytes)

Agranulocytes (a GRAN yoo loh sites) are WBCs named for their lack of granules. The alternative name, **mononuclear leukocytes,** is so given because they have one nucleus. The two names are used interchangeably. Although these cells originate in the bone marrow, they mature after entering the lymphatic system. There are two types of these WBCs:

1. **Monocytes** (MON oh sites): These cells, named for their single, large nucleus, transform into **macrophages** (MACK roh fay jehs), which eat pathogens (phagocytosis) and are effective against severe infections.
2. **Lymphocytes** (LIM foh sites) (lymphs): These cells are key in what is called the **immune response,** which involves the "recognition" of dangerous, foreign (viral) substances, and the manufacture of their neutralizers. The

 Be Careful!

Granulocytes are also known as **polymorphonucleocytes,** *abbreviated* **PMNs** *or* **polys.** *However, one type of granulocyte, the neutrophil, is also commonly referred to as a* **polymorph (PMN, poly)** *because it has the greatest degree of nuclear polymorphism, in addition to being the most common type of leukocyte.*

 Be Careful!

Don't confuse **cyt/o** *meaning cell with* **cyst/o** *meaning a bladder or a sac.*

Be Careful!

Don't confuse **hemostasis** *meaning control of blood flow with* **homeostasis** *meaning a steady state.*

foreign substances are called **antigens** (AN tih juns), and the neutralizers are called **antibodies** (AN tih bod ees).

Thrombocytes (Platelets)

Platelets (plats; also known as *thrombocytes*) have a round or oval shape and are so named because they look like small plates. Platelets aid in **coagulation** (koh agg yoo LAY shun), the process of changing a liquid to a solid. When blood cells escape their normal vessels, they **agglutinate** (ah GLOO tih nate), or clump together, by the following process:

1. First, they activate clotting factors (such as, Factor X) that produce prothrombin activator (PTA).
2. Next, in the presence of calcium (Ca), the PTA reacts with the blood protein, **prothrombin** (proh THROM bin), to form **thrombin.**
3. Thrombin then converts another blood protein, **fibrinogen** (fye BRIN ah jen), to **fibrin** (FYE brin), which eventually forms a mesh-like fibrin clot (blood clot), achieving **hemostasis** (hee moh STAY sis) (control of blood flow; that is, stopping the bleeding).

See Fig. 9-5 for a visual explanation of the clotting process.

Plasma

Plasma, the liquid portion of blood, is composed of the following:

- Water (90%)
- Inorganic substances (Ca, potassium [K], sodium [Na])
- Organic substances (glucose, amino acids, fats, cholesterol, hormones)
- Waste products (urea, uric acid, ammonia, creatinine)
- Plasma proteins (serum albumin, serum globulin, and two clotting proteins: fibrinogen and prothrombin)

Serum (SEER um) (*pl.* sera) is plasma minus the clotting proteins. **Serology** is the branch of laboratory medicine that studies blood serum for evidence of infection by evaluating antigen-antibody reactions in vitro.

Serum = Plasma − (Prothrombin + Fibrinogen)

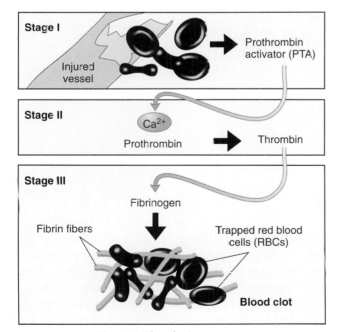

Fig. 9-5 The clotting process.

---

thrombocyte
thromb/o = clot, clotting
-cyte = cell

prothrombin
pro- = before
-thrombin = clotting substance

fibrinogen
fibrin/o = fiber substance
-gen = producing

hemostasis
hem/o = blood
-stasis = stopping, controlling

plasma = plasm/o

serum = ser/o

EXERCISE 1: The Hematic System

Match the following combining forms with their meanings.

_____ 1. blood

_____ 2. red

_____ 3. same

_____ 4. clotting, clot

_____ 5. fiber

_____ 6. disease

_____ 7. little grain

_____ 8. lymph

_____ 9. shape, form

_____ 10. white

_____ 11. safety, protection

_____ 12. rosy, dawn-colored

_____ 13. eat, swallow

_____ 14. bone marrow

A. thromb/o
B. phag/o
C. leuk/o
D. morph/o
E. home/o
F. lymph/o, lymphat/o
G. eosin/o
H. immun/o
I. hem/o, hemat/o
J. erythr/o
K. path/o
L. granul/o
M. fibr/o
N. myel/o

Match the following suffixes with their meanings.

_____ 15. -stasis

_____ 16. -cyte

_____ 17. -poiesis

_____ 18. -lysis

_____ 19. -poietin

_____ 20. -phil

_____ 21. -globin

_____ 22. -gen

_____ 23. -siderin

_____ 24. -thrombin

A. cell
B. attraction
C. iron substance
D. producing
E. formation
F. clotting substance
G. protein substance
H. breakdown
I. forming substance
J. controlling, stopping

Decode the terms.

25. polynuclear _____

26. agranulocytic _____

27. lymphatic _____

28. anuclear _____

29. polymorphic _____

Blood Groups

antigen
anti- = against
-gen = producing

agglutinogen
agglutin/o = clumping
-gen = producing

Human blood is divided into four major different types: A, B, AB, and O. See Fig. 9-6 for a table of blood types, agglutinogens, and agglutinins. The differences are due to antigens present on the surface of the RBCs. **Antigens** (ANN tih jens) are substances that produce an immune reaction by their nature of being perceived as foreign to the body. In response, the body produces substances called **antibodies** that nullify or neutralize the antigens. In blood, these antigens are called **agglutinogens** (ah gloo TIN oh jens) because their presence can

Blood Type	Antigen (RBC membrane)	Antibody (plasma)	Can receive blood from	Can donate blood to
A (40%)	A antigen	Anti-B antibodies	A, O	A, AB
B (10%)	B antigen	Anti-A antibodies	B, O	B, AB
AB (4%)	A antigen, B antigen	No antibodies	A, B, AB, O	AB
O (46%)	No antigen	Both Anti-A and Anti-B antibodies	O	O, A, B, AB

Fig. 9-6 ABO blood groups.

cause the blood to clump. The antibody is termed an **agglutinin** (ah GLOO tin nin). For example, type A blood has A antigen, type B has B antigen, type AB has both A and B antigens, and type O has neither A nor B antigens. If an individual with type A blood is transfused with type B blood, the A antigens will form anti-B antibodies, because they perceive B blood as being foreign. Following the logic of each of these antigen-antibody reactions, an individual with type AB blood is a **universal recipient,** and an individual with type O blood is a **universal donor.**

Another antigen, the **Rh factor,** is important in pregnancy because a mismatch between the fetus and the mother can cause erythroblastosis fetalis, or **hemolytic** (hee moh LIT ick) **disease of the newborn (HDN).** In this disorder, a mother with a negative Rh factor will develop antibodies to an Rh+ fetus during the first pregnancy. If another pregnancy occurs with an Rh+ fetus, the antibodies will destroy the fetal blood cells.

agglutinin
agglutin/o = clumping
-in = substance

hemolytic
hem/o = blood
-lytic = pertaining to breaking down

EXERCISE 2: Blood Groups

1. The four blood types are _____.

2. Blood types are different because of _____ on the surface of the RBCs.

3. A person with type A blood can donate blood to people with which blood type?

   _____

4. Type O blood type is the *(universal donor, universal recipient),* whereas type AB is the *(universal donor, universal recipient)* (underline one).

5. HDN is an example of an antigen-antibody reaction of what blood factor?

   _____

Lymphatic System

The lymphatic system is responsible for the following:

- Cleansing the cellular environment
- Returning proteins and tissue fluids to the blood
- Providing a pathway for the absorption of fats into the bloodstream
- Defending the body against disease

lymph = lymph/o, lymphat/o

lymph vessel = lymphangi/o

lymph gland = lymphaden/o

macrophage
  macro- = large
  phag/o = eat, swallow
  -e = noun ending

The lymphatic system (Fig. 9-7) is composed of **lymph** (or **interstitial fluid**), **lymph vessels, lymph nodes** or lymph glands, lymph organs (e.g., tonsils, adenoids, appendix, spleen, thymus gland, patches of tissue in the intestines called *Peyer patches*), and lymphoid tissue. Monocytes and lymphocytes pass from the bloodstream through the blood capillary walls into the spaces between the cells in body tissue. When they pass into this lymph, or interstitial fluid, that surrounds cells, they perform their protective functions. Monocytes change into **macrophages** (MACK roh fay jehs), destroy pathogens, and collect debris from damaged cells. Lymphocytes are much more complicated and are essential to the immune response, so they are discussed in the next section. Once monocytes and lymphocytes pass into the lymphatic capillaries, the fluid is termed *lymph* or *lymphatic fluid*.

Lymph moves in one direction to prevent pathogens from flowing through the entire body. The system filters out the microorganisms as the lymph passes through its various capillaries, vessels, and nodes. Lymph travels in the following sequence:

1. From the interstitial spaces between the cells.
2. Then toward the heart through lymphatic capillaries.
3. To lymphatic vessels that carry lymph via valves (one-way vessels).

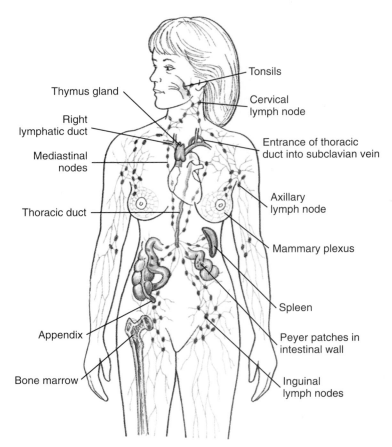

Thymus gland

Tonsils

Cervical lymph node

Right lymphatic duct

Entrance of thoracic duct into subclavian vein

Mediastinal nodes

Axillary lymph node

Thoracic duct

Mammary plexus

Spleen

Appendix

Peyer patches in intestinal wall

Bone marrow

Inguinal lymph nodes

Fig. 9-7 The lymphatic system.

You can review the anatomy of the lymphatic systems by clicking on **Body Spectrum Electronic Anatomy Coloring Book → Lymphatic.**

4. To the lymphatic nodes, which are also called **lymph glands,** that filter the debris produced by macrophages. These nodes can become enlarged when pathogens are present. Note the major lymph nodes in Fig. 9-7, including the **cervical, axillary, inguinal,** and **mediastinal** nodes.
5. Then to either the **right lymphatic duct** or the **thoracic duct,** both of which empty into the large subclavian veins in the neck.
6. Once in the venous blood, the lymph is recycled through the body through the circulatory system.

The organs in the lymphatic system are the **spleen,** the **thymus gland,** the **tonsils,** the **appendix,** and Peyer patches. The spleen is located in the upper left quadrant of the abdomen and serves to filter, store, and produce blood cells; remove RBCs; and activate B lymphocytes. The thymus gland is located in the mediastinum and is instrumental in the development of T lymphocytes (T cells). The tonsils are lymphatic tissue (lingual, pharyngeal, and palatine) that helps protect the entrance to the respiratory and digestive systems. The vermiform appendix and Peyer patches are lymphoid tissue in the intestines.

neck = cervic/o	
axilla, armpit = axill/o	
groin = inguin/o	
mediastinum = mediastin/o	
spleen = splen/o	
thymus = thym/o	
tonsil = tonsill/o	
appendix = append/o, appendic/o	

 Be Careful!

*Don't confuse **thym/o,** which means thymus, with **thyr/o,** which means thyroid.*

 EXERCISE 3: Lymphatic System

Match the following combining forms with their meanings.

_____ 1. spleen

_____ 2. lymph vessel

_____ 3. armpit

_____ 4. tonsil

_____ 5. groin

_____ 6. space between

_____ 7. lymph gland

_____ 8. mediastinum

_____ 9. thymus

_____ 10. appendix

A. lymphangi/o
B. thym/o
C. interstit/o
D. splen/o
E. inguin/o
F. mediastin/o
G. lymphaden/o
H. axill/o
I. appendic/o, append/o
J. tonsill/o

Build the terms.

11. pertaining to the armpit _____

12. pertaining to the groin _____

13. pertaining to the neck _____

EXERCISE 4: Lymphatic System

Label the drawing using the terms provided.

spleen
mediastinal nodes
inguinal nodes
thymus gland
axillary node
bone marrow
tonsils
appendix
thoracic duct
Peyer patches

cytokine
 cyt/o = cell
 -kine = movement

lymphokine
 lymph/o = lymph
 -kine = movement

monokine
 mono- = one
 -kine = movement

interleukin
 inter- = between
 -leukin = white substance

Immune System

The immune system is composed of organs, tissues, cells, and chemical messengers that interact to protect the body from external invaders and its own internally altered cells. The chemical messengers are **cytokines** (SYE toh kynez), which are secreted by cells of the immune system that direct immune cellular interactions. Lymphocytes (leukocytes that are categorized as either **B cells** or **T cells**) secrete **lymphokines** (LIM foh kynez). Monocytes and macrophages secrete **monokines** (MAH noh kynez). **Interleukins** (in tur LOO kinz) are a type of cytokine that sends messages among leukocytes to direct protective action.

The best way to understand this system is through the body's various levels of defense. The goal of pathogens is to breach these levels to enter the body, reproduce, and, subsequently, exploit healthy tissue, causing harm. The immune system's task is to stop them.

Fig. 9-8 illustrates the levels of defense. The two outside circles represent **nonspecific immunity** and its two levels of defense. The inner circle represents the various mechanisms of **specific immunity,** which can be **natural (genetic)** or **acquired** in four different ways. Most pathogens can be contained by the first two lines of nonspecific defense. However, some pathogens deserve a "special" means of protection, which is discussed in the Specific Immunity section.

Fig. 9-8 The levels of defense.

Nonspecific Immunity

The term *nonspecific immunity* refers to the various ways that the body protects itself from many types of pathogens without having to "recognize" them. The *first line of defense* in nonspecific immunity (the outermost layer) consists of the following methods of protection:

- **Mechanical:** Examples include the skin, which acts as a barrier, and the sticky mucus on mucous membranes, which serves to trap pathogens.
- **Physical:** Examples include coughing, sneezing, vomiting, and diarrhea. Although not pleasant, these serve to expel pathogens that have gotten past the initial barriers.
- **Chemical:** Examples include tears, saliva, and perspiration. These have a slightly acidic nature that deters pathogens from entering the body while also washing them away. In addition, stomach acids and enzymes serve to kill germs.

The *second line of defense* in nonspecific immunity comes into play if the pathogens make it past the first line. Defensive measures include certain processes, proteins, and specialized cells.

Defensive processes include the following:

- **Phagocytosis** (fag oh sye TOH sis): Phagocytosis is the process of cells "eating" and destroying microorganisms. Pathogens that make it past the first line of defense and enter into the bloodstream may be consumed by neutrophils and monocytes.
- **Inflammation:** Acquiring its name from its properties, inflammation is a protective response to irritation or injury. The characteristics (heat, swelling, redness, and pain) arise in response to an immediate vasoconstriction, followed by an increase in vascular permeability. These provide a good environment for healing. If caused by a pathogen, the inflammation is called an **infection.**
- **Pyrexia** (pye RECK see uh): Pyrexia is the medical term for fever. When infection is present, fever may serve a protective function by increasing the action of phagocytes and decreasing the viability of certain pathogens.

The **protective proteins** are part of the second line of defense. These include **interferons** (in tur FEER ons), which get their name from their ability to "interfere" with viral replication and limit a virus's ability to damage the body. The **complement proteins,** a second protein type, exist as inactive forms in blood circulation that become activated in the presence of bacteria, enabling them to lyse (destroy) the organisms.

Finally the last of the "team" in the second line of defense are the **natural killer (NK) cells.** This special kind of lymphocyte acts nonspecifically to kill cells that have been infected by certain viruses and cancer cells.

phagocytosis
phag/o = eat, swallow
cyt/o = cell
-osis = abnormal condition

pyrexia
pyr/o = fever, fire
-exia = condition

Specific Immunity

Specific immunity may be either **genetic**—an inherited ability to resist certain diseases because of one's species, race, sex, or individual genetics—or **acquired.** Specific immunity is dependent on the body's ability to identify a pathogen and prepare a specific response (antibody) to only that invader (antigen). Antibodies are also referred to as **immunoglobulin (Ig)** (ih myoo noh GLOB you lin). There are five distinct classes of immunoglobulins (IgA, IgD, IgE, IgG, and IgM), each of which responds to a specific antigen. The acquired form can be further divided into natural and artificial forms, which in turn can each be either active or passive. After the specific immune process is described, each of the four types is discussed.

Specific immunity is dependent on the agranulocytes (lymphocytes and monocytes) for its function. The monocytes metamorphose into macrophages, which dispose of foreign substances. The lymphocytes differentiate into either T lymphocytes (which mature in the thymus) or B lymphocytes (which mature in the bone marrow or fetal liver). Although both types of lymphocytes take part in specific immunity, they do so in different ways.

The T cells neutralize their enemies through a process of **cell-mediated immunity.** This means that they attack antigens directly. They are effective against fungi, cancer cells, protozoa, and, unfortunately, organ transplants. B cells use a process of **humoral immunity** (also called **antibody-mediated immunity**). This means that they secrete antibodies to "poison" their enemies.

humoral
humor/o = liquid
-al = pertaining to

Types of Acquired Immunity

Acquired immunity is categorized as *active* or *passive* and then is further subcategorized as *natural* or *artificial*. All of these describe ways that the body has acquired antibodies to specific diseases.

Active acquired immunity can take either of the following two forms:

- **Natural:** Development of memory cells to protect the individual from a second exposure.
- **Artificial:** Vaccination (immunization) that uses a greatly weakened form of the antigen, thus enabling the body to develop antibodies in response to this intentional exposure. Examples are the DTP and MMR vaccines.

Passive acquired immunity can take either of the following two forms:

- **Natural:** Passage of antibodies through the placenta or breast milk.
- **Artificial:** Use of immunoglobulins harvested from a donor who developed resistance against specific antigens.

EXERCISE 5: Immune System

1. How do nonspecific and specific immunity differ?

_____

2. List the first-line defenses, and give examples of each.

_____

3. List the second-line defenses.

_____

Choose from the following types of acquired immunity to fill in the blanks:

active natural, active artificial, passive natural, passive artificial

4. If a child has an immunization against measles, he/she has what type of immunity? _____

5. If an individual receives maternal antibodies, then this is a type of _____ immunity.

6. If an individual receives a mixture of antibodies from a donor, he/she has received _____ immunity.

7. Acquiring a disease and producing memory cells for that disease is a type of _____ immunity.

Match the following word parts with their meanings.

_____ 8. fever	_____ 13. liquid	A. humor/o
		B. pyr/o
_____ 9. eat	_____ 14. not	C. leuk/o
		D. -in
_____ 10. substance	_____ 15. movement	E. inter-
		F. phag/o
_____ 11. between	_____ 16. one	G. non-
		H. -kine
_____ 12. white	_____ 17. cell	I. mono-
		J. cyt/o

 *Choose **Hear It, Spell It** to practice spelling the anatomy and physiology terms you have learned in this chapter.*

Combining and Adjective Forms for the Anatomy and Physiology of the Blood, Lymphatic, and Immune Systems

Meaning	Combining Form	Adjective Form
appendix	append/o, appendic/o	appendicular
axilla, armpit	axill/o	axillary
base	bas/o	basal
blood	hem/o, hemat/o	hematic
bone marrow	myel/o	
clotting, clot	thromb/o	thrombic
clumping	agglutin/o	agglutinous
disease	path/o	
eat, swallow	phag/o	
fever, fire	pyr/o	pyretic
fiber	fibr/o	fibrous
groin	inguin/o	inguinal
little grain	granul/o	granular
lymph	lymph/o, lymphat/o	lymphatic
lymph gland (node)	lymphaden/o	
lymph vessel	lymphangi/o	lymphangial

Continued

Combining and Adjective Forms for the Anatomy and Physiology of the Blood, Lymphatic, and Immune Systems—cont'd

Meaning	Combining Form	Adjective Form
mediastinum	mediastin/o	mediastinal
neck	cervic/o	cervical
neutral	neutr/o	neutral
nucleus	nucle/o	nuclear
plasma	plasm/o	
red	erythr/o	
rosy-colored	eosin/o	
safety, protection	immun/o	
same	home/o	
serum	ser/o	serous
shape	morph/o	morphous
spleen	splen/o	splenic
thymus	thym/o	thymic
tonsil	tonsill/o	tonsillar
white	leuk/o	

Prefixes for the Anatomy and Physiology of the Blood, Lymphatic, and Immune Systems

Prefix	Meaning
a-	without
anti-	against
inter-	between
macro-	large
mono-	one
poly-	many
pro-	before

Suffixes for the Anatomy and Physiology of the Blood, Lymphatic, and Immune Systems

Suffix	Meaning	Suffix	Meaning
-cyte	cell	-lytic	pertaining to breaking down
-exia	condition		
-gen	producing	-osis	abnormal condition
-globin	protein substance	-phil	attraction
-in	substance	-poiesis	formation
-kine	movement	-poietin	forming substance
-leukin	white substance	-siderin	iron substance
-logy	study of	-stasis	controlling, stopping
-lysis	breaking down	-thrombin	clotting substance

Click on Label It to practice labeling the lymphatic system.

PATHOLOGY

Dyscrasia (dis KRAY zsa), a term that means a bad *(dys-)* mixture *(-crasia)*, is used more specifically to describe diseases of the blood or bone marrow. Many disorders of the blood have to do with too many or too few of certain types of blood cells. **Anemia** is a decrease in RBCs, hemoglobin, and/or hematocrit. Many others have to do with abnormalities of cell morphology or shape.

Terms Related to Deficiency Anemias

Term	Word Origin	Definition
acute posthemorrhagic anemia post heh moh RAJ ick ah NEE mee uh	*post-* after *hem/o* blood *-rrhagic* pertaining to bursting forth *an-* no, not *-emia* blood condition	RBC deficiency caused by blood loss.
B_{12} deficiency		Insufficient blood levels of cobalamin, a so called vitamin B_{12}, which is essential for RBC maturation. Condition may be caused by inadequate dietary intake, as in some extreme vegetarian diets, or it may result from absence of **intrinsic factor**, a substance in the gastrointestinal (GI) system essential to vitamin B_{12} absorption.
chronic blood loss		Long-term internal bleeding. May cause anemia.
folate deficiency FOH late		Anemia as a result of a lack of folate from dietary, drug-induced, congenital, or other causes.
hypovolemia hye poh voh LEE me ah	*hypo-* deficient *vol/o* volume *-emia* blood condition	Deficient volume of circulating blood.
sideropenia sih dur roh PEE nee ah	*sider/o* iron *-penia* deficiency	Condition of having reduced numbers of healthy RBCs because of chronic blood loss, inadequate iron intake, or unspecified causes. A type of **iron deficiency** anemia.
pernicious anemia pur NIH shush	*an-* no, not *-emia* blood condition	Progressive anemia that results from a lack of intrinsic factor essential for the absorption of vitamin B_{12} (also known as cobalamin).

Terms Related to Aplastic and Hemolytic Anemias

Term	Word Origin	Definition
aplastic anemia a PLAS tick	*a-* no, not *plast/o* formation *-ic* pertaining to *an-* no, not *-emia* blood condition	Suppression of bone marrow function leading to a reduction in RBC production. Although causes of this often fatal type of anemia may be hepatitis, radiation, or cytotoxic agents, most causes are idiopathic. Also called **hypoplastic anemia.**
hemolytic anemia hee moh LIH tick	*hem/o* blood *-lytic* pertaining to destruction	A group of anemias caused by destruction of RBCs.
autoimmune acquired hemolytic anemia hee moh LIT ick	*auto-* self *immune* safety, protection *hem/o* blood *-lytic* pertaining to destruction *an-* no, not *-emia* blood condition	Anemia caused by the body's destruction of its own RBCs by serum antibodies.
non-autoimmune acquired hemolytic anemia	*non-* not *hem/o* blood *-lytic* pertaining to destruction *an-* no, not *-emia* blood condition	Anemia that may be drug induced or may be caused by an infectious disease, in which the RBCs are destroyed.
sickle cell anemia	*an-* no, not *-emia* blood condition	Inherited anemia characterized by crescent-shaped RBCs. This abnormality in morphology causes RBCs to block small-diameter capillaries, thereby decreasing the oxygen supply to the cells (Fig. 9-9). A **sickle cell crisis** is an acute, painful exacerbation of sickle cell anemia.
thalassemia thal ah SEE mee ah	*thalass/o* sea *-emia* blood condition	Group of inherited disorders of people of Mediterranean, African, and Southeast Asian descent, in which the anemia is the result of a decrease in the synthesis of hemoglobin, resulting in decreased production and increased destruction of RBCs.
pancytopenia pan sye toh PEE nee ah	*pan-* all *cyt/o* cell *-penia* deficiency	Deficiency of all blood cells caused by dysfunctional stem cells (Fig. 9-10).

A Normal red blood cells (RBCs)

B RBCs in sickle cell disease

Fig. 9-9 A, Normal, donut-shaped red blood cells (RBCs) bend to fit through capillaries. **B,** Sickled RBCs cannot bend and therefore block the flow of blood through the vessel.

Fig. 9-10 A, Normal cellularity.
B, Hypocellularity in pancytopenia.

EXERCISE 6: Anemias

Fill in the blank with one of the following terms:

pancytopenia, thalassemia, aplastic anemia, sickle-cell anemia, autoimmune acquired hemolytic anemia, pernicious anemia, acute posthemorrhagic anemia

1. What type of inherited anemia has misshapen blood cells that block blood vessels, causing oxygen deprivation to the cells? _____

2. What type of anemia is caused by the body destroying its own blood cells? _____

3. What type of inherited anemia may affect people of Mediterranean, African, and Southeast Asian descent? _____

4. What type of anemia is caused by bone marrow suppression? _____

5. Deficiency of all types of blood cells caused by dysfunctional stem cells is called _____.

6. Lack of intrinsic factor causes this type of progressive anemia.

7. Anemia caused by sudden blood loss is called _____.

Decode the terms.

8. hypovolemia _____

9. hemolytic _____

10. sideropenia _____

Case Study   Mary Kate Knowles

Twelve-year-old Mary Kate Knowles is admitted for acute exacerbation of sickle cell anemia. Mary Kate is in acute distress, complaining of pain in her hands, feet, and shins. Upon examination, she is found to have hepatomegaly, splenomegaly, and jaundice. Treatment includes analgesics, evaluation for infectious disease, and possible blood transfusion.

1. Sickle cell anemia is characterized by crescent-shaped _____.

2. What is an acute exacerbation of sickle cell disease called? _____

3. Hepatomegaly is enlargement of the _____ _____.

4. Splenomegaly is enlargement of the _____ _____.

5. Mary Kate has jaundice. What color are the sclera of her eyes and skin?
   a. blue
   b. yellow
   c. red
   d. white

Terms Related to Coagulation Disorders, Purpura, and Other Hemorrhagic Conditions

Term	Word Origin	Definition
hemophilia hee moh FEE lee ah	*hem/o* blood *-philia* attraction condition	Group of inherited bleeding disorders characterized by a deficiency of one of the factors necessary for the coagulation of blood. Excessive bleeding and **hemarthrosis** (blood in a joint) can result from even a minor injury.
polycythemia vera pah lee sye THEE mee ah VARE ah	*poly-* many *cyt/o* cell *-emia* blood condition *vera* true	Chronic increase in the number of RBCs and the concentration of hemoglobin. "Vera" signifies that this is not a sequela of another condition.
purpura PURR purr uh	*purpur/o* purple *-a* noun ending	Bleeding disorder characterized by hemorrhage into the tissues (Fig. 9-11).
thrombocytopenia throm boh sye toh PEE nee ah	*thromb/o* clot, clotting *cyt/o* cell *-penia* deficiency	Deficiency of platelets that causes an inability of the blood to clot. The most common cause of bleeding disorders.

Fig. 9-11 Purpura.

Septic/o *means infection, but* sept/o *means septum, wall, or partition.*

Terms Related to Systemic Infections of the Blood

Term	Word Origin	Definition
septicemia sep tih SEE mee ah	*septic/o* infection *-emia* blood condition	Systemic infection with pathologic microbes in the blood as a result of an infection that has spread from elsewhere in the body. The term "sepsis" means infection.
septic shock SEP tick	*septic/o* infection *-ic* pertaining to	Inadequate blood flow to the body caused by an overwhelming infection and resultant low blood pressure. Organs fail and death may occur.
systemic inflammatory response syndrome (SIRS)	*system/o* system	A type of septic shock, SIRS is an inflammatory state affecting the whole body. SIRS can be caused by infection, trauma, ischemia, or inflammation.

Terms Related to Leukocytic Disorders

Term	Word Origin	Definition
leukocytosis loo koh sye TOH sis	*leuk/o* white blood cell *-cytosis* abnormal increase in cells	Abnormal increase in WBCs. Abnormal increases in each type of granulocyte are termed **eosinophilia, basophilia,** or **neutrophilia,** where the suffix *-philia* denotes a slight increase. Abnormal increases in the number of each type of agranulocyte are termed **lymphocytosis** or **monocytosis.**
leukopenia loo koh PEE nee ah	*leuk/o* white blood cell *-penia* deficiency	Abnormal decrease in WBCs. Specific deficiencies are termed **neutropenia, eosinopenia, monocytopenia,** and **lymphocytopenia.** Also called **leukocytopenia.**
neutropenia noo troh PEE nee ah	*neutr/o* neutral *-penia* deficiency	Abnormal decrease in neutrophils due to disease process. Formerly called **agranulocytosis.**

Terms Related to Lymphatic Disorders

Term	Word Origin	Definition
edema eh DEE muh		Abnormal accumulation of fluid in the interstitial spaces of tissues.
hypersplenism hye purr SPLEE niz um	*hyper-* excessive *splen/o* spleen *-ism* condition	Increased function of the spleen, resulting in hemolysis.
lymphadenitis lim fad uh NYE tis	*lymphaden/o* lymph gland *-itis* inflammation	Inflammation of a lymph node.
lymphadenopathy lim fad uh NOP puh thee	*lymphaden/o* lymph gland *-pathy* disease process	Disease of the lymph nodes or vessels that may be localized or generalized.
lymphangitis lim fan JYE tis	*lymphangi/o* lymph vessel *-itis* inflammation	Inflammation of lymph vessels.
lymphedema lim fuh DEE muh	*lymph/o* lymph *-edema* swelling	Accumulation of lymphatic fluid and resultant swelling caused by obstruction, removal, or hypoplasia of lymph vessels (Fig. 9-12).
lymphocytopenia lim foh sye toh PEE nee ah	*lymphocyt/o* lymphocyte *-penia* deficiency	Deficiency of lymphocytes caused by infectious mononucleosis, malignancy, nutritional deficiency, or a hematologic disorder.
lymphocytosis lim foh sye TOH sis	*lymph/o* lymph *-cytosis* abnormal increase of cells	Abnormal increase in lymphocytes.
mononucleosis mah noh noo klee OH sis	*mono-* one *nucle/o* nucleus *-osis* abnormal condition	Increase in the number of mononuclear cells (monocytes and lymphocytes) in the blood caused by the Epstein-Barr virus (EBV) (Fig. 9-13). Can result in **splenomegaly** (enlarged spleen) (see Fig. 1-6).

Fig. 9-12 Lymphedema. The patient had to bind her feet so that she could wear shoes.

Fig. 9-13 Mononucleosis. The blood smear has been stained to differentiate between the blood cells. The cell on the left is a typical small lymphocyte with the nucleus almost filling the cell. The larger atypical lymphocyte on the right has much more cytoplasm and a larger nucleus.

EXERCISE 7: Coagulation, Leukocytic, and Lymphatic Disorders

Match the disorders with their definitions.

_____ 1. mononucleosis   _____ 5. leukopenia

_____ 2. hemophilia   _____ 6. edema

_____ 3. purpura   _____ 7. hypovolemia

_____ 4. polycythemia

A. deficient volume of circulating blood
B. hereditary bleeding disorder
C. deficiency of WBCs
D. excessive RBCs
E. hemorrhagic bleeding disorder of tissues
F. abnormal accumulation of fluid in tissues
G. disorder caused by the EBV

Build the terms.

8. deficiency of lymph cells _____

9. abnormal increase in white blood cells _____

10. inflammation of lymph vessels _____

11. excessive spleen condition _____

Decode the terms.

12. lymphadenopathy _____

13. lymphangitis _____

14. thrombocytopenia _____

15. lymphocytosis _____

Case Study   Christian Halvorson

Christian Halvorson is a hemophiliac who has been out of a job for a year. Because he has very little money, he has been skipping the medication that he needs to take to treat his condition. But severe pain due to hemarthroses in his knees and a cut that won't stop bleeding has sent him to the emergency department (ED). Prothrombin time (PT) and partial thromboplastin time (PTT) are ordered, and the ED doctor works to stop the cut from bleeding. He also suspects that Christian will need a blood transfusion.

1. The term that means the stopping or controlling of bleeding is _____.

2. Hemarthrosis is bleeding in a _____ _____.

3. Hemophilia is characterized by a deficiency of one of the necessary for the _____ of blood.

4. What does the combining form *hem/o* mean? _____

5. What does the suffix *-philia* mean? _____ _____

Terms Related to Immune Disorders

Term	Word Origin	Definition
acquired immunodeficiency syndrome (AIDS) ih myoo noh deh FIH shun see		Syndrome caused by the **human immunodeficiency virus (HIV)** and transmitted through body fluids via sexual contact or intravenous exposure. HIV attacks the helper T cells, which diminishes the immune response (Fig. 9-14).
allergy AL ur jee	*allo-* other, different *erg/o* work *-y* condition	Immune system's overreaction to irritants that are perceived as antigens. The substance that causes the irritation is called an **allergen.** Also called **hypersensitivity.**
anaphylaxis an uh fuh LACK sis	*ana-* without *-phylaxis* protection	Extreme form of allergic response in which the patient suffers severely decreased blood pressure and constriction of the airways.
delayed response allergy	*allo-* other, different *erg/o* work *-y* condition	Immune system hypersensitivity caused by activated T cells that respond to an exposure of the skin to a chemical irritant up to 2 days later. An example would be poison ivy. The resulting rash is called *contact dermatitis.*
immediate response allergy	*allo-* other, different *erg/o* work *-y* condition	Hypersensitivity of the immune system caused by IgE. Examples are tree and grass pollens.
autoimmune disease	*auto-* self *immun/o* safety, protection	Condition in which a person's T cells attack his/her own cells, causing extensive tissue damage and organ dysfunction. Examples of resultant **autoimmune diseases** include myasthenia gravis, rheumatoid arthritis, systemic lupus erythematosus, and multiple sclerosis.

Systemic:
• Pyrexia
• Weight loss

Mouth:
• Aphthous stomatitis
• Candidiasis

Pharyngitis

Esophagus:
• Ulcers

Muscles:
• Myalgia

Central:
• Fatigue
• Headache

Lymph nodes:
• Lymphadenopathy

Skin:
• Exanthem

Liver and spleen:
• Hepatomegaly
• Splenomegaly

Gastric:
• Nausea
• Vomiting
• Diarrhea

Fig. 9-14 Physiological manifestations of AIDS.

Fighting Future Diseases

The National Institute of Allergy and Infectious Diseases (NIAID) is one of the branches of the National Institutes of Health (NIH). Because its mission is to conduct and support research on immunologic and infectious diseases, students may be interested in visiting its website at http://www.niaid.nih.gov/strategicplan and reading about its plans to combat emerging infectious diseases in the twenty-first century.

For those interested in a more global view, another website that may be of interest is that of the World Health Organization (WHO) at http://www.who.int. Links include "Disease Outbreak News" and "Emergencies and Disasters."

EXERCISE 8: Abnormal Immune Responses

Match the immune system terms with their definitions.

_____ 1. allergy

_____ 2. autoimmune disease

_____ 3. anaphylaxis

_____ 4. AIDS

_____ 5. delayed allergy

_____ 6. immediate allergy

A. extreme form of allergic response
B. condition in which a person's T cells attack his or her own cells
C. hypersensitivity caused by T cells
D. hypersensitivity
E. hypersensitivity caused by IgE
F. syndrome caused by HIV

Case Study Rebekah Robbins

Eleven-year-old Rebekah was stung on the hand by a bee while on a family picnic. Her mother removed the stinger, and after a few tears, Rebekah seemed fine and went on playing with her cousins. However, 20 minutes later she tells her mother that she can't breathe very well and she feels "hot." Her mother rushes her to the local urgent healthcare center, where it is discovered that Rebekah has an irregular heartbeat and low blood pressure, along with swelling at the site of the sting, around her lips and tongue, and in the oropharynx.

1. Rebekah is experiencing _____, an extreme form of allergic response.

2. The _____ that caused this allergic response was bee venom.

3. Rebekah's condition is a type of _____ allergy, a hypersensitivity of the immune system caused by IgE.

4. What is the term that means an abnormal accumulation of fluid in the interstitial spaces of tissues?
_____

5. How do you break down the term *anaphylaxis*?
_____

Terms Related to Benign Neoplasms

Term	Word Origin	Definition
thymoma thigh MOH mah	*thym/o* thymus gland *-oma* tumor	Noncancerous tumor of epithelial origin that is often associated with myasthenia gravis.

Terms Related to Malignant Neoplasms

Term	Word Origin	Definition
acute lymphocytic leukemia (ALL) limf oh SIH tick loo KEE mee ah	*lymph/o* lymph *cyt/o* cell *-ic* pertaining to *leuk/o* white *-emia* blood condition	Also termed **acute lymphoblastic leukemia**, this cancer is characterized by the uncontrolled proliferation of immature lymphocytes. It is the most common type of leukemia for individuals under the age of 19 (Fig. 9-15).
acute myelogenous leukemia (AML) mye ah LAJ en us loo KEE mee ah	*myel/o* bone marrow *-genous* pertaining to originating from *leuk/o* white *-emia* blood condition	This rapidly progressive form of leukemia develops from immature bone marrow stem cells.
chronic lymphocytic leukemia (CLL) limf oh SIH tick loo KEE me ah	*lymph/o* lymph *cyt/o* cell *-ic* pertaining to *leuk/o* white *-emia* blood condition	A slowly progressing form of leukemia in which immature lymphocytes proliferate. Occurs most frequently in middle age (or older) adults; rarely occurs in children.
chronic myelogenous leukemia (CML) mye ah LAJ en us loo KEE me ah	*myel/o* bone marrow *-genous* pertaining to originating from *leuk/o* white *-emia* blood condition	A slowly progressing form of leukemia in which immature bone marrow cells proliferate. Like CLL, CML occurs most frequently in middle age (or older) adults; it rarely occurs in children.
Hodgkin lymphoma limf OH mah	*lymph/o* lymph *-oma* tumor, mass	Also termed **Hodgkin disease**, this cancer is diagnosed by the detection of Reed-Sternberg cells, a type of cell specific only to Hodgkin lymphoma.

Fig. 9-16 Diffuse punched-out osteolytic lesions are scattered throughout the skull in this patient with multiple myeloma.

Fig. 9-15 Micrograph of leukemia.

Terms Related to Malignant Neoplasms—cont'd

Term	Word Origin	Definition
myeloma, multiple mye eh LOH mah	*myel/o* bone marrow *-oma* tumor, mass	Also termed **plasma cell dyscrasia** or **myelomatosis,** this rare malignancy of the plasma cells is formed from B lymphocytes. It is called "multiple" myeloma because the tumors are found in many bones. If it occurs in only one bone, the tumor is referred to as a *plasmacytoma* (Fig. 9-16).
non-Hodgkin lymphoma limf OH mah	*lymph/o* lymph *-oma* tumor, mass	A collection of all other lymphatic cancers but Hodgkin lymphomas. This type is the more numerous of the two lymphomas and is the sixth most common type of cancer in the United States.
thymoma, malignant thigh MOH mah	*thym/o* thymus gland *-oma* tumor, mass	Also termed **thymic carcinoma,** this rare malignancy of the thymus gland is particularly invasive and, unlike its benign form, is not associated with autoimmune disorders.

EXERCISE 9: Neoplasms

Match the neoplasms with their definitions.

_____ 1. non-Hodgkin lymphoma

_____ 2. ALL

_____ 3. thymoma

_____ 4. CLL

_____ 5. CML

_____ 6. multiple myeloma

_____ 7. AML

_____ 8. malignant thymoma

_____ 9. Hodgkin lymphoma

A. rapidly progressive form of leukemia due to immature bone marrow cells
B. benign tumor of thymus gland
C. cancer of lymphatic system detected by presence of Reed-Sternberg cells
D. slowly progressing form of leukemia with proliferation of immature lymphocytes
E. thymic carcinoma
F. slowly progressing form of leukemia in which immature bone marrow cells proliferate
G. a collection of all lymphatic cancers except Hodgkin lymphoma
H. plasma cell dyscrasia; tumors are found in many bones
I. rapidly progressing form of leukemia developing from immature lymphocytes

Case Study Cooper Billings

Cooper Billings had been a bubbly, busy, 4-year-old until his parents noticed that he seemed tired all the time and he was bruising easily. His appetite had also decreased, and he was losing weight. Cooper's family doctor orders a complete blood cell count (CBC) and peripheral blood smear. Pancytopenia and a proliferation of immature WBCs (lymphoblasts) confirm what she suspects, and after more testing, Cooper is diagnosed with ALL.

1. ALL stands for _____ _____.

2. ALL is characterized by uncontrolled proliferation of _____ lymphocytes.

3. Pancytopenia means a deficiency of _____ _____ cells.

4. The suffix *-blast* in lymphoblast means _____ _____.

5. CLL occurs most commonly in older adults. What does the C in CLL stand for? _____ _____

 Click on **Hear It, Spell It** to practice spelling the pathology terms you have learned in this chapter. To review the pathology terms in this chapter, play **Medical Millionaire.**

Age Matters

Pediatrics

Childhood disorders of the blood, lymphatic, and immune systems range from hypersensitivities (allergies) to congenital disorders (HDN) to ALL.

Geriatrics

Unlike the children, seniors will have a host of diagnoses from this chapter on their charts. Anemias are common, along with a lack of blood volume (hypovolemia), which may be due to internal bleeding, trauma, or disease process. Cancers of these systems also appear in fairly significant numbers. Non-Hodgkin lymphoma and AML account for thousands of hospitalizations every year.

DIAGNOSTIC PROCEDURES

Terms Related to Imaging

Term	Word Origin	Definition
lymphadenography lim fad uh NAH gruh fee	*lymphaden/o* lymph gland *-graphy* process of recording	Radiographic visualization of the lymph gland after injection of a radiopaque substance. Also called **lymphography.**
lymphangiography lim fan jee AH gruh fee	*lymphangi/o* lymph vessel *-graphy* process of recording	Radiographic visualization of a part of the lymphatic system after injection with a radiopaque substance (Fig. 9-17).
splenic arteriography SPLEH nik ar teer ee AH gruh fee	*splen/o* spleen *arteri/o* artery *-graphy* process of recording	Radiographic visualization of the spleen with the use of a contrast medium.

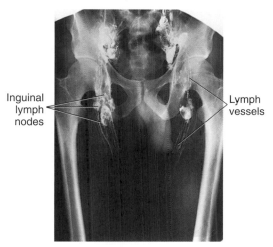

Fig. 9-17 Lymphangiogram of inguinal region and upper thighs.

Fig. 9-18 Western blot test. A technician is placing a Western blot strip in a test tray. If present, antigens will bind to this sheet and later be detected. (From the CDC.)

Terms Related to Laboratory Tests

Term	Word Origin	Definition
AIDS tests— enzyme-linked immunosorbent assay (ELISA), Western blot		Tests to detect the presence of HIV types 1 and 2 (Fig. 9-18).
allergy testing	*allo-* other, different *erg/o* work *-y* condition	Series of tests involving a patch, scratch, or intradermal injection of an attenuated amount of an allergen to test for hypersensitivity (Fig. 9-19).
basic metabolic panel (BMP)		Group of blood tests to measure Ca, glucose, electrolytes, such as Na, K, and chloride (Cl), creatinine, and blood urea nitrogen (BUN).
blood cultures		Blood samples are submitted to propagate microorganisms that may be present. Cultures may be indicated for bacteremia or septicemia, or to discover other pathogens (fungi, viruses, or parasites) (Fig. 9-20).
complete blood cell count (CBC)		Twelve tests, including RBC count, WBC count, hemoglobin (Hb), hematocrit/packed-cell volume (Hct/PCV), and diff (WBC differential).
comprehensive metabolic panel (CMP)		Set of 14 blood tests that add protein and liver function tests to the BMP. Glucose is also measured with a different method than in the basic panel.
Coombs antiglobulin test koomz an tee GLOB yoo lin	*anti-* against *-globulin* protein substance	Blood test to diagnose HDN, acquired hemolytic anemia, or a transfusion reaction.
differential (diff) count		Measure of the numbers of the different types of WBCs.
erythrocyte sedimentation rate (ESR) eh RITH roh syte seh dih men TAY shun	*erythr/o* red *-cyte* cell	Measurement of time for mature RBCs to settle out of a blood sample after an anticoagulant is added. An increased ESR indicates inflammation.

Continued

Terms Related to Laboratory Tests—cont'd

Term	Word Origin	Definition
hematocrit/packed-cell volume (Hct/PCV) hee MAT oh krit	*hemat/o* blood -*crit* separate	Measure of the percentage of RBCs in the blood.
hemoglobin (Hgb, Hb) HEE moh gloh bin	*hem/o* blood -*globin* protein substance	Measure of iron-containing pigment of RBCs that carries oxygen to tissues.
mean corpuscular hemoglobin (MCH) kor PUS kyoo lur	*hem/o* blood -*globin* protein substance	Test to measure the average weight of hemoglobin per RBC. Useful in diagnosing anemia.
mean corpuscular hemoglobin concentration (MCHC)	*hem/o* blood -*globin* protein substance	Test to measure the concentration of hemoglobin in RBCs. This test is useful for measuring a patient's response to treatment for anemia.
monospot MAH noh spot		Test for infectious mononucleosis.
partial thromboplastin time (PTT) THROM boh plas tin	*thromb/o* clot, clotting -*plastin* forming substance	Test of blood plasma to detect coagulation defects of the intrinsic system; used to detect hemophilia.
prothrombin time (PT) proh THROM bin	*pro-* before -*thrombin* clotting substance	Test that measures the amount of time taken for clot formation. It is used to determine the cause of unexplained bleeding, to assess levels of anticoagulation in patients taking warfarin or with vitamin K deficiency, and to assess the ability of the liver to synthesize blood-clotting proteins.
Schilling test SHILL ing		Nuclear medicine test used to diagnose vitamin B_{12} deficiency and pernicious anemia.
white blood cell (WBC) count		Measurement of the number of leukocytes in the blood. An increase may indicate the presence of an infection; a decrease may be caused by radiation or chemotherapy.

Fig. 9-19 A, Allergen patch test impregnated with individual allergens is applied to the back of the patient. **B,** Positive allergy reactions of varying intensity.

Fig. 9-20 Blood culture.

EXERCISE 10: Diagnostic Procedures

Matching. Some answers may be used more than once.

_____ 1. Coombs antiglobulin	_____ 9. Western blot	A. percentage of RBCs in the blood
		B. if increased, inflammation indicated
_____ 2. Schilling test	_____ 10. Hct	C. anemia
		D. HIV
_____ 3. PTT	_____ 11. ELISA	E. response to anemia treatment
		F. determines cause of bleeding
_____ 4. PCV	_____ 12. MCH	G. hemophilia
		H. pernicious anemia
_____ 5. monospot	_____ 13. MCHC	I. infectious mononucleosis
		J. hypersensitivity
_____ 6. ESR	_____ 14. allergy test	K. HDN, transfusion reaction
		L. microorganisms
_____ 7. blood culture	_____ 15. PT	M. number of leukocytes in the blood
_____ 8. WBC		

Build the terms.

16. process of recording the lymph vessels _____

17. process of recording a splenic artery _____

18. process of recording a lymph gland (node) _____

Case Study **Ramon Alvarez**

Ramon Alvarez is a 43-year-old product manager being seen today in the emergency room for a cut that has not healed. While trying to fix his motorcycle last week, he managed to gash his palm with a screwdriver. He says that he hadn't thought it was a problem at the time, but now his hand is red, hot, swollen, oozing, and there seems to be a "red line" on his arm. He said he thinks that he might also be unlucky enough to be coming down with the flu, because he has a fever, chills, and feels "just plain awful." Lab testing includes blood cultures, PT, PTT, a CBC, and platelet count. Ramon is surprised to find that he isn't going to be treated and released, but is instead admitted for SIRS.

1. What do blood cultures detect? _____

2. What does PT stand for? _____

3. What does PTT stand for? _____

4. What is another term for platelet? _____

5. What does SIRS stand for? _____

Medical Record *Libby Taylor*

TAYLOR, LIBBY T. - 478502 Opened by JONES-LITTLE, ANNA

Task   Edit   View   Time Scale   Options   Help

As Of 09:05

| TAYLOR, LIBBY T. | Age: 45 years | Sex: Female | Loc: BLKHK |
| | DOB: 02/05/1970 | MRN: 478502 | FIN: 3506004 |

Reference Text Browser | Form Browser | Medication Profile

Orders | Last 48 Hours | ED | **Lab** | Radiology | Assessments | Surgery | Clinical Notes | Pt. Info | Pt. Schedule | Task List | I & O | MAR

Flowsheet: Lab   ...   Level: Lab Report   ○ Table ○ Group ○ List

Navigator
✓   Lab Report

Basic Metabolic Panel
[Na]	Sodium	142	mEq/L	(L=134	H=145)	]
[K]	Potassium	3.7	mEq/L	(L=3.50	H=145)	]
[Cl]	Chloride	104	mEq/L	(L=93	H=145)	]
[CO]	CO2	27	mEq/L	(L=23	H=145)	]
[GL]	Glucose	88	mg/dL	(L=80	H=145)	]
[BU]	BUN	15	mg/dL	(L=7	H=145)	]
[CR]	Creatinine	0.7	mg/dL	(L=0.50	H=145)	]
[	Age	45	yrs			]
[	Non-aa gfr	87	mL/min			]
[	Afr Amer gfr	105	mL/min			]
[	Bun/creat	21	H	(L=10	H=20)	]
[Ca]	Calcium	8.8	mg/dL	(L=8.40	H=10.40)	]
[	Anion gap	11		(L=5	H=15)	]

PROD MAHAFC   26 Feb 2015   09:05

EXERCISE 11: Lab Report

Using the preceding lab report, answer the following questions.

1. What is the patient's K level? _____

2. What is the Na level? _____

3. What is the patient's BUN? _____

THERAPEUTIC INTERVENTIONS

Terms Related to Blood and Bone Marrow Interventions

Term	Word Origin	Definition
apheresis aff ur EE sis	*-apheresis* removal	Temporary removal of blood from a donor, in which one or more components are removed, and the rest of the blood is reinfused into the donor. Examples include **leukapheresis**, removal of WBCs; **plasmapheresis**, removal of plasma; and **plateletpheresis**, removal of thrombocytes. Also called **pheresis**.
bone marrow transplant (BMT)		The transplantation of bone marrow to stimulate production of normal blood cells.
autologous BMT ah TALL uh gus	*auto-* self *log/o* study *-ous* pertaining to	Harvesting of patient's own healthy bone marrow before treatment for reintroduction later.
homologous BMT hoh MALL uh gus	*homo-* same (species) *log/o* study *-ous* pertaining to	Transplantation of healthy bone marrow from a donor to a recipient to stimulate formation of new blood cells.
blood transfusion	*trans-* across *-fusion* pouring	Intravenous transfer of blood from a donor to a recipient, giving either whole blood or its components.
autologous transfusion ah TALL uh gus	*auto-* self *log/o* study *-ous* pertaining to *trans-* across *-fusion* pouring	Process in which the donor's own blood is removed and stored in anticipation of a future need (Fig. 9-21).
autotransfusion	*auto-* self *trans-* across *-fusion* pouring	Process in which the donor is transfused with his/her own blood, after anticoagulation and filtration, from an active bleeding site in cases of major surgery or trauma.
hemostasis	*hem/o* blood *-stasis* stopping, controlling	The control of bleeding by mechanical or chemical means.

Fig. 9-21 Autologous blood transfusion.

Be Careful!
Do not confuse -apheresis meaning removal with -poiesis, which means formation.

Fig. 9-22 Adenoidectomy.

Terms Related to Lymphatic and Immune System Interventions

Term	Word Origin	Definition
adenoidectomy ad eh noyd ECK tuh mee	*adenoid/o* adenoid *-ectomy* removal	Removal of the adenoids. Also called the **pharyngeal tonsils** (Fig. 9-22).
biopsy (bx) of lymphatic structures	*bi/o* life *-opsy* process of viewing *lymphat/o* lymph *-ic* pertaining to	Removal of the lymph nodes or lymphoid tissue as a means to diagnosis and treatment.
lymphadenectomy lim fad uh NECK tuh mee	*lymphaden/o* lymph gland *-ectomy* removal	Removal of a lymph node.
splenectomy spleh NECK tuh mee	*splen/o* spleen *-ectomy* removal	Removal of the spleen.

⟳ EXERCISE 12: Therapeutic Interventions

Match the interventions with their definitions.

_____ 1. autologous transfusion

_____ 2. homologous BMT

_____ 3. apheresis

_____ 4. autologous BMT

_____ 5. biopsy of lymphatic structures

_____ 6. autotransfusion

A. harvesting of patient's own bone marrow to be reintroduced later
B. donor is transfused with his own blood from an active bleeding site
C. temporary removal of blood from donor with removal of one or more components and subsequent reinfusion
D. transplantation of healthy bone marrow from donor
E. donor is reinfused with his/her own stored blood
F. removal of lymph nodes for examination

Build the terms.

7. removal of the spleen _____

8. removal of the pharyngeal tonsils _____

9. removal of platelets _____

10. removal of a lymph node _____

Case Study *Donna LeMasters*

Donna is a 59-year-old post mastectomy patient who presents to her physician with left unilateral axillary node swelling. Donna had a positive sentinel node biopsy with a resulting modified total left mastectomy last year. Chronic lymphedema has recently progressed to lymphangitis.

1. What is the first node to receive lymphatic drainage from a malignant tumor? _____

2. Where are the axillary nodes? _____ _____

3. What is removed in a lymphadenectomy? _____ _____

4. What is lymphangitis? _____ _____

5. What is the word that means one side? _____ _____

Medical Record *Manny Ochoa*

Black Hawk Hospital
1400 Washington Ave.
Waterloo, IA 50707

MEDICAL LETTER

Sally C. Quinn, MD
Student Health Center
Black Hawk Hospital
1400 Washington Avenue
Waterloo, IA 50707

Allen B. Corwin, MD
River City Physician Practice
7777 S. Shore Dr.
Mason City, IA 50428

Re: Manny Ochoa

Dear Dr. Quinn,

Please find the enclosed summary of treatment for Manny Ochoa, date of birth 8/3/1991, a college student whom I treated in my office last month. He requested that I forward this to you as his primary care physician in his home town; I understand he will be returning home this summer.

This 21-year-old college student had a 2-week history of a sore throat, stiffness and tenderness of his neck, and extreme fatigue. On examination, he had mild pyrexia with posterior cervical lymphadenopathy, palatal petechiae, and pharyngeal inflammation without an exudate. Abdominal examination showed marked splenomegaly. There was no evidence of a skin rash or jaundice.

The clinical diagnosis of infectious mononucleosis was confirmed on investigation with more than 50% of the lymphocytes showing atypical lymphocytosis. His serum contained IgM antibodies to the Epstein-Barr viral antigen. Liver function test results were normal.

He was treated symptomatically and was advised to avoid strenuous activity until his splenomegaly has completely resolved because of the danger of splenic rupture. He was also advised to abstain from alcohol for at least 6 months because many patients show clinical or biochemical evidence of liver involvement.

Sincerely,
Allen B. Corwin, MD

EXERCISE 13: Medical Letter

Using the preceding medical letter, answer the following questions.

1. How do you know that the patient had a slight fever? _____

2. On examination, what phrase might explain why his throat was sore? _____

3. Decode "cervical lymphadenopathy." _____

4. How do you know that the patient's spleen was enlarged? _____

5. What term tells you that test results showed an increase in the number of lymphocytes?

    _____

6. How do you know that he had been exposed to the EBV? _____

---

*Click on **Hear It, Spell It** to practice spelling the diagnostic and therapeutic terms that you have learned in this chapter.*

PHARMACOLOGY

Circulatory Drugs

anti- = against

anticoagulants: Prevent or delay the coagulation of blood and the formation of thrombi. Examples include heparin, warfarin (Coumadin), enoxaparin (Lovenox), and apixaban (Eliquis).

antiplatelets: Inhibit the function of platelets or destroy them. Examples include aspirin, clopidogrel (Plavix), dipyridamole (Persantine), ticlopidine (Ticlid), and abciximab (ReoPro).

blood-flow modifiers: Promote blood flow by keeping platelets from clumping or decreasing blood viscosity. Examples include the prescription medications cilostazol (Pletal) and pentoxifylline (Trental) and the herbal product ginkgo biloba.

colony-stimulating factors (CSFs): Stimulate the production of WBCs in the bone marrow. The two kinds are granulocyte CSF (G-CSF) and granulocyte-macrophage CSF (GM-CSF). Available synthetic agents of each type are filgrastim (Neupogen) and sargramostim (Leukine), respectively.

erythropoietic
erythr/o = red
-poietic = pertaining to formation

erythropoietic agents: Increase production of RBCs by stimulating erythropoiesis. Two available agents are epoetin alfa (Epogen, Procrit) and darbepoetin alfa (Aranesp).

hematinics (hee muh TIN icks): Increase the number of erythrocytes and/or hemoglobin concentration in the erythrocytes usually to treat iron-deficiency anemia. Examples are iron supplements and B-complex vitamins.

hematopoietic
hemat/o = blood
-poietic = pertaining to formation

hematopoietic (hem uh toh poy EH tick) **agents:** Stimulate blood cell production. Subdivisions of this class include CSFs, erythropoietic agents, and thrombopoietic factors.

hemostatic
hem/o = blood
-static = pertaining to stopping or controlling

hemostatics: Help stop the flow of blood. Examples include aminocaproic acid (Amicar) and tranexamic acid (Cyklokapron).

thrombopoietic factors: Stimulate the production of thrombocytes or platelets. Oprelvekin (Neumega) is an available agent.

Lymphatic and Immune Drugs

antihistamines: Block histamine (H_1) receptors to manage allergy symptoms. Examples include clemastine (Tavist), diphenhydramine (Benadryl), loratadine (Claritin), and fexofenadine (Allegra).

anti-IgE agents: Monoclonal antibodies that treat allergic asthma and allergic rhinitis. Omalizumab (Xolair) is the first available agent in this class.

antineoplastics: Treat cancer by preventing growth or promoting destruction of neoplastic (tumor) cells. Numerous drugs, including methotrexate and rituximab (Rituxan), fall into this category.

antiretrovirals: Minimize the replication of HIV and its progression into AIDS. Examples include zidovudine or azidothymidine (AZT) (Retrovir) and efavirenz (Sustiva).

corticosteroids: Steroids that suppress the immune system and reduce inflammation. Examples include fluticasone (Flovent, Flonase), hydrocortisone (Cortizone), and prednisone (Rayos).

cytotoxic agents: Damage or destroy cells to treat cancer; often act as immunosuppressants or antineoplastics.

immune modulators: Reduce the impact of immune system disorders. Dimethyl fumarate (Tecfidera) is an example of a drug used to treat multiple sclerosis.

immunosuppressants: Minimize the immune response. Examples include azathioprine (Imuran), cyclophosphamide (Cytoxan), cyclosporine (Sandimmune), and tacrolimus (Prograf).

leukotriene receptor antagonists: Block leukotrienes to manage later stages of allergic reactions; especially used to manage allergic asthma. Examples are montelukast (Singulair) and zafirlukast (Accolate).

protease (PRO tee aze) **inhibitors:** Antiretrovirals used to treat HIV infection. By blocking the production of an essential enzyme called *protease*, these drugs keep the virus from replicating. Examples are indinavir (Crixivan), nelfinavir (Viracept), and saquinavir (Invirase).

vaccines: Modified disease-causing microbial components administered to induce immunity or reduce the pathologic effects of a disease. Examples are the measles, mumps, rubella vaccine, and the chickenpox vaccine. A **vaccination** is an injection or oral solution derived from dead or weakened (attenuated) virus.

EXERCISE 14: Pharmacology

Match each drug group with its action.

_____ 1. erythropoietic agents

_____ 2. antiplatelets

_____ 3. hematopoietic agents

_____ 4. hematinics

_____ 5. anticoagulants

_____ 6. antihistamines

_____ 7. immunosuppressants

_____ 8. antineoplastics

_____ 9. hemostatics

_____ 10. vaccines

A. treat allergic reactions
B. delay clotting of blood
C. inhibit clotting, destroy thrombocytes
D. help induce immunity
E. increase blood cell production
F. stop the flow of blood
G. decrease tumor cells
H. lessen the immune response
I. increase RBC or Hgb concentration
J. increase production of RBCs

Abbreviations

Abbreviation	Definition	Abbreviation	Definition
A, B, AB, O	blood types	Hct	hematocrit
AIDS	acquired immunodeficiency syndrome	HDN	hemolytic disease of the newborn
ALL	acute lymphocytic leukemia	Hgb	hemoglobin
AML	acute myelogenous leukemia	HIV	human immunodeficiency virus
ANA	antinuclear antibody	Ig	immunoglobulin
basos	basophils	K	potassium
BMP	basic metabolic panel	lymphs	lymphocytes
BMT	bone marrow transplant	MCH	mean corpuscular hemoglobin
BUN	blood urea nitrogen	MCHC	mean corpuscular hemoglobin concentration
bx	biopsy	Na	sodium
Ca	calcium	neuts	neutrophils
CBC	complete blood cell count	NK	natural killer (cells)
Cl	chloride	PCV	packed-cell volume
CLL	chronic lymphocytic leukemia	plats	platelets, thrombocytes
CML	chronic myelogenous leukemia	PMNs, polys	polymorphonucleocytes
CMP	comprehensive metabolic panel	PT	prothrombin time
CO_2	carbon dioxide	PTT	partial thromboplastin time
diff	differential (WBC count)	RBC	red blood cell (count)
EBV	Epstein-Barr virus	Rh	Rhesus
eosins	eosinophils	SIRS	systemic immune response syndrome
ESR	erythrocyte sedimentation rate	WBC	white blood cell (count)
Hb	hemoglobin		

EXERCISE 15: Abbreviations

Write out the term for the following abbreviations.

1. Karl was admitted with a diagnosis of EBV. _____

2. The patient's blood sample was tested for Hct and Hb. _____

3. The AIDS patient was HIV positive. _____

4. The patient was sent for a CMP. _____

5. The patient was admitted for a BMT with his twin as the donor. _____

Chapter Review

Match the word parts to their definitions.

Word Parts

Suffix

| -cyte |
| -cytosis |
| -edema |
| -emia |
| -gen |
| -globin |
| -penia |
| -philia |
| -poiesis |
| -siderin |

Definition

1. _____ cell
2. _____ producing
3. _____ abnormal increase in cells
4. _____ protein substance
5. _____ formation
6. _____ swelling
7. _____ attraction condition
8. _____ deficiency
9. _____ iron substance
10. _____ blood condition

Combining Form

| axill/o |
| cyt/o |
| eosin/o |
| erythr/o |
| granul/o |
| hemat/o |
| inguin/o |
| leuk/o |
| lymphaden/o |
| lymphangi/o |
| lymph/o |
| morph/o |
| myel/o |
| neutr/o |
| nucle/o |
| plasm/o |
| pyr/o |
| ser/o |
| splen/o |
| thromb/o |
| thym/o |
| tonsill/o |

Definition

11. _____ blood
12. _____ rosy-colored
13. _____ groin
14. _____ nucleus
15. _____ lymph vessel
16. _____ bone marrow
17. _____ spleen
18. _____ fever, fire
19. _____ red
20. _____ clotting, clot
21. _____ lymph gland (node)
22. _____ cell
23. _____ neutral
24. _____ armpit
25. _____ white
26. _____ serum
27. _____ little grain
28. _____ plasma
29. _____ thymus
30. _____ lymph
31. _____ shape
32. _____ tonsil

Wordshop

Prefixes	Combining Forms	Suffixes
an-	adenoid/o	-cytosis
dys-	cyt/o	-ectomy
hyper-	erythr/o	-edema
hypo-	hem/o	-graphy
pan-	leuk/o	-ia
par-	lymphaden/o	-ic
	lymphangi/o	-in
	lymph/o	-ism
	phag/o	-itis
	sider/o	-lysis
	splen/o	-penia
	thromb/o	-stasis

Build the following terms by combining the preceding word parts. Some word parts may be used more than once. Some may not be used at all. The number in parentheses is the number of word parts needed to correctly build the term.

Definition	Term
1. deficiency of all cells (3)	_____
2. abnormal increase of white blood cells (2)	_____
3. inflammation of a lymph gland/node (2)	_____
4. deficiency of clotting cells (3)	_____
5. process of recording a lymph gland (2)	_____
6. abnormal increase of red blood cells (2)	_____
7. removal of the adenoids (2)	_____
8. swelling (due to) lymph (fluid) (2)	_____
9. stopping/controlling bleeding (2)	_____
10. break down of blood (2)	_____
11. blood iron substance (3)	_____
12. iron deficiency anemia (2)	_____
13. process of recording a lymph vessel (2)	_____
14. condition of excessive spleen (3)	_____
15. removal of the spleen (2)	_____

Sort the terms below into the correct categories.

Term Sorting

Anatomy and Physiology	Pathology	Diagnostic Procedures	Therapeutic Interventions

adenoidectomy

agglutination

anaphylaxis

antibody

antiretrovirals

apheresis

blood transfusion

BMP

BMT

CBC

CMP

coagulation

diff count

dyscrasia

edema

ELISA

eosinophil

Hct

hematinic

hematopoiesis

hemoglobin

hemostasis

hemostatics

hypovolemia

leukocytosis

lymphangiography

lymphangitis

MCHC

mononucleosis

monospot

plasma

plateletpheresis

Schilling test

septicemia

sideropenia

splenectomy

thalassemia

thrombocyte

thymus

vaccine

Replace the highlighted words with the correct terms.

Translations

1. On physical examination, Ms. Cooper's physician observed **an enlarged spleen** and she was scheduled for a **removal of the spleen.**

2. Laboratory findings indicated **deficiency of all blood cells** and Mrs. Hamilton was diagnosed with **suppression of bone marrow function leading to a reduction in RBC production.**

3. Laboratory testing revealed that Marc Douglas had an **abnormal increase in WBCs** and **blood samples submitted to propagate microorganisms that may be present** was positive for staphylococci.

4. Tyra was stung by a bee and suffered **an extreme form of allergic response.**

5. The patient underwent a **transplantation of bone marrow to stimulate production of normal blood cells** to treat his **rapidly progressive form of leukemia that develops from immature bone marrow stem cells.**

6. Mr. Washington was admitted with **an acute, painful exacerbation of sickle-cell anemia** that was complicated by **an increased function of the spleen that results in hemolysis.**

7. **Removal of thrombocytes from a donor** was used to treat Mrs. Alverez' **deficiency of platelets that causes an inability of the blood to clot.**

8. The patient was diagnosed with **RBC deficiency caused by blood loss** and needed **an intravenous transfer of blood from a donor to a recipient.**

9. Tommy was seen for cervical **disease of the lymph nodes** and was diagnosed with **an increase in the number of mononuclear cells.**

10. The physician suspected that Alex had **a deficiency of one of the factors necessary for the coagulation of blood** and ordered **a test of blood plasma to detect coagulation defects of the intrinsic system.**

11. Dr. Martinez thought Amanda had **progressive anemia that results from a lack of intrinsic factor** ordered a **nuclear medicine test used to diagnose B$_{12}$ deficiency.**

12. Francis had **a bleeding disorder characterized by hemorrhage into the tissues** and was diagnosed with **a systemic infection with pathologic microbes in the blood.**

13. Greta's doctor ordered blood tests to see if she had **an abnormal decrease in WBCs** or **an abnormal decrease in neutrophils due to disease process.**

14. The patient was diagnosed with **a group of inherited bleeding disorders characterized by a deficiency of one of the factors necessary for the coagulation of blood.**

Medical Record Ozzie Samuelson

SAMUELSON, OZZIE P. - 499483 Opened by WATERFIELD, WENDY

Task   Edit   View   Time Scale   Options   Help

SAMUELSON, OZZIE P.

| Age: 42 years | Sex: Male | Loc: WHC-SMMC |
| DOB: 01/27/1972 | MRN: 499483 | FIN: 3506004 |

Reference Text Browser   Form Browser   Medication Profile

Orders | Last 48 Hours | ED | Lab | Radiology | Assessments | Surgery | **Clinical Notes** | Pt. Info | Pt. Schedule | Task List | I & C | MAR

Flowsheet: Clinical Notes   Level: Discharge Summary   ○ Table ○ Group ○ List

Navigator

✓ Clinical Notes

Principal Diagnosis: Sickle-Cell Crisis
Surgical Procedure: None
History of Present Illness: On the above date, the patient was admitted via the emergency room, with a chief complaint of pain all over his body since the night before.
    The patient, a 42-year-old African American male with a history of sickle-cell anemia, stated that he started having pain all over his body, especially at the back of the legs. He also notes having chills, but denies sweats.
    Medical History: The patient has a medical history of sickle-cell anemia and pneumonia in 2004.
Surgical History: Surgical history includes a total hip replacement and an appendectomy.
Allergies: The patient has no history of allergies.
Medications: Motrin and Darvon.
Occupation: The patient is unemployed, on disability. The patient is a nonsmoker and a nondrinker.
Family History: The patient's family history reveals mother and father with sickle-cell trait; otherwise unremarkable.
Review of Systems: Unremarkable except for global body pain.
Physical Examination: Temperature was 98.1 degrees, blood pressure was 155/90, heart rate of 75, respiratory rate of 23.
Consultations: The consultations included Dr. Smith for sickle-cell disease.
Pertinent Laboratory Studies: Reticulocyte count of 13.8; white blood cell count of 12.9 hemoglobin and hematocrit of 12.0 and 29.4, respectively; albumin of 2.1.
Hospital Course: The patient was admitted on 11/01/2011 and progressed steadily with intravenous analgesic support until discharge on 11/05/2011, when the patient was deemed stable.
Condition on Discharge: Stable.
Discharge Instructions: The patient is to limit activity and should follow up with Dr. Rohr in his office in 1 week.
Medications on Discharge: Biaxin, Suprax, Trental, folic acid, Toradol, and vitamin E.

PROD | MAHAFC | 11 Nov 2014 | 12:52

⟳ CLINICAL NOTES

1. What statement in the discharge summary indicates that the patient was in sickle-cell crisis?

    _____

2. What medications were used to treat the patient's symptoms?

    _____

3. The patient's past healthcare history mentions a resection of his _____.

10 Cardiovascular System

CHAPTER OUTLINE

OBJECTIVES

- Recognize and use terms related to the anatomy and physiology of the cardiovascular system.
- Recognize and use terms related to the pathology of the cardiovascular system.
- Recognize and use terms related to the diagnostic procedures for the cardiovascular system.
- Recognize and use terms related to the therapeutic interventions for the cardiovascular system.

For interactive learning, click on:
- **Match the Word Parts** to review cardiovascular word parts.
- **Word Shop** to practice word building.
- **Tournament of Terminology** to test your knowledge of cardiovascular terms.
- **Term Sorting** to practice sorting cardiovascular terms in categories.

*Click on **Chapter at a Glance** to print off a list of key terms and word parts for this chapter.*

FUNCTIONS OF THE CARDIOVASCULAR SYSTEM

The primary function of the **cardiovascular** (kar dee oh VAS kyoo lur) **system,** also called the **circulatory system,** is to provide transportation of oxygen (O_2), nutrients, water, body salts, hormones, and other substances to every cell in the body. It also acts to carry waste products, such as carbon dioxide (CO_2), away from the cells, eventually to be excreted. The **heart** functions as a pump; the blood **vessels** act as "pipes;" and the blood is the transportation medium. If the system does not function properly, causing O_2 or the other critical substances to be withheld from the cells, dysfunction results, and the cells (and the person) may be injured or die.

SPECIALISTS/SPECIALTIES

Cardiology is the diagnosis, treatment, and prevention of disorders of the heart. The specialist in this field is called a **cardiologist.**

ANATOMY AND PHYSIOLOGY

Pulmonary and Systemic Circulation

To accomplish its task of pumping substances to and from the cells of the body, the heart is in the center of two overlapping cycles of circulation: **pulmonary** and **systemic.**

Pulmonary Circulation

In short, pulmonary circulation goes from the heart to the lungs and then back to the heart. Pulmonary circulation begins with the right side of the heart, sending blood to the lungs to absorb O_2 and release CO_2. Note in Fig. 10-1 that the vessels that carry blood to the lungs from the heart are blue to show the blood as being **deoxygenated** (dee OCK sih juh nay tid), or oxygen deficient. Once the O_2 is absorbed, the blood is considered **oxygenated,** or oxygen rich. Note in Fig. 10-1 that the vessels traveling away from the lungs are red to show oxygenation. The blood then progresses back to the left side of the heart, where it is pumped out to begin its route through the systemic circulatory system.

Systemic Circulation

The systemic circulation carries blood from the heart to the cells of the body, where nutrient and waste exchange takes place; the wastes, such as CO_2, are carried back to the heart on the return trip. This blood is then pumped out of the right side of the heart to the lungs to dispose of its CO_2, absorb O_2, and repeat the cycle. In systemic circulation, the blood traveling away from the heart first passes through the largest artery in the body called the **aorta** (a ORE tuh). From the aorta, the vessels branch into conducting **arteries** (AR tur reez), then into smaller **arterioles** (ar TEER ee olez), and finally to the **capillaries** (CAP ih lair eez). Arteries are blood vessels that carry blood *away* from the heart (Fig. 10-2, *A*). Note in Fig. 10-3 that the color has changed from the red of oxygenated blood to a purple color at the capillaries. This is the site of exchange between the cells' fluids and the plasma of the circulatory system. O_2 and other substances are supplied, and CO_2 is collected, along with a number of other wastes. Once the blood begins its journey back to the heart, it first goes through **venules** (VEEN yools), then **veins** (vayns), and finally into one of the two largest veins, either the **superior** or the **inferior vena cava** (VEE nuh KAY vuh). Veins are blood vessels that carry blood *toward* the heart (see Fig. 10-2, *B*). Fig. 10-4 illustrates

cardiovascular
cardi/o = heart
vascul/o = vessel
-ar = pertaining to

heart = cardi/o, coron/o, cordi/o

vessel = vascul/o, angi/o, vas/o

cardiology
cardi/o = heart
-logy = study of

pulmonary = pulmon/o

systemic
system/o = system
-ic = pertaining to

oxygen = ox/i, ox/o

carbon dioxide = capn/o

lung = pulmon/o, pneum/o, pneumat/o

aorta = aort/o

artery = arteri/o, arter/o

arteriole = arteriol/o

capillary = capillar/o

venule = venul/o

vein = ven/o, phleb/o

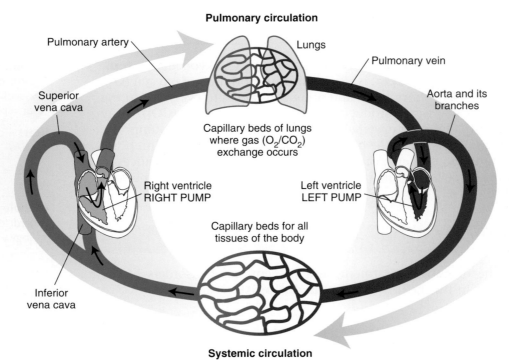

Fig. 10-1 Pulmonary and systemic circulation.

the muscular, thick nature of arteries; the valvular, thinner nature of veins; and the delicate exchange function of capillaries. Arteries are generally thicker than veins, because they must withstand the force of the heart's pumping action. Veins do not have the thick muscle coat of the arteries to propel the blood on its journey through the circulatory system but instead rely on one-way valves that prevent the backflow of blood. In addition, skeletal muscle contraction provides pumping action. The capillaries' diameters are so tiny that only one blood cell at a time can pass through them.

EXERCISE 1: Pulmonary and Systemic Circulation

Match the following combining forms with their meanings. More than one answer may be correct.

_____ 1. vein   _____ 6. lung   A. vas/o   G. cardi/o
                                             B. pulmon/o   H. capillar/o
_____ 2. artery   _____ 7. aorta   C. angi/o   I. vascul/o
                                             D. phleb/o   J. arteriol/o
_____ 3. heart   _____ 8. arteriole   E. arteri/o   K. aort/o
                                             F. ven/o   L. venul/o
_____ 4. venule   _____ 9. vessel

_____ 5. capillary

Decode the terms.

10. endovascular _____

11. intravenous _____

12. pericardial _____

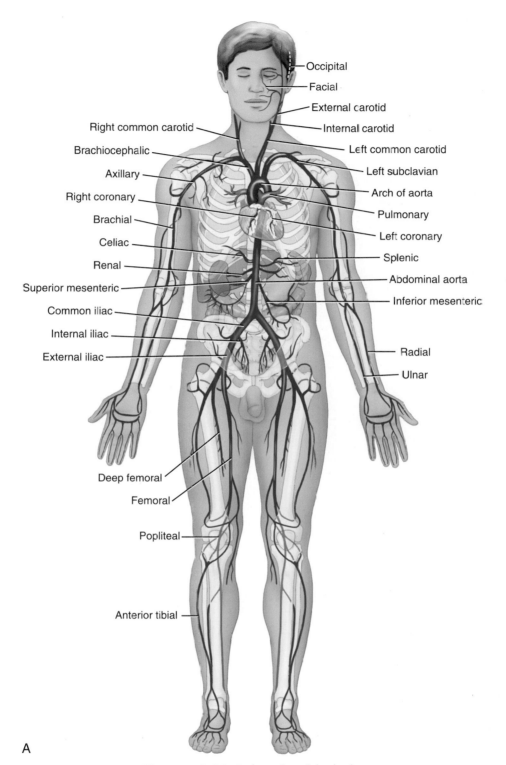

Occipital
Facial
External carotid
Internal carotid
Right common carotid
Brachiocephalic
Left common carotid
Axillary
Left subclavian
Right coronary
Arch of aorta
Brachial
Pulmonary
Celiac
Left coronary
Renal
Splenic
Superior mesenteric
Abdominal aorta
Common iliac
Inferior mesenteric
Internal iliac
External iliac
Radial
Ulnar
Deep femoral
Femoral
Popliteal
Anterior tibial

A

Fig. 10-2 A, Principal arteries of the body.

Continued

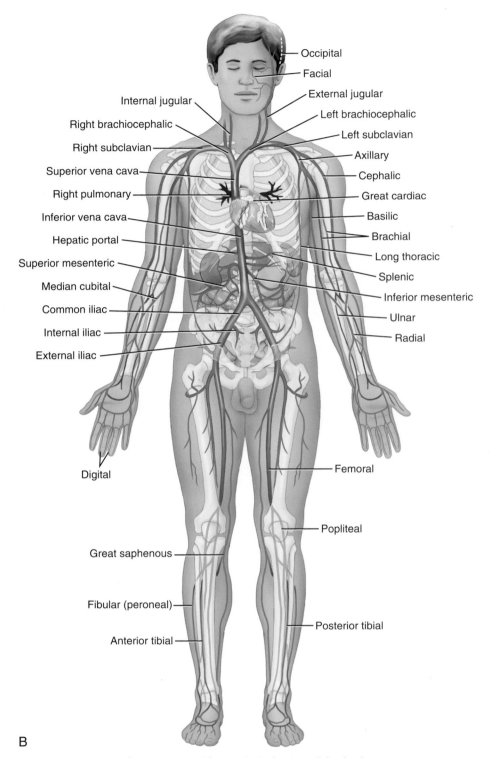

Occipital

Facial

External jugular

Internal jugular

Left brachiocephalic

Right brachiocephalic

Left subclavian

Right subclavian

Axillary

Superior vena cava

Cephalic

Right pulmonary

Great cardiac

Inferior vena cava

Basilic

Hepatic portal

Brachial

Superior mesenteric

Long thoracic

Median cubital

Splenic

Common iliac

Inferior mesenteric

Internal iliac

Ulnar

External iliac

Radial

Digital

Femoral

Popliteal

Great saphenous

Fibular (peroneal)

Posterior tibial

Anterior tibial

B

Fig. 10-2, cont'd B, Principal veins of the body.

Fig. 10-3 Oxygenated/deoxygenated status.

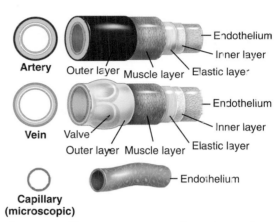

Fig. 10-4 Differences among arteries, veins, and capillaries.

Anatomy of the Heart

The human heart is about the size of a fist. It is located in the mediastinum of the thoracic cavity, slightly left of the midline. Its pointed tip, the **apex,** rests just above the diaphragm. The area of the chest wall anterior to the heart and lower thorax is referred to as the **precordium** (pree KORE dee um). The heart muscle has its own dedicated system of blood supply, the **coronary** (KORE ih nair ee) **arteries** (Fig. 10-5, *A*). The two main coronary arteries are called the *left* and *right coronary arteries (LCA, RCA)*. They supply a constant, uninterrupted blood flow to the heart. The areas of the heart wall that they feed are designated as *inferior, lateral, anterior,* and *posterior.*

The heart has four chambers (see Fig. 10-5, *B*). The upper chambers are called **atria** (A tree uh) (*sing.* atrium). The lower chambers are called **ventricles** (VEN trih kuls). Between the atria and ventricles, and between the ventricles and vessels, are valves that allow blood to flow through in one direction. Those values are opened and closed with the assistance of the papillary muscles and their connecting cords, the chordae tendineae. The tissue walls between the chambers are called **septa** (SEP tuh) (*sing.* septum). The heart wall is constructed of three layers. The **endocardium** (en doh KAR dee um) is the thin tissue that acts as a lining of each of the chambers and **valves.** The **myocardium** (mye oh KAR dee um) is the cardiac muscle surrounding each of these chambers. The **pericardium** (pare ee KAR dee um) is the double-folded layer of connective tissue that surrounds the heart. The inner surface of this double fold is called the **visceral** (VIS uh rul) **pericardium,** and the outer membrane, closest to the body wall, is the **parietal** (puh RYE uh tul) **pericardium.** Another name for the visceral pericardium is the **epicardium** (eh pee KAR dee um) because it is the structure on top of the heart.

apex = apic/o

precordium
  pre- = before
  cordi/o = heart
  -um = structure

atrium = atri/o

ventricle = ventricul/o

septum = sept/o

valve = valvul/o

endocardium = endocardi/o

myocardium = myocardi/o

visceral = viscer/o

parietal = pariet/o

pericardium = pericardi/o

epicardium
  epi- = above, on top of
  cardi/o = heart
  -um = structure

 Be Careful! *Do not confuse* **aort/o** *meaning aorta,* **atri/o** *meaning atrium,* **arteri/o** *meaning artery, and* **arteriol/o** *meaning arteriole.*

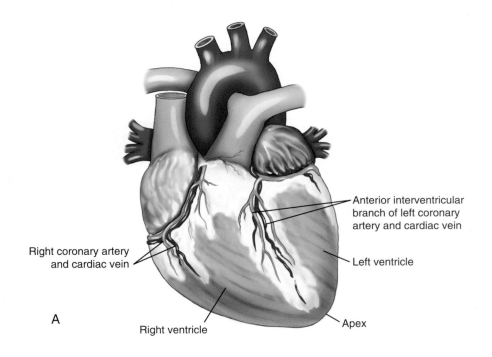

Anterior interventricular branch of left coronary artery and cardiac vein

Left ventricle

Right coronary artery and cardiac vein

Apex

Right ventricle

A

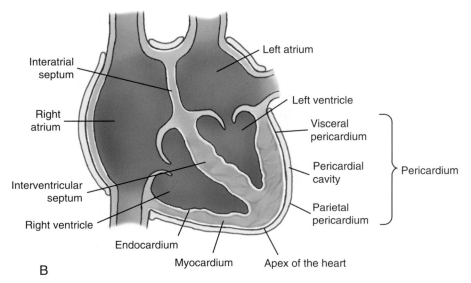

Interatrial septum

Left atrium

Right atrium

Left ventricle

Visceral pericardium

Pericardial cavity

Pericardium

Interventricular septum

Parietal pericardium

Right ventricle

Endocardium

Myocardium

Apex of the heart

B

Fig. 10-5 A, The heart and great vessels. **B,** Chambers of the heart.

EXERCISE 2: Anatomy of the Heart

Match the combining form with the correct body part.

_____ 1. sept/o

_____ 2. valvul/o

_____ 3. atri/o

_____ 4. ventricul/o

_____ 5. aort/o

_____ 6. cardi/o, cordi/o, coron/o

_____ 7. apic/o

_____ 8. endocardi/o

_____ 9. myocardi/o

_____ 10. pericardi/o

_____ 11. pulmon/o

_____ 12. arteri/o

A. upper chamber of the heart
B. lower chamber of the heart
C. heart
D. largest artery
E. inner lining of chambers of heart
F. outer sac surrounding the heart
G. lung
H. muscle layer of the heart
I. valve
J. vessel that carries blood away from the heart
K. wall between chambers
L. the pointed extremity of a conical structure

Build the terms.

13. pertaining to between the ventricles _____

14. pertaining to surrounding the tip (of the heart) _____

15. pertaining to before the heart _____

16. pertaining to through the heart muscle _____

EXERCISE 3: Anatomy of the Heart

Label the drawing using the terms provided.

pericardium
interventricular septum
right atrium
right ventricle
myocardium
endocardium
left ventricle
left atrium
interatrial septum

Blood Flow Through the Heart

Using Fig. 10-6 as a guide, follow the route of the blood through the heart. The pictures and words in this diagram are shaded red and blue to represent oxygenated and deoxygenated blood. Blood is squeezed from the **right atrium (RA)** to the **right ventricle (RV)** through the **tricuspid** (try KUSS pid) **valve (TV).** Valves are considered to be competent if they open and close properly, letting through or holding back an expected amount of blood. Once in the RV, the blood is squeezed out through the **pulmonary semilunar valve** through the short, wide **pulmonary trunk** and into the **pulmonary arteries (PAs),** which carry blood to the lungs and are the only arteries that carry deoxygenated blood. In the capillaries of the lungs, the CO_2 is passed out of the blood and O_2 is taken in. The now-oxygenated blood continues its journey back to the left side of the heart through the **pulmonary veins.** These are the only veins that carry oxygenated blood. The blood then enters the heart through the **left atrium (LA)** and has to pass the **mitral** (MYE trul) **valve (MV),** also termed the **bicuspid valve,** to enter the **left ventricle (LV).** When the LV contracts, the blood is finally pushed out through the **aortic semilunar valve** into the **aorta** and begins yet another cycle through the body.

The amount of blood expelled from the LV compared with the total volume of blood filling the ventricle is referred to as the *stroke volume* and is a measure of the **ejection fraction** of cardiac output. Typically around 65%, this amount is reduced in certain types of heart disease.

If a woman's heart rate is 80 beats per minute (bpm), then that means her heart contracts almost 5000 times per hour and more than 100,000 beats per day, every day, for a lifetime. Truly an amazing amount of work is accomplished by an individual's body without a bit of conscious thought!

ejection

e- = out
ject/o = throwing
-ion = process of

Fig. 10-6 Route of the blood through the heart.

⟳ EXERCISE 4: Blood Flow Through the Heart

Fill in the correct answer.

1. _____ are the only arteries that carry deoxygenated blood.

2. The _____ valve is between the RA and RV.

3. The _____ valve is between the LA and LV.

4. _____ valves open and close properly.

5. The amount of blood expelled from the LV compared with total heart

   volume is a measure of the _____ .

The Cardiac Cycle

Systemic and pulmonary circulations occur as a result of a series of coordinated, rhythmic pulsations, called **contractions** and **relaxations,** of the heart muscle. The normal *rate* of these pulsations in humans is 60 to 100 bpm and is noted as a patient's **heart rate.** Fig. 10-7 illustrates various pulse points, places where heart rate can be measured in the body. **Blood pressure (BP)** is the resulting *force* of blood against the arteries. The contractive phase is **systole** (SIS toh lee), and the relaxation phase is **diastole** (dye AS toh lee). BP is recorded in millimeters of mercury (Hg) as a fraction representing the systolic pressure over the diastolic pressure. Optimum BP is a systolic reading less than 120 and a diastolic reading less than 80. This is written as 120/80. Normal BP is represented by a range. See the following table for BP guidelines.

contraction
 con- = together
 tract/o = pull
 -ion = process of

Blood Pressure Guidelines			
	Systolic		Diastolic
Normal	under 120	and	under 80
Prehypertension	121-139	or	80-89
Stage 1 hypertension	140-159	or	90-99
Stage 2 hypertension	over 160	or	over 100

Modified from US Department of Health and Human Services.

The cues for the timing of the heartbeat come from the electrical pathways in the muscle tissue of the heart (Fig. 10-8). The heartbeat begins in the RA in the tissue referred to as the **sinoatrial** (sin oh A tree ul) **(SA) node,** also called the *natural pacemaker of the heart.* The initial electrical signal causes the atria to undergo electrical changes that signal contraction. This electrical signal is sent to the **atrioventricular** (a tree oh ven TRICK yoo lur) **(AV) node,** which is located at the base of the RA proximal to the interatrial septum. From the AV node, the signal travels next to the **bundle of His** (also called the **atrioventricular bundle**). This bundle, a band of specialized cardiac muscle fibers, is in the interatrial septum, and its right and left bundle branches transmit the impulse to the **Purkinje** (poor KIN jee) **fibers** in the RV and LV. Once the Purkinje fibers receive stimulation, they cause the ventricles to undergo electrical changes that signal contraction to force blood out to the PAs and the aorta. If the electrical activity is normal, it is referred to as a **normal sinus rhythm (NSR)** or **heart rate.** Any deviation of this electronic signaling may lead to an **arrhythmia** (ah RITH mee ah), which is an abnormal heart rhythm that compromises an individual's cardiovascular functioning by pumping too much or too little blood during that segment of the cardiac cycle.

sinoatrial
 sin/o = sinus
 atri/o = atrium
 -al = pertaining to

atrioventricular
 atri/o = atrium
 ventricul/o = ventricle
 -ar = pertaining to

arrhythmia
 a- = without
 rhythm/o = rhythm
 -ia = condition

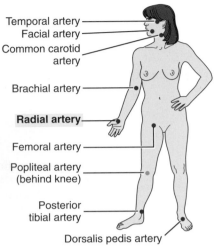

Temporal artery
Facial artery
Common carotid artery
Brachial artery
Radial artery
Femoral artery
Popliteal artery (behind knee)
Posterior tibial artery
Dorsalis pedis artery

Fig. 10-7 Pulse points. The radial artery is the most commonly used pulse point.

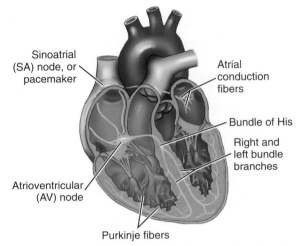

Sinoatrial (SA) node, or pacemaker
Atrioventricular (AV) node
Purkinje fibers
Atrial conduction fibers
Bundle of His
Right and left bundle branches

Fig. 10-8 Electrical conduction pathways of the heart.

*Choose **Hear It, Spell It** to practice spelling the anatomy and physiology terms you have learned in this chapter. You can review the anatomy of the cardiovascular system by clicking on **Body Spectrum Electronic Anatomy Coloring Book** → **Circulatory**.*
*Click on **Label It** to practice labeling the heart.*

Medical Record William Woodward

WOODWARD, WILLIAM W - 52243

Task   Edit   View   Time Scale   Options   Help

| WOODWARD, WILLIAM W | Age: 58 years DOB: 06/06/1956 | Sex: Male MRN: 52243 | Loc: VVH FIN: 884401 |

Reference Text Browser | Form Browser | Medication Profile

Orders | Last 48 Hours | ED | Lab | **Radiology** | Assessments | Surgery | Clinical Notes | Pt. Info | Pt. Schedule | Task List | I & O | MAR

Flowsheet: Radiology   Level: Radiology Report   ⊙ Table ○ Group ○ List

Navigator
✓ Radiology

Intraoperative Left Carotid Arteriogram

A single intraoperative left carotid arteriogram is submitted. The catheter tip is located within the distal common carotid artery. The injection has opacified a widely patent endarterectomy site. The former stenosis located at the origin of the right internal carotid artery has been completely reduced. The left internal carotid artery is widely patent into the intracranial circulation. The external carotid artery is also widely patent.

Impression: Intraoperative arteriogram demonstrating a widely patent left carotid endarterectomy site.

PROD | MAHAFC | 26 March 2015 | 12:37

⟳ EXERCISE 5: Imaging Report

Fill in the correct answer in the following questions using the report provided earlier.

1. "Intraoperative" tells you that the procedure was done _____ the operation.

2. The carotid arteries are located in the _____ and supply blood to the _____.

3. An "endarterectomy" site would refer to an area _____ an artery.

4. The term *stenosis* in the report refers to a _____ of the artery.

Combining and Adjective Forms for the Anatomy and Physiology of the Cardiovascular System

Meaning	Combining Form	Adjective Form
aorta	aort/o	aortic
apex	apic/o	apical
arteriole	arteriol/o	
artery	arteri/o, arter/o	arterial
atrium	atri/o	atrial
carbon dioxide	capn/o	
endocardium	endocardi/o	endocardial
epicardium	epicardi/o	epicardial
heart	cardi/o, coron/o, cordi/o	cardiac, coronary, cordial
lung	pulmon/o, pneum/o, pneumat/o	pulmonary, pneumatic
myocardium	myocardi/o	myocardial
oxygen	ox/i, ox/o	
pericardium	pericardi/o	pericardial
pull	tract/o	
rhythm	rhythm/o	rhythmic
septum, wall	sept/o	septal
sinus	sin/o	
system	system/o	systemic
valve	valvul/o	valvular
vein	ven/o, phleb/o	venous
ventricle	ventricul/o	ventricular
venule	venul/o	
vessel	vascul/o, angi/o, vas/o	vascular
viscera	viscer/o	visceral
wall	pariet/o	parietal

Prefixes for Anatomy and Physiology of the Cardiovascular System

Prefix	Meaning
a-	without
con-	together
e-	out
pre-	before

Suffixes for Anatomy and Physiology of the Cardiovascular System

Suffix	Meaning
-ar, -ary, -ic, -al	pertaining to
-ia	condition
-ion	process of
-logy	study of
-um	structure

PATHOLOGY

Terms Related to Cardiac Signs and Symptoms

Term	Word Origin	Definition
bradycardia brad dee KAR dee ah	*brady-* slow *-cardia* heart condition	Slow heartbeat with ventricular contractions less than 60 bpm (Fig. 10-9, *B*).
bruit BROO ee		Abnormal sound heard when an artery is auscultated. Usually a blowing or swishing sound, higher pitched than a murmur.
cardiodynia kar dee oh DIN ee uh	*cardi/o* heart *-dynia* pain	Heart pain that may be described as atypical or ischemic. **Atypical pain** is a stabbing or burning pain that is variable in location and intensity and unrelated to exertion. **Ischemic pain** is a pressing, squeezing, or weight-like cardiac pain caused by decreased blood supply that usually lasts only minutes. **Precordial pain** is pain in the area over the heart. Also called **cardialgia**.
cardiomegaly kar dee oh MEG uh lee	*cardi/o* heart *-megaly* enlargement	Enlargement of the heart.
claudication klah dih KAY shun		Cramplike pains in the calves caused by poor circulation in the leg muscles.
cyanosis sye uh NOH sis	*cyan/o* blue *-osis* abnormal condition	A bluish or grayish discoloration of skin, nail beds, and/or lips caused by a lack of oxygen in the blood.
diaphoresis dye uh foh REE sis		Profuse secretion of sweat.
dyspnea; dyspnea on exertion (DOE) DISP nee uh	*dys-* difficult *-pnea* breathing	Difficult and/or painful breathing; if DOE, it is experienced when effort is expended.
edema eh DEE muh		Abnormal accumulation of fluid in interstitial spaces of tissues.
emesis EM uh sis	*emesis* to vomit	Forcible or involuntary emptying of the stomach through the mouth.
ischemia	*isch/o* to hold back *-emia* blood condition	Lack of blood in a body part due to a blockage or functional constriction.

Continued

Terms Related to Cardiac Signs and Symptoms—cont'd

Term	Word Origin	Definition
murmur		Abnormal heart sound heard during systole, diastole, or both, which may be described as a gentle blowing, fluttering, or humming sound.
nausea NAH zsa		Sensation that accompanies the urge to vomit but does not always lead to vomiting.
orthopnea or THOP nee uh	*orth/o* straight, upright *-pnea* breathing	Condition in which a person must sit or stand to breathe comfortably.
pallor PAL ur		Paleness of skin and/or mucous membranes. On darker pigmented skin, it may be noted on the inner surfaces of the lower eyelids or the nail beds.
palpitations pal pih TAY shuns		Pounding or racing of the heart, such that the patient is aware of his/her heartbeat.
pulmonary congestion	*pulmon/o* lung *-ary* pertaining to	Excessive amount of blood in the pulmonary vessels. Usually associated with heart failure (HF).
shortness of breath (SOB)		Breathlessness, air hunger.
syncope SING kuh pee		Fainting, loss of consciousness.
tachycardia tack ee KAR dee ah	*tachy-* rapid *-cardia* heart condition	Rapid heartbeat, more than 100 bpm (see Fig. 10-9, *C*).
thrill		Fine vibration felt by the examiner on palpation.
venous distention	*ven/o* vein *-ous* pertaining to	Enlarged or swollen veins.

⊗ Be Careful!

Do not confuse **palpation,** *which means examination by touch,* **palpebration,** *which means blinking, and* **palpitation,** *which means a pounding or racing of the heart.*

Fig. 10-9 Electrocardiograms (ECGs). **A,** Normal. **B,** Bradycardia. **C,** Tachycardia.

EXERCISE 6: Cardiac Signs and Symptoms

Matching.

_____ 1. claudication	_____ 8. ischemia	A. fainting
_____ 2. syncope	_____ 9. nausea	B. paleness of skin
_____ 3. diaphoresis	_____ 10. pallor	C. air hunger
		D. fine vibration felt on palpation
_____ 4. bruit	_____ 11. palpitations	E. difficult breathing
_____ 5. murmur	_____ 12. dyspnea	F. abnormal sound heard upon auscultation of an artery
		G. cramplike pains in legs
_____ 6. thrill	_____ 13. cyanosis	H. abnormal heart sound
_____ 7. emesis	_____ 14. SOB	I. blue color due to lack of oxygen

A. fainting
B. paleness of skin
C. air hunger
D. fine vibration felt on palpation
E. difficult breathing
F. abnormal sound heard upon auscultation of an artery
G. cramplike pains in legs
H. abnormal heart sound
I. blue color due to lack of oxygen
J. urge to vomit
K. vomiting
L. decreased blood supply
M. profuse sweating
N. pounding of the heart

Decode the terms.

15. bradycardia _____

16. tachycardia _____

17. cardiomegaly _____

Terms Related to Congenital Disorders of the Heart

Term	Word Origin	Definition
coarctation of the aorta koh ark TAY shun		Congenital cardiac anomaly characterized by a localized narrowing of the aorta. **Coarctation** is another term for a narrowing (Fig. 10-10).
patent ductus arteriosus (PDA) PAY tent DUCK tus ar teer ee OH sis		Abnormal opening between the PA and the aorta caused by failure of the fetal ductus arteriosus to close after birth, most often in premature infants. **Patent** means *open.* **Occluded** means *closed.*
septal defect SEP tul	*sept/o* septum, wall *-al* pertaining to	Any congenital abnormality of the walls between the heart chambers. **Atrial septal defect (ASD)** is a hole in the wall between the upper chambers of the heart. **Ventricular septal defect (VSD)** is a hole in the wall between the lower two chambers of the heart.
tetralogy of Fallot teh TROL uh jee fah LOH	*tetra-* four *-logy* study of	Congenital cardiac anomaly that consists of four defects: pulmonic stenosis; VSD; malposition of the aorta, so that it arises from the septal defect or the RV; and right ventricular hypertrophy (Fig. 10-11).

Fig. 10-10 Coarctation of the aorta.

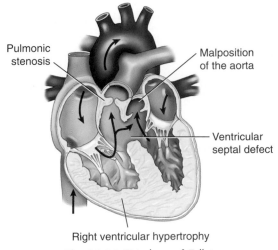

Fig. 10-11 Tetralogy of Fallot.

EXERCISE 7: Congenital Disorders

Match the congenital disorders with their definitions.

_____ 1. patent ductus arteriosus

_____ 2. septal defect

_____ 3. coarctation of the aorta

_____ 4. tetralogy of Fallot

A. cardiac anomaly of four defects
B. narrowing of the largest artery of the body
C. abnormal opening between the PA and the aorta
D. hole in the wall between the upper or lower chambers of the heart

---

Case Study Julio Montez

Julio Montez was born prematurely at 34 weeks. He had cyanosis at birth and exhibited dyspnea while feeding later that day. An echocardiogram confirmed a diagnosis of tetralogy of Fallot. Julio was scheduled for corrective surgery in a few months to repair his VSD and other cardiac anomalies.

1. What is the medical term for difficulty breathing? _____

2. *Cyanosis* is a term that indicates a lack of oxygen and is evidenced by what color of skin, nail beds, and lips? _____

3. How may separate heart defects accompany tetralogy of Fallot? _____

4. What does VSD stand for? _____ _____

5. Dyspnea means difficult _____.

The following valvular heart diseases (VHDs) present as incompetent or insufficient valvular function as a result of **stenosis** (narrowing), **regurgitation** (backflow), or **prolapse** (drooping). The causes are either congenital or acquired.

Terms Related to Valvular Heart Disease

Term	Word Origin	Definition
aortic stenosis (AS) a OR tick sten OH sis	*aort/o* aorta *-ic* pertaining to stenosis narrowing	Narrowing of the aortic valve, which may be acquired or congenital (Fig. 10-12).
mitral regurgitation (MR) MYE trul ree gur jih TAY shun		Backflow of blood from the LV into the LA in systole across a diseased valve. It may be the result of congenital valve abnormalities, rheumatic fever, or mitral valve prolapse (MVP).
mitral stenosis (MS) MYE trul sten OH sis	*stenosis* narrowing	Narrowing of the valve between the LA and LV caused by adhesions on the leaflets of the valve, usually the result of recurrent episodes of rheumatic endocarditis. Left atrial hypertrophy develops and may be followed by right-sided HF and pulmonary edema (cor pulmonale) (see Fig. 10-12).
mitral valve prolapse (MVP) MYE trul valv PRO laps	*pro-* forward *-lapse* fall	Protrusion of one or both cusps of the MV back into the LA during ventricular systole (Fig. 10-13).
tricuspid stenosis (TS) try KUSS pid sten OH sis	*stenosis* narrowing	Relatively uncommon narrowing of the tricuspid valve associated with lesions of other valves caused by rheumatic fever. Symptoms include jugular vein distention and pulmonary congestion (see Fig. 10-12).
valvulitis val vyoo LYE tis	*valvul/o* valve *-itis* inflammation	Inflammatory condition of a valve, especially a cardiac valve, caused most commonly by rheumatic fever and less frequently by bacterial endocarditis or syphilis. Results are stenoses and obstructed blood flow.

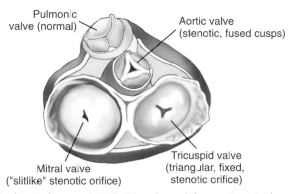

Fig. 10-12 Valvular heart disease (VHD). Disorders of the aortic, mitral, and tricuspid valves.

Be Careful!

Do not confuse **stenosis,** *which means a narrowing, with* **sclerosis,** *which means a hardening.*

Fig. 10-13 Mitral valve prolapse (MVP).

Mitral valve prolapse
Normal mitral valve

 EXERCISE 8: Valvular Heart Disorders

Matching.

_____ 1. stenosis   _____ 3. prolapse   A. drooping, falling forward
                                                  B. narrowing
_____ 2. regurgitation   _____ 4. valvulitis   C. backflow
                                                  D. inflammation of a valve

A **dysrhythmia** is an abnormal heartbeat (*dys-* means abnormal, *rhythm/o* means rhythm, and *-ia* means condition). Remember that a normal heart rate is referred to as a *normal sinus rhythm (NSR)*.

Terms Related to Cardiac Dysrhythmias (Arrhythmias)

Term	Word Origin	Definition
arrhythmia ah RITH mee ah	*a-* without *rhythm/o* rhythm *-ia* condition	Abnormal variation from the normal heartbeat rhythm. Also called **dysrhythmia**.
atrioventricular (AV) block a tree oh ven TRICK yoo lur	*atri/o* atrium *ventricul/o* ventricle *-ar* pertaining to	Partial or complete heart block that is the result of a lack of electrical communication between the atria and the ventricles. Also termed *heart block*.
bundle branch block (BBB) eck TOP ick		Incomplete electrical conduction in the bundle branches, either left or right.
	ec- out of *top/o* place *-ic* pertaining to	Heartbeats that occur outside of a normal rhythm.
	atri/o atrium *-al* pertaining to	Atrial ectopic beats (AEBs) are irregular contractions of the atria. Also termed **premature atrial contractions (PACs)**.

Terms Related to Cardiac Dysrhythmias (Arrhythmias)—cont'd

Term	Word Origin	Definition
ectopic beats eck TOP ick	*ec-* out of *top/o* place *-ic* pertaining to	Heartbeats that occur outside of a normal rhythm.
atrial	*atri/o* atrium *-ic* pertaining to	**Atrial ectopic beats (AEBs)** are irregular contractions of the atria. Also called **premature atrial contractions (PACs)**.
ventricular	*ventricul/o* ventricle *-ar* pertaining to	**Ventricular ectopic beats (VEBs)** are irregular contractions of the ventricles. Also called **premature ventricular contractions (PVCs)**. PVCs are not always considered pathologic.
fibrillation fibrill LAY shun		Extremely rapid and irregular contractions (300 to 600 bpm) occurring with or without an underlying cardiovascular disorder, such as coronary artery disease (CAD).
atrial	*atri/o* atrium *-al* pertaining to	**Atrial fibrillation (AF)** is the most common type of cardiac arrhythmia.
ventricular	*ventricul/o* ventricle *-ar* pertaining to	Rapid, irregular ventricular contractions; may be fatal unless reversed.
flutter		Extremely rapid but regular heartbeat (250 to 350 bpm). **Atrial flutter** is a rapid, regular atrial rhythm.
sick sinus syndrome (SSS)		Any abnormality of the sinus node that may include the necessity of an implantable pacemaker.
ventricular tachycardia ven TRICK yoo lur tack ee KAR dee ah	*ventricul/o* ventricle *-ar* pertaining to *tachy-* rapid *-cardia* heart condition	Condition of ventricular contractions that are more than 100 bpm.

EXERCISE 9: Cardiac Dysrhythmias

Fill in the blank.

1. Another general term for an arrhythmia is a/an _____.

2. Extremely rapid and irregular contractions are _____.

3. An extremely rapid but regular heartbeat is _____.

4. The general term for a lack of electrical communication is heart _____.

5. Any abnormality of the sinus node is termed _____.

6. Another term for premature ventricular contractions is _____.

7. The term for ventricular contractions over 100 bpm is _____.

Case Study   Cynthia Frost

Cynthia Frost was getting out of her car at the mall when she felt her heart pounding, and she couldn't catch her breath. She immediately sat down and thought she was going to pass out. A passerby called 911. The local paramedics took her to an emergency department (ED) where she was diagnosed with atrial fibrillation and prescribed antiarrhythmic drugs.

1. Fibrillation is a type of _____.
   a. arrhythmia
   b. infection
   c. inflammation
   d. murmur

2. Atrial fibrillation occurs in the _____ chambers of the heart.
   a. upper
   b. lower

3. Fibrillation is a regular but rapid rhythm of _____ 300 bpm.
   a. less than
   b. greater than

4. What does SOB stand for? _____ _____

5. A pounding or racing of the heart so that the person is aware of her heartbeat is called _____ _____.

Terms Related to Other Disorders of Coronary Circulation

Term	Word Origin	Definition
angina pectoris an JYE nuh PECK tore us	*pector/o* chest *-is* structure	Paroxysmal chest pain that is often accompanied by SOB and a sensation of impending doom (Fig. 10-14).
coronary artery disease (CAD) KORE uh nare ee	*coron/o* heart, crown *-ary* pertaining to	Accumulation and hardening of plaque in the coronary arteries that eventually can deprive the heart muscle of oxygen, leading to **angina (heart pain).**
myocardial infarction (MI) mye oh KAR dee ul in FARCK shun	*myocardi/o* heart muscle *-al* pertaining to	Cardiac tissue death that occurs when the coronary arteries are occluded (blocked) by an **atheroma** (ath uh ROH mah), a mass of fat or lipids on the wall of an artery, or a blood clot caused by an atheroma; and thus are unable to carry enough oxygenated blood to the heart muscle. Depending on the area affected, the patient may die if enough of the heart muscle is destroyed (Fig. 10-15). Also called a **heart attack.** When a person is in the process of having a heart attack, it is called an **acute myocardial infarction (AMI).**

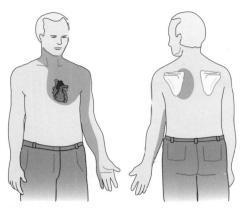

Fig. 10-14 Common sites of pain in angina pectoris.

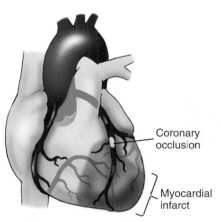

Coronary occlusion

Myocardial infarct

Fig. 10-15 Myocardial infarction.

Inflammation and Heart Disease

Research has uncovered a link between higher levels of a protein present in the blood when blood vessels are inflamed and cardiovascular disease risk. Elevated C-reactive protein (CRP) levels are associated with a dramatically increased risk for heart attack and stroke, independent of an individual's cholesterol levels, obesity, smoking history, or BP. Although the research indicates that diagnosis and treatment of the inflammation may reduce one's risk of heart disease, the American Heart Association continues to recommend that individuals stop smoking, eat a healthy diet, exercise, maintain a healthy BP, and manage diabetes if present for optimal cardiovascular health.

Terms Related to Other Cardiac Conditions

Term	Word Origin	Definition
cardiac tamponade tam pon ADE		Compression of the heart caused by fluid in the pericardial sac.
cardiomyopathy kar dee oh mye AH puh thee	*cardiomy/o* myocardium *-pathy* disease	Progressive disorder of the ventricles of the heart.
endocarditis en doh kar DYE tis	*endocardi/o* endocardium *-itis* inflammation	Inflammation of the endocardium and heart valves, characterized by lesions and caused by a number of different microbes (Fig. 10-16).
heart failure (HF)		Inability of the heart muscle to pump blood efficiently so that it becomes overloaded. The heart enlarges with unpumped blood, and the lungs fill with fluid. Previously referred to as **congestive heart failure (CHF)**.
pericarditis pair ee kar DYE tis	*pericardi/o* pericardium *-itis* inflammation	Inflammation of the sac surrounding the heart with the possibility of **pericardial effusion** (the escape of blood into the pericardium).

Fig. 10-16 Acute bacterial endocarditis. The valve is covered with large irregular vegetations *(arrow)*.

Endothelium
Vessel wall
A   Atherosclerotic plaque

B

C

Fig. 10-17 Atherosclerosis. **A,** Artery is blocked by an atheroma. **B,** Fatty deposits on wall of artery. **C,** Image of the resultant narrowed coronary artery.

EXERCISE 10: Other Disorders of Coronary Circulation and Cardiac Conditions

Fill in the blank.

1. The medical term for a heart attack is a/an (2 words) _____.

2. The inability for the heart muscle to pump blood efficiently is (2 words)

    _____.

3. A compression of the heart caused by fluid in the pericardial sac is (2 words)

    _____.

4. Paroxysmal chest pain accompanied by shortness of breath is (2 words)

    _____.

5. An accumulation and hardening of plaque in the coronary arteries is (3 words) _____

    _____, abbreviated CAD.

Build the terms.

6. inflammation of the pericardium _____

7. inflammation of the endocardium _____

8. disease of the heart muscle _____

Terms Related to Vascular Disorders

Term	Word Origin	Definition
aneurysm AN yoo rizz um		Localized dilation of an artery caused by a congenital or acquired weakness in the wall of the vessel. The acquired causes may be arteriosclerosis, trauma, infection, and/or inflammation.
arteriosclerosis ar teer ee oh sklah ROH sis	*arteri/o* artery *-sclerosis* abnormal condition of hardening	Disease in which the arterial walls become thickened and lose their elasticity, without the presence of atheromas.
atherosclerosis ath uh roh sklah ROH sis	*ather/o* fat, plaque *-sclerosis* abnormal condition of hardening	Form of arteriosclerosis in which medium and large arteries have atheromas, which can reduce or obstruct blood flow. Patients with peripheral atherosclerosis complain of intermittent claudication (Fig. 10-17).
esophageal varices eh sof uh JEE ul VARE ih seez	*esophag/o* esophagus *-eal* pertaining to *varic/o* dilated vein	Varicose veins that appear at the lower end of the esophagus as a result of portal hypertension; they are superficial and may cause ulceration and bleeding.
hemorrhoid HEM uh royd		Varicose condition of the external or internal rectal veins that causes painful swellings at the anus.
hypertension (HTN) hye pur TEN shun	*hyper-* excessive *tens/o* stretching *-ion* process of	Condition of high or elevated BP, also known as **arterial hypertension**; occurs in two forms—**primary** (or **essential**) **hypertension,** which has no identifiable cause; and **secondary hypertension,** which occurs in response to another disorder. **Malignant hypertension** is very high BP that results in organ damage.
hypotension hye poh TEN shun	*hypo-* below, deficient *tens/o* stretching *-ion* process of	Condition of below normal BP. **Orthostatic hypotension** occurs when a patient experiences an episode of low BP upon rising to a standing position.
peripheral arterial occlusion puh RIFF uh rul ar TEER ree ul oh KLOO zhun	*arteri/o* artery *-al* pertaining to *occlus/o* blockage *-ion* process of	Blockage of blood flow to the extremities. Acute or chronic conditions may be present, but patients with both types of conditions are likely to have underlying atherosclerosis. *Occlusion* means blockage.
peripheral vascular disease (PVD) puh RIFF uh rul VAS kyoo lur	*vascul/o* vessel *-ar* pertaining to	Any vascular disorder limited to the extremities; may affect not only the arteries and veins but also the lymphatics.
Raynaud disease ray NODE		**Idiopathic** disease—that is, of unknown cause—of the peripheral vascular system that causes intermittent cyanosis/erythema of the distal ends of the fingers and toes, sometimes accompanied by numbness; occurs almost exclusively in young women. Presentation is bilateral. **Raynaud phenomenon** is secondary to rheumatoid arthritis, scleroderma, or trauma. Presentation is unilateral.
thrombophlebitis throm boh fluh BYE tis	*thromb/o* clotting, clot *phleb/o* vein *-itis* inflammation	Inflammation of either deep veins (**deep vein thrombosis, or DVT**) or superficial veins (**superficial vein thrombosis, or SVT**) with the formation of one or more blood clots (Fig. 10-18).

Continued

Terms Related to Vascular Disorders—cont'd

Term	Word Origin	Definition
varicose veins VARE ih kose	*varic/o* varices *-ose* pertaining to	Elongated, dilated superficial veins (varices) with incompetent valves that permit reverse blood flow. These veins may appear in various parts of the anatomy, but the term varicose vein(s) has been reserved for those in the lower extremities.
vasculitis vas kyoo LYE tis	*vascul/o* vessel *-itis* inflammation	Inflammation of the blood vessels. Also called **angiitis**.

Fig. 10-18 A, Deep vein thrombophlebitis (DVT). **B,** Large embolus derived from a lower extremity DVT and now located in a pulmonary artery (PA) branch.

 EXERCISE 11: Vascular Disorders

Fill in the blanks with one of the following terms:

essential, primary, secondary, varicose veins, claudication, hemorrhoids, esophageal varices, aneurysm, peripheral artery occlusion, Raynaud disease

1. A localized dilation of an artery caused by a weakness in the vessel wall is a/an

    _____.

2. Cramplike pain in the calves caused by poor circulation is called _____.

3. If hypertension is idiopathic, it is called _____ or _____hypertension.

4. _____ hypertension is due to another disorder.

5. Swollen, twisted veins in the region of the anus are called _____.

6. Varicose veins of the lower end of the tube from the throat to the stomach are called

    _____.

7. A blockage of blood flow to the extremities is called _____.

8. An idiopathic disease of the peripheral vascular system is called _____.

9. Elongated superficial dilated veins are called _____.

Decode the terms.

10. vasculitis _____

11. hypotension _____

12. hypertension _____

13. thrombophlebitis _____

Case Study   Anne Louise Potts

Anne Louise Potts is a 62-year-old, two-pack-a-day smoker who complains of cramplike pains in her legs when she walks. She says the pain is so bad that she has to sometimes use a cane. After examining Anne Louise, her physician suspects peripheral atherosclerosis. He orders a lipid profile and vascular sonography.

1. If Anne Louise has atherosclerosis, she has masses of fat in her arteries called _____.

2. Atherosclerosis is a form of _____.
   a. hypertension
   b. aneurysm
   c. arteriosclerosis
   d. varicose vein

3. The suffix *-sclerosis* refers to an abnormal condition of _____.

4. A lipid profile measures the amount of _____ and triglycerides in circulating blood.

5. What is the term that means cramplike pains in the legs due to poor circulation? _____

Terms Related to Benign Neoplasms

Term	Word Origin	Definition
atrial myxoma A tree uhl mick SOH mah	*atri/o* atrium *-al* pertaining to *myx/o* mucus *-oma* tumor, mass	Benign growth usually occurring on the interatrial septum (Fig. 10-19).
hemangioma heh man jee OH mah	*hemangi/o* blood vessel *-oma* tumor, mass	Noncancerous tumor of the blood vessels. May be congenital ("stork bite") or may develop later in life.

Terms Related to Malignant Neoplasms

Term	Word Origin	Definition
angiosarcoma an jee oh sar KOH mah	*angi/o* vessel *-sarcoma* connective tissue cancer	Rare cancer of the cells that line the blood vessels. Also called a **hemangiosarcoma.**
cardiac myxosarcoma mick soh sar KOH mah	*myx/o* mucus *-sarcoma* connective tissue cancer	Rare cancer of the heart usually originating in the LA (Fig. 10-20).

Fig. 10-19 Left atrial myxoma.

Fig. 10-20 Myxosarcoma of the heart.

EXERCISE 12: Neoplasms

Fill in the blank.

1. What is a benign tumor of the blood vessels? _____.

2. What is a rare malignant tumor of the heart? _____.

3. What is a benign tumor that originates in the atria of the heart? _____.

4. What is a rare malignant tumor of the lining of the blood vessels? _____.

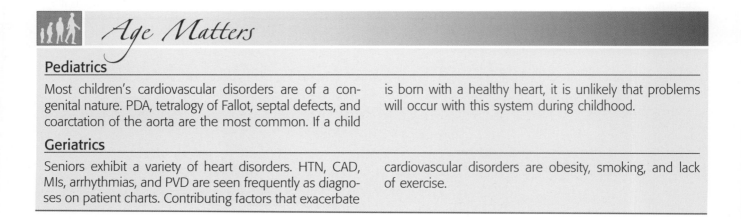

Age Matters

Pediatrics

Most children's cardiovascular disorders are of a congenital nature. PDA, tetralogy of Fallot, septal defects, and coarctation of the aorta are the most common. If a child is born with a healthy heart, it is unlikely that problems will occur with this system during childhood.

Geriatrics

Seniors exhibit a variety of heart disorders. HTN, CAD, MIs, arrhythmias, and PVD are seen frequently as diagnoses on patient charts. Contributing factors that exacerbate cardiovascular disorders are obesity, smoking, and lack of exercise.

Medical Record Helen Podrasky

PODRASKY, HELEN P - 612347 Opened by ADAMS, JOHANNA MD   _ ⊡ ☒

Task   Edit   View   Time Scale   Options   Help

As Of 15:09

PODRASKY, HELEN P

Age: 63 years	Sex: Female	Loc: WHC-SMMC
DOB: 06/02/1952	MRN: 612347	FIN: 3506004

Reference Text Browser   Form Browser   Medication Profile

Orders | Last 48 Hours | ED | Lab | Radiology | Assessments | Surgery | **Clinical Notes** | Pt. Info | Pt. Schedule | Task List | I & O | MAR

Flowsheet: Clinical Notes   Level: Progress Note   ⦿ Table   ○ Group   ○ List

Navigator ☒

✔ Progress Note

Patient is status post coronary bypass grafting approximately 1 year ago. Today, she developed a rapid pulse of approximately 145, no chest pain, and no SOB, but indicated she felt weak as a result.

PAST MEDICAL HISTORY:	As above
MEDICATIONS:	verapamil, digoxin, Coumadin, iron
PHYSICAL EXAM:	
Vital signs:	BP 150/66, pulse 136 and irregular, temp. 97.2º F
Chest:	Clear
Heart:	Rhythm is irregular
Abdomen:	Soft and nontender
LABORATORY FINDINGS:	ECG showed atrial flutter 125-145. Chest x-ray showed cardiomegaly. Patient given 5 mg verapamil and converted to sinus rhythm at a rate of 85 almost immediately. Patient will be admitted to Cardiology Services at the hospital.
DIAGNOSIS:	Atrial flutter, converted. Cardiomegaly.

PROD | MAHAFC | 07 May 2015 | 15:09

 EXERCISE 13: Progress Note

Using the preceding report, answer the following questions by circling the correct answer:

1. Which vessels in the cardiovascular system were operated on 1 year ago? *(heart vessels/veins/intracranial vessels)*

2. "Sinus rhythm" refers to *(irregular heartbeat/normal heartbeat).*

3. "Flutter" is an example of a/an *(arrhythmia/valve disorder/occlusion).*

4. "Atrial" refers to *(the pericardium/the upper chambers of the heart/the lower chambers of the heart).*

5. "Cardiomegaly" means that the heart is *(inflamed/prolapsed/enlarged).*

6. An "ECG" is an *(electroencephalogram/electrocardiogram/electromyogram).*

*Click on **Hear It, Spell It** to practice spelling the pathology terms you have learned in this chapter. To review pathology terms play **Medical Millionaire**.*

Heart Disease in Women

Heart disease is not just a man's disease. In fact 1 in 4 women in the United States will die from heart disease. Heart disease is the number one killer of women in the United States, killing more women every year than men. The Office of Research on Women's Health at the National Institutes of Health (NIH) is charged with understanding how biologic and physiologic differences between the sexes affect health. As a result of this research, hormonal fluctuations are now believed to account for the variations in the results of a number of diagnostic tests and the optimal time for certain types of treatments. Visit www.womenshealth.gov to view the latest results of studies that examine the differences gender makes in cardiovascular and other diseases.

DIAGNOSTIC PROCEDURES

Terms Related to General Diagnostic Procedures

Term	Word Origin	Definition
blood pressure (BP)		A measure of the systolic over the diastolic pressure. The instrument used is a **sphygmomanometer.**
auscultation and percussion (A&P) oss kull TAY shun pur KUH shun		Listening to internal sounds in the body, usually with a **stethoscope,** or by tapping (percussing).

Terms Related to Imaging

Term	Word Origin	Definition
angiocardiography an jee oh kar dee AH gruh fee	*angi/o* vessel *cardi/o* heart *-graphy* process of recording	Injection of a radiopaque substance during cardiac catheterization for the purpose of imaging the heart and related structures (Fig. 10-21).
cardiac catheterization KAR dee ack kath ih tur ih ZAY shun	*cardi/o* heart *-ac* pertaining to	Threading of a catheter (thin tube) into the heart under fluoroscopic guidance to collect diagnostic information about structures in the heart, coronary arteries, and great vessels; also used to aid in treatment of CAD, congenital abnormalities, and HF (Fig. 10-22).
digital subtraction angiography (DSA) an jee AH gruh fee	*sub-* under *tract/o* pulling *-ion* process of *angi/o* vessel *-graphy* process of recording	Digital imaging process wherein contrast images are used to "subtract" the noncontrast image of surrounding structures, leaving only a clear image of blood vessels (Fig. 10-23).

Continued

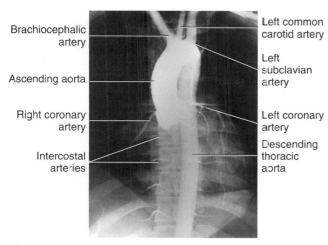

Brachiocephalic artery
Ascending aorta
Right coronary artery
Intercostal arteries
Left common carotid artery
Left subclavian artery
Left coronary artery
Descending thoracic aorta

Fig. 10-21 Angiocardiography. Aorta and right and left coronary arteries (RCA, LCA) are shown.

RVA
RCC
LVA
RSA
IN LCC LSA

Fig. 10-23 Digital subtraction image of the aorta.

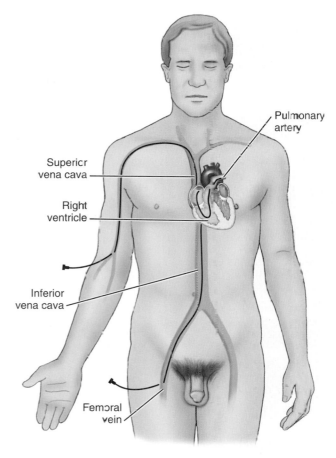

Pulmonary artery
Superior vena cava
Right ventricle
Inferior vena cava
Femoral vein

Fig. 10-22 Right-sided heart catheterization. The catheter is inserted into the femoral or brachial vein and advanced through the inferior vena cava through the superior vena cava, right atrium (RA), and right ventricle (RV) and then into the pulmonary artery (PA).

Fig. 10-24 A, Person undergoing echocardiography (ECHO). **B,** Color Doppler image of the heart.

Terms Related to Imaging—cont'd

Term	Word Origin	Definition
echocardiography (ECHO) eck oh kar dee AH gruh fee	*echo-* sound *cardi/o* heart *-graphy* process of recording	Use of ultrasonic waves directed through the heart to study the structure and motion of the heart (Fig. 10-24). **Transesophageal echocardiography (TEE)** images the heart through a transducer introduced into the esophagus.
electrocardiography (ECG, EKG) ee leck troh kar dee AH gruf ee	*electr/o* electricity *cardi/o* heart *-graphy* process of recording	Recording of electrical impulses of the heart as wave deflections of a needle on an instrument called an **electrocardiograph.** The record, or recording, is called an **electrocardiogram.**
exercise stress test (EST)		Imaging of the heart during exercise on a treadmill; may include the use of radioactive substance. Also called an **exercise electrocardiogram.**
fluoroscopy	*fluor/o* to flow *-scopy* process of viewing	Special kind of x-ray procedure that allows visualization of structures in real time directly on a monitor screen.
Holter monitor HOLE tur		Portable electrocardiograph that is worn to record the reaction of the heart to daily activities (Fig. 10-25).
magnetic resonance imaging (MRI)		Computerized imaging that uses radiofrequency pulses in a magnetic field to detect areas of MI, stenoses, and areas of blood flow.
MUGA scan MOO guh		**Mu**ltiple-**g**ated **a**cquisition scan is a noninvasive method of imaging a beating heart by tagging RBCs with a radioactive substance. A gamma camera captures the outline of the chambers of the heart as the blood passes through them.
myocardial perfusion imaging mye oh KAR dee ul pur FYOO zhun	*myocardi/o* myocardium *-al* pertaining to *per-* through *-fusion* process of pouring	Use of radionuclide to diagnose CAD, valvular or congenital heart disease, and cardiomyopathy.
phlebography fleh BAH gruh fee	*phleb/o* vein *-graphy* process of recording	X-ray imaging of a vein after the introduction of a contrast dye.
positron emission tomography (PET) POZ ih tron ee MIH shun toh MAH gruh fee	*e-* out *-mission* sending *tom/o* slice *-graphy* process of recording	Computerized nuclear medicine procedure that uses inhaled or injected radioactive substances to help identify how much a patient will benefit from revascularization procedures.
radiography	*radi/o* rays *-graphy* process of recording	Posteroanterior and lateral chest x-rays may be used to evaluate the size and shape of the heart.
Swan-Ganz catheter swann ganz		Long, thin cardiac catheter with a tiny balloon at the tip that is fed into the femoral artery near the groin and extended up to the LV. This instrument then is used to determine left ventricular function by measuring pulmonary capillary wedge pressure.

Fig. 10-25 **A,** Holter monitor. **B,** Placement of the leads on the chest.

Terms Related to Laboratory Tests

Term	Word Origin	Definition
cardiac enzymes test		Blood test that measures the amount of cardiac enzymes characteristically released during a MI; determines the amount of lactate dehydrogenase (LDH) and creatine phosphokinase (CPK) in the blood.
lipid profile		Blood test to measure the lipids (cholesterol and triglycerides) in the circulating blood (see a sample lipid profile in the following table).
phlebotomy fleh BAH tuh mee	*phleb/o* vein *-tomy* incision	The opening of a vein to withdraw a blood sample. Also called **venipuncture.**

Sample Lipid Profile

Test	Your results	Date	Normal Range
Total cholesterol	171	11/02/2011	Under 200
HDL ("good cholesterol")	55	11/02/2011	Over 40
Triglycerides	84	11/02/2011	Under 150
LDL ("bad cholesterol")	99	11/02/2011	Under 100
TSH (Thyroid)	2.470	11/03/2011	0.35-5.50
Blood count	Normal		
Vitamin D	30.8		32-100

HDL, High-density lipoprotein; *LDL,* low-density lipoprotein; *TSH,* thyroid-stimulating hormone.

EXERCISE 14: Diagnostic Procedures

Fill in the blanks with one of the following terms.

cardiac enzymes test, cardiac catheterization, lipid profile, radiography, myocardial perfusion imaging, PET scan, exercise stress test, MUGA scan, digital subtraction angiography

1. What test uses a gamma camera to view the heart chambers? _____

2. What test measures cholesterol and triglycerides? _____

3. What test measures the enzymes released during a heart attack? _____

4. What technique "subtracts" background structures to image vessels? _____

5. What test uses a radionuclide to diagnose heart disease? _____

6. Heart size and shape can be evaluated with _____.

7. The reaction of the heart to exercise is measured through what type of test? _____

8. An invasive technique that is commonly used either to help diagnose or to treat disorders of the

    heart is called _____.

9. A computerized nuclear medicine procedure to help identify the extent to which a patient will

    benefit from a vessel repair procedure is called _____.

Build the terms.

10. incision of a vein _____

11. process of recording a heart vessel _____

12. process of recording a vein _____

13. process of recording electrical activity of the heart _____

14. process of recording the heart using sound _____

Case Study   Jennifer Cahill

Jennifer Cahill woke up this morning with crushing chest pain and diaphoresis. A few minutes later, she collapses in her kitchen. Her husband performs cardiopulmonary resuscitation (CPR), and she is admitted to the hospital. Her cardiac enzymes test and ECG confirm that Jennifer has had an MI.

1. MI stands for _____.

2. The muscle layer of the heart is called the _____.

3. What is the term that means chest pain? _____

4. ECG stands for _____.

5. A/an _____ looks for enzymes that are released during a MI.

THERAPEUTIC INTERVENTIONS

Terms Related to Cardiac Procedures

Term	Word Origin	Definition
angioplasty AN gee oh plas tee	*angi/o* vessel *-plasty* surgical repair	Reconstruction of blood vessels damaged by disease or injury, often performed by inflating a balloon within a vessel at the site of narrowing to restore blood flow.
atherectomy ath uh RECK tuh mee	*ather/o* fat, plaque *-ectomy* removal	Removal of plaque from the coronary artery (or other arteries) through a catheter with a rotating shaver or a laser.
cardiac defibrillator dee FIB ruh lay tur		Either external or implantable device that provides an electric shock to the heart to restore a normal sinus rhythm.
automatic implantable cardioverter-defibrillator (AICD)		A device that is implanted in the chest to monitor the heartbeat and correct it if needed (speed it up or slow it down).
carotid endarterectomy kuh RAH tid en dar tur ECK tuh mee	*end-* within *arter/o* artery *-ectomy* removal	Removal of the atheromatous plaque lining the carotid artery to increase blood flow and leave a smooth surface. Done to prevent thrombotic occlusions (Fig. 10-26).
cardiac pacemaker		Small, battery-operated device that helps the heart beat in a regular rhythm; can be either internal (permanent) or external (temporary) (Fig. 10-27).

Continued

Fig. 10-26 Carotid endarterectomy.

- Internal carotid artery
- External carotid artery
- Incision reveals atherosclerotic plaque
- Common carotid artery
- Aortic arch

Fig. 10-27 **A,** Pacemakers. **B,** Chest radiography of patient with permanent pacemaker implanted.

Terms Related to Cardiac Procedures—cont'd

Term	Word Origin	Definition
cardiopulmonary resuscitation (CPR) kar dee oh PULL muh nare ee reh suss ih TAY shun	*cardi/o* heart *pulmon/o* lung *-ary* pertaining to	Manual external cardiac massage and artificial respiration used to restart the heartbeat and breathing of a patient.
cardioversion		Pharmacologic or electrical procedure to restore a fast or irregular heartbeat to a normal sinus rhythm. In electrical cardioversion, the heart is given low-energy shocks using a **cardioverter.**
commissurotomy kom ih shur AH tuh mee	*commissur/o* connection *-tomy* incision	Surgical division of a fibrous band or ring connecting corresponding parts of a body structure. Commonly performed to separate the thickened, adherent leaves of a stenosed MV.
coronary artery bypass graft (CABG)	*coron/o* heart, crown *-ary* pertaining to	Open-heart surgery in which a piece of a blood vessel from another location is grafted onto one of the coronary arteries to reroute blood around a blockage (Fig. 10-28).
extracorporeal circulation (ECC) ecks truh kore PORE ee ul	*extra-* outside *corpor/o* body *-eal* pertaining to	Use of a cardiopulmonary machine to do the work of the heart during open-heart procedures.
heart transplantation		Removal of a diseased heart and transplantation of a donor heart when cardiac disease can no longer be treated by any other means.
left ventricular assist device (LVAD)		Mechanical pump device that assists a patient's weakened heart by pulling blood from the LV into the pump and then ejecting it out into the aorta. LVADs may be used on those patients awaiting a transplant.

Did You Know?

Heart transplantation is a reality for more than 2000 Americans every year. Many more of these candidates die each year for lack of donor organs. Research continues in the development of an artificial heart.

Fig. 10-28 Coronary artery bypass graft (CABG). **A,** A section of vein is harvested from the right leg and is anastomosed to a coronary artery to bypass an occlusion of the right coronary artery (RCA). **B,** Bypass of the left coronary artery (LCA) with a mammary artery.

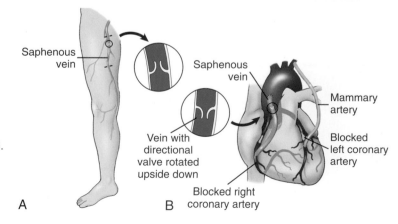

- Saphenous vein
- Saphenous vein
- Mammary artery
- Vein with directional valve rotated upside down
- Blocked left coronary artery
- Blocked right coronary artery

A

B

Terms Related to Cardiac Procedures—cont'd

Term	Word Origin	Definition
minimally invasive direct coronary artery bypass (MIDCAB)		Surgical procedure in which the heart is still beating while a minimal incision is made over the blocked coronary artery and an artery from the chest wall is used as the bypass.
percutaneous transluminal coronary angioplasty (PTCA) pur kyoo TAY nee us trans LOO mih nul KOR in nare ee AN jee oh plas tee	*per-* through *cutane/o* skin *-ous* pertaining to *trans-* across *lumin/o* lumen *-al* pertaining to *coron/o* heart, crown *-ary* pertaining to *angi/o* vessel *-plasty* surgical repair	Surgical procedure in which a catheter is threaded into the coronary artery affected by atherosclerotic heart disease. The balloon at the tip of the catheter is inflated and deflated to compress the plaque against the wall of the artery and increase blood flow. **Stents,** wire mesh tubes, are placed in the arteries and used to prop them open after the angioplasty (Fig. 10-29). Recent studies show cases of in-stent stenosis, a narrowing of the lumen of a stent.
pericardiocentesis pair ee kar dee oh sen TEE sis	*pericardi/o* pericardium *-centesis* surgical puncture	Aspiration of fluid from the pericardium to treat cardiac tamponade (Fig. 10-30).
port-access coronary artery bypass (PACAB)		Procedure in which the heart is stopped and bypass surgery is accomplished through small incisions in the chest.

Continued

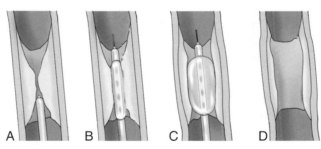

Fig. 10-29 Percutaneous transluminal coronary angioplasty (PTCA). **A,** Catheter is threaded into artery where the atheroma occludes blood flow. **B,** Balloon is inflated. **C,** Plaque is compressed against the artery wall. **D,** Balloon is deflated and withdrawn from the artery.

Lung

Pericardial space

18-gauge thin wall needle

Fig. 10-30 Pericardiocentesis for aspiration of pericardial fluid.

Terms Related to Cardiac Procedures—cont'd

Term	Word Origin	Definition
radiofrequency catheter ablation (RFCA) ray dee oh FREE kwen see uh BLAY shun		Destruction of abnormal cardiac electrical pathways causing arrhythmias.
thromboendarterectomy (TEA) throm boh en dar tur ECK tuh mee	*thromb/o* clot, clotting *end-* within *arter/o* artery *-ectomy* removal	Removal of a blood clot along with part of the lining of the obstructed artery.
transmyocardial revascularization (TMR) trans mye oh KAR dee ul ree vas kyoo lair ih ZAY shun	*trans-* through *myocardi/o* myocardium *-al* pertaining to *re-* again *vascul/o* vessel *-ization* process	Procedure used to relieve severe angina in a patient who cannot tolerate a CABG or PTCA. With a laser, a series of holes is made in the heart tissue in the hope of increasing blood flow by stimulating new blood vessels to grow (**angiogenesis**).
valvuloplasty VAL vyoo loh plas tee	*valvul/o* valve *-plasty* surgical repair	Repair of a stenosed heart valve with the use of a balloon-tipped catheter.

Terms Related to Vascular Procedures

Term	Word Origin	Definition
endovenous laser ablation (EVLT) ah BLAY shun	*endo-* within *ven/o* vein *-ous* pertaining to	Thermal destruction of varicose veins using laser fibers within a vein.
hemorrhoidectomy hem uh royd ECK tuh mee	*hemorrhoid/o* hemorrhoids *-ectomy* removal	Excision of hemorrhoids.
peripherally inserted central catheter (PICC)		A means of allowing intravenous (IV) access for delivery of chemotherapy, antibiotics, IV fluids, and feeding for a prolonged time.
phlebectomy fleh BECK tuh mee	*phleb/o* vein *-ectomy* removal	Removal of a vein.
sclerotherapy skleh roh THAIR uh pee	*scler/o* hard *-therapy* treatment	Injection of chemical solution into varicosities to cause inflammation, resulting in an obliteration of the lining of the vein; blood flow then is rerouted through adjoining vessels. **Microsclerotherapy** is a treatment to remove spider veins.

EXERCISE 15: Therapeutic Interventions

Fill in the blanks with one of the following terms.

RFCA, CABG, PICC, PTCA, EVLT, commissurotomy, CPR, LVAD, AICD, MIDCAB, PACAB

1. What surgery stops the heart so surgery can be performed? _____

2. What procedure detours a blockage in a coronary artery to reestablish blood flow around the

    blockage? _____

3. What emergency procedure restarts the heartbeat and breathing? _____

4. What is IV access for delivery of chemotherapy? _____

5. What is the procedure to correct mitral stenosis? _____

6. What procedure introduces a balloon into a coronary artery via a catheter to reestablish patency?

    _____

7. A minimal incision made over a blocked artery so that an artery bypass can be performed is

    _____.

8. Destruction of abnormal cardiac electrical pathways is called _____.

9. A mechanical pump device implanted in the lower left chamber of the heart to lessen the work of

    the heart is called a/an _____.

10. Thermal destruction of veins with the use of a laser is called _____.

11. A device implanted in the chest to monitor and correct the heartbeat is called a/an

    _____.

Decode the term.

12. phlebectomy _____

13. pericardiocentesis _____

14. hemorrhoidectomy _____

15. sclerotherapy _____

16. valvuloplasty _____

17. atherectomy _____

 *Click on **Hear It, Spell It** to practice spelling the diagnostic and therapeutic terms you have learned in this chapter.*

PHARMACOLOGY

As in other body systems, medications may be described as over the counter (OTC) or prescribed (Rx). An example of an OTC drug used in this system is chewable baby (81 mg) aspirin, which is sometimes given to patients who are at high risk for having a MI. Prescription drugs used to treat the cardiovascular system may be grouped as follows:

angiotensin-converting enzyme (ACE) inhibitors: Relax blood vessels by preventing the formation of the vasoconstrictor angiotensin II. This inhibition causes a decrease in water retention and BP and an improvement in cardiac output. ACE inhibitors are commonly used to treat HTN and HF. Examples are lisinopril (Prinivil), enalapril (Vasotec), and quinapril (Accupril).

angiotension II receptor blockers (ARBs): Lower BP by inhibiting the vasoconstrictor angiotension II from binding its action sites. Examples include irbesartan (Avapro) and valsartan (Diovan).

antiarrhythmic drugs: Restore NSR via various mechanisms to treat cardiac arrhythmias. Examples are digoxin (Lanoxin), amiodarone (Pacerone), and flecainide (Tambocor).

anticoagulants: Prevent the formation of blood clots. Examples are warfarin (Coumadin) and heparin.

antihyperlipidemics: Lower LDL and/or raise HDL cholesterol levels to reduce the risk of heart attack or stroke. There are five different types: fibrates (gemfibrozil; Lopid), HMG-CoA reductase inhibitors or "statins" (simvastatin; Zocor), bile acid sequestrants (cholestyramine; Prevalite), niacin, and ezetimibe (Zetia).

antihypertensives: Lower blood pressure. Types include ACE inhibitors, ARBs, beta-blockers, CCBs, and renin inhibitors.

beta-blockers: Depress the heart rate and force of heart contractions by decreasing the effectiveness of the nerve impulses to the cardiovascular system. They typically are prescribed to treat angina pectoris, HTN, and cardiac arrhythmias. Examples are propranolol (Inderal), atenolol (Tenormin), and metoprolol (Lopressor).

calcium channel blockers (CCBs): Decrease myocardial oxygen demand by inhibiting the flow of calcium to smooth muscle cells of the heart, which causes arterial relaxation. CCBs are used to treat angina, HTN, and HF. Examples are diltiazem (Cardizem), verapamil (Calan), amlodipine (Norvasc), and nifedipine (Procardia).

diuretics (dye ur REH ticks): Promote the excretion of sodium and water as urine; they are used in the treatment of HTN and HF. Examples of diuretics are furosemide (Lasix), hydrochlorothiazide (HydroDIURIL), and triamterene (Dyrenium).

nitrates (antianginals): Relax blood vessels and reduce myocardial oxygen consumption to lessen the pain of angina pectoris; also used to treat HTN and HF. Examples include isosorbide dinitrate (Isordil) and nitroglycerin (Nitro, Nitro-dur).

renin inhibitors: relax blood vessels by decreasing renin conversion of angiotensinogen to angiotensin I. An example is aliskiren (Tekturna).

thrombolytics: Aid in the dissolution of blood clots. "Clot busters" are used to treat obstructing coronary thrombi (clots). Examples are tissue plasminogen activator (tPA), steptokinase (Streptase), alteplase (Activase) reteplase (Retevase) and tenecteplase (TNKase).

EXERCISE 16: Pharmacology

Match the type of drug with the disease(s) it treats. There may be more than one answer.

_____ 1. antiarrhythmic

_____ 2. beta-blocker

_____ 3. ACE inhibitor

_____ 4. antianginal

_____ 5. CCB

_____ 6. diuretic

_____ 7. thrombolytic

_____ 8. anticoagulant

_____ 9. HMG-CoA reductase
         inhibitor

A. hypertension
B. existing thrombosis
C. dysrhythmia
D. angina
E. HF
F. formation of thromboses
G. high LDL cholesterol

Case Study Micah Sutton

Micah Sutton is a 62-year-old newspaper editor who was recently diagnosed with mitral stenosis. Today he is being admitted for a commissurotomy. His symptoms include fatigue and orthopnea, and he is currently on medication for hypertension.

1. Mitral stenosis is a _____
    _____ of the MV.

2. Another name for the mitral valve is the _____
    _____ valve.

3. The term for difficulty with breathing unless in an upright position is _____.

4. A commissurotomy is a/an _____ of the adhesions in a valve.
    a. new opening   b. excision
    c. incision   d. fixation

5. Hypertension is the term for _____ blood pressure.
    a. high   b. low
    c. normal

Case Study   Bradley Chadwick

Bradley Chadwick is a 78-year-old senior visiting his doctor for continuing treatment of HF. His ankles are swollen, and he admits to no longer taking his diuretics. His other medications include digitalis and an ACE inhibitor, which he says that he takes "pretty often." He asks about LVAD surgery, but is told that it is not an option for him at this time.

1. HF stands for _____.

2. What is the medical term for swelling? _____

3. What drugs are prescribed to remove fluids from the body? _____

4. LVAD stands for _____ _____.

5. What does ACE stand for in ACE inhibitor? _____ _____

Abbreviations (Anatomic)

Abbreviation	Definition	Abbreviation	Definition
AV	atrioventricular	O_2	oxygen
BP	blood pressure	PA	pulmonary artery
CO_2	carbon dioxide	PV	pulmonary vein
CV	cardiovascular	RA	right atrium
LA	left atrium	RV	right ventricle
LV	left ventricle	SA	sinoatrial
MV	mitral valve	TV	tricuspid valve
NSR	normal sinus rhythm		

Abbreviations (Pathology)

Abbreviation	Definition	Abbreviation	Definition
AEB	atrial ectopic beat	MR	mitral regurgitation
AF	atrial fibrillation	MS	mitral stenosis
AMI	acute myocardial infarction	MVP	mitral valve prolapse
AS	aortic stenosis	PAC	premature atrial contraction
ASD	atrial septal defect	PDA	patent ductus arteriosus
ASHD	arteriosclerotic heart disease	PVC	premature ventricular contraction
BBB	bundle branch block	PVD	peripheral vascular disease
CAD	coronary artery disease	SOB	shortness of breath
CHF	congestive heart failure	SSS	sick sinus syndrome
DOE	dyspnea on exertion	SVT	superficial vein thrombosis
DVT	deep vein thrombosis	TS	tricuspid stenosis
HF	heart failure	VEB	ventricular ectopic beat
HTN	hypertension	VSD	ventricular septal defect
MI	myocardial infarction	VT	ventricular tachycardia

Abbreviations (Diagnostic)

Abbreviation	Definition	Abbreviation	Definition
A&P	auscultation and percussion	ECHO	echocardiography
BP	blood pressure	EST	exercise stress test
bpm	beats per minute	HDL	high-density lipoprotein
Cath	(cardiac) catheterization	LDH	lactate dehydrogenase
CO_2	carbon dioxide	LDL	low-density lipoprotein
CPK	creatine phosphokinase	PET	positron emission tomography
DSA	digital subtraction angiography	TEE	transesophageal echocardiography
ECG, EKG	electrocardiography, electrocardiogram		

Abbreviations (Therapeutic Interventions)

Abbreviation	Definition	Abbreviation	Definition
AICD	automatic implantable cardiac-defibrillator	PACAB	port-access coronary artery bypass
CABG	coronary artery bypass graft	PICC	peripherally inserted central catheter
CCB	calcium channel blocker	PTCA	percutaneous transluminal coronary angioplasty
CPR	cardiopulmonary resuscitation		
ECC	extracorporeal circulation	RFCA	radiofrequency catheter ablation
EVLT	endovenous laser ablation	SK	streptokinase
		TEA	thromboendarterectomy
LVAD	left ventricular assist device	TMR	transmyocardial revascularization
MIDCAB	minimally invasive direct coronary artery bypass		

EXERCISE 17: Abbreviations

Matching.

_____ 1. upper right chamber of the heart

_____ 2. pertaining to upper and lower chambers of the heart

_____ 3. valve on right side of heart

_____ 4. valve on left side of heart

_____ 5. ultrasound procedure to examine the heart through the esophagus

_____ 6. heart attack

_____ 7. narrowing of largest artery in body

_____ 8. hole between top chambers of the heart

_____ 9. circulation of blood outside body during surgery

_____ 10. noninvasive test that indicates possible artery blockage

A. TEE
B. MI
C. ASD
D. TV
E. ECC
F. MV
G. EST
H. RA
I. AS
J. AV

Match the word parts to their definitions.

Word Parts

Prefix/Suffix

brady-	
-cardia	
echo-	
-graphy	
-megaly	
-pathy	
-sclerosis	
tachy-	
tetra-	
-um	

Definition

1. _____ heart condition
2. _____ four
3. _____ disease
4. _____ slow
5. _____ abnormal condition of hardening
6. _____ sound
7. _____ rapid
8. _____ process of recording
9. _____ structure
10. _____ enlargement

Combining Form

angi/o	
aort/o	
arteri/o	
ather/o	
atri/o	
cardi/o	
coron/o	
corpor/o	
cyan/o	
endocardi/o	
epicardi/o	
hemangi/o	
isch/o	
lumin/o	
myocardi/o	
pariet/o	
pericardi/o	
phleb/o	
pulmon/o	
sept/o	
thromb/o	
vascul/o	

Definition

11. _____ artery
12. _____ heart
13. _____ lung
14. _____ vessel
15. _____ lumen
16. _____ endocardium
17. _____ vessel
18. _____ wall
19. _____ myocardium
20. _____ vein
21. _____ blood vessel
22. _____ aorta
23. _____ body
24. _____ heart
25. _____ fat, plaque
26. _____ epicardium
27. _____ clotting, clot
28. _____ atrium
29. _____ wall, septum
30. _____ to hold back
31. _____ blue
32. _____ pericardium

Wordshop

Prefixes	Combining Forms	Suffixes
brady-	angi/o	-al
echo-	arteri/o	-ar
extra-	ather/o	-ary
tachy-	cardi/o	-cardia
trans-	corpor/o	-eal
	myocardi/o	-ectomy
	pericardi/o	-graphy
	pulmon/o	-ia
	rhythm/o	-itis
	thromb/o	-plasty
		-sclerosis
		-tomy

Build the following terms by combining the preceding word parts. Some word parts may be used more than once. Some may not be used at all. The number in parentheses is the number of word parts needed to build the term.

Definition	Term
1. inflammation of the sac surrounding the heart (2)	_____
2. inflammation of a vein with a clot (3)	_____
3. condition of a rapid heart (beat) (2)	_____
4. process of recording the heart using sound (3)	_____
5. process of recording a vessel (2)	_____
6. surgical repair of a vessel (2)	_____
7. condition of abnormal rhythm (3)	_____
8. abnormal condition of hardening of the arteries (2)	_____
9. heart pain (2)	_____
10. removal of fatty plaque (2)	_____
11. pertaining to the heart and lungs (3)	_____
12. removal of a vein (2)	_____
13. pertaining to the outside of the body (3)	_____
14. pertaining to through the heart muscle (3)	_____
15. process of recording a vein (2)	_____

Sort the terms into the correct categories.

Term Sorting

Anatomy and Physiology	Pathology	Diagnostic Procedures	Therapeutic Interventions

aneurysm	CABG	EST	phlebography
angiocardiography	CAD	EVLT	phlebotomy
aorta	capillary	fluoroscopy	PTCA
arrhythmia	claudication	hemangiosarcoma	Purkinje fibers
atrium	commissurotomy	HTN	septum
auscultation	diastole	lipid profile	SOB
BP	ECC	LVAD	systole
bradycardia	ECG	MIDCAB	TEA
bruit	endocarditis	MUGA scan	valvuloplasty
bundle of His	endocardium	pericardiocentesis	ventricle

Replace the highlighted words with the correct terms.

Translations

1. Monique LaPlante was born with **an abnormal opening between the pulmonary artery and the aorta** that was originally detected by her pediatrician, who noted the presence of a **continuous abnormal heart sound heard during systole, diastole, or both.**

2. The child's **congenital cardiac anomaly that consists of four defects** was noted on **use of ultrasonic waves directed through the heart to study the structure and motion of the heart.**

3. Mrs. Williams had **an excessive amount of blood in the pulmonary vessels** and was diagnosed with **the inability of the heart muscle to pump blood efficiently.**

4. The 72-year-old man had an advanced case of **accumulation and hardening of plaque in the coronary arteries.** He had a history of cigarette smoking and **heart pain.**

5. The patient underwent **an x-ray imaging of a vein after the introduction of a contrast dye** to diagnose **his inflammation and formation of clots of either deep veins or superficial veins.**

6. Mr. Singh was admitted with **profuse secretion of sweat** and **rapid heartbeat.**

7. **A blood test that measures the amount of cardiac enzymes characteristically released during an MI** and **a recording of electrical impulses of the heart** was performed on the patient.

8. **Thermal destruction of veins using laser fibers within a vein** was used to treat Maria Lope's **elongated, dilated superficial veins.**

9. The patient was diagnosed with **paroxysmal chest pain** and was prescribed **drugs that relax blood vessels and reduce myocardialoxygen consumption.**

10. The cardiologist ordered **an aspiration of fluid from the pericardium** to treat Hugo's **compression of the heart caused by fluid in the pericardial sac.**

11. **A small, battery-operated device that helps the heart beat in a regular rhythm** was implanted in Mrs. Dawson's left chest to treat her **abnormality of the sinus node.**

12. Because Mr. Lin was unable to tolerate **a surgical procedure in which a catheter is threaded into the coronary artery,** his cardiologist ordered **a procedure in which a series of holes in made in the heart tissue using a laser.**

13. Malcolm's **narrowing of the tricuspid valve caused by rheumatic fever** was treated with **a repair of a stenosed heart valve with the use of a balloon-tipped catheter.**

Medical Record — Cheryl Miller

MILLER, CHERYL Y - 644497 Opened by TRUSKOWSKI, ABIGAIL MD

Task   Edit   View   Time Scale   Options   Help

As Of 17:16

MILLER, CHERYL Y
Age: 45 years   Sex: Female   Loc: WHC-SMMC
DOB: 10/10/1970   MRN: 644497   FIN: 3506004

Reference Text Browser | Form Browser | Medication Profile

Orders | Last 48 Hours | ED | Lab | Radiology | Assessments | Surgery | **Clinical Notes** | Pt. Info | Pt. Schedule | Task List | I & O | MAR

Flowsheet: Clinical Notes   ...   Level: Discharge Summary   ● Table ○ Group ○ List

Navigator

✓ Discharge Summary

Principal Diagnosis: Inferolateral myocardial infarction
Secondary Diagnoses: Coronary artery disease; hypertension
Procedure: Coronary artery bypass graft
History of Present Illness: The patient, a 45-year-old African-American female, has a history of substernal chest pain, nausea, dyspnea, and diaphoresis for 1½ hours before being seen in the ED.
Medical History: Significant for hypertension.
Social History: Positive for social alcohol use, and patient has smoked 1 pack per day for the past 30 years.
Medications: The patient is not currently taking any medication.
Physical Examination: On physical examination, the patient's vital signs showed a blood pressure of 165/105, a pulse rate of 88, and a temperature of 98.6 degrees. The patient was a well-developed, well-nourished, African-American female in mild distress. The patient's head, eyes, ears, nose, and throat were unremarkable. The neck was supple, with no jugular venous distension. Heart showed regular rhythm. The lungs were clear to auscultation and percussion. The abdominal examination was soft and nontender. Extremities had no cyanosis, clubbing, or edema. The neurologic examination was nonfocal.
Laboratory Studies: White blood cell count 19, hematocrit 39.9, platelets 385. Differential included 89 neutrophils, 2 bands, 5 lymphocytes, and 1 mono. Sodium 142, potassium 4.3, BUN 11, creatinine 1.0, glucose 229, calcium 7.8, magnesium 1.9, phosphorus 8.4, CPK 375. Urinalysis revealed no abnormal findings. ECG revealed normal sinus rhythm at 85 bpm.
Hospital Course: The patient was admitted and started on intravenous nitroglycerin, heparin, aspirin, and Lopressor. Cardiac catheterization demonstrated 94% occlusion of the RCA. Echo-cardiogram showed an ejection fraction of 29%.
     Patient underwent the bypass without incident and has progressed at a moderate pace through postoperative physical rehabilitation. At the time of discharge, she was ambulating well and demonstrated a good understanding of necessary lifestyle changes to maintain her health.
Medications on Discharge: Ascriptin, 325 mg po daily; atenolol, 50 mg daily; clodripogel 75 mg daily; pravastatin 40 mg daily.

PROD | MAHAFC | 10 Sept 2015 | 17:16

⟳ DISCHARGE SUMMARY

Using the medical report for Cheryl Miller, answer the following questions.

1. Which term means Cheryl had difficulty breathing? _____

2. Which term means Cheryl was sweating profusely? _____

3. Where was the chest pain perceived? _____

4. How do you know that Ms. Miller did not lack oxygen in her extremities? _____

5. What was the name of the ultrasound procedure performed to assess her cardiac function?

    _____

6. What procedure was done to treat her CAD? _____

11

Respiratory System

OBJECTIVES

- Recognize and use terms related to the anatomy and physiology of the respiratory system.
- Recognize and use terms related to the pathology of the respiratory system.
- Recognize and use terms related to the diagnostic procedures for the respiratory system.
- Recognize and use terms related to the therapeutic interventions for the respiratory system.

For more interactive learning, click on:
- **Match the Word Part** to review respiratory word parts.
- **Word Shop** to practice word building.
- **Tournament of Terminology** to test your knowledge of respiratory terms.
- **Term Sorting** to practice sorting respiratory terms into categories.

*Click on **Chapter at a Glance** to print out a list of key word parts and terms.*

FUNCTIONS OF THE RESPIRATORY SYSTEM

The respiratory system handles the following functions for the body:

- Delivering oxygen (O_2) to the blood for transport to cells in the body.
- Excreting the waste product of cellular respiration, carbon dioxide (CO_2).
- Filtering, cleansing, warming, and humidifying air taken into the lungs.
- Helping to regulate blood pH.
- Helping the production of sound for speech and singing.
- Providing the tissue that receives the stimulus for the sense of smell, olfaction.

Analyzing the name for this system gives a clue as to its first two functions. The word **respiratory** (RES pur uh tore ee) comes from the combining form *spir/o,* which means to breathe. As a matter of fact, to breathe in is to **inspire,** and to breathe out is to **expire.** When one dies, one breathes out and no longer breathes in again—hence the expression that the patient has "expired." **Inhalation** (in hull LAY shun) and **exhalation** (ex hull LAY shun) are alternative terms for **inspiration** and **expiration.**

The next two functions—filtering air and regulating blood pH—take place during breathing. The function of producing sound for speech and singing is accomplished by the interaction of air and the structures of the voice box, the larynx, and the hollow cavities (the sinuses) connected to the nasal passages.

Although the sense of smell, **olfaction** (ohl FACK shun), is not strictly a function of respiration, it is accomplished by the tissue in the nasal cavity, which receives the stimulus for smell and routes it to the brain through the nervous system.

SPECIALTIES/SPECIALISTS

Pulmonology is the diagnosis, treatment, and prevention of disorders of the respiratory tract. The specialist in this field is called a **pulmonologist.**

ANATOMY AND PHYSIOLOGY

The respiratory system is anatomically divided into the upper respiratory tract—the nose, pharynx, and larynx—and the lower respiratory tract—the trachea, bronchial tree, and lungs (Fig. 11-1). Physiologically, it is divided into conduction passageways and gas exchange surfaces.

There are two forms of respiration: **external respiration** and **internal respiration.** External respiration is the process of exchanging O_2 and CO_2 between the external environment and the lungs. Internal respiration is the exchange of gases between the lungs and the blood.

Upper Respiratory Tract

The upper respiratory system encompasses the area from the nose to the larynx (Fig. 11-2). Air can enter the body through the mouth, but for the most part, it enters the body through the two **nares** (NAIR eez) (nostrils) of the **nose** that are separated by a partition called the **nasal septum** (NAY zul SEP tum). The hairs in the nose serve to filter out large particulate matter, and the mucous membrane and **cilia** (SEE lee uh) (small hairs) of the respiratory tract provide a further means of keeping air clean, warm, and moist as it travels to the lungs. The cilia continually move in a wavelike motion to push mucus and debris out of the respiratory tract. The air then travels up and backward, where it is filtered, warmed, and humidified by the environment in the upper portion of the nasal cavity. Fig. 11-3 illustrates the route of air into the body. The receptors

respiratory
re- = again
spir/o = to breathe
-atory = pertaining to

inspiration
in- = in
spir/o = to breathe
-ation = process of

expiration
ex- = out
(s)pir/o = to breathe
-ation = process of

inhalation
in- = in
hal/o = to breathe
-ation = process of

exhalation
ex- = out
hal/o = to breathe
-ation = process of

air = pneum/o, aer/o

pulmonologist
pulmon/o = lung
-logist = one who specializes in the study of

oxygen (O_2) = ox/i, ox/o

carbon dioxide (CO_2) = capn/o

nose = nas/o, rhin/o

septum
sept/o = wall
-um = structure

Be Careful!

*The plural of **sinus** is not sini, but **sinuses**.*

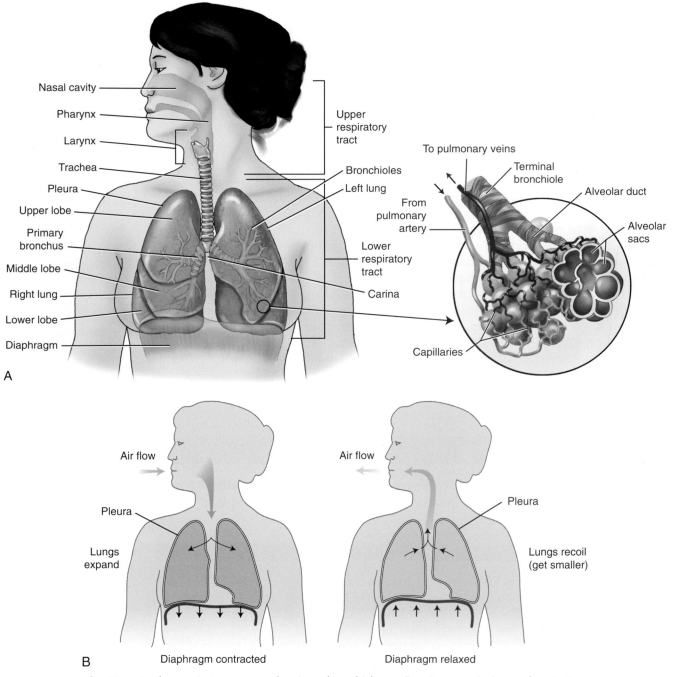

Fig. 11-1 A, The respiratory system showing a bronchial tree *(inset)*. **B,** Inspiration and expiration.

paranasal
  para- = near
  nas/o = nose
  -al = pertaining to

sinus = sinus/o, sin/o

mucus = muc/o

nasopharynx
  nas/o = nose
  pharyng/o = throat, pharynx
  pharynx = pharyng/o

eustachian tube = salping/o

for olfaction are located in the nasal cavity. The nasal cavity is connected to the **paranasal sinuses** (pair uh NAY zul SYE nus suhs), named for their proximity to the nose.

These sinuses, divided into the frontal, maxillary, sphenoid, and ethmoid cavities, acquire their names from the bones in which they are located. The function of sinus cavities in the skull is to warm and filter the air taken in and to assist in the production of sound. They are lined with a mucous membrane that drains into the nasal cavity and can be the site of painful inflammation.

Air continues to travel past into the **nasopharynx** (NAY zoh fair inks), which is the part of the throat **(pharynx)** behind the nasal cavity. The **eustachian** (yoo STAY shun) **tubes** from the ears connect with the throat at this point to equalize pressure between the ears and the throat. This is the site of lymphatic tissue, the **pharyngeal tonsils** (fur IN jee ul TAHN suls), which are also

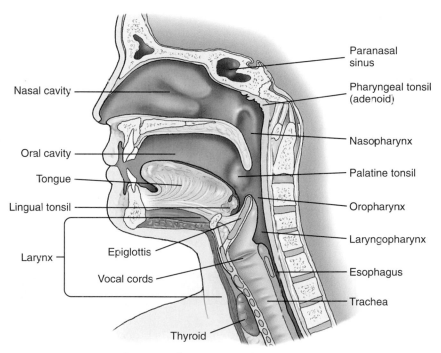

Fig. 11-2 The upper respiratory system.

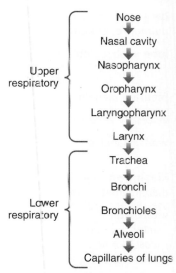

Fig. 11-3 Schematic of the order in which air passes through the upper respiratory system and into the lower respiratory system.

termed the **adenoids** (AD uh noyds). These pharyngeal tonsils help to protect against pathogens. The next structure, the **oropharynx** (or oh FAIR inks), is the part of the throat posterior to the oral cavity and also the location of more lymphatic tissue, the **palatine tonsils** (PAL ah tyne TAHN suls), which are so named because they are continuous with the roof of the mouth (the palate). These tonsils, just like the adenoids, are made up of protective lymphatic tissue. The lingual tonsil, located on the posterior aspect of the tongue, also serves a protective function. The oropharynx is also part of the digestive system; food and air pass through it. Below the oropharynx is the part of the throat referred to as the **laryngopharynx** (luh ring goh FAIR inks) because of its proximity to the adjoining structure, the **larynx** (LAIR inks), or voice box. As air passes back out through the opening of the larynx, the **vocal cords,** which are paired bands of cartilaginous tissue, vibrate to produce speech. The **epiglottis** (eh pee GLOT is) is a flap of cartilage at the opening to the larynx that closes access to the **trachea** (TRAY kee uh) during swallowing so that food is routed into the esophagus and is kept from entering the trachea. Though this is an effective protection most of the time, it can be overridden accidentally if the individual tries to talk and eat at the same time. When this happens, food can be pulled into the trachea with possible serious consequences.

Lower Respiratory Tract

The lower respiratory tract begins with the **trachea** (or windpipe), which extends from the larynx into the chest cavity. The trachea lies within the space between the lungs called the **mediastinum** (mee dee uh STY num). Air travels into the lungs as the trachea bifurcates (branches) at the **carina** (kuh RIH nuh), where the right and left airways called **bronchi** (BRONG kee) (*sing.* bronchus) divide into smaller branches called **bronchioles** (BRONG kee ohls). These bronchioles end in microscopic ducts capped by air sacs called **alveoli** (al VEE oh lye) (*sing.* alveolus). Each alveolus is in contact with a blood capillary to provide a means of exchange of gases. It is at this point that O_2 is diffused across cell membranes into the blood cells, and CO_2 is diffused out to be expired. Each alveolus is coated with a substance called **surfactant** (sur FACK tunt) that keeps it from collapsing.

adenoids = adenoid/o

oropharynx

or/o = mouth
pharyng/o = throat,
pharynx

tonsils = tonsill/o

larynx, voice box =
laryng/o

laryngopharynx
laryng/o = larynx
pharyng/o = pharynx

epiglottis = epiglott/o

trachea, windpipe =
trache/o

mediastinum =
mediastin/o

chest = thorac/o, steth/o,
pector/o

bronchus = bronch/o,
bronchi/o

bronchiole = bronchiol/o

alveolus = alveol/o

lung = pneumon/o, pulmon/o, pneum/o

lobe = lob/o, lobul/o

pleura = pleur/o

viscera = viscer/o

wall = pariet/o

diaphragm = diaphragm/o, diaphragmat/o, phren/o

intercostal
  inter- = between
  cost/o = rib
  -al = pertaining to

Each **lung** is composed of sections called **lobes.** The right lung is made up of three sections, whereas the left has only two. The abbreviations for the lobes of the lungs are RUL (right upper lobe), RML (right middle lobe), RLL (right lower lobe), LUL (left upper lobe), and LLL (left lower lobe).

Each lung is also enclosed by a double-folded, serous membrane called the **pleura** (PLOOR uh) (*pl.* pleurae). The side of the membrane that coats the lungs is the **visceral pleura** (VIH sur ul PLOOR ah); the side that lines the inner surface of the rib cage is the **parietal pleura** (puh RYE uh tul PLOOR ah). The two sides of the pleural membrane contain fluid that facilitates the expansion and contraction of the lungs with each breath.

The muscles responsible for normal, quiet respiration are the **diaphragm** (DYE uh fram), the large dome-shaped muscle between the thoracic and abdominal cavities, and the **intercostal** (in tur KOS tul) **muscles,** which are located between the ribs. On inspiration, the diaphragm is pulled down as it contracts and the intercostal muscles expand, pulling air into the lungs (see Fig. 11-1, *B*).

⊗ Be Careful!	⊗ Be Careful!	⊗ Be Careful!
Salping/o means both eustachian tubes and fallopian tubes.	*Don't confuse the combining form ox/i, which means oxygen, with the prefix oxy-, which means rapid.*	*Don't confuse bronchi/o, which means the bronchial tubes, with brachi/o, which means the arm.*

⟳ EXERCISE 1: Anatomy and Physiology of the Respiratory System

Match the respiratory structure with its combining form or prefix. More than one letter may be correct.

_____ 1. pleura

_____ 2. lobe

_____ 3. tonsil

_____ 4. mucus

_____ 5. diaphragm

_____ 6. windpipe

_____ 7. adenoids

_____ 8. eustachian tube

_____ 9. bronchiole

_____ 10. rib

_____ 11. breathe

_____ 12. throat

_____ 13. alveolus

_____ 14. lung

_____ 15. sinus

_____ 16. bronchus

_____ 17. voice box

_____ 18. mouth

_____ 19. nose

_____ 20. mediastinum

_____ 21. in

_____ 22. air

_____ 23. out

_____ 24. epiglottis

_____ 25. wall

_____ 26. carbon dioxide

_____ 27. oxygen

A. ox/o
B. bronch/o, bronchi/o
C. salping/o
D. pneum/o, pneumon/o
E. phren/o
F. hal/o, spir/o
G. pharyng/o
H. adenoid/o
I. sept/o
J. rhin/o
K. pneum/o, aer/o
L. pulmon/o
M. capn/o
N. lob/o, lobul/o
O. diaphragm/o, diaphragmat/o
P. nas/o
Q. trache/o

R. alveol/o
S. tonsill/o
T. pleur/o
U. sin/o, sinus/o
V. muc/o
W. epiglott/o
X. laryng/o
Y. in-
Z. bronchiol/o
AA. cost/o
BB. mediastin/o
CC. ex-
DD. or/o

Decode the terms.

28. intercostal _____

29. inspiratory _____

30. paranasal _____

31. endotracheal _____

 *You can review the anatomy of the respiratory system by clicking on **Body Spectrum Electronic Anatomy Coloring Book → Respiratory**. Choose **Hear It, Spell It** to practice spelling the anatomy and physiology terms that you have learned in this chapter.*

EXERCISE 2: Respiratory System

Label the drawings below using the terms provided.

diaphragm
trachea
nasal cavity
pharynx
primary bronchus
lower lobe
larynx
middle lobe

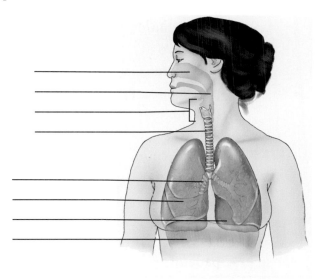

palatine tonsil
trachea
nasal cavity
oral cavity
epiglottis
oropharynx
larynx
pharyngeal tonsil
nasopharynx
vocal cords
laryngopharynx
lingual tonsil

Combining and Adjective Forms for the Anatomy and Physiology of the Respiratory System

Meaning	Combining Form	Adjective Form
adenoid	adenoid/o	adenoidal
air	pneum/o, aer/o	pneumatic
alveolus	alveol/o	alveolar
bronchiole	bronchiol/o	bronchiolar
bronchus	bronch/o, bronchi/o	bronchial
carbon dioxide	capn/o	
chest	steth/o, thorac/o, pector/o	thoracic, pectoral
diaphragm	diaphragm/o, diaphragmat/o, phren/o	diaphragmatic
eustachian tube	salping/o	salpingeal
larynx (voice box)	laryng/o	laryngeal
lobe	lob/o, lobul/o	lobular, lobar
lung	pulmon/o, pneumon/o, pneum/o	pulmonary, pneumatic
mediastinum	mediastin/o	mediastinal
mouth	or/o, stomat/o	oral
mucus	muc/o	mucous
nose	nas/o, rhin/o	nasal, rhinal
oxygen	ox/i, ox/o	
pharynx (throat)	pharyng/o	pharyngeal
pleura	pleur/o	pleural
rib	cost/o	costal
septum, wall	sept/o	septal
sinus	sinus/o, sin/o	
to breathe	spir/o, hal/o	
tonsil	tonsill/o	tonsillar
trachea (windpipe)	trache/o	tracheal
viscera	viscer/o	visceral
wall	pariet/o	parietal

Prefixes for Anatomy and Physiology of the Respiratory System

Prefix	Meaning
ex-	out
in-	in
inter-	between
para-	near
re-	again

Suffixes for Anatomy of the Respiratory System

Suffix	Meaning
-atory, -al	pertaining to
-ation	process of
-logist	one who specializes in the study of
-um	structure

 *Click on **Label It** to practice labeling respiratory structures.*

PATHOLOGY

Terms Related to Respiratory Symptoms

Term	Word Origin	Definition
aphonia ah FOH nee ah	*a-* without *phon/o* sound *-ia* condition	Loss of ability to produce sounds. **Dysphonia** is difficulty making sounds.
Cheyne-Stokes respiration chayne stokes		Deep, rapid breathing followed by a period of apnea.
clubbing KLUH bing		Abnormal enlargement of the distal phalanges as a result of diminished O_2 in the blood (Fig. 11-4).
cyanosis sye uh NOH sis	*cyan/o* blue *-osis* abnormal condition	Lack of O_2 in blood seen as bluish or grayish discoloration of the skin, nail beds, and/or lips (Fig. 11-5).
dyspnea DISP nee ah	*dys-* difficult *-pnea* breathing	Difficult and/or painful breathing. **Eupnea** is good, normal breathing (*eu-* means healthy, normal).
apnea AP nee ah	*a-* without *-pnea* breathing	Abnormal, periodic cessation of breathing.
bradypnea brad IP nee ah	*brady-* slow *-pnea* breathing	Abnormally slow breathing.
hyperpnea hye PURP nee ah	*hyper-* excessive *-pnea* breathing	Excessively deep breathing. **Hypopnea** is extremely shallow breathing.
orthopnea or THOP nee ah	*orth/o* straight *-pnea* breathing	Condition of difficult breathing unless in an upright position.
tachypnea tack ip NEE ah	*tachy-* fast *-pnea* breathing	Rapid, shallow breathing.
epistaxis ep ih STACK sis		Nosebleed. Also called **rhinorrhagia.**
hemoptysis heh MOP tih sis	*hem/o* blood *-ptysis* spitting	Coughing up blood or blood-stained sputum.
hypercapnia hye pur KAP nee ah	*hyper-* excessive *capn/o* carbon dioxide *-ia* condition	Condition of excessive CO_2 in the blood.

Continued

Fig. 11-4 Clubbing.

Fig. 11-5 Cyanosis of the lower foot and great toe.

Terms Related to Respiratory Symptoms—cont'd

Term	Word Origin	Definition
hyperventilation hye pur ven tih LAY shun	*hyper-* excessive	Abnormally increased breathing.
hypoxemia hye pock SEE mee ah	*hypo-* deficient *ox/o* oxygen *-emia* blood condition	Condition of deficient O_2 in the blood. **Hypoxia** is the condition of deficient O_2 in the tissues.
pleurodynia ploor oh DIN ee ah	*pleur/o* pleura *-dynia* pain	Pain in the chest caused by inflammation of the intercostal muscles.
pyrexia pye RECK see ah	*pyr/o* fire *-exia* condition	Fever.
rhinorrhea rye noh REE ah	*rhin/o* nose *-rrhea* discharge	Discharge from the nose.
shortness of breath (SOB)		Breathlessness; air hunger.
sputum SPYOO tum		Mucus coughed up from the lungs and expectorated through the mouth. If abnormal, it may be described as to its amount, color, or odor.
thoracodynia thor uh koh DIN ee ah	*thorac/o* chest *-dynia* pain	Chest pain.

Terms Related to Abnormal Chest Sounds

Term	Word Origin	Definition
friction sounds		Sounds made by dry surfaces rubbing together.
hiccup HICK up		Sound produced by the involuntary contraction of the diaphragm, followed by rapid closure of the glottis. Also called **hiccough,** or **singultus.**
rales rayls		Also called **crackles,** an abnormal lung sound heard on auscultation, characterized by discontinuous bubbling noises.
rhonchi RON kye		Abnormal rumbling sound heard on auscultation, caused by airways blocked by secretions or muscle contractions.
stridor STRY dur		High-pitched inspiratory sounds from the larynx; a sign of upper airway obstruction.
tympany, chest TIM puh nee	*tympan/o* drum	Low-pitched resonant sound from the chest.
wheezing WHEE zeeng		Whistling sound made during breathing.

EXERCISE 3: Symptoms of Respiratory Disease and Abnormal Chest Sounds

Fill in the blank.

1. Ms. Sims visits her physician's office complaining of orthopnea. She has _____.

2. A person who has a bout of epistaxis has _____.

3. Singultus is another name for _____.

4. Rapid, shallow breathing is called _____.

5. When Samuel Wrightson had laryngitis, he experienced aphonia. He could not _____.

6. A temporary lack of breathing is called _____.

7. What is the term that means blue color of the skin due to lack of O_2?

   _____

8. Another name for rales is _____.

9. Pain caused by inflamed intercostal muscles and their points of attachment to the diaphragm is

   referred to as _____.

10. A whistling sound made during inhalation is called _____.

11. The distal phalanges are abnormally enlarged in which symptom of advanced chronic pulmonary

    disease? _____.

Build the terms.

12. nose discharge _____

13. chest pain _____

14. spitting blood _____

15. good breathing _____

16. excessive (deep) breathing _____

Terms Related to Disorders of the Upper Respiratory Tract

Term	Word Origin	Definition
coryza koh RYE zah		The common cold.
croup croop		Acute viral infection of early childhood, marked by stridor caused by spasms of the larynx, trachea, and bronchi.
deviated septum DEE vee a tid SEP tum	*sept/o* wall, septum *-um* structure	Deflection of the nasal septum that may obstruct the nasal passages, resulting in infection, sinusitis, SOB, headache, or recurring epistaxis.
epiglottitis eh pee glah TYE tis	*epiglott/o* epiglottis *-itis* inflammation	Inflammation of the epiglottis (Fig. 11-6).
laryngitis lair in JYE tis	*laryng/o* voice box (larynx) *-itis* inflammation	Inflammation of the voice box.
obstructive sleep apnea (OSA) APP nee ah	*a-* without *-pnea* breathing	A temporary lack of breathing that occurs during sleep when the posterior pharynx relaxes and covers the trachea.
pharyngitis fair in JYE tis	*pharyng/o* throat (pharynx) *-itis* inflammation	Inflammation or infection of the pharynx, usually causing symptoms of a sore throat.
polyp, nasal and vocal cord PAWL up		Small, tumorlike growth that projects from a mucous membrane surface, including the inside of the nose, the paranasal sinuses, and the vocal cords (Fig. 11-7).
rhinitis rye NYE tis	*rhin/o* nose *-itis* inflammation	Inflammation of the mucous membrane of the nose.
rhinomycosis rye noh mye KOH sis	*rhin/o* nose *myc/o* fungus *-osis* abnormal condition	Abnormal condition of fungus in the nose.
rhinosalpingitis rye noh sal pin JYE tis	*rhin/o* nose *salping/o* eustachian tube *-itis* inflammation	Inflammation of the mucous membranes of the nose and eustachian tubes.
sinusitis sye nuh SYE tis	*sinus/o* sinus *-itis* inflammation	Inflammation of one or more of the paranasal sinuses.

Fig. 11-6 Epiglottitis. The epiglottis is red and swollen.   **Fig. 11-7** Polypoid nodules of the vocal cords.

Terms Related to Disorders of the Upper Respiratory Tract—cont'd

Term	Word Origin	Definition
tracheomalacia tray kee oh mah LAY see ah	*trache/o* windpipe (trachea) *-malacia* softening	Softening of the tissues of the trachea.
tracheostenosis tray kee oh sten OH sis	*trache/o* windpipe (trachea) *-stenosis* narrowing	Narrowing of the windpipe.
upper respiratory infection (URI)		Inflammation and/or infection of structures of the upper respiratory tract.

Case Study Sara McClellan

Sara McClellan is a 25-year-old third grade teacher who is visiting her doctor on Friday for suspected laryngitis. She whispers that she has barely made it through her first week of class at her new school and that she has now totally "lost her voice." She needs something to help her heal quickly so that she can get back to her class on Monday.

1. Laryngitis is _____ of the larynx.

2. The nonmedical term for the larynx is the _____.

3. What is the term that means difficulty in making sounds? _____

4. What is the medical term for a lack of the ability to make sound? _____

Terms Related to Disorders of the Lower Respiratory Tract

Term	Word Origin	Definition
acute respiratory failure (ARF)		A sudden inability of the respiratory system to provide O_2 and/or remove CO_2 from the blood.
asthma AZ muh		Respiratory disorder characterized by recurring episodes of **paroxysmal** (sudden, episodic) dyspnea. Patients exhibit coughing, wheezing, and SOB. If the attack becomes continuous (termed **status asthmaticus**), it may be fatal (Fig. 11-8).

Continued

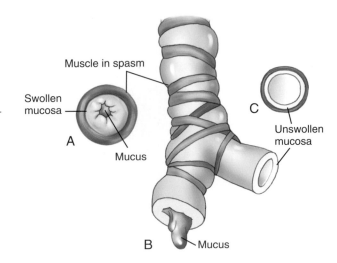

Fig. 11-8 Factors causing expiratory obstruction in asthma. **A,** Cross-section of a bronchiole occlude by muscle spasm, swollen mucosa, and mucus. **B,** Longitudinal section of an obstructed bronchiole. **C,** Cross-section of a clear bronchiole.

Terms Related to Disorders of the Lower Respiratory Tract—cont'd

Term	Word Origin	Definition
atelectasis at ih LECK tuh sis	*a-* not *tel/o* complete *-ectasis* dilation	Collapse of lung tissue or an entire lung.
bronchiectasis brong kee ECK tuh sis	*bronchi/o* bronchus *-ectasis* dilation	Chronic dilation of the bronchi. Symptoms include dyspnea, expectoration of foul-smelling sputum, and coughing.
bronchiolitis brong kee oh LYE tis	*bronchiol/o* bronchiole *-itis* inflammation	Viral inflammation of the bronchioles; more common in children younger than 18 months.
bronchitis brong KYE tis	*bronchi/o* bronchus *-itis* inflammation	Inflammation of the bronchi. May be acute or chronic.
bronchospasm brong koh SPAZZ um	*bronch/o* bronchus *-spasm* sudden, involuntary contraction	A sudden involuntary contraction of the bronchi, as in an asthma attack.
chronic obstructive pulmonary disease (COPD)	*pulmon/o* lung *-ary* pertaining to	Respiratory disorder characterized by a progressive and irreversible diminishment in inspiratory and expiratory capacity of the lungs. Patient experiences **dyspnea on exertion (DOE),** difficulty inhaling or exhaling, and a chronic cough.
cystic fibrosis (CF) SIS tick fye BROH sis		Inherited disorder of the exocrine glands resulting in abnormal, thick secretions of mucus that cause COPD.
diphtheria diff THEER ee ah		Bacterial respiratory infection characterized by a sore throat, fever, and headache.
emphysema em fah SEE mah		Abnormal condition of the pulmonary system characterized by distention and destructive changes of the alveoli. The most common cause is tobacco smoking, but exposure to environmental particulate matter may also cause the disease.

Fig. 11-9 Flail chest. **A,** Fractured rib sections are unattached to the rest of the chest wall. **B,** On inspiration, the flail segment of ribs is sucked inward, causing the lung to shift inward. **C,** On expiration, the flail segment of ribs bellows outward, causing the lung to shift outward. Air moves back and forth between the lungs instead of through the upper airway.

Terms Related to Disorders of the Lower Respiratory Tract—cont'd

Term	Word Origin	Definition
flail chest		A condition in which multiple rib fractures cause instability in part of the chest wall and in which the lung under the injured area contracts on inspiration and bulges out on expiration (Fig. 11-9).
hemothorax hee moh THOR acks	*hem/o* blood *-thorax* chest (pleural cavity)	Blood in the pleural cavity (Fig. 11-10).
influenza in floo EN zah		Also known as the **flu.** Acute infectious disease of the respiratory tract caused by a virus. **Avian (bird) flu** is caused by type A influenza virus. **Swine flu** is caused by H1N1 virus.
pertussis pur TUSS is		Bacterial infection of the respiratory tract with a characteristic high-pitched "whoop." Also called **whooping cough.**
pleural effusion PLOOR ul eh FYOO zhun	*pleur/o* pleura *-al* pertaining to	Abnormal accumulation of fluid in the intrapleural space.
pleurisy PLOOR ih see	*pleur/o* pleura	Inflammation of the parietal pleura of the lungs. May be caused by cancer, pneumonia, or tuberculosis (TB).
pneumoconiosis noo moh koh nee OH sis	*pneum/o* lung *coni/o* dust *-osis* abnormal condition	Loss of lung capacity caused by an accumulation of dust in the lungs. Types may include **asbestosis** (abnormal condition of asbestos in the lungs), **silicosis** (sil ih KOH sis) (abnormal accumulation of glass dust in the lungs), and **anthracosis** (abnormal accumulation of coal dust in the lungs—also known as **black lung disease** or **coal workers' pneumoconiosis [CWP]**) (Fig. 11-11).
pneumonia noo MOH nya	*pneumon/o* lung *-ia* condition	Inflammation of the lungs caused by a variety of pathogens. If infectious, it is termed *pneumonia;* if noninfectious, it is termed **pneumonitis.** The name(s) of the lobes are used to describe the extent of the disease (e.g., **RML pneumonia** is pneumonia of the right middle lobe). If both lungs are affected, it is termed **double pneumonia.**

Continued

Fig. 11-10 Hemothorax. Blood below the left lung causes the lung to collapse.

Fig. 11-11 Coal workers' pneumoconiosis (CWP). The lungs show increased black pigmentation.

Fig. 11-12 Pneumothorax. The lung collapses as air gathers in the pleural space.

Terms Related to Disorders of the Lower Respiratory Tract—cont'd

Term	Word Origin	Definition
pneumothorax noo moh THOR acks	*pneum/o* air *-thorax* chest (pleural cavity)	Air or gas in the pleural space causing the lung to collapse (Fig. 11-12).
pulmonary abscess PULL mun nair ee AB ses	*pulmon/o* lung *-ary* pertaining to	Localized accumulation of pus in the lung.
pulmonary edema PULL mun nair ee eh DEE mah	*pulmon/o* lung *-ary* pertaining to	Accumulation of fluid in the lung tissue. Often present in congestive heart failure, it is caused by the inability of the heart to pump blood.
pyothorax pye oh THOR acks	*py/o* pus *-thorax* chest (pleural cavity)	Pus in the pleural cavity. Also called **empyema.**
respiratory syncytial virus (RSV) RES pur uh tore ee sin SISH uhl VYE rus		Acute respiratory disorder usually occurring in the lower respiratory tract in children and the upper respiratory tract in adults. Most common cause of bronchiolitis and pneumonia in infants and highly contagious in young children.
severe acute respiratory syndrome (SARS)	*syn-* together, with *-drome* to run	Viral respiratory disorder caused by a coronavirus. Usually results in pneumonia.
tuberculosis (TB) too bur kyoo LOH sis		Chronic infectious disorder caused by an acid-fast bacillus, *Mycobacterium tuberculosis.* Transmission is normally by inhalation or ingestion of infected droplets. **Multidrug-resistant tuberculosis (MDRTB)** is fatal in 80% of cases.

Case Study Mario Castellanto

Mario Castellanto is a 23-year-old extreme biker. At the end of one of his rides, he falls and breaks three adjacent ribs on his right side, which causes his lung to contract on inspiration and bulge out on expiration. He is scheduled for surgery, but before it can be performed, Mario experiences hypotension, tachycardia, and sudden breathing difficulty. His lips and fingernails turn blue. X-rays confirm that Mario's lung has collapsed.

1. Mario's original injury, in which his lung contracts and bulges through the weakened chest wall is called _____ _____.

2. Chest pain is called _____ _____.

3. Mario's collapsed lung is called _____ _____.

4. The term that means difficulty breathing is _____ _____.

5. Mario's blue lips and fingernails are a condition known as _____.

⟳ EXERCISE 4: Disorders of the Upper and Lower Respiratory Tract

Fill in the blank with one of the following terms:

atelectasis, vocal polyps, URI, asthma, cystic fibrosis, pleurisy, croup, pertussis, deviated septum, coryza, emphysema, pneumoconiosis, flail chest, pulmonary abscess

1. A term for the common cold is _____.

2. An inflammation and/or infection of the structures of the upper respiratory tract is

    _____.

3. A deflection of the nasal wall that may result in nosebleeds, SOB, infection, and/or headaches is

    _____.

4. Growths that occur on the mucous membranes of the larynx are referred to as

    _____.

5. An inflammation of the parietal pleura is _____.

6. An acute, infectious viral disease of the respiratory tract is _____.

7. The term for collapse of a lung is _____.

8. A chronic pulmonary disease marked by distention of the alveoli is

    _____.

9. A respiratory disorder characterized by episodes of paroxysmal dyspnea is

    _____.

10. Localized accumulation of pus in the lung is _____.

11.   Loss of lung capacity caused by dust in the lung is _____ .

12.   An inherited disorder of the exocrine glands that causes COPD is _____ .

13.   Patients with chest trauma who experience breathing in which the lung contracts on inspiration

and expands on expiration have _____ .

14.   This is also called *whooping cough:* _____

Decode the terms.

15.   pneumonia _____ .

16.   pneumothorax _____ .

17.   pyothorax _____ .

Build the terms.

18.   blood in the pleural cavity _____

19.   inflammation of the bronchi _____

20.   spasm of the bronchi _____

Case Study   Allen Roher

Allen Roher, a 57-year-old formercoal miner, has been enjoying early retirement when a constant but minor cough becomes worse. His wife insists that Allen visit the family doctor, and he reluctantly agrees. Allen tells his physician that he has been feeling tired even though he has been getting more sleep each night now than he had in decades, and he seems to be short of breath when climbing stairs. His physician listens to his lungs and sends him for a chest x-ray (CXR). He is diagnosed with CWP later that week.

1. CWP stands for _____ _____ _____ .

2. What is a synonym for CWP? _____
   _____

3. The combining form *coni/o* in the term *pneumoconiosis* means:
   a. coal
   b. asbestosis
   c. sand
   d. dust

4. Allen says he is short of breath. What is the abbreviation for this symptom? _____

5. What is the term that means abnormal condition of asbestos in the lungs?_____

Neoplasms

Because organs are composed of tissues and tissues are constructed from a variety of cell types, cancer of an organ can occur in a number of different varieties, depending on which types of cells mutate. Fig. 11-13 shows the three main categories of lung cancer along with the types of cells from which they originate.

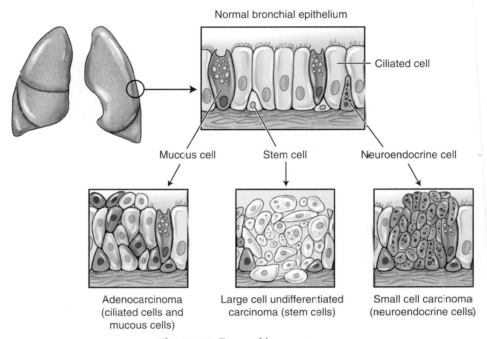

Normal bronchial epithelium

Ciliated cell

Mucous cell   Stem cell   Neuroendocrine cell

Adenocarcinoma
(ciliated cells and
mucous cells)

Large cell undifferentiated
carcinoma (stem cells)

Small cell carcinoma
(neuroendocrine cells)

Fig. 11-13 Types of lung cancer.

Terms Related to Benign Neoplasms

Term	Word Origin	Definition
hamartoma, pulmonary ham ar TOH mah	*hamart/o* defect *-oma* tumor, mass	A benign tumor of limited abnormal tissue formed in the respiratory tract. Also called a **chondroadenoma**.
mucous gland adenoma ad ih NOH mah	*muc/o* mucus *-ous* pertaining to *aden/o* gland *-oma* tumor, mass	A benign tumor of the mucous glands of the respiratory system.
papilloma pap ih LOH mah	*papill/o* nipple *-oma* tumor, mass	A benign tumor of epithelial origin named for its nipple-like appearance.

Fig. 11-14 Mesothelioma.

Terms Related to Malignant Neoplasms

Term	Word Origin	Definition
mesothelioma mee soh thee lee OH ma	*-oma* tumor, mass	A rare malignancy of the pleura or other protective tissues that cover the internal organs of the body. Often caused by exposure to asbestos (Fig. 11-14).
non–small cell lung cancer (NSCLC)		Most prevalent type of lung cancer.
adenocarcinoma ad ih noh kar sih NOH mah	*aden/o* gland *-carcinoma* cancer of epithelial origin	NSCLC derived from the mucus-secreting glands in the lungs.
large cell carcinoma	*carcinoma* cancer of epithelial origin	NSCLC originating in the lining of the smaller bronchi.
squamous cell carcinoma SKWAY muss	*squam/o* scaly *-ous* pertaining to *carcinoma* cancer of epithelial origin	NSCLC originating in the squamous epithelium of the larger bronchi.
small cell lung cancer (carcinoma) (SCLC)	*carcinoma* cancer of epithelial origin	Second most common type of lung cancer. Associated with smoking. Derived from neuroendocrine cells in the bronchi. Also called **oat cell carcinoma.**

EXERCISE 5: Neoplasms

Fill in the blank.

1. Hamartomas, adenomas, and papillomas are examples of _____ lung tumors.

2. Another name for a hamartoma is a/an _____.

3. Squamous cell carcinoma is an example of a/an _____.

4. Another name for small cell carcinoma is _____.

Age Matters

Pediatrics

Respiratory disorders account for three of the top ten reasons for hospitalization among children and adolescents. These top three include pneumonia, asthma, and acute bronchitis—all disorders of the lower respiratory system. Five of the top ten diagnoses for newborns are also respiratory problems or infections.

Geriatrics

Although pneumonia is one of the most common diagnoses for elderly patients, pulmonary edema, COPD, respiratory failure, and cancer have become the other most common disorders.

Click on **Hear It, Spell It** *to practice spelling the pathology terms that you have learned in this chapter. To review the pathology terms in this chapter, play* **Medical Millionaire.**

Medical Record Josiah Montgomery

MONTGOMERY, JOSIAH N - 707418 Opened by OLNACK, PAUL MD

Task   Edit   View   Time Scale   Options   Help

As Of 11:20

| MONTGOMERY, JOSIAH N | Age: 39 years | Sex: Male | Loc: WHC-SMMC |
| | DOB: 04/23/1976 | MRN: 707418 | FIN: 3506004 |

Reference Text Browser | Form Browser | Medication Profile

Orders | Last 48 Hours | **ED** | Lab | Radiology | Assessments | Surgery | Clinical Notes | Pt. Info | Pt. Schedule | Task List | I & O | MAR

Flowsheet: ED   Level: ED Note   ⦿ Table ○ Group ○ List

Navigator

✓ ED Note

Patient comes to the emergency room complaining of fever off and on since 7 days ago. He states he has also had some chills and urinary urgency. Denies sore throat, nausea, vomiting, diarrhea, and cough. Also states has been having some low back pain and headache occasionally with fever.

PMH:	HTN
MEDICATION:	None
ALLERGIES:	Penicillin
SH:	Nonsmoker, married
PHYSICAL EXAM:	
Vitals:	Temp 103.6, pulse 96, respirations 20, BP 168/88
Lungs:	Clear to auscultation, no wheezes or crackles
Heart:	Regular rate and rhythm
Abdomen:	Nondistended, positive bowel sounds, nontender
LABORATORY FINDINGS:	Chest x-ray shows left lower lobe atelectasis, urinalysis shows findings compatible with urinary tract infection.
DIAGNOSIS:	Left lower lobe atelectasis
	Patient will be treated with Cipro for his left lower lobe atelectasis and urinary tract infection symptoms.

PROD | MAHAFC | 2 Dec 2015 | 11:20

EXERCISE 6: Emergency Department Note

Using the preceding emergency department (ED) note, answer the following questions.

1. What phrase in the ED note tells you that the patient's chest is free of fluid or exudates?

    _____

2. What term tells you that the patient has not exhibited a whistling sound made during breathing?

    _____

3. What term tells you that the patient has not exhibited any discontinuous bubbling noises in his chest?

    _____

4. What was the diagnostic imaging procedure used? _____

5. What term tells you that the patient has a collapsed lung? _____

 Be Careful!

A **stethoscope** *is used to listen, not to look.*

DIAGNOSTIC PROCEDURES

The physical examination includes listening to the patient's chest by the process of **auscultation** (os kull TAY shun) (listening) **and percussion** (pur KUH shun) (tapping) **(A&P).** If the patient's chest is free of fluid or exudates, it is considered *clear to auscultation (CTA).* Further examination of chest sounds may be accomplished through the use of a **stethoscope** (STETH oh scope).

Terms Related to Diagnostic Procedures

Term	Word Origin	Definition
arterial blood gas (ABG)	*arteri/o* artery *-al* pertaining to	Blood test that measures the amount of O_2 and CO_2 in the blood.
bronchoscopy brong KOS skuh pee	*bronch/o* bronchus *-scopy* process of viewing	Endoscopic procedure used to examine the bronchial tubes visually (Fig. 11-15).
chest x-ray (CXR)		One of the most common imaging techniques for the respiratory system; used to visualize abnormalities of the respiratory system (Fig. 11-16). X-rays may also include the use of a contrast medium, as in **pulmonary angiography,** which uses a dye injected into the blood vessels of the lung, followed by subsequent x-ray imaging to demonstrate the flow of blood through these vessels.
computed tomography (CT)	*tom/o* slice *-graphy* process of recording	Imaging technique that can image the respiratory system and associated structures by creating cross-sections or "slices" of tissue.
laryngoscopy lair ing GOS skuh pee	*laryng/o* larynx, voice box *-scopy* process of viewing	Endoscopic procedure used to visualize the interior of the larynx.

Fiberoptic bronchoscope

Smaller bronchus

Fig. 11-15 Bronchoscopy.

Fig. 11-16 A, Normal posteroanterior (PA) chest x-ray (CXR). The backward "L" in the upper right corner is placed on the film to indicate the left side of the patient's chest. A, Diaphragm. B, Costophrenic angle. C, Left ventricle. D, Right atrium. E, Aortic arch. F, Superior vena cava. G, Trachea. H, Right bronchus. I, Left bronchus. J, Breast shadows. **B,** X-ray of lung with pneumonia.

Terms Related to Diagnostic Procedures—cont'd

Term	Word Origin	Definition
lung perfusion scan		Nuclear medicine test that produces an image of blood flow to the lungs; used to detect pulmonary embolism.
lung ventilation scan		Test using radiopharmaceuticals to produce a picture of how air is distributed in the lungs; measures the ability of the lungs to take in air (Fig. 11-17).
magnetic resonance imaging (MRI)		Computerized imaging that uses radiofrequency pulses to detect lung tumors, embolisms, and chest trauma.
Mantoux skin test mon TOO		Intradermal injection of purified protein derivative (PPD) used to detect the presence of TB antibodies.
mediastinoscopy mee dee ah stih NAH skuh pee		Endoscopic procedure used for visual examination of the structures contained within the space between the lungs.
peak flow meter		Instrument used in a pulmonary function test (PFT) to measure breathing capacity (Fig. 11-18).
pulmonary function tests (PFT)	*pulmon/o* lung *-ary* pertaining to	Procedures for determining the capacity of the lungs to exchange O_2 and CO_2 efficiently. See the table on the following page for examples of PFTs.
pulse oximetry ock SIM uh tree	*ox/i* oxygen *-metry* process of measurement	Noninvasive test to measure O_2 in arterial blood in which a noninvasive, clip-like device is attached to either the earlobe or the fingertip (Fig. 11-19).
QuantiFERON-TB (QFT) Gold test		Definitive blood test to diagnose TB.
sonography	*son/o* sound *-graphy* process of recording	Use of high-frequency sound waves to image structures within the body.
spirometry spy ROM uh tree	*spir/o* breathing *-metry* process of measurement	Test to measure the air capacity of the lungs with a **spirometer.**

Continued

Terms Related to Diagnostic Procedures—cont'd

Term	Word Origin	Definition
sputum culture and sensitivity SPYOO tum		Cultivation of microorganisms from sputum that has been collected from expectoration (spitting).
stethoscope STEH tho skohp	*steth/o* chest -*scope* instrument to view	An instrument commonly used to listen to sounds within the body, especially the chest.
sweat test		Method of evaluating sodium and chloride concentration in sweat as a means of diagnosing CF.
thoracoscopy thor ah KOSS kuh pee	*thorac/o* chest -*scopy* process of viewing	Visual exam of the chest cavity.
throat culture		Cultivation of microorganisms from a throat swab to determine the type of organism that is causing a disorder.

Fig. 11-17 Lung ventilation image of normal lungs.

Fig. 11-18 Peak flow meter.

Fig. 11-19 Pulse oximetry.

Examples of Pulmonary Function Tests

Function	Abbreviation	Description
Forced expiratory volume	FEV	Amount of air that can be exhaled with force in one breath.
Forced residual capacity	FRC	Amount of air remaining after a normal exhalation.
Forced vital capacity	FVC	Amount of air that can be exhaled with force after one inhales as deeply as possible.
Inspiratory capacity	IC	Amount of air that can be inspired after a normal expiration.
Tidal volume	TV	Amount of air normally inspired and expired in one respiration.
Total lung capacity	TLC	Amount of air in the lungs after one inhales as deeply as possible.

EXERCISE 7: Diagnostic Procedures

Fill in the blank.

1. A test for TB using purified protein derivation is called _____.

2. A blood test that measures O_2 and CO_2 is a/an _____.

3. A _____ is used to diagnose CF.

4. A _____ is a test of how air is distributed in the lung.

5. An imaging technique that shows the flow of blood through the vessels of the lungs is called

   _____.

Build the terms.

6. process of viewing the bronchi _____

7. process of viewing the voice box _____

8. process of measurement of breathing _____

Case Study   Mikasa Roven

Mikasa Roven is in the middle of her weekly outdoor yoga class at her local senior center when she suddenly feels extremely winded and can't catch her breath. She feels better after resting but does make an appointment for her internist, Dr. Thurston. He performs pulse oximetry and spirometry, which leads to a diagnosis of COPD.

1. What does pulse oximetry measure? _____
   _____

2. What does spirometry measure? _____
   _____

3. What does COPD stand for? _____
   _____

EXERCISE 8: Progress Note

Using the preceding progress note, answer the following questions.

1. The patient has a history of infection of which organs? _____

2. The term *inspiratory* refers to what? _____

3. What was the recent endoscopic procedure that the patient had? _____

4. Where is the site of the infection? _____

5. What is the abbreviation for the respiratory disorder that this patient is diagnosed with?

_____

THERAPEUTIC INTERVENTIONS

Therapeutic interventions for the respiratory system involve removal (*-ectomy*), repair (*-plasty*), a new opening (*-stomy*), a surgical puncture to remove fluid (*-centesis*), or intubation. See examples in the following table.

Patients who need assistance in attaining adequate O_2 levels may need a mechanical device called a **ventilator** to provide positive-pressure breathing (PPB). The device delivers the O_2 in different ways. If a low level of O_2 is required, a nasal **cannula** (KAN you lah) (tube) may be adequate. Face masks are another option. The amount of O_2 may be monitored more accurately with a **Venturi mask.** If high O_2 concentrations are necessary, a nonrebreathing or partial **rebreathing mask** may be used.

Positive-pressure breathing (PPB) is a respiratory therapy technique designed to deliver air at greater than atmospheric pressure to the lungs. **Continuous positive airway pressure (CPAP)** may be delivered through a ventilator and endotracheal tube or a nasal cannula, face mask, or hood over the patient's head. See Fig. 11-20 for several examples of oxygenation therapy.

Fig. 11-20 Routes of oxygen (O_2) therapy. **A,** Simple face mask. **B,** Venturi mask. **C,** Nasal cannula. **D,** Continuous positive airway pressure (CPAP).

Terms Related to Therapeutic Interventions

Term	Word Origin	Definition
adenoidectomy ad uh noyd ECK tuh mee	*adenoid/o* adenoid *-ectomy* removal, excision	Excision of the pharyngeal tonsils, or adenoids.
bronchoplasty BRONG koh plas tee	*bronch/o* bronchus *-plasty* surgical repair	Surgical repair of a bronchial defect.
endotracheal intubation en doh TRAY kee ul in too BAY shun	*endo-* within *trache/o* windpipe (trachea) *-al* pertaining to	Passage of a tube through the mouth into the trachea to ensure a patent (open) airway.
laryngectomy lair in JECK tuh mee	*laryng/o* voice box (larynx) *-ectomy* removal, excision	Excision of the voice box.
pulmonary resection		Excision of a portion or a lobe of the lung or the entire lung. Called a **lobectomy** when an entire lobe is excised and a **pneumonectomy** when the entire lung is excised (Fig. 11-21).
rhinoplasty RYE noh plas tee	*rhin/o* nose *-plasty* surgical repair	Surgical repair of the nose for healthcare or cosmetic reasons.

Continued

Terms Related to Therapeutic Interventions—cont'd

Term	Word Origin	Definition
septoplasty SEP toh plas tee	*sept/o* wall, septum *-plasty* surgical repair	Surgical repair of the wall between the nares.
sinusotomy sye nuh SOT tuh mee	*sinus/o* sinus *-tomy* incision	Incision of a sinus.
thoracocentesis thor ack koh sen TEE sis	*thorac/o* thorax *-centesis* surgical puncture	Aspiration of a fluid from the pleural cavity. Also called **pleurocentesis** or **thoracentesis.**
thoracotomy thor uh KOT uh mee	*thorac/o* chest *-tomy* incision	Incision of the chest as a means of approach for surgery.
tonsillectomy ton sih LECK tuh mee	*tonsill/o* tonsil *-ectomy* removal, excision	Excision of the palatine tonsils.
tracheostomy tray kee OS tuh mee	*trache/o* trachea (windpipe) *-stomy* new opening	Opening through the neck into the trachea, through which an indwelling tube may be inserted temporarily or permanently (Fig. 11-22).
tracheotomy tray kee AH tuh mee	*trache/o* trachea (windpipe) *-tomy* incision	Incision made into the trachea below the larynx to gain access to the airway; usually performed as an emergency procedure.

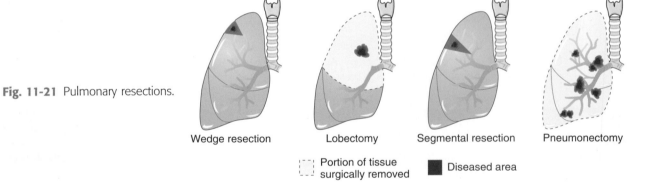

Fig. 11-21 Pulmonary resections.

Wedge resection   Lobectomy   Segmental resection   Pneumonectomy

Portion of tissue surgically removed   Diseased area

Thyroid cartilage

Cricoid cartilage

Second, third, and fourth tracheal rings

A   B   C

Fig. 11-22 A, Vertical tracheal incision for a tracheostomy. **B,** Tracheostomy tube. **C,** Placement of gauze and tie around a tracheostomy tube.

EXERCISE 9: Therapeutic Interventions

Match the terms with their definitions.

_____ 1. excision of the palatine tonsils

_____ 2. surgical repair of the wall between the nares

_____ 3. incision of a sinus

_____ 4. removal of a lobe of the lung

_____ 5. removal of the pharyngeal tonsils

_____ 6. surgical repair of a bronchus

_____ 7. aspiration of fluid from the pleural cavity

_____ 8. incision of the windpipe

_____ 9. tube within the windpipe

A. thoracocentesis
B. tracheotomy
C. endotracheal intubation
D. bronchoplasty
E. tonsillectomy
F. adenoidectomy
G. lobectomy
H. septoplasty
I. sinusotomy

Build the terms.

10. excision of the voice box _____

11. surgical repair of the nose _____

12. new opening in the windpipe _____

Case Study Morgan Butterfield

Morgan Butterfield works as a waitress at a chain restaurant to help pay for school. Although she's been feeling under the weather for a few days, she thought that it was from her busy schedule of waitressing at night and attending classes during the day. Today, however, she has a horribly sore throat and difficulty breathing. While visiting her doctor, Dr. Hahn, she sees that "inspiratory stridor" and "tachypnea" are noted on her chart. When asked, Dr. Hahn says that they describe the abnormal sound and rate of her breathing. She suspects that Morgan has epiglottitis, and she's worried that Morgan may need a tracheostomy if the inflammation gets worse and the swelling closes her airway.

1. What is the term that means difficulty breathing?
   a. hypoxemia
   b. aphonia
   c. dyspnea
   d. eupnea

2. A continuous high-pitched sound that is heard when a person inhales is called _____.

3. Abnormally rapid breathing is called _____.

4. An inflammation of the epiglottis is called _____.

5. What does the suffix -*stomy* mean in the term *tracheostomy?*
   a. cutting
   b. making an opening
   c. removing
   d. suturing

*Click on **Hear It, Spell It** to practice spelling the diagnostic and therapeutic terms that you have learned in this chapter.*

PHARMACOLOGY

Routes of administration for respiratory pharmaceuticals include the use of **ventilators,** devices that serve to assist respiration, and intensive PPB. A **hand-held nebulizer (HHN)** is a powered device that converts liquids into a fine spray, such as for inhaled medications. An **inhaler** is a nonmechanical device for administering medications that are inhaled, such as vapors or fine powders. A **spacer**, a device connected to the inhaler that contains the mist expelled from the inhaler until the user can breathe it, usually is used for children and individuals who have difficulty using the inhaler device alone.

antihistamines: Block histamine receptors to manage allergies associated with allergic rhinitis or allergy-induced asthma. Examples are clemastine (Tavist), diphenhydramine (Benadryl), loratadine (Claritin), and fexofenadine (Allegra).

antitussives: Suppress the cough reflex. Examples include dextromethorphan (Delsym), codeine (Robitussin AC), and benzonatate (Tessalon).

bronchodilators: Relax bronchi to improve ventilation to the lungs. Examples include theophylline (Theo-Dur), ipratropium (Atrovent), and albuterol (Proventil, Ventolin), often administered through inhalers or nebulizers.

decongestants: Reduce congestion or swelling of mucous membranes. Examples are pseudoephedrine (Sudafed) and phenylephrine (Sudafed PE).

expectorants: Promote the expulsion of mucus from the respiratory tract. An example is guaifenesin (Mucinex).

inhaled corticosteroids: Reduce airway inflammation to improve ventilation or reduce nasal congestion. Administered via oral or nasal inhalation accordingly. Examples include fluticasone (Flovent, Flonase), mometasone (Nasonex), and beclomethasone (Qvar).

mucolytics: Break up thick mucus in the respiratory tract. An example is N-acetylcysteine (Mucomyst).

EXERCISE 10: Pharmacology

Matching.

_____ 1. relaxes the bronchi

_____ 2. expels mucus

_____ 3. reduces congestion

_____ 4. blocks histamine receptors to manage allergies

_____ 5. suppresses coughs

A. antihistamine
B. antitussive
C. bronchodilator
D. decongestant
E. expectorant

Answer the following questions.

6.   What type of mechanical device is used to produce a fine spray for inhaled medications?

7. What type of nonmechanical device is used to administer medications that are inhaled, such as fine powders or vapors? _____

8. A/n _____ is a device designed to assist in respiration and intensive PPB.

Abbreviations

Abbreviation	Definition	Abbreviation	Definition
ABG	arterial blood gas	MDRTB	multidrug-resistant tuberculosis
A&P	auscultation and percussion	MRI	magnetic resonance imaging
AP	anteroposterior	NSCLC	non–small cell lung cancer
ARF	acute respiratory failure	O_2	oxygen
CF	cystic fibrosis	OSA	obstructive sleep apnea
CO_2	carbon dioxide	PPB	positive-pressure breathing
COPD	chronic obstructive pulmonary disease	PPD	purified protein derivative
CPAP	continuous positive airway pressure	QFT	quantiFERON-TB Gold test
		RAD	reactive airway disease
CT	computed tomography	RLL	right lower lobe (of the lung)
CTA	clear to auscultation	RML	right middle lobe (of the lung)
CWP	coal workers' pneumoconiosis	RSV	respiratory syncytial virus
CXR	chest x-ray	RUL	right upper lobe (of the lung)
DOE	dyspnea on exertion	SARS	severe acute respiratory syndrome
HHN	hand-held nebulizer		
LLL	left lower lobe (of the lung)	SCLC	small cell lung cancer
LUL	left upper lobe (of the lung)	SOB	shortness of breath
MDI	metered dose inhaler	TB	tuberculosis
		URI	upper respiratory infection

EXERCISE 11: Abbreviations

Write out the following abbreviations.

1. A CXR revealed RML pneumonia in the 43-year-old teacher. _____

2. The patient was tested with PPD for suspected TB. _____

3. Solange had rhinorrhea and a productive cough, and she was diagnosed with a URI.

   _____

4. The patient with COPD had dyspnea, DOE, and a chronic cough.

   _____

5. Years of work in the mines resulted in the patient's diagnosis of CWP. _____

6. The child came to the ED and was diagnosed with RSV. _____

Chapter Review

Match the word parts to their definitions.

Word Parts Definitions

Prefix/Suffix		Definition
a-	1. _____	healthy, normal
dys-	2. _____	excessive
-ectasis	3. _____	deficient
eu-	4. _____	without
hyper-	5. _____	breathing
hypo-	6. _____	spitting
-metry	7. _____	discharge
-pnea	8. _____	difficult
-ptysis	9. _____	process of measurement
-rrhea	10. _____	dilation

Combining Form		Definition
capn/o	11. _____	carbon dioxide
cost/o	12. _____	lung
laryng/o	13. _____	chest
muc/o	14. _____	to breathe
nas/o	15. _____	straight
orth/o	16. _____	pleura
ox/i	17. _____	nose
pector/o	18. _____	septum, wall
pharyng/o	19. _____	chest
phren/o	20. _____	pus
pleur/o	21. _____	throat
pneum/o	22. _____	mucus
pulmon/o	23. _____	oxygen
py/o	24. _____	diaphragm
rhin/o	25. _____	lung
salping/o	26. _____	chest
sept/o	27. _____	rib
sin/o	28. _____	sinus
spir/o	29. _____	tonsil
steth/o	30. _____	eustachian tube
thorac/o	31. _____	voice box
tonsill/o	32. _____	nose

Wordshop

Prefixes	Combining Forms	Suffixes
a-	coni/o	-al
brady-	cost/o	-ation
dys-	hem/a	-eal
endo-	laryng/o	-itis
eu-	my/o	-osis
ex-	myc/o	-plasty
hyper-	pleur/o	-pnea
in-	pneum/o	-rrhea
inter-	py/o	-scopy
para-	rhin/o	-stenosis
tachy-	spir/o	-stomy
	troche/a	-thorax
	thorac/o	-tomy

Build the following terms by combining the preceding word parts. Some word parts may be used more than once. Some may not be used at all. The number in parenthesis is the number of word parts needed to build the term.

Definition	Term
1. difficult breathing (2)	_____
2. rapid breathing (2)	_____
3. abnormal condition of dust in the lungs (3)	_____
4. discharge from the nose (2)	_____
5. process of breathing out (3)	_____
6. pus in the chest (pleural cavity) (2)	_____
7. inflammation of the pleurae (2)	_____
8. surgical repair of the nose (2)	_____
9. blood in the chest (pleural cavity) (2)	_____
10. abnormal condition of narrowing of the windpipe (2)	_____
11. incision of the windpipe (2)	_____
12. pertaining to between the ribs (3)	_____
13. pertaining to within the windpipe (3)	_____
14. abnormal condition of fungus in the nose (3)	_____
15. process of viewing the chest (2)	_____

Sort the terms into the correct categories.

Term Sorting

Anatomy and Physiology	Pathology	Diagnostic Procedures	Therapeutic Interventions

ABG	CXR	mediastinum	SARS
alveolus	diaphragm	olfaction	septoplasty
aphonia	emphysema	oropharynx	sinusotomy
apnea	epiglottis	pleurisy	spirometry
bronchiectasis	epistaxis	PFT	thoracocentesis
bronchodilator	eustachian tube	pleura	throat culture
bronchoplasty	hemoptysis	pulse oximetry	tonsillectomy
bronchoscopy	inhalation	QFT	trachea
CPAP	laryngectomy	rhinomycosis	tracheostomy
CT	mediastinoscopy	rhonchi	tracheotomy

Replace the highlighted words with the correct terms.

Translations

1. **Difficult and/or painful breathing** and **whistling sound made during breathing** were signs that Sari had asthma.

2. The patient's **difficulty making sounds** and **inflammation of the voice box** were associated with an upper respiratory infection.

3. The baby had **a high-pitched inspiratory sound from the larynx,** which was a sign of **acute viral infection of early childhood marked by stridor caused by spasms of the larynx, trachea, and bronchi.**

4. Dr. Hollander told Ryan's mother that her son's fever and **chest pain** were symptoms of **abnormal accumulation of fluid in the intrapleural space.**

5. The patient underwent a **CXR** to see if she had **an infectious inflammation of the lungs.**

6. After 3 days of **severe inflammation or infection of the pharynx,** Abby had **a cultivation of microorganisms from a throat swab** to determine the pathogen.

7. **A noninvasive test to measure oxygen in arterial blood** and **a test to measure the air capacity of the lungs** were performed on the patient.

8. Marketta's **deflection of the nasal septum** was treated with **a surgical repair of the wall between the nares.**

9. **An aspiration of a fluid from the pleural cavity** was necessary to treat the patient's **blood in the pleural cavity.**

10. The pulmonologist diagnosed Mr. Borasky with **chronic dilation of the bronchi** and **respiratory disorder characterized by a progressive and irreversible diminishment in capacity of the lungs.**

11. After the patient's treatment for **pertaining to the larynx** cancer, she had a temporary **opening through the neck into the trachea.**

12. Monique had **an intradermal injection of PPD,** which revealed that she had **a chronic infectious disorder caused by an acid-fast bacillus.**

13. Mr H. was treated for **abnormal accumulation of coal dust in the lungs,** a type of **loss of lung capacity caused by an accumulation of dust in the lungs** that developed after years of work in a coal mine.

14. The child had a **method of evaluation sodium and chloride concentration in sweat** to see if she had **an inherited disorder of the exocrine glands, resulting in abnormal, thick secretions of mucus.**

Medical Record   *Casey Sandoval*

SANDOVAL, CASEY C - 557248 Opened by HAMILTON, WILLIAM RRT

Task   Edit   View   Time Scale   Options   Help

| SANDOVAL, CASEY C | Age: 8 years | Sex: Female | Loc: WHC-SMMC |
| | DOB: 03/31/2006 | MRN: 557248 | FIN: 3506004 |

Reference Text Browser | Form Browser | Medication Profile

Orders | Last 48 Hours | ED | Lab | Radiology | Assessments | Surgery | Clinical Notes | Pt. Info | Pt. Schedule | Task List | I & O | MAR

Flowsheet: ED   Level: ED Record   ⦿ Table   ○ Group   ○ List

Navigator

✓ ED Record

Casey Sandoval, an 8-year-old female, came to the ED in moderately severe respiratory distress. She was accompanied by her mother. Pt appeared pale, anxious, and slightly diaphoretic, and had slight nail bed cyanosis. Casey was unable to speak more than two or three word phrases between breaths. She was placed on oxygen per face mask and connected to cardiac monitor and pulse oximetry. HR was 125, RR was 33, and labored; pulse oximetry measured 89% on 6 L/min O_2. Wheezes were auscultated in all lung fields, with prolonged expiratory phase. Pt has frequent nonproductive cough. Physical exam revealed intercostal retractions and use of accessory muscles on inspiration.

Pt was given an immediate nebulization treatment via hand-held nebulizer containing 5 mg Albuterol and 3 mL NS solution driven by 8 L/min O_2. Pulse oximetry increased to 95% by end of nebulization. Peak flows were measured at 100 L/min post-HHN. Respirations had decreased to 25; heart rate was 95. Breath sounds revealed mild, scattered expiratory wheezes and rhonchi bilaterally. Repeat nebulizer treatment was performed 15 minutes later. Peak flow measurements had increased to 175 L/min, and pt was able to wean off supplemental oxygen and maintained oxygen saturation of 94% on room air.

A third HHN was ordered 30 minutes later, and repeat peak flows measured 210 L/min. Breath sounds were clear, and pt respiratory rate had decreased to 18 breaths/min, heart rate to 87, and saturation was 97% on room air.

Oral prednisone was prescribed. Pt and parent were instructed on use of metered dose inhaler with spacer and peak flow meter. MDIs containing Albuterol and Flovent 88 mcg b.i.d. were prescribed. Child and parent were instructed to use 4 puffs Albuterol every 4 hours, and 2 puffs Flovent b.i.d. Peak flows were to be measured three times daily pre Albuterol and post Albuterol and graphed on the diary card.

| PROD | MAHAFC | 25 May 2014 | 17:43 |

⟳ EMERGENCY DEPARTMENT RECORD

Using the preceding ED record, answer the following questions.

1. In your own words, explain the meaning of the symptoms "slightly diaphoretic" and "slight nail bed cyanosis." _____

2. How is O_2 measured in pulse oximetry? _____

3. Name and define the two abnormal sounds heard on auscultation in this report.

   _____

4. What is the purpose of a peak flow meter? _____

5. What does the abbreviation HHN mean? _____

Nervous System

12

OBJECTIVES

- Recognize and use terms related to the anatomy and physiology of the nervous system.
- Recognize and use terms related to the pathology of the nervous system.

- Recognize and use terms related to the diagnostic procedures for the nervous system.
- Recognize and use terms related to the therapeutic interventions for the nervous system.

For interactive learning, click on:
- **Match the Word Parts** to review nervous system word parts.
- **Word Shop** to practice word building.
- **Tournament of Terminology** to test your knowledge of nervous system terms.
- **Term Sorting** to practice sorting nervous system terms into categories.

*Click on **Chapter at a Glance** to print off a list of key terms and word parts for this chapter.*

homeostasis
home/o = same
-stasis = stopping, controlling

nerve = neur/o

FUNCTIONS OF THE NERVOUS SYSTEM

Possibly the most complex and poorly understood system, the nervous system plays a major role in **homeostasis** (hoh mee oh STAY sis), keeping the other body systems coordinated and regulated to achieve optimum performance. It accomplishes this goal by helping the individual respond to his or her internal and external environments.

The nervous and endocrine systems are responsible for communication and control throughout the body. There are three main **neural** functions, which are as follows:

1. Collecting information about the external and internal environment *(sensing)*.
2. Processing this information and making decisions about action *(interpreting)*.
3. Directing the body to put into play the decisions made *(acting)*.

For example, the sensory function begins with a stimulus (e.g., the uncomfortable pinch of tight shoes). That information travels to the brain, where it is interpreted. The return message is sent to react to the stimulus (e.g., remove the shoes).

SPECIALTIES/SPECIALISTS

neurology
neur/o = nerve
-logy = study of

Physicians who specialize in the diagnosis, treatment, and prevention of neurologic disorders are called **neurologists.** The specialty is **neurology.**

ANATOMY AND PHYSIOLOGY

Organization of the Nervous System

To carry out its functions, the nervous system is divided into two main subsystems. Fig. 12-1 shows a schematic of the divisions. The **central nervous system (CNS)** is composed of the brain and the spinal cord. It is the only site of nerve cells called **interneurons** (in tur NOOR ons), which connect sensory and motor neurons. The **peripheral nervous system (PNS)** is composed of the nerves that extend from the brain and spinal cord to the tissues of the body. These are organized into 12 pairs of cranial nerves and 31 pairs of spinal nerves. The PNS is further divided into voluntary and involuntary nerves, which may be **afferent** (or **sensory**), carrying impulses to the brain and spinal cord, or **efferent** (or **motor**), carrying impulses from the brain and spinal cord to either voluntary or involuntary muscles.

interneuron
inter- = between
neur/o = nerve
-on = structure

PNS nerves are further categorized into two subsystems:

body = somat/o

somatic (soh MAT ick) **system:** This system is *voluntary* in nature. These nerves collect information from and return instructions to the skin, muscles, and joints.
autonomic (ah toh NAH mick) **system:** Mostly *involuntary* functions are controlled by this system as sensory information from the internal environment is sent to the CNS, and, in return, motor impulses from the CNS are sent to involuntary muscles: the heart, glands, and organs.

 Be Careful! *Remember that **efferent** means to carry away, whereas **afferent** means to carry toward. In the nervous system, these terms are used to refer to away from and toward the brain.*

Fig. 12-1 The nervous system. Afferent nerves carry nervous impulses from a stimulus toward the central nervous system (CNS). Efferent nerves carry the impulse away from the CNS to affect a response to the stimulus.

EXERCISE 1: Organization of the Nervous System

Fill in the blanks.

1. The two main divisions of the nervous system are the _____ and the

    _____.

Circle the correct answer.

2. Sensory neurons *(transmit, receive)* information *(to, from)* the CNS.
3. Motor neurons, also called *(efferent, afferent)* neurons, transmit information *(to, from)* the CNS.
4. The *(somatic, autonomic)* nervous system is voluntary in nature, whereas the *(somatic, autonomic)* nervous system is largely involuntary.

Cells of the Nervous System

The nervous system is made up of the following two types of cells:

1. Parenchymal cells, or **neurons,** the cells that carry out the work of the system.
2. Stromal cells, or **glia** (GLEE uh), the cells that provide a supportive function.

neuron
  neur/o = nerve
  -on = structure

Neurons

The basic unit of the nervous system is the nerve cell, or neuron (Fig. 12-2). Not all neurons are the same, but they all have features in common. **Dendrites** (DEN drytes), projections from the cell body, receive **neural impulses,** also called **action potentials,** from a **stimulus** of some kind. This impulse travels along the dendrite and into the cell body, which is the control center of the cell. This cell body contains the nucleus and surrounding cytoplasm.

From the cell body, the impulse moves out along the **axon** (AX on), a slender, elongated projection that carries the nervous impulse toward the next neuron. The **terminal fibers** result from the final branching of the axon and the site

dendrite = dendr/o

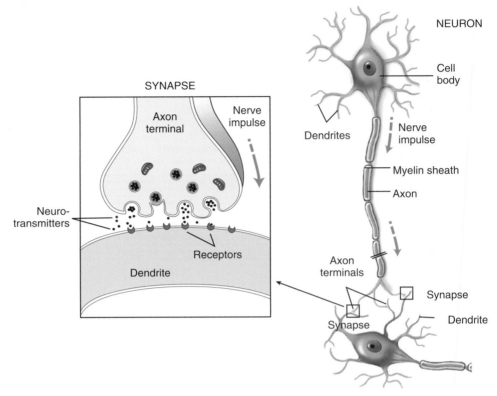

Fig. 12-2 The nerve cell (neuron) with an inset of a synapse.

neuroglia
  neur/o = nerve
  -glia = glue

astrocyte
  astr/o = star
  -cyte = cell

of the **axon terminals** that store the chemical **neurotransmitters.** In neurons *outside* the CNS, the axon is coated by the **myelin** (MY uh lin) **sheath,** which is a substance produced by **Schwann** (shvahn) **cells** that coat the axons.

From the axon's terminal fibers, the neurotransmitter is released from the cell to travel across the space between these terminal fibers and the dendrites of the next cell. This space is called the **synapse** (SIN aps) (see Fig. 12-2). The impulse continues in this manner until its destination is reached.

Glia

These supportive, or stromal, cells are also called **neuroglia** (noo RAH glee ah). They accomplish their supportive function by physically holding the neurons together and also protecting them. One type of neuroglia, the **astrocytes** (AS troh sites), connect neurons and blood vessels and form a structure called the **blood-brain barrier (BBB),** which prevents or slows the passage of some drugs and disease-causing organisms to the CNS.

 EXERCISE 2: Cells of the Nervous System

1. List words connected by arrows to show the path of the action potential from initial stimulus to synapse.

_____

Match the terms with their word parts.

_____ 2. star   _____ 5. glue   A. -glia
                                                B. somat/o
_____ 3. body   _____ 6. dendrite   C. dendr/o
                                                D. astr/o
_____ 4. nerve   E. neur/o

Decode the terms.

7. perineural _____

8. oligodendric _____

9. microglial _____

The Central Nervous System

As stated previously, the CNS is composed of the **brain** and the **spinal cord.**

The Brain

The brain is one of the most complex organs of the body. It is divided into four parts: the **cerebrum** (suh REE brum), the **cerebellum** (sair ih BELL um), the **diencephalon** (dye en SEF fuh lon), and the **brainstem** (Fig. 12-3).

Cerebrum

The largest portion of the brain, the cerebrum, is divided into two halves, or hemispheres (Fig. 12-4). It is responsible for thinking, reasoning, and memory. The surfaces of the hemispheres are covered with **gray matter** and are called the **cerebral cortex.** Arranged into folds, the valleys are referred to as **sulci** (SULL sye) (*sing.* sulcus), and the ridges are **gyri** (JYE rye) (*sing.* gyrus). The cerebrum is further divided into sections called **lobes,** each of which has its own functions:

1. The **frontal lobe** contains the functions of speech and the motor area that controls voluntary movement on the contralateral side of the body.
2. The **temporal** (TEM pur rul) **lobe** contains the auditory and olfactory areas.
3. The **parietal** (puh RYE uh tul) **lobe** controls the sensations of touch and taste.
4. The **occipital** (ock SIP ih tul) **lobe** is responsible for vision.

brain = encephal/o	
cerebrum = cerebr/o	
cerebellum = cerebell/o	
cortex = cortic/o	
lobe = lob/o	

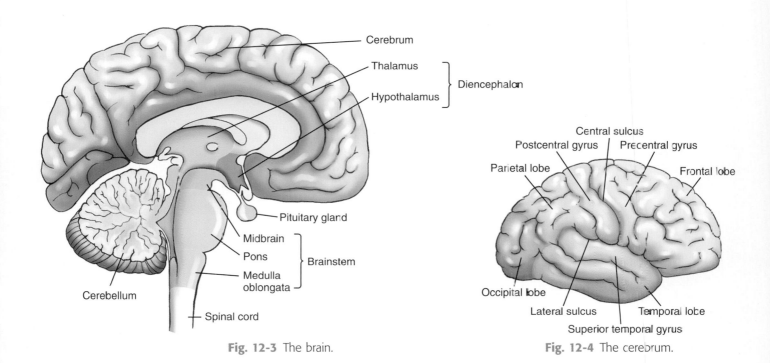

Fig. 12-3 The brain.

Fig. 12-4 The cerebrum.

Cerebellum

Located inferior to the occipital lobe of the cerebrum, the **cerebellum** coordinates voluntary movement but is involuntary in its function. For example, walking is a voluntary movement. The coordination needed for the muscles and other body parts to walk smoothly is involuntary and is controlled by the cerebellum.

Diencephalon

The diencephalon is composed of the **thalamus** (THAL uh mus) and the structure inferior to it, the **hypothalamus** (HYE poh thal uh mus). The thalamus is responsible for relaying sensory information (with the exception of smell) and translating it into sensations of pain, temperature, and touch. The hypothalamus activates, integrates, and controls the peripheral autonomic nervous system (ANS), along with many functions, such as body temperature, sleep, and appetite.

Brainstem

The brainstem connects the cerebral hemispheres to the spinal cord. It is composed of three main parts: **midbrain, pons** (ponz), and **medulla oblongata** (muh DOO lah ob lon GAH tah). The midbrain connects the pons and cerebellum with the hemispheres of the cerebrum. It is the site of reflex centers for eye and head movements in response to visual and auditory stimuli. The second part of the brainstem, the pons, serves as a bridge between the medulla oblongata and the cerebrum. Finally, the lowest part of the brainstem, the medulla oblongata, regulates heart rate, blood pressure, and breathing.

The Spinal Cord

The **spinal cord** extends from the medulla oblongata to the first lumbar vertebra (Fig. 12-5). It then extends into a structure called the **cauda equina** (KAH

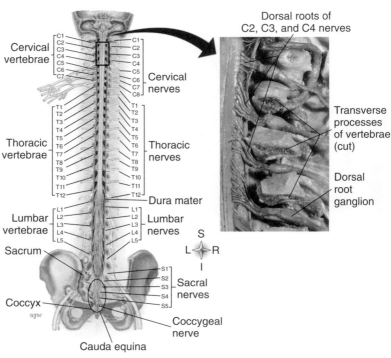

Fig. 12-5 The spinal cord with an inset of a cervical segment showing emerging cervical nerves.

⊗ Be Careful!

Myel/o *can mean bone marrow or spinal cord; memorization and context will be the student's only methods to determine which meaning applies.*

spinal cord = cord/o, chord/o, myel/o

dah eh KWY nah). The spinal cord is protected by the bony vertebrae surrounding it and the coverings unique to the CNS called **meninges** (meh NIN jeez). The spinal cord is composed of **gray matter,** the cell bodies of motor neurons, and **white matter,** the myelin-covered axons or nerve fibers that extend from the nerve cell bodies. The 31 pairs of spinal nerves emerge from the spinal cord at the **nerve roots.**

Meninges

Meninges act as protective coverings for the CNS and are composed of three layers separated by spaces (Fig. 12-6). The **dura mater** (DUR ah MAY tur) is the tough, fibrous, outer covering of the meninges; its literal meaning is *hard mother.* The space between the dura mater and arachnoid membrane is called the **subdural space.** Next comes the **arachnoid** (uh RACK noyd) **membrane,** a thin, delicate membrane that takes its name from its spidery appearance. The **subarachnoid space** is the space between the arachnoid membrane and the pia mater, containing **cerebrospinal fluid (CSF).** CSF is also present in cavities in the brain called **ventricles.** Finally, the **pia mater** (PEE uh MAY tur) is the thin, vascular membrane that is the innermost of the three meninges; its literal meaning is *soft mother.*

The Peripheral Nervous System

The peripheral nervous system is divided into 12 pairs of **cranial nerves** that conduct impulses between the brain and the head, neck, thoracic, and abdominal areas, and 31 pairs of **spinal nerves** that closely mimic the organization of the vertebrae and provide innervation to the rest of the body. If the nerve

meninges = mening/o, meningi/o

nerve root = rhiz/o, radicul/o

dura mater = dur/o

ventricle = ventricul/o

Fig. 12-6 The meninges.

fibers from several spinal nerves form a network, it is termed a **plexus** (PLECK sus). Spinal nerves are named by their location (cervical, thoracic, lumbar, sacral, and coccygeal) and by number (Fig. 12-7). Cranial nerves are named by their number and also their function or distribution.

The Cranial Nerves

Number	Name	Origin of Sensory Fibers	Effector Innervated by Motor Fibers
I	Olfactory	Olfactory epithelium of nose (smell)	None
II	Optic	Retina of eye (vision)	None
III	Oculomotor	Proprioceptors* of eyeball muscles	Muscles that move eyeball; muscles that change shape of lens; muscles that constrict pupil
IV	Trochlear	Proprioceptors* of eyeball muscles	Muscles that move eyeball
V	Trigeminal	Teeth and skin of face	Some muscles used in chewing
VI	Abducens	Proprioceptors* of eyeball muscles	Muscles that move eyeball
VII	Facial	Taste buds of anterior part of tongue	Muscles used for facial expression; submaxillary and sublingual salivary glands
VIII	Vestibulocochlear (auditory)		None
	Vestibular branch	Semicircular canals of inner ear (senses of movement, balance, and rotation)	
	Cochlear branch	Cochlea of inner ear (hearing)	
IX	Glossopharyngeal	Taste buds of posterior third of tongue and lining of pharynx	Parotid salivary gland; muscles of pharynx used in swallowing
X	Vagus	Nerve endings in many of the internal organs (e.g., lungs, stomach, aorta, larynx)	Parasympathetic fibers to heart, stomach, small intestine, larynx, esophagus, and other organs
XI	Spinal accessory	Muscles of shoulder	Muscles of neck and shoulder
XII	Hypoglossal	Muscles of tongue	Muscles of tongue

*Proprioceptors are receptors located in muscles, tendons, or joints that provide information about body position and movement.

dermatome
dermat/o = skin
-tome = instrument used to cut

Dermatomes (DUR mah tomes) are skin surface areas supplied by a single afferent spinal nerve. These areas are so specific that it is actually possible to map the body by dermatomes (Fig. 12-8). This specificity can be demonstrated in patients with shingles, who show similar patterns as specific peripheral nerves are affected (see Fig. 12-17).

The **autonomic nervous system (ANS)** consists of nerves that regulate involuntary function. Examples include cardiac muscle and smooth muscle. The motor portion of this system is further divided into the sympathetic nervous system and the parasympathetic nervous system, two opposing systems that provide balance in the rest of the body systems:

- The **sympathetic nervous system** is capable of producing a "fight-or-flight" response. This is the one part of the nervous system that helps the individual respond to perceived stress. The heart rate and blood pressure increase, digestive processes slow, and sweat and adrenal glands increase their secretions.

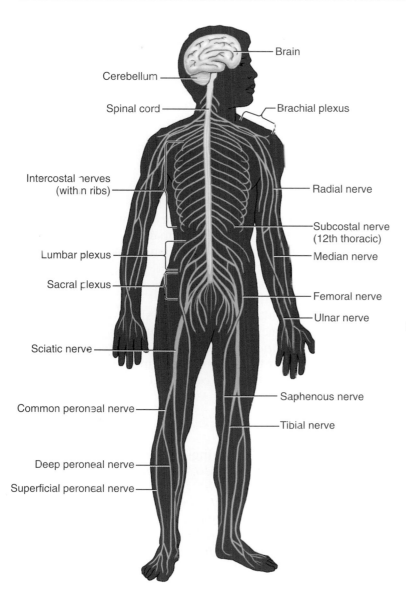

Fig. 12-7 Spinal nerves.

- The **parasympathetic nervous system** tends to do the opposite of the sympathetic nervous system—slowing the heart rate, lowering blood pressure, increasing digestive functions, and decreasing adrenal and sweat gland activity. This is sometimes called the "rest and digest" system.

Here is an example of a sensory response:

Eight-year-old Joey is hungry. He decides to sneak some cookies before dinner. Afraid that his mother will see him, he surreptitiously takes a handful into the hall closet and shuts the door. As he begins to eat, the closet door flies open. Joey's heart begins to race as he whips the cookies out of sight. When he sees it's only his sister, he relaxes and offers her a cookie as a bribe not to tell on him.

Joey's afferent (sensory) somatic neurons carried the message to his brain that he was hungry. This message was interpreted by his brain as a concern, and the response was to sneak cookies from the jar and hide himself as he ate them. When the closet door flew open, his sensory neurons perceived a danger and triggered a sympathetic "fight-or-flight" response, which raised his heart rate and blood pressure and stimulated his sweat glands. When the intruder was perceived to be harmless, his parasympathetic nervous system took over and reduced his heart rate, bringing it back to normal. The same afferent fibers perceived the intruder in two different ways with two different sets of autonomic motor responses (sympathetic and parasympathetic).

Fig. 12-8 Dermatomes. Each dermatome is named for the spinal nerve that serves it.

> ⊗ **Be Careful!**
> The term **dermatome** can be used to describe an instrument that cuts thin slices of skin for grafting, and the term also signifies a mesodermal layer in early development, which becomes the dermal layers of the skin.

 EXERCISE 3: Central and Peripheral Nervous System

Match the following parts of the brain with their functions.

_____ 1. pons

_____ 2. parietal cerebral lobe

_____ 3. hypothalamus

_____ 4. temporal cerebral lobe

_____ 5. midbrain

_____ 6. cerebellum

_____ 7. occipital cerebral lobe

_____ 8. thalamus

_____ 9. frontal cerebral lobe

_____ 10. medulla oblongata

A. auditory and olfactory activity
B. relays sensory information
C. reflex center for eye and head movements
D. sensation of vision
E. regulates heart rate, blood pressure, and breathing
F. regulates temperature, sleep, and appetite
G. speech and motor activity
H. connects medulla oblongata with cerebrum
I. coordinates voluntary movement
J. sensation of touch and taste

Match the CNS part with its combining form.

_____ 11. cerebellum

_____ 12. spinal cord

_____ 13. meninges

_____ 14. nerve root

_____ 15. dura mater

_____ 16. cerebrum

_____ 17. brain

_____ 18. skin

_____ 19. spine

_____ 20. ventricle

A. meningi/o, mening/o
B. myel/o, cord/o, chord/o
C. dur/o
D. rhiz/o, radicul/o
E. dermat/o
F. cerebr/o
G. spin/o
H. cerebell/o
I. encephal/o
J. ventricul/o

Decode the terms.

21. intraventricular _____

22. epidural _____

23. parasinal _____

24. infracerebellar _____

EXERCISE 4: Central and Peripheral Nervous System

Label the drawings using the terms provided.

neurotransmitters
cell body
synapse
axon terminal
dendrites
receptors
nerve impulse
axon

temporal lobe
parietal lobe
frontal lobe
occipital lobe

Combining and Adjective Forms for the Anatomy and Physiology of the Nervous System

Meaning	Combining Form	Adjective Form
body	somat/o	somatic
brain	encephal/o	
cerebellum	cerebell/o	cerebellar
cerebrum	cerebr/o	cerebral
cortex	cortic/o	cortical
dendrite	dendr/o	dendritic
dura mater	dur/o	dural
lobe	lob/o	lobular, lobar
meninges	mening/o, meningi/o	meningeal
nerve	neur/o	neural
nerve root	rhiz/o, radicul/o	radicular
same	home/o	
skin	dermat/o	dermatic
spinal cord	cord/o, chord/o, myel/o	cordal, chordal
star	astr/o	astral
ventricle	ventricul/o	ventricular

Suffixes for the Anatomy and Physiology of the Nervous System

Suffix	Meaning
-cyte	cell
-glia	glue
-logy	study of
-on	structure
-stasis	stopping, controlling
-tome	instrument used to cut

 *Click on **Label It** to practice labeling structures of the nervous system.*
*You can review the anatomy of the nervous system by clicking on **Body Spectrum Electronic Anatomy Coloring Book → Nervous**. Choose **Hear It, Spell It** to practice spelling the anatomy and physiology terms that you have learned in this chapter.*

 Be Careful!

*Don't confuse **dysarthria** (difficulty with speech) and **dysarthrosis** (any disorder of a joint).*

PATHOLOGY

The signs and symptoms for this system encompass many systems because of the nature of the neural function: communicating, or failing to communicate, with other parts of the body.

Terms Related to Signs and Symptoms

Term	Word Origin	Definition
amnesia am NEE zsa		Loss of memory caused by brain damage or severe emotional trauma.
aphasia ah FAY zsa	*a-* without *phas/o* speech *-ia* condition	Lack or impairment of the ability to form or understand speech. Less severe forms include **dysphasia** (dis FAY zsa) and **dysarthria** (dis AR three ah); dysarthria refers to difficulty in the articulation (pronunciation) of speech.
athetosis ath uh TOH sis		Continuous, involuntary, slow, writhing movement of the extremities.
aura OR uh		Premonition; sensation of light or warmth that may precede an epileptic seizure or the onset of some types of headache.
dysphagia dis FAY zsa	*dys-* difficult *phag/o* eat *-ia* condition	Condition of difficulty with swallowing.
dyssomnia dih SAHM nee ah	*dys-* difficult *somn/o* sleep *-ia* condition	Disorders of the sleep-wake cycles. **Insomnia** is the inability to sleep or stay asleep. **Hypersomnia** is excessive depth or length of sleep, which may be accompanied by daytime sleepiness.
fasciculation fah sick yoo LAY shun		Involuntary contraction of small, local muscles.
gait, abnormal		Disorder in the manner of walking. An example is **ataxia** (uh TACK see uh), a lack of muscular coordination, as in cerebral palsy (CP).
hypokinesia hye poh kih NEE sza	*hypo-* deficient *kinesi/o* movement *-ia* condition	Decrease in normal movement; may be due to paralysis.
neuralgia noor AL jah	*neur/o* nerve *-algia* pain	Nerve pain. If described as a "burning pain," it is called **causalgia**.
paresthesia pair uhs THEE zsa	*para-* abnormal *esthesi/o* feeling *-ia* condition	Feeling of prickling, burning, or numbness.
seizure SEE zhur		Neuromuscular reaction to abnormal electrical activity within the brain. Causes include fever or epilepsy, a recurring seizure disorder; also called **convulsions**.
spasm SPAZ um		Involuntary muscle contraction of sudden onset. Examples are hiccoughs, tics, and stuttering.
syncope SINK oh pee		Fainting. A **vasovagal** (VAS soh VAY gul) **attack** is a form of syncope that results from abrupt emotional stress involving the vagus nerve's effect on blood vessels.
tremors TREH murs		Rhythmic, quivering, purposeless skeletal muscle movements seen in some elderly individuals and in patients with various neurodegenerative disorders.
vertigo VUR tih goh		Dizziness; abnormal sensation of movement when there is none—either of oneself moving, or of objects moving around oneself.

Terms Related to Learning and Perceptual Difficulties

Term	Word Origin	Definition
acalculia ay kal KYOO lee ah	*a-* no, not, without *calcul/o* stone *-ia* condition	Inability to perform mathematical calculations.
ageusia ah GOO zsa	*a-* no, not, without *geus/o* taste *-ia* condition	Absence of the ability to taste. **Parageusia** (pair ah GOO zsa) is an abnormal sense of taste or a bad taste in the mouth.
agnosia ag NOH zsa	*a-* no, not, without *gnos/o* knowledge *-ia* condition	Inability to recognize objects visually, auditorily, or with other senses.
agraphia a GRAFF ee ah	*a-* no, not, without *graph/o* record *-ia* condition	Inability to write.
anosmia an NAHS mee ah	*an-* no, not, without *osm/o* sense of smell *-ia* condition	Lack of sense of smell.
apraxia ah PRACK see ah	*a-* no, not, without *prax/o* purposeful movement *-ia* condition	Inability to perform purposeful movements or to use objects appropriately.
dyslexia dis LECK see ah	*dys-* difficult *lex/o* word *-ia* condition	Inability or difficulty with reading and/or writing.

EXERCISE 5: Neurologic Signs, Symptoms, and Perceptual Difficulties

Match the terms with their meanings.

_____ 1. syncope

_____ 2. vertigo

_____ 3. amnesia

_____ 4. spasm

_____ 5. athetosis

_____ 6. aura

_____ 7. fasciculation

_____ 8. hypokinesia

_____ 9. paresthesia

A. dizziness
B. involuntary contraction of small muscles
C. loss of memory
D. fainting
E. premonition
F. slow, writhing movement of extremities
G. sudden, involuntary muscle contraction
H. decrease in normal movement
I. prickling or burning feeling

Build the terms.

10. Condition of without sense of smell _____

11. Condition of without taste _____

12. Condition of without knowledge _____

13. Condition of difficult sleep _____

14. Condition of difficult eating _____

15. Condition of without speech _____

Terms Related to Congenital Disorders

Term	Word Origin	Definition
cerebral palsy (CP) SAIR uh brul PAWL zee	*cerebr/o* cerebrum *-al* pertaining to	Motor function disorder as a result of permanent, nonprogressive brain defect or lesion caused perinatally. Neural deficits may include paralysis, ataxia, athetosis, seizures, and/or impairment of sensory functions.
Huntington chorea koh REE ah		Inherited disorder that manifests itself in adulthood as a progressive loss of neural control, uncontrollable jerking movements, and dementia.
hydrocephalus hye droh SEFF uh lus	*hydr/o* water *-cephalus* head	Condition of abnormal accumulation of fluid in the ventricles of the brain; may or may not result in mental retardation (Fig. 12-9). Although usually diagnosed in babies, may also occur in adults as a result of stroke, trauma, or infection.
spina bifida SPY nah BIFF uh dah	*spin/o* spine *bi-* two *-fida* split	Condition in which the spinal column has an abnormal opening that allows protrusion of the meninges and/or the spinal cord. This is termed a **meningocele** (meh NIN goh seel) (meninges only) or **meningomyelocele** (meh nin goh MYE eh loh seel) (meninges and spinal cord) (Fig. 12-10). **Spina bifida occulta** is a congenital malformation of the bony spinal canal without involvement of the spinal cord (*occulta* means "hidden").
Tay-Sachs disease tay sacks		Inherited disease that occurs mainly in people of Eastern European Jewish origin; caused by an enzyme deficiency, which results in CNS deterioration.

Fig. 12-9 Hydrocephalus.

Fig. 12-10 Meningomyelocele.

Terms Related to Traumatic Conditions

Term	Word Origin	Definition
coma KOH mah		Deep, prolonged unconsciousness from which the patient cannot be aroused; usually the result of a head injury, neurologic disease, acute hydrocephalus, intoxication, or metabolic abnormalities.
concussion kun KUH shun		Serious head injury characterized by one or more of the following: loss of consciousness, amnesia, seizures, or a change in mental status.

Continued

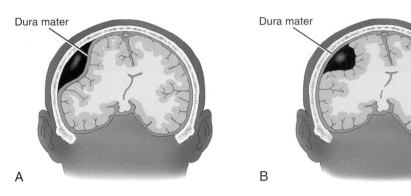

Dura mater   Dura mater

A   B

Fig. 12-11 A, Epidural hematoma. **B,** Subdural hematoma.

Be Careful!

Although the word origin of the term **hematoma** *means a blood tumor, this is a misnomer. A hematoma is a mass of blood that has leaked out of a vessel and pooled.*

Terms Related to Traumatic Conditions—cont'd

Term	Word Origin	Definition
contusion, cerebral kun TOO zhun		Head injury of sufficient force to bruise the brain. Bruising of the brain often involves the brain surface and causes extravasation of blood without rupture of the pia-arachnoid; often associated with a concussion.
hematoma hee muh TOH mah	*hemat/o* blood *-oma* tumor, mass	Localized collection of blood, usually clotted, in an organ, tissue, or space, due to a break in the wall of a blood vessel (Fig. 12-11). A **subdural hematoma** is an accumulation of blood in the subdural space. An **epidural hematoma** is an accumulation of blood in the epidural space.
herniated intervertebral disk (HIVD)	*inter-* between *vertebr/o* vertebra *-al* pertaining to	A displacement of an intervertebral disk so that it presses on a nerve, causing pain and/or numbness.

EXERCISE 6: Congenital and Traumatic Conditions

Fill in the blanks with the correct congenital disorder or trauma term listed below.

Tay-Sachs, cerebral contusion, cerebral palsy, coma, Huntington chorea, concussion, herniated intervertebral disk

1. An inherited disorder resulting in dementia and a progressive loss of neural control beginning in

    adulthood. _____

2. An inherited disease of people of Eastern European descent that results in deterioration of the brain

    and spinal cord as a result of an enzyme deficiency. _____

3. Permanent motor function disorder as a result of brain damage during the perinatal period. _____

    _____

4. Prolonged unconsciousness from which the patient cannot be aroused is termed _____.

5. Head injury accompanied by amnesia, loss of consciousness, seizures, and/or change in mental status

    is called a/an _____.

6.   Bruising of the brain with hemorrhage and swelling is a/an _____.

7.   Displacement of an intervertebral disk is _____.

Build the terms.

8.   mass of blood _____

9.   spine split in two _____

10.   water in the head _____

Case Study   Amelia Jones-Burgh

Twenty-three-year-old Amelia Jones-Burgh was in a car accident yesterday and suffered a serious head injury. She experienced amnesia, cephalgia, cerebral contusion, and a concussion. Her symptoms are worse today, and she has lost consciousness. Emergency imaging reveals that she has a subdural hematoma. She is rushed to surgery.

1. A loss of memory is called _____ _____.

2. What is the medical term for a headache? _____ _____

3. A cerebral contusion is a _____ _____ of the brain.

4. A subdural hematoma is a mass of _____ that can cause neurologic defects.

5. The *sub-* in subdural means _____ the dura mater.
   a. under
   b. over

Terms Related to Degenerative Disorders

Term	Word Origin	Definition
Alzheimer disease (AD) AHLZ hye mur		Progressive, neurodegenerative disease in which patients exhibit an impairment of cognitive functioning. As the brain degenerates and begins to atrophy, ventricles dilate, sulci widen, and gyri narrow. AD is the most common cause of dementia (Fig. 12-12).
amyotrophic lateral sclerosis (ALS) ay mye oh TROH fick LAT ur ul sklih ROH sis	*a-* no *my/o* muscle *troph/o* development *-ic* pertaining to *later/o* side *-al* pertaining to sclerosis condition of hardening	Degenerative, fatal disease of the motor neurons, in which patients exhibit progressive muscle weakness and atrophy; also called **Lou Gehrig disease.**
Guillain-Barré syndrome GEE on bar AY		Autoimmune disorder of acute polyneuritis producing profound **myasthenia** (muscle weakness) that may lead to paralysis.
multiple sclerosis (MS) skleh ROH sis	*sclerosis* condition of hardening	Neurodegenerative disease characterized by destruction of the myelin sheaths on the CNS neurons (demyelination) and their abnormal replacement by the gradual accumulation of hardened plaques. The disease may be progressive or characterized by remissions and relapses. Cause is unknown (Fig. 12-13).

Continued

Fig. 12-12 Alzheimer disease (AD). As the brain degenerates and begins to atrophy, ventricles dilate, sulci widen, and gyri narrow, affecting language and memory functions.

Fig. 12-13 Nerve sheath demyelination seen in multiple sclerosis (MS).

> ⊗ **Be Careful!** | **MS** *stands for musculoskeletal system, mitral stenosis, and multiple sclerosis.*

Terms Related to Degenerative Disorders—cont'd

Term	Word Origin	Definition
Parkinson disease (PD) PAR kin sun		Progressive neurodegenerative disease characterized by tremors, fasciculations, slow shuffling gait, hypokinesia, dysphasia, and dysphagia.
trigeminal neuralgia try JEM ih nuhl noo RAL jun	*neur/o* nerve *-algia* pain	Disorder of the fifth cranial nerve (trigemina) characterized by stabbing pain that radiates along the nerve. Also called **tic douloureux** or **prosopalgia** (Fig. 12-14).

Terms Related to Non-Degenerative Disorders

Term	Word Origin	Definition
Bell palsy PALL zee		Paralysis of the facial nerve. Unknown in cause, the condition usually resolves on its own within 6 months (Fig. 12-15).
epilepsy EP ih lep see	*epi-* above *-lepsy* seizure	Group of disorders characterized by some or all of the following: recurrent seizures, sensory disturbances, abnormal behavior, and/or loss of consciousness. Types of seizures include **tonic clonic (grand mal),** accompanied by temporary loss of consciousness and severe muscle spasms; **absence seizures (petit mal),** accompanied by loss of consciousness exhibited by unresponsiveness for short periods without muscle involvement. **Status epilepticus** (STA tis eh pih LEP tih kuss) is a condition of intense, unrelenting, life-threatening seizures. **Pseudoseizures** are false seizures. Causes may be trauma, tumor, intoxication, chemical imbalance, or vascular disturbances.
narcolepsy NAR koh lep see	*narc/o* sleep *-lepsy* seizure	Disorder characterized by sudden attacks of sleep.
Tourette syndrome tur ETT		Abnormal condition characterized by facial grimaces, tics, involuntary arm and shoulder movements, and involuntary vocalizations, including **coprolalia** (kop pro LAYL yah) (the use of vulgar, obscene, or sacrilegious language).

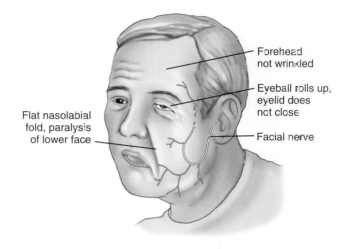

Fig. 12-14 Trigeminal neuralgia; distribution of trigger zones.

Fig. 12-15 The facial characteristics of Bell palsy.

 EXERCISE 7: Degenerative and Non-Degenerative Disorders

Fill in the blank with the correct disorder listed below.

Alzheimer disease, Guillain-Barré syndrome, epilepsy, Bell palsy, amyotrophic lateral sclerosis, multiple sclerosis, Parkinson disease, Tourette syndrome, narcolepsy

1. A paralysis of a facial nerve. _____

2. A disease characterized by tics, facial grimaces, and involuntary vocalizations. _____

3. A progressive disease characterized by a shuffling gait, tremors, and dysphasia. _____

4. A degenerative fatal disorder of motor neurons. _____

5. A progressive, degenerative disorder of impairment of cognitive functioning. _____

6. An autoimmune disorder causing severe muscle weakness, often leading to paralysis.

    _____

7. Group of disorders characterized by seizures. _____

8. Neurogenic disease characterized by demyelination. _____

9. Disorder characterized by sudden attacks of sleep. _____

Terms Related to Infectious Diseases and Inflammations

Term	Word Origin	Definition
encephalitis en seff uh LYE tis	*encephal/o* brain *-itis* inflammation	Inflammation of the brain, most frequently caused by a virus transmitted by the bite of an infected mosquito.
meningitis men in JYE tis	*mening/o* meninges *-itis* inflammation	Any infection or inflammation of the membranes covering the brain and spinal cord, most commonly due to viral infection, although more severe strains are bacterial or fungal in nature.

Continued

Terms Related to Infectious Diseases and Inflammations—cont'd

Term	Word Origin	Definition
neuritis noo RYE tis	*neur/o* nerve *-itis* inflammation	Inflammation of the nerves.
poliomyelitis poh lee oh mye uh LYE tiss	*polio-* gray *myel/o* spinal cord *-itis* inflammation	Inflammation of the gray matter of the spinal cord caused by a poliovirus. Severe forms cause paralysis.
polyneuritis pahl ee noo RYE tis	*poly-* many *neur/o* nerve *-itis* inflammation	Inflammation of several peripheral nerves.
radiculitis rad ick kyoo LYE tis	*radicul/o* nerve root *-itis* inflammation	Inflammation of the root of a spinal nerve.
sciatica sye AT ick kah		Inflammation of the sciatic nerve. Symptoms include pain and tenderness along the path of the nerve through the thigh and leg (Fig. 12-16).
shingles SHIN guls		Acute infection caused by the reactivation of the latent varicella zoster virus (chickenpox), characterized by the development of vesicular skin eruption underlying the route of cranial or spinal nerves; also called **herpes zoster** (HER pees ZAH ster) (Fig. 12-17).

Fig. 12-16 Sciatica.

Fig. 12-17 Shingles on dermatome T4.

Terms Related to Vascular Disorders

Term	Word Origin	Meaning
cerebrovascular accident (CVA) seh ree broh VAS kyoo lır	*cerebr/o* cerebrum *vascul/o* vessel *-ar* pertaining to	Ischemia of cerebral tissue due to an occlusion (blockage) from a thrombus (*pl.* thrombi) or embolus (*pl.* emboli), or as a result of a cerebral hemorrhage. Results of a stroke depend on the duration and location of the ischemia. These sequelae may include paralysis, weakness, speech defects, sensory changes that last longer than 24 hours, or death. Also called **stroke, brain attack,** and **cerebral infarction** (*infarction* means tissue death) (Fig. 12-18).
migraine MYE grain		Headache of vascular origin. May be classified as migraine with aura or migraine without aura.
transient ischemic attack (TIA) TRANS ee ent is KEE mick	*ischem/o* hold back *-ic* condition pertaining to	TIA has the same mechanisms as a CVA, but the sequelae resolve and disappear within 24 hours; also known as a **mini stroke.**

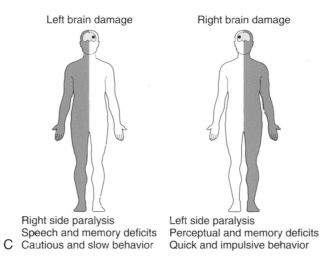

Fig. 12-18 Cerebrovascular accident (CVA). **A,** Events causing stroke. **B,** Magnetic resonance imaging (MRI) scan showing hemorrhagic stroke in the right cerebrum. **C,** Areas of the body affected by CVA.

Case Study   Martin Milagro

Martin Milagro comes to the clinic with rash that runs horizontally along one side of his back and left side. He is in a lot of pain and the rash has started to itch. The physician on duty diagnoses shingles.

1. What virus causes shingles? _____ _____

2. Which nervous system is affected by shingles?
   a. PNS
   b. CNS

3. Which of the patient's illnesses caused the shingles?
   a. measles
   b. mumps
   c. chickenpox
   d. pneumonia

4. What is the synonym for shingles? _____ _____

Paralysis

Paralysis (puh RAL ih sis) is the loss of muscle function, sensation, or both. It may be described according to which side is affected and whether it is the dominant or nondominant side (Fig. 12-19).

Terms Related to Paralytic Conditions

Term	Word Origin	Meaning
diplegia dye PLEE jee ah	*di-* two *-plegia* paralysis	Paralysis of the same body part on both sides of the body.
hemiparesis hem mee pah REE sis	*hemi-* half *-paresis* slight paralysis	Muscular weakness or slight paralysis on the left or right side of the body.
hemiplegia hem mee PLEE jee ah	*hemi-* half *-plegia* paralysis	Paralysis on the left or right side of the body (see Fig. 12-19).
monoparesis mah noh pah REE sis	*mono-* one *-paresis* slight paralysis	Weakness or slight paralysis of one limb on the left or right side of the body.
monoplegia mah noh PLEE jee ah	*mono-* one *-plegia* paralysis	Paralysis of one limb on the left or right side of the body.
paraparesis pair uh pah REE sis	*para-* abnormal *-paresis* slight paralysis	Slight paralysis of the lower limbs and trunk.
paraplegia pair uh PLEE jee ah	*para-* abnormal *-plegia* paralysis	Paralysis of the lower limbs and trunk (see Fig. 12-19).
quadriparesis kwah drih pah REE sis	*quadri-* four *-paresis* slight paralysis	Weakness or slight paralysis of the arms, legs, and trunk.
quadriplegia kwah drih PLEE jee ah	*quadri-* four *-plegia* paralysis	Paralysis of arms, legs, and trunk (see Fig. 12-19).

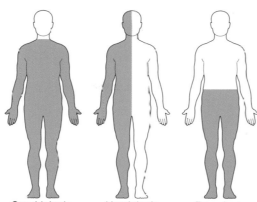

Quadriplegia   Hemiplegia   Paraplegia

Fig. 12-19 Types of paralysis.

EXERCISE 8: Infectious, Inflammatory, Vascular, and Paralytic Disorders

Fill in the correct answers.

1. An acute infection caused by the latent varicella zoster virus is _____.

2. A headache of vascular origin is a/an _____.

3. An inflammation of a nerve in the thigh and leg is called _____.

4. Paralysis on the left or right half of the body is called _____.

5. A mini stroke is a _____.

6. A slight paralysis from the waist down is called _____.

7. CVA stands for _____, the medical term for a stroke.

Match the suffixes and prefixes with their correct meanings.

_____ 8. hemi-	_____ 12. para-	A. one
		B. slight paralysis
_____ 9. -plegia	_____ 13. -paresis	C. half
		D. abnormal
_____ 10. mono-	_____ 14. di-	E. paralysis
		F. four
_____ 11. quadri-		G. two

Decode the terms.

15. radiculitis _____.

16. encephalitis _____.

17. hemiparesis _____.

18. quadriplegia _____.

Build the terms.

19. inflammation of the meninges _____.

20. inflammation of a nerve _____.

21. inflammation of many nerves _____.

Case Study   Cressida Whittier

Sixty-three-year-old Cressida Whittier fell after experiencing a bout of dizziness. Her son brings her to the emergency department (ED), even though Cressida says she feels fine now. Cressida's medical history includes a TIA with aphasia and right-sided paralysis. She also has high blood pressure and epilepsy. The nurse notes Cressida's newest symptoms in the electronic health record (EHR) and tells her that the physician will be in soon to examine her.

1. What is the medical term that means dizziness? ___ _____

2. TIA stands for _____ ischemic attack.

3. What is the term that means paralysis of one side of the body? _____

4. *Aphasia* refers to an inability to form or understand _____.

5. The suffix *-lepsy* in the term *epilepsy* means _____ _____.

Terms Related to Benign Neoplasms

Term	Word Origin	Meaning
meningioma meh nin jee OH mah	*meningi/o* meninges *-oma* tumor, mass	Slow growing, usually benign tumor of the meninges. Although benign, may cause problems because of their size and location (Fig. 12-20).
neurofibroma noor oh fye BROH mah	*neur/o* nerve *fibr/o* fiber *-oma* tumor, mass	Benign fibrous tumors composed of nervous tissue.
neuroma noor OH mah	*neur/o* nerve *-oma* tumor, mass	Benign tumor of the nerves.

Terms Related to Malignant Neoplasms

Term	Word Origin	Definition
astrocytoma as troh sye TOH mah	*astr/o* star *cyt/o* cell *-oma* tumor, mass	Tumor arising from star-shaped glial cells that is malignant in higher grades. A grade IV astrocytoma is referred to as a **glioblastoma multiforme**, which is the most common primary brain cancer (Fig. 12-21).
medulloblastoma med yoo loh blass TOH mah	*medull/o* medulla *blast/o* embryonic *-oma* tumor, mass	Tumor arising from embryonic tissue in the cerebellum. Most commonly seen in children.
neuroblastoma noor oh blass TOH mah	*neur/o* nerve *blast/o* embryonic *-oma* tumor, mass	Highly malignant tumor arising from either the ANS or the adrenal medulla. Usually affects children younger than 10 years of age.

Fig. 12-20 Meningioma.

Fig. 12-21 A glioblastoma appearing as a necrotic, hemorrhagic, infiltrating mass in the center of the brain.

EXERCISE 9: Neoplasms

Match the neoplasms with their definitions.

_____ 1. Benign tumor of the meninges

_____ 2. Benign tumor of the nerves

_____ 3. Malignant tumor of star-shaped glial cells

_____ 4. Malignant tumor of embryonic nervous tissue that arises from the ANS or the adrenal medulla in children

_____ 5. Benign fibrous tumor composed of nerve tissue

_____ 6. Malignant tumor arising from embryonic cerebellar tissue

A. neurofibroma
B. astrocytoma
C. medulloblastoma
D. neuroma
E. meningioma
F. neuroblastoma

Medical Record Celeste Thibeaux

THIBEAUX, CELESTE S - 601106 Opened by BIRDSONG, LINDA MD

Task   Edit   View   Time Scale   Options   Help

As Of 10:54

THIBEAUX, CELESTE S   Age: 19 years   Sex: Female   Loc: WHC-SMMC
DOB: 02/22/1996   MRN: 601106   FIN: 3506004

| Reference Text Browser | Form Browser | Medication Profile |

| Orders | Last 48 Hours | **ED** | Lab | Radiology | Assessments | Surgery | Clinical Notes | Pt. Info | Pt. Schedule | Task List | I & O | MAR |

Flowsheet: ED   Level: ED Report   ⦿ Table   ◯ Group   ◯ List

Navigator
✓   ED Report

Physician's Report: 19-year-old female comes in today brought by ambulance with tonic clonic seizure times four. She has been seizing every 1-2 minutes for 30 seconds. Had upper extremity jerking. Gave her some Valium to start an IV and switched to IV Ativan. Seizures do not appear normal. Jerks to the upper extremities in an oddlike fashion with forward flexion and extension of her arms. Talked to her mom out in the hall and questioned whether the seizures were real. Does have some psychological issues. Psych just took her off antidepressants because of drug interactions. Vital signs are stable. Cranial nerves II through XII intact. TMs clear. Pharynx is clear.

IMPRESSION: Pseudoseizures
Diagnosis: Pseudoseizures

PROD   MAHAFC   28 Feb 2015   10:54

EXERCISE 10: Emergency Room Note

Using the preceding emergency room note, fill in the blanks.

1. This physician is using the term *tonic-clonic seizure*. What is another term for that? _____

2. What is a pseudoseizure? _____

3. What action is described by flexion and extension of her arms? _____

4. How do you know that she has no problems with her throat? _____

5. Which cranial nerves are functioning normally? _____

Age Matters

Pediatrics

Most children's neurologic disorders are congenital ones. CP is usually the result of birth trauma, whereas Tay-Sachs is an inherited condition. Hydrocephalus may be detected on an ultrasound before delivery, and intrauterine prenatal procedures can be done to lessen the effects of the disorder. It should be noted that this disorder may, although infrequently, occur in adults after trauma or disease. Spina bifida is yet another congenital disorder that may be detected before birth through prenatal testing. Two pathologic conditions that are not congenital but that are a concern to parents are viral and bacterial meningitis. Although viral meningitis is less severe and usually resolves without treatment, bacterial meningitis can be fatal. The vaccine that is now available and recommended is the Hib, which stands for the bacteria it protects against, *Haemophilus influenzae*, type b.

Geriatrics

The two major neurologic disorders of concern as we age are cerebrovascular disease and AD. The first disorder manifests itself in two forms: mini strokes (TIAs) and strokes (CVAs). The other disorder is AD, a progressive cognitive mental deterioration. It is estimated that by the age of 65, one in ten individuals will be diagnosed with the disease. By age 85, more than half of the population will carry the diagnosis.

ℯ *Click on* **Hear It, Spell It** *to practice spelling the pathology terms that you have learned in this chapter. To review the pathology terms in this chapter, play* **Medical Millionaire.**

DIAGNOSTIC PROCEDURES

Terms Related to Imaging

Term	Word Origin	Definition
brain scan		Nuclear medicine procedure involving intravenous injection of radioisotopes to localize and identify intracranial masses, lesions, tumors, or infarcts. Photography is done by a scintillator or scanner.
cerebral angiography	*cerebr/o* cerebrum *-al* pertaining to *angi/o* vessel *-graphy* process of recording	X-ray of the cerebral arteries, including the internal carotids, taken after the injection of a contrast medium (Fig 12-22); also called **cerebral arteriography.**
computed tomography (CT) scan	*tom/o* slice *-graphy* process of recording	Transverse sections of the CNS are imaged, sometimes after the injection of a contrast medium (unless there is suspected bleeding). Used to diagnose strokes, edema, tumors, and hemorrhage resulting from trauma.
echoencephalography eh koh en seh fan LAH gruh fee	*echo-* sound *encephal/o* brain *-graphy* process of recording	Sonography exam of the brain, usually done only on newborns because sound waves do not readily penetrate mature bone.
magnetic resonance imaging (MRI)		Medical imaging that uses radiofrequency pulses in a powerful magnetic field. **Magnetic resonance angiography (MRA)** is imaging of the carotid arteries using injected contrast agents. Fig 12-23 shows reconstructed data using MRI, MRA, and sonography.

Continued

Terms Related to Imaging—cont'd

Term	Word Origin	Definition
myelography mye eh LAH gruh fee	*myel/o* spinal cord *-graphy* process of recording	X-ray of the spinal canal after the introduction of a radiopaque substance.
positron emission tomography (PET)		Use of radionuclides to visualize brain function. Measurements can be taken of blood flow, volume, and oxygen and glucose uptake, enabling radiologists to determine the functional characteristics of specific parts of the brain (Fig. 12-24). PET scans are used to assist in the diagnosis of AD and stroke.
single-photon emission computed tomography (SPECT)		An injection of a radioactive sugar substance that is metabolized by the brain, which is then scanned for abnormalities (Fig. 12-25).

Fig. 12-22 Cerebral angiography. **A,** Insertion of dye through a catheter in the common carotid artery outlines the vessels of the brain. **B,** Angiogram showing vessels. *1,* Internal carotid artery; *2,* middle cerebral artery; *3,* middle meningeal artery.

Fig. 12-23 Reconstructed data from three-dimensional (3D) power Doppler, magnetic resonance imaging (MRI), and magnetic resonance angiography (MRA) scans demonstrating proximal and distal bifurcations of the middle cerebral artery *(arrows).*

Fig. 12-24 Positron emission tomography (PET) scan of the brain of a 6-month-old male with seizures, demonstrating focal area.

Fig. 12-25 Single-photon emission computed tomography (SPECT) of a normal brain.

Fig. 12-26 Electroencephalography (EEG).

Terms Related to Electrodiagnostic Procedures

Term	Word Origin	Definition
electroencephalography (EEG) ee leck troh en seff fah LAH gruh fee	*electr/o* electricity *encephal/o* brain *-graphy* process of recording	Recording of the electrical activity of the brain. May be used in the diagnosis of epilepsy, infection, and coma (Fig. 12-26). The resultant record is called an **electrocardiogram**.
evoked potential (EP) ee VOHKT		Electrical response from the brainstem or cerebral cortex that is produced in response to specific stimuli. This results in a distinctive pattern on an EEG.
multiple sleep latency test (MSLT)		Test that consists of a series of short, daytime naps in the sleep lab to measure daytime sleepiness and how fast the patient falls asleep; used to diagnose or rule out narcolepsy.
nerve conduction test		Test of the functioning of peripheral nerves. Conduction time (impulse travel) through a nerve is measured after a stimulus is applied; used to diagnose polyneuropathies.
polysomnography (PSG) pah lee som NAH gruh fee	*poly-* many *somn/o* sleep *-graphy* process of recording	Measurement and record of a number of functions while the patient is asleep (e.g, cardiac, muscular, brain, ocular, and respiratory functions). Most often used to diagnose sleep apnea.

Terms Related to Other Diagnostic Tests

Term	Word Origin	Definition
activities of daily living (ADLs)		An ADL assessment may be used to evaluate a patient's ability to live independently after an illness or event (such as, a CVA).
Babinski reflex bah BIN skee		In normal conditions, the dorsiflexion of the great toe when the plantar surface of the sole is stimulated. **Babinski sign** is the loss or diminution of the Achilles tendon reflex seen in sciatica.
cerebrospinal fluid (CSF) analysis	*cerebr/o* cerebrum *spin/o* spine *-al* pertaining to	Examination of fluid from the CNS to detect pathogens and abnormalities. Useful in diagnosing hemorrhages, tumors, and various diseases.

Continued

Terms Related to Other Diagnostic Tests—cont'd

Term	Word Origin	Definition
deep tendon reflex (DTR)		Assessment of an automatic motor response by striking a tendon. Useful in the diagnosis of stroke.
gait assessment rating scale (GARS)		Inventory of 16 aspects of gait (how one walks) to determine abnormalities. May be used as one method to evaluate cerebellar function.
lumbar puncture (LP)	*lumb/o* lower back *-ar* pertaining to	Procedure to aspirate CSF from the lumbar subarachnoid space. A needle is inserted between two lumbar vertebrae to withdraw the fluid for diagnostic purposes. Also called a **spinal tap** (Fig. 12-27).
neuroendoscopy noor oh en DOSS kuh pee	*neur/o* nerve *endo-* within *-scopy* process of viewing	Use of a fiberoptic camera to visualize neural structures. Used for placing a shunt in hydrocephalic patients.

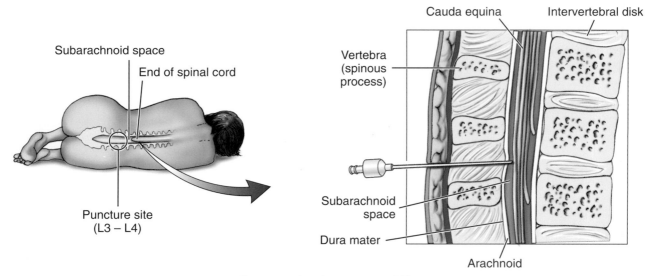

Fig. 12-27 Lumbar puncture (LP).

EXERCISE 11: Diagnostic Procedures

Fill in the blank.

1. Walking abnormalities are measured by a _____.

2. Examination of fluid from the CNS is a/an _____.

3. Aspiration of CSF for diagnostic purposes is a _____.

4. A finding that indicates loss of Achilles tendon reflex is _____.

5. _____ is used to diagnose narcolepsy.

6. An x-ray study of cerebral arteries is called _____.

7. _____ is an injection of a radioactive sugar substance to scan for abnormalities.

8. _____ is the use of radionuclides to visualize brain function.

Decode the terms.

9. electroencephalography _____

10. echoencephalography _____

11. neuroendoscopy _____

Build the terms.

12. process of recording the spinal cord _____

13. process of recording the brain using sound _____

14. process of recording many (functions of) sleep _____

Case Study Naomi Waterman

Naomi Waterman, a 54-year-old editor, has noticed that she seems to be more clumsy than usual. Her left leg feels weak, and her speech "stumbles" at times. Her physician sends her for testing that includes an EEG, a lumbar puncture to examine her CSF, and an MRA. After the results come back, he explains to Naomi that she has MS, a disease characterized by destruction of the myelin sheaths on her CNS neurons.

1. What does MS stand for? _____
   _____

2. What does CSF stand for? _____
   _____

3. What is another name for lumbar puncture?
   _____

4. What does MRA stand for? _____
   _____

5. What is the term that means destruction of the myelin sheaths? _____

Medical Record *Nellie Shumaker*

SHUMAKER, ELEANOR R - 673016 Opened by RAIS, ROBERT MD

Task   Edit   View   Time Scale   Options   Help

As Of 12:58

SHUMAKER, ELEANOR R	Age: 81 years DOB: 08/16/1934	Sex: Female MRN: 673016	Loc: WHC-SMMC FIN: 3506004

Reference Text Browser | Form Browser | Medication Profile

Orders | Last 48 Hours | **ED** | Lab | Radiology | Assessments | Surgery | Clinical Notes | Pt. Info | Pt. Schedule | Task List | I & O | MAR

Flowsheet: Clinical Notes ▼ ...   Level: ED Record ▼   ⦿ Table ○ Group ○ List

Navigator
✓ ED Record

Description: Fall with questionable associated loss of consciousness. Left parietal epidural hematoma.

Chief Complaint: Fall with questionable associated loss of consciousness.

History: This 81 y/o female fell down 20 steps on the evening of admission, 8/27/11. She was evaluated locally and had amnesia about the event at the time of examination. A CT scan was obtained and she was transferred to neurosurgery.

Meds: Lasix 40mg daily, Zantac 150mg daily, Lanoxin 0.125mg daily, Capoten 2.5mg bid, Salsalate 750mg tid, ASA 325mg daily, "Ginsana" (Ginseng) 100mg bid.

Past medical history: 1)Atrial fibrillation, 2) Right hemisphere stroke, 11/22/98, with associated left hemiparesis. This was followed by a right carotid endarterectomy.

EXAM: BP: 157/86; HR: 100 and irregular; RR: 20; Temp: 36.7C; O2 Sat:100%

Mental Status: A&O to person, place, time. Speech fluent and without dysarthria.

CN: Pupils 3/3 decreasing to 2/2 on exposure to light. EOM intact. Optic disks were flat. Face was symmetric with symmetric movement. The remainder of the CN exam was unremarkable.

Motor: 5/5 strength throughout with normal muscle tone and bulk.

Sensory: unremarkable.

Coord: unremarkable.

Reflexes: symmetric. Plantar responses were flexor, bilaterally.

COURSE: 8/27/11, CT was reviewed; it revealed a left parietal epidural hematoma. X-ray revealed a fracture of the right lateral malleolus for which she was casted. Repeat CTs showed no change in the epidural hematoma and she was discharged home on DPH.

PROD | MAHAFC | 27 Aug 2015 | 12:58

⊘ EXERCISE 12: Emergency Room Record

Using the preceding emergency room record, answer the following questions.

1. This patient has a history of what disorder? _____

2. What term tells you that she has had no prickling, burning, or numbness in her legs? _____

3. In the Review of Systems, what term tells you that she had no lack of muscular coordination?

   _____

4. How did her aphasia manifest itself? _____

5. Why would a CT be done emergently if her neurologic symptoms worsen or reemerge?

   _____

THERAPEUTIC INTERVENTIONS

Terms Related to Brain and Skull Interventions

Term	Word Origin	Definitions
craniectomy kray nee ECK tuh mee	*crani/o* skull, cranium *-ectomy* removal	Removal of part of the skull.
craniotomy kray nee AH tuh mee	*crani/o* skull, cranium *-tomy* incision	Incision into the skull as a surgical approach or to relieve intracranial pressure; also called **trephination** (treff fin NAY shun).
stereotaxic radiosurgery stair ee oh TACK sick	*stere/o* three-dimensional (3D) *tax/o* order, arrangement *-ic* pertaining to	Surgery using radio waves to localize structures within 3D space.
ventriculoperitoneal shunt ven trick yoo loh pair ih tuh nee uhl	*ventricul/o* ventricle *peritone/o* peritoneum *-al* pertaining to	A tube used to drain fluid from brain ventricles into the abdominal cavity (Fig. 12-28).
ventriculostomy, endoscopic ven trick yoo LAH stuh mee	*endo-* within *-scopic* pertaining to viewing *ventricul/o* ventricle *-stomy* new opening	A new opening between the third ventricle and the subarachnoid space used to relieve pressure and to treat one type of hydrocephalus.

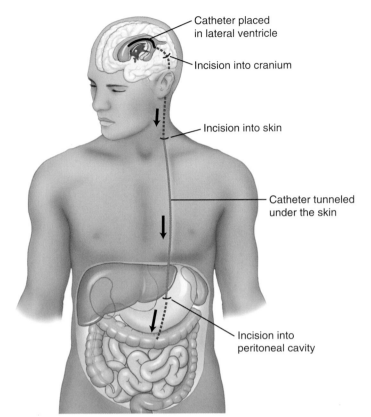

Fig. 12-28 Ventriculoperitoneal shunt.

Catheter placed in lateral ventricle

Incision into cranium

Incision into skin

Catheter tunneled under the skin

Incision into peritoneal cavity

Case Study   *Samantha and Max Bryson*

Samantha and Max Bryson are the twins of one of the staff nurses. Samantha was born with spina bifida occulta, and Max was born with hydrocephalus. Samantha's condition has caused her no trouble, but Max has a ventriculoperitoneal shunt to manage his congenital disorder. The twins are very close, and Samantha has become Max's "protector."

1. Some children with spina bifida have protrusion of the spinal cord and meninges. What is the term for this condition? _____

2. What is the term for the spina bifida condition in which only the meninges are protruding? _____
_____

3. Hydrocephalus is an abnormal accumulation of fluid in the _____ of the brain.

4. A ventriculoperitoneal shunt drains excess fluid into the _____ cavity.

5. The word *occulta* means _____
_____.

Terms Related to General Interventions

Term	Word Origin	Definition
microsurgery	*micro-* small, tiny	Surgery in which magnification is used to repair delicate tissues.
neurectomy noo RECK tuh mee	*neur/o* nerve *-ectomy* removal	Excision of part or all of a nerve.
neurolysis noo RAH lih sis	*neur/o* nerve *-lysis* destruction	Destruction of a nerve.
neuroplasty NOO roh plas tee	*neur/o* nerve *-plasty* surgical repair	Surgical repair of a nerve.
neurorrhaphy noo ROAR ah fee	*neur/o* nerve *-rrhaphy* suture	Suture of a severed nerve.
neurotomy noo RAH tuh mee	*neur/o* nerve *-tomy* incision	Incision of a nerve.
vagotomy vay GAH tuh mee	*vag/o* vagus nerve *-tomy* incision	Cutting of a branch of the vagus nerve to reduce the secretion of gastric acid (Fig. 12-29).

Fig. 12-29 Vagotomy.

Fig. 12-30 Transcutaneous electrical nerve stimulation (TENS) treatment.

Terms Related to Pain Management

Term	Word Origin	Definition
cordotomy kore DAH tuh mee	*cord/o* spinal cord *-tomy* incision	Incision of the spinal cord to relieve pain. Also spelled **chordotomy.**
nerve block		Use of anesthesia to prevent sensory nerve impulses from reaching the CNS.
rhizotomy rye ZAH tuh mee	*rhiz/o* spinal nerve root *-tomy* incision	Resection of the dorsal root of a spinal nerve to relieve pain.
sympathectomy sim puh THECK tuh mee	*sympath/o* to feel with *-ectomy* removal	Surgical interruption of part of the sympathetic pathways for the relief of chronic pain or to promote vasodilation.
transcutaneous electrical nerve stimulation (TENS)	*trans-* through *cutane/o* skin *-ous* pertaining to	Method of pain control affected by the application of electrical impulses to the skin (Fig. 12-30).

⊘ EXERCISE 13: Therapeutic Interventions

Match the terms with their meanings.

_____ 1. neuroplasty

_____ 2. TENS

_____ 3. sympathectomy

_____ 4. rhizotomy

_____ 5. neurotomy

_____ 6. microsurgery

_____ 7. nerve block

_____ 8. endoscopic ventriculostomy

_____ 9. stereotaxic radiosurgery

_____ 10. craniotomy

_____ 11. neurectomy

A. surgical repair of a nerve
B. pain control using electronic impulses
C. incision of a nerve
D. incision of the skull
E. excision of a dorsal nerve root
F. anesthesia to prevent sensory impulses from reaching the CNS
G. new opening in brain to relieve the pressure of CSF fluid in hydrocephalus
H. surgery using radio waves within 3D space
I. excision of a sympathetic pathway
J. surgery in which magnification is used to repair delicate tissues
K. removal of a nerve

Decode the terms.

12. cordotomy _____

13. neurolysis _____

14. ventriculoperitoneal shunt _____

Build the terms.

15. suture of a severed nerve _____

16. incision of the vagus nerve _____

17. removal of part or all of the skull _____

PHARMACOLOGY

analgesics: Reduce pain. Narcotic analgesics have a CNS effect and include NSAIDs, opioids, or cyclooxygenase-2 (COX-2) inhibitors. Examples include morphine (MS Contin), hydrocodone (Vicodin or Lortab, in combination with acetaminophen), sumatriptan (Imitrex), acetaminophen (Tylenol), and naproxen (Anaprox).

anesthetics: Cause a loss of feeling or sensation. They can act either locally (local anesthetic) or systemically (general anesthetic), and a general anesthetic can induce unconsciousness. Examples include propofol (Diprivan) and lidocaine (Xylocaine, Lidoderm).

anticonvulsants: Reduce the frequency and severity of epileptic or other convulsive seizures. Examples include clonazepam (Klonopin), carbamazepine (Tegretol), and phenytoin (Dilantin).

antiparkinsonian drugs: Effective in treating Parkinson disease. Examples include levodopa and carbidopa (Sinemet) and tolcapone (Tasmar).

antipyretics: Reduce fever. Examples include aspirin (Bayer), acetaminophen (Tylenol), and ibuprofen (Advil, Motrin).

hypnotics: Promote sleep. They may also be referred to as *soporifics* or *somnifacients*. Many hypnotics have a sedative effect also. Examples include temazepam (Restoril), zolpidem (Ambien), and flurazepam (Dalmane).

neuromuscular blockers: Drugs that block the action of acetylcholine at the motor nerve end plate to cause paralysis. May be used in surgery to minimize patient movement. Examples include pancuronium (Pavulon), vecuronium (Norcuron), and succinylcholine (Anectine).

sedatives: Inhibit neuronal activity to calm and relax. Many sedatives also have hypnotic effects. Examples include alprazolam (Xanax), lorazepam (Ativan), and phenobarbital (Luminal).

stimulants: Increase synaptic activity of targeted neurons in the CNS to treat narcolepsy, attention-deficit disorder with hyperactivity, and fatigue and to suppress the appetite. Examples include dextroamphetamine (Dexedrine), methylphenidate (Ritalin), caffeine, and phentermine (Adipex-P).

 EXERCISE 14: Pharmacology

Match the drug type with its effect.

_____ 1. treats PD

_____ 2. relieves pain

_____ 3. calms and relaxes

_____ 4. induces sleep

_____ 5. reduces fever

_____ 6. reduces severity of seizures

_____ 7. causes paralysis

_____ 8. causes loss of sensation

A. anesthetic
B. antipyretic
C. soporific
D. anticonvulsant
E. sedative
F. neuromuscular blocker
G. analgesic
H. antiparkinsonian drug

Case Study Brent Holliday

Brent Holliday is a 26-year-old personal trainer who has lately been experiencing shooting pains in his lower back, down his hip, and into his left leg. He said that he first noticed the pain when he was lifting weights, but he doesn't remember injuring himself. His medical history includes a herniated intervertebral disk that resolved 6 years ago. His doctor diagnoses him with sciatica and prescribes an analgesic. He is also advised not to lift weights until the pain resolves.

1. The _____ nerve is affected in sciatica.

2. What is the abbreviation for a herniated intervertebral disk? _____

3. What is the general term that means nerve pain? _____

4. An intervertebral disk is located _____ the vertebrae.
   a. above
   b. under
   c. between

5. If his pain does not resolve, Brent wonders if he could be a candidate for _____, an incision into the dorsal root of a spinal nerve to relieve pain.

*Click on **Hear It, Spell It** to practice spelling the diagnostic and therapeutic terms that you have learned in this chapter.*

Abbreviations

Abbreviation	Definition
AD	Alzheimer disease
ADL	activity of daily living
ALS	amyotrophic lateral sclerosis
ANS	autonomic nervous system
BBB	blood-brain barrier
C1-C8	cervical nerves
CNS	central nervous system
CP	cerebral palsy
CSF	cerebrospinal fluid
CT scan	computerized tomography scan
CVA	cerebrovascular accident
DTR	deep tendon reflex
EEG	electroencephalogram, electroencephalography
EP	evoked potential
GARS	gait assessment rating scale
HIVD	herniated intervertebral disk

Abbreviation	Definition
L1-L5	lumbar nerves
LP	lumbar puncture
MRI	magnetic resonance imaging
MS	multiple sclerosis
MSLT	multiple sleep latency test
PD	Parkinson disease
PET scan	positron emission tomography scan
PNS	peripheral nervous system
PSG	polysomnography
S1-S5	sacral nerves
SNS	somatic nervous system
SPECT	single-photon emission computed tomography
T1-T12	thoracic nerves
TENS	transcutaneous electrical nerve stimulation
TIA	transient ischemia

EXERCISE 15: Abbreviations

Spell out the following abbreviations.

1. Barry had an LP to analyze his CSF for meningitis.

   _____

2. Maria became a quadriplegic when she sustained a C2 fracture while diving into the shallow end of a swimming pool.

   _____

3. Ms. Damjanov had an MRI to aid in the diagnosis of her MS.

   _____

4. The patient underwent PSG to detect abnormalities related to hypersomnia.

   _____

5. Walter needed help with his ADL after a CVA that left him with right hemiparesis.

   _____

Chapter Review

Match the word parts to their definitions.

Word Parts Definitions

Prefix/Suffix

Prefix/Suffix
-esthesia
hemi-
-lepsy
mono-
-oma
para-
-paresis
-plegia
poly-
quadri-

Definition

1. _____ four
2. _____ slight paralysis
3. _____ half
4. _____ many
5. _____ one
6. _____ seizure
7. _____ tumor, mass
8. _____ abnormal
9. _____ feeling
10. _____ paralysis

Combining Form

Combining Form
blast/o
cerebell/o
cerebr/o
cord/o
cortic/o
dendr/o
dur/o
encephal/o
esthesi/o
geus/o
gnos/o
mening/o
myel/o
narc/o
neur/o
osm/o
phag/o
phas/o
radicul/o
rhiz/o
somn/o
ventricul/o

Definition

11. _____ cortex
12. _____ eat
13. _____ taste
14. _____ nerve root
15. _____ cerebellum
16. _____ feeling
17. _____ embryonic
18. _____ spinal cord
19. _____ dura mater
20. _____ speech
21. _____ ventricle
22. _____ brain
23. _____ spinal cord
24. _____ dendrite
25. _____ sleep
26. _____ nerve
27. _____ cerebrum
28. _____ knowledge
29. _____ nerve root
30. _____ sleep
31. _____ sense of smell
32. _____ meninges

Word Shop

Prefixes	Combining Forms	Suffixes
a-	ambul/o	-algia
an-	encepha/o	-graphy
di-	esthesi/o	-ia
dys-	geus/o	-ism
echo-	gnos/o	-itis
hemi-	mening/o	-lysis
hyper-	myel/o	-paresis
in-	neur/o	-plegia
mono-	osm/o	-somnia
par-	radicul/o	-stomy
para-	rhiz/o	-tomy
poly-	somn/o	
quadri-	vag/a	
	ventricul/o	

Build the following terms by combining the preceding word parts. Some word parts may used more than once. Some may not be used at all. The number in parentheses is the number of word parts needed to build the terms.

Definition	Term
1. inflammation of many nerves (3)	_____
2. inflammation of the brain (2)	_____
3. paralysis of four (limbs) (2)	_____
4. process of recording the brain using sound (3)	_____
5. incision of a nerve (2)	_____
6. condition of no recognition (3)	_____
7. condition of without sense of smell (3)	_____
8. nerve pain (2)	_____
9. condition of abnormal sensation (3)	_____
10. process of (many) sleep recording (3)	_____
11. resection of the dorsal root of a spinal nerve (2)	_____
12. destruction of a nerve to relieve pain (2)	_____
13. condition of no ability to taste (3)	_____
14. condition of difficult sleep (3)	_____
15. slight paralysis of four (limbs) (2)	_____

Sort the terms into the correct categories.

Term Sorting

Anatomy and Physiology	Pathology	Diagnostic Procedures	Therapeutic Interventions

ADL	craniectomy	meninges	rhizotomy
agraphia	CSF	MRI	sciatica
ALS	echoencephalography	nerve block	SPECT
amnesia	EP	neuroendoscopy	spina bifida
axon	fasciculation	neurolysis	synapse
Babinski reflex	GARS	neuron	syncope
cauda equina	HIVD	neuroplasty	TENS
cerebellum	hydrocephalus	neurorrhaphy	TIA
CNS	hypnotic	neurotransmitter	vagotomy
cordotomy	LP	PSG	ventricle

Replace the highlighted words with the correct terms.

Translations

1. Mr. Sharif had a right-sided **ischemia of cerebral tissue due to an occlusion or a cerebral hemorrhage** that affected the **pertaining to the opposite side.**

2. After Roberto's CVA, he suffered **slight paralysis on the left or right side of the body** and **condition of lack of the ability to form or understand speech.**

3. As a result of a blow to the head, the patient sustained an epidural **localized collection of blood** and **resultant loss of memory caused by brain damage.**

4. Ms. C reported **dizziness** and **fainting** before her arrival at the emergency department.

5. The baby's **condition in which there is an abnormal opening in the spinal column** resulted in a **saclike protrusion of the meninges.**

6. The neonate's **condition of abnormal accumulation of fluid in the ventricles of the brain** was treated with a **tube used to drain fluid from brain ventricles into the abdominal cavity.**

7. Mrs. Aubrum was experiencing **rhythmic, quivering, purposeless skeletal muscle movements** and **decrease in normal movement** and was ultimately diagnosed with Parkinson disease.

8. The physician suspected that the patient had **a disorder characterized by sudden attacks of sleep** and ordered a **test that measures daytime sleepiness and how fast the patient falls asleep.**

9. A **procedure to aspirate CSF from the lumbar subarachnoid space** was done to rule out **an infection or inflammation of the membranes covering the brain and spinal cord.**

10. Helen O'Neal underwent **measurement and record of a number of functions while patient is asleep** to determine why she was experiencing **excessive depth or length of sleep.**

11. Alice underwent a **resection of the dorsal root of a spinal nerve to relieve pain** to stop the pain resulting from **a disorder of the 5th cranial nerve.**

12. Hector told his doctor that his **headache of vascular origin** was preceded by a/an **sensation of light.**

13. The neurologist asked Bella if she was experiencing **nerve pain** or **a feeling or prickling, burning, or numbness.**

14. Mike's doctor told him that his **inflammation of the sciaticnerve** was caused by **a displacement of an intervertebral disk so that it presses on a nerve.**

Medical Record *Max Janovski*

JANOVSKI, MARTIN W - 693269 Opened by SMYTHE JM, MD

Task   Edit   View   Time Scale   Options   Help

JANOVSKI, MARTIN W

| Age: 65 years | Sex: Male | Loc: WHC-SMMC |
| DOB: 01/12/1950 | MRN: 693269 | FIN: 3506004 |

Reference Text Browser | Form Browser | Medication Profile

Orders | Last 48 Hours | ED | Lab | Radiology | Assessments | Surgery | **Clinical Notes** | Pt. Info | Pt. Schedule | Task List | I & O | MAR

Flowsheet [Clinical Notes]   Level: [Discharge Summary]   ● Table ○ Group ○ List

Navigator

✓ Discharge Summary

Admission Diagnosis: Rule out cerebrovascular accident
Discharge Diagnoses: (1) TIA (2) emphysema; (3) CAD.

History
This patient is a 65-year-old white male with a history of emphysema, coronary artery disease, and benign prostatic hyperplasia. His BPH was treated with a TURP in 2005. He had a triple CABG in 2007. Patient reports smoking two packs per day until 2 years ago. Denies any recent tobacco or alcohol use. He has benefited from oxygen therapy for the past 2 months.

He was admitted for an episode of vertigo and several episodes of syncope that occurred as he was visiting his son's family over the fourth of July holiday. His son brought him to the ED when he reported a loss of feeling on his right side and aphasia. These symptoms resolved before he arrived at the hospital. He has no history of headaches, but has admitted to continued dizziness.

Physical Examination on Admission
Physical examination was largely negative. The patient is quiet, mildly anxious yet cooperative. Pupils are equal and reactive. Neck is negative. There is a normal sinus rhythm with no significant murmurs. Abdomen is negative. There is no peripheral edema. Patient exhibits a minimal amount of ataxia on walking, but there are no other neurologic findings.

The neurologist ordered and reviewed CT scans of head, MRIs, intracranial and extracranial MRAs, and Holter monitor readings. Cerebral hemorrhage was ruled out.

Laboratory findings included mild hypercholesterolemia and a hemoglobin of 12.1. Chest x-ray demonstrated hyperinflation, with vascular markings diminished at the apices. EEG was normal.

Patient appears to be stable at the present time and is discharged to his son's home.

An appointment has been scheduled for follow-up in 2 weeks.

PROD | MAHAFC | 04 July 2015 | 21:01

⟳ DISCHARGE SUMMARY

Using the preceding report, answer the following questions.

1. The patient was admitted for vertigo and syncope. Define each.

   _____

2. What is an MRA? _____

3. On what part of the head were the MRAs performed? _____

4. Ataxia refers to _____.

13

Eye and Ear

OBJECTIVES

- Recognize and use terms related to the anatomy and physiology of the eyes and ears.
- Recognize and use terms related to the pathology of the eyes and ears.
- Recognize and use terms related to the diagnostic procedures for the eyes and ears.
- Recognize and use terms related to the therapeutic interventions for the eyes and ears.

For interactive learning go to the Shiland Evolve website, and click on:
- **Match the Word Parts** to review eye and ear word parts.
- **Word Shop** to practice word building.
- **Tournament of Terminology** to test your knowledge of eye and ear terms.
- **Term Sorting** to practice sorting eye and ear terms into categories.

*Click on **Chapter at a Glance** to print off a list of key terms and word parts for this chapter.*

FUNCTIONS OF THE SPECIAL SENSES

When we want to relate our understanding of how someone is feeling, we say, "I hear you," or even, "I see what you're saying!" Our experience in the world is filtered through our senses and our interpretations of them.

The senses include vision, hearing, taste, smell, and touch. They allow us to experience our environment through specific nervous tissue that transmits, processes, and then acts on our perceptions. This chapter covers the eyes and ears. Disorders of taste and touch are covered in Chapter 12, and olfaction (smell) is discussed in Chapter 11.

SPECIALTIES/SPECIALISTS

Ophthalmology (Ophth) is the diagnosis and treatment of disorders and diseases of the eye. The specialist is an **ophthalmologist.** An **optometrist** is a healthcare professional who measures vision and prescribes corrective solutions as needed. Although glasses and contact lenses used to be the only options to correct vision, corrective surgery is now accepted practice.

Audiology is the diagnosis, treatment, and prevention of hearing disorders. An **audiologist** is the healthcare specialist in this field.

Otorhinolaryngology is the diagnosis and treatment of disorders of the ears, nose, and throat (ENT). The specialist is an **otorhinolaryngologist.**

THE EYE

ANATOMY AND PHYSIOLOGY

The **eye** can be divided into the ocular adnexa—the structures that surround and support the function of the eyeball—and the structures of the globe of the eye itself.

Ocular Adnexa

Each of our paired eyes is encased in a protective, bony socket called the **orbit.** Our **binocular** vision sends two slightly different images to the brain that produce depth of vision. The right eye is called the *oculus dextra,* the left eye is called the *oculus sinistra,* and the term for "each eye" is *oculus uterque.* Within the orbit, the eyeball is protected by a cushion of fatty tissue. The **eyebrows** mark the supraorbital area and provide a modest amount of protection from perspiration and sun glare. Further protection is provided by the upper and lower eyelids and the eyelashes that line their edges (Fig. 13-1).

The corners of the eyes are referred to as the **canthi** (KAN thy) (*sing.* canthus); the inner canthus is termed *medial* (toward the middle of the body), and the outer canthus is *lateral.* The area where the upper and lower eyelids meet is referred to as the **palpebral fissure** (PAL puh brul FISH ur). This term comes from the function of blinking, called **palpebration** (pal puh BRAY shun). The eyelids are lined with a protective, thin mucous membrane called the **conjunctiva** (kun jungk TYE vuh) (*pl.* conjunctivae) that spreads to coat the anterior surface of the eyeball as well.

Also surrounding the eye are two types of glands. Sebaceous glands in the eyelid secrete oil to lubricate the eyelashes, and lacrimal glands above the eyes produce **tears.** The sebaceous glands for the eyelashes are called **meibomian** (mye BOH mee un) **glands.** These glands can be a source of complaint when they become blocked or infected. The other type of gland, the **lacrimal** (LACK

vision = opt/o, optic/o

hearing = audi/o, acous/o

otorhinolaryngology
  ot/o = ear
  rhin/o = nose
  laryng/o = throat
  -logy = study of

eye = ocul/o, ophthalm/o

orbit = orbit/o

binocular
  bin- = two
  ocul/o = eye
  -ar = pertaining to

supraorbital
  supra- = above
  orbit/o = orbit
  -al = pertaining to

eyelid = blephar/o, palpebr/o

canthus = canth/o

conjunctiva = conjunctiv/o

tears = lacrim/o, dacry/o

Fig. 13-1 Ocular adnexa.

Be Careful!

*The term **palpebrate** means to blink or wink. Do not confuse this with the terms **palpate** or **palpitate**.*

lacrimal gland = dacryoaden/o

lacrimal sac = dacryocyst/o

nasolacrimal
nas/o = nose
lacrim/o = tear
-al = pertaining to

extraocular
extra- = outside
ocul/o = eye
-ar = pertaining to

rih mul) **gland,** or tear gland, provides a constant source of cleansing and lubrication for the eye. The process of producing tears is termed **lacrimation** (lack rih MAY shun). The lacrimal glands are located in the upper outer corners of the orbit. The constant blinking of the eyelids spreads the tears across the eyeball. They then drain into two small holes (the lacrimal puncta) in the medial canthus, into the **lacrimal sacs,** and then into the **nasolacrimal ducts,** which carry the tears to the nasal cavity.

The **extraocular** (eck strah OCK yoo lur) **muscles** attach the eyeball to the orbit and, on impulse from the cranial nerves, move the eyes. These six voluntary (skeletal) muscles are made up of four rectus (straight) and two oblique (diagonal) muscles.

 EXERCISE 1: Accessory Eye Structures

Match the term with its correct combining form or prefix. More than one answer may be correct.

_____ 1. membrane that lines eyelids and covers the surface of the eyes

_____ 2. eyelid

_____ 3. tear

_____ 4. vision

_____ 5. two

_____ 6. eye

_____ 7. outside

_____ 8. above

A. lacrim/o
B. conjunctiv/o
C. optic/o, opt/o
D. ophthalm/o
E. palpebr/o
F. ocul/o
G. blephar/o
H. bin-
I. dacry/o
J. supra-
K. extra-

Build the terms.

9. pertaining to two eyes _____

10. pertaining to above the orbit _____

11. pertaining to outside the eye _____

EXERCISE 2: Accessory Eye Structures

Label the drawing using the terms provided.

medial canthus
lateral canthus
nasolacrimal duct
lacrimal puncta
lacrimal gland
lacrimal sac

The Eyeball

The anatomy of the eyeball itself is traditionally described as being three layers or **tunics** (TOO nicks) (Fig. 13-2). The outer layer, or **fibrous tunic,** consists of the **sclera** (SKLAIR uh) and **cornea** (KOR nee uh). The middle layer, or **vascular tunic,** consists of the **uvea** (YOO vee uh), which is made up of the **choroid** (KOR oyd), **ciliary** (SILL ih air ee) **body,** and **iris** (EYE ris). The inner layer, or **nervous tunic,** consists of the **retina** (RET in uh). These three layers are essential to the process of seeing. All parts work together with impressive

sclera = scler/o

cornea = corne/o, kerat/o

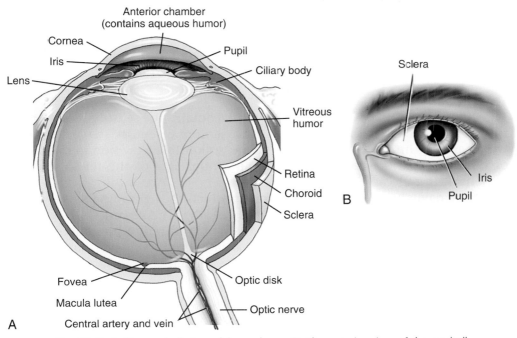

Fig. 13-2 A, The eyeball viewed from above. **B,** The anterior view of the eyeball.

harmony. The eye muscles coordinate their movements with one another; the cornea and pupil control the amount of light that enters the eye; the lens focuses the image on the retina; and the optic nerve transmits the image to the brain.

Two important mechanisms also contribute to the ability to see. As light hits the eye, it passes first through the cornea, which bends the rays of light **(refraction)** so that they are projected properly onto receptor cells in the eye. Then, muscles in the ciliary body adjust the shape of the lens to aid in this refraction. The lens flattens to adjust to something seen at a distance, or thickens for close vision—a process called **accommodation.** Errors of refraction are the most common reason for lens prescriptions.

The Sclera

The outermost lateral and posterior portion of the eye, the white of the eye, is called the **sclera,** which means *hard*. The portion of the sclera that covers the anterior section of the eye is transparent and is called the **cornea.** The border of the cornea, between it and the sclera, is called the **limbus** (LIM bus). The cornea is where refraction (the bending of light) begins.

The Uvea

The **uvea** is the middle, highly vascular layer of the eye. It includes the **iris,** the **ciliary body,** and the **choroid.** The iris (*pl.* irides), pupil, lens (*pl.* lenses), and ciliary body are located directly behind the cornea. The iris is a smooth muscle that contracts and relaxes to moderate the amount of light that enters the eye. In most individuals, this is the colored part of the eye (brown, gray, hazel, or blue) because of its pigmentation. Individuals with albinism, however, have reddish-pink irides (*sing.* iris) because a lack of pigment makes visible the blood cells traveling through the vessels supplying the iris.

The **pupil** is the dark area in the center of the iris where the light continues its progress through to the lens. The **lens** is an avascular structure made of protein and covered by an elastic capsule. It is held in place by the thin strands of muscle that make up the ciliary body. The fluid produced by the capillaries of the ciliary body is called the **aqueous** (AY kwee us) **humor.** It nourishes the cornea, gives shape to the anterior eye, and maintains an optimum intraocular pressure (IOP). It normally drains through tiny veins called the canals of Schlemm. The aqueous humor circulates in both the anterior chamber, between the cornea and the iris, and the posterior chamber, behind the iris and in front of the lens. Between the lens and the retina is a jellylike substance, the **vitreous** (VIT ree us) **humor** (also called the **vitreous body**), which holds the choroid membrane against the retina to ensure an adequate blood supply. The choroid is the vascular membrane between the sclera and the retina.

The Retina

The inner layer of the eye, called the **retina,** contains the sensory receptors for the images carried by the light rays. These sensory receptors are either **rods,** which appear throughout the retina and are responsible for vision in dim light, or **cones,** which are concentrated in the central area of the retina and are responsible for color vision.

During daylight, the area of the retina on which the light rays focus is called the **macula lutea** (MACK yoo lah LOO tee uh). The **fovea** (FOH vee uh) **centralis** is an area within the macula that contains only cones and provides the sharpest image. The area that allows a natural blind spot in our vision is the **optic disk,** where the optic nerve leaves the retina to travel to the brain. There are no light receptors there.

 Be Careful!

Core/o, *meaning pupil of the eye,* and **corne/o,** *meaning cornea, are easy to confuse.*

uvea = uve/o

choroid = choroid/o

ciliary body = cycl/o

iris = ir/o, irid/o

pupil = pupill/o, core/o, cor/o

lens = phak/o, phac/o

vitreous humor = vitre/o

retina = retin/o

macula lutea = macul/o

optic disk = papill/o

EXERCISE 3: The Eyeball

Match the parts of the eye with the correct combining forms. More than one answer may be correct.

_____ 1. ir/o, irid/o   _____ 8. choroid/o

_____ 2. papill/o   _____ 9. cycl/o

_____ 3. retin/o   _____ 10. uve/o

_____ 4. cor/o, core/o   _____ 11. kerat/o

_____ 5. pupill/o   _____ 12. scler/o

_____ 6. macul/o   _____ 13. vitre/o

_____ 7. phac/o, phak/o

A. hard, outer covering of the eye
B. dark center of iris
C. substance between retina and lens
D. middle, highly vascular layer of the eye
E. choroid
F. ciliary body
G. transparent, anterior portion of sclera
H. lens
I. made up of rods and cones
J. pigmented muscle that allows light in eye
K. light focuses on this retinal structure
L. optic disk
M. inner layer of eye

Decode the adjective forms.

14. extraocular _____

15. preretinal _____

16. intrascleral _____

 EXERCISE 4: the Eyeball

Label the drawings using the terms provided.

ciliary body
sclera
optic disk
fovea
pupil
cornea
lens
vitreous humor
retina
optic nerve
macula lutea
iris
anterior chamber
choroid

 You can review the anatomy of the eye by going to the Evolve website at http:// evolve.elsevier.com/Shiland and clicking on **Body Spectrum Electronic Anatomy Coloring Book** → **Senses** → **Eye**. *Choose* **Hear It, Spell It** *to practice spelling the anatomy and physiology terms for the eye.*

Combining and Adjective Forms for the Anatomy and Physiology of the Eye

Meaning	Combining Form	Adjective Form
canthus	canth/o	canthal
choroid	choroid/o	choroidal
ciliary body	cycl/o	cyclic
conjunctiva	conjunctiv/o	conjunctival
cornea	corne/o, kerat/o	corneal, keratic
eye	ocul/o, ophthalm/o	ocular, ophthalmic
eyelid	blephar/o, palpebr/o	palpebral
iris	ir/o, irid/o	iridic
lacrimal gland	dacryoaden/o	dacryoadenal
lacrimal sac	dacryocyst/o	dacryocystic
lens	phak/o, phac/o	
macula lutea	macul/o	macular
optic disk	papill/o	papillary
orbit	orbit/o	orbital
pupil	pupill/o, core/o, cor/o	pupillary
retina	retin/o	retinal
sclera	scler/o	scleral
tears	lacrim/o, dacry/o	lacrimal
uvea	uve/o	uveal
vision	opt/o, optic/o	optic, optical
vitreous humor	vitre/o, vitr/o	vitreous

Prefixes for Anatomy of the Eye

Prefix	Meaning
bin-	two
extra-	outside
supra-	above

 *Click on **Label It** to practice labeling the structures of the eye.*

PATHOLOGY

Terms Related to Eyelid Disorders

Term	Word Origin	Definition
blepharedema bleff ah ruh DEE mah	*blephar/o* eyelid -*edema* swelling	Swelling of the eyelid.
blepharitis bleff ah RYE tis	*blephar/o* eyelid -*itis* inflammation	Inflammation of the eyelid.

Terms Related to Eyelid Disorders—cont'd

Term	Word Origin	Definition
blepharochalasis bleff ah roh KAL luh sis	*blephar/o* eyelid *-chalasis* relaxation, slackening	Hypertrophy of the skin of the eyelid.
blepharoptosis bleff ah rop TOH sis	*blephar/o* eyelid *-ptosis* drooping	Drooping of the upper eyelid.
ectropion eck TROH pee on	*ec-* out *trop/o* turning *-ion* process of	Turning outward (eversion) of the eyelid, exposing the conjunctiva (Fig. 13-3).
entropion en TROH pee on	*en-* in *trop/o* turning *-ion* process of	Turning inward of the eyelid toward the eye (Fig. 13-4).

Fig. 13-3 Ectropion of the lower lid.

Fig. 13-4 Entropion of the lower lid. Note that this patient has undergone corneal transplantation.

Terms Related to Eyelash Disorders

Term	Word Origin	Definition
chalazion kuh LAY zee on		Hardened swelling of a meibomian gland resulting from a blockage. Also called **meibomian cyst** (Fig. 13-5).
hordeolum hor DEE uh lum		Stye; infection of one of the sebaceous glands of an eyelash (Fig. 13-6).

Fig. 13-5 Chalazion.

Fig. 13-6 Acute hordeolum of upper eyelid.

Terms Related to Tear Gland Disorders

Term	Word Origin	Definition
dacryoadenitis dack ree oh add eh NYE tis	*dacryoaden/o* lacrimal gland *-itis* inflammation	Inflammation of a lacrimal gland.
dacryocystitis dack ree oh sis TYE tis	*dacryocyst/o* lacrimal sac *-itis* inflammation	Inflammation of a lacrimal sac (Fig. 13-7).
epiphora eh PIFF or ah		Overflow of tears; excessive lacrimation.
xerophthalmia zeer off THAL mee ah	*xer/o* dry *ophthalm/o* eye *-ia* condition	Dry eye; lack of adequate tear production to lubricate the eye. Usually the result of vitamin A deficiency.

Terms Related to Conjunctiva Disorders

Term	Word Origin	Definition
conjunctivitis kun junk tih VYE tis	*conjunctiv/o* conjunctiva *-itis* inflammation	Inflammation of the conjunctiva, commonly known as **pinkeye,** a highly contagious disorder (Fig. 13-8).
ophthalmia neonatorum off THAL mee uh nee oh nay TORE um	*ophthalm/o* eye *-ia* condition *neo-* new *nat/o* born *-um* structure	Severe, purulent conjunctivitis in the newborn, usually due to gonorrheal or chlamydial infection. Routine introduction of an antibiotic ophthalmic ointment (erythromycin) prevents most cases.

⊗ Be Careful!

Do not confuse these similar terms: **esotropia,** **exotropia,** **entropion,** *and* **ectropion.**

Fig. 13-7 Dacryocystitis.

Fig. 13-8 Acute purulent conjunctivitis.

Terms Related to Eye Muscle and Orbital Disorders

Term	Word Origin	Definition
amblyopia am blee OH pee ah	*ambly/o* dull, dim *-opia* vision condition	Dull or dim vision due to disuse.
diplopia dih PLOH pee ah	*dipl/o* double *-opia* vision condition	Double vision. **Emmetropia** (EM, Em) means normal vision.
esotropia eh soh TROH pee ah	*eso-* inward *trop/o* turning *-ia* condition	Turning inward of one or both eyes (Fig. 13-9).
exophthalmia eck soff THAL mee ah	*ex-* out *ophthalm/o* eye *-ia* condition	Protrusion of the eyeball from its orbit; may be congenital or the result of an endocrine disorder.
exotropia eck so TROH pee ah	*exo-* outward *trop/o* turning *-ia* condition	Turning outward of one or both eyes (Fig. 13-10).
photophobia foh toh FOH bee ah	*phot/o* light *-phobia* condition of fear	Extreme sensitivity to light. The suffix *-phobia* here means "aversion," not fear.
strabismus strah BISS mus		General term for a lack of coordination between the eyes, usually due to a muscle weakness or paralysis. Sometimes called a "squint," which refers to the patient's effort to correct the disorder.

Fig. 13-9 Esotropia.

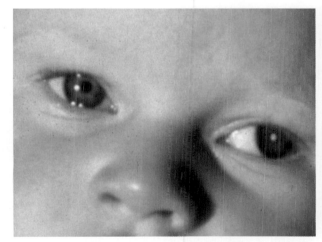

Fig. 13-10 Exotropia in left eye.

EXERCISE 5: Disorders of the Ocular Adnexa

Match the disorders with their definitions.

_____ 1. epiphora   _____ 7. chalazion

_____ 2. strabismus   _____ 8. exotropia

_____ 3. hordeolum   _____ 9. conjunctivitis

_____ 4. ectropion   _____ 10. exophthalmia

_____ 5. diplopia   _____ 11. blepharedema

_____ 6. amblyopia   _____ 12. ophthalmia
                                    neonatorum

A. severe conjunctivitis in the newborn
B. eversion of the eyelid
C. swelling of the eyelid
D. excessive lacrimation
E. dull or dim vision
F. stye
G. meibomian cyst
H. outward protrusion of the eyeball
I. squint
J. outward turning of the eye
K. pinkeye
L. double vision

Decode the terms.

13. xerophthalmia _____

14. esotropia _____

15. blepharochalasis _____

16. dacryocystitis _____

Build the terms.

17. inflammation of the eyelids _____

18. inflammation of a tear gland _____

19. drooping of an eyelid _____

20. process of inward turning (of the eyelid) _____

Case Study   Michael Schwartz

Michael Schwartz is a 79-year-old retired jeweler who has noticed a definite drooping and slackening of the skin of his eyelids. He tells his optometrist that he thinks his vision has been affected. After a thorough eye exam, he is referred to a plastic surgeon to treat his blepharochalasis and blepharoptosis.

1. The combining form *blephar/o* means _____.
   a. eyelash   b. pupil
   c. eyelid   d. eyebrow

2. Blepharoptosis means a _____ of the eyelids.
   a. hardening   b. swelling
   c. slackening   d. drooping, sagging

3. Blepharochalasis means a _____ of the eyelids.
   a. hardening   b. softening
   c. slackening, relaxation   d. drooping, sagging

4. If Michael had had blepharedema, he would have had _____ of the eyelids.
   a. swelling   b. softening
   c. slackening   d. drooping, sagging

Terms Related to Refraction and Accommodation Disorders

Term	Word Origin	Definition
astigmatism (Astig, As, Ast) ah STIG mah tiz um		Malcurvature of the cornea leading to blurred vision. If uncorrected, asthenopia (a condition in which the eyes tire easily) may result (Fig. 13-11, *A*).
hyperopia hye pur OH pee ah	*hyper-* excessive *-opia* vision condition	Farsightedness; refractive error that does not allow the eye to focus on nearby objects (see Fig. 13-11, *B*).
myopia (MY) mye OH pee ah	*my/o* to shut *-opia* vision condition	Nearsightedness; refractive error that does not allow the eye to focus on distant objects (see Fig. 13-11, *C*).
presbyopia press bee OH pee ah	*presby-* old age *-opia* vision condition	Progressive loss of elasticity of the lens (usually accompanies aging), resulting in hyperopia.

Fig. 13-11 Refraction errors. **A,** Myopia (MY; nearsightedness). **B,** Hyperopia (farsightedness). **C,** Astigmatism.

Terms Related to Sclera Disorders

Term	Word Origin	Definition
corneal ulcer KORE nee uhl UHL sur	*corne/o* cornea *-al* pertaining to	Trauma to the outer covering of the eye, resulting in an abrasion.
keratitis kair uh TYE tis	*kerat/o* cornea *-itis* inflammation	Inflammation of the cornea.

Terms Related to Uvea Disorders

Term	Word Origin	Definition
anisocoria an nye soh KORE ee ah	*an-* no, not, without *is/o* equal *cor/o* pupil *-ia* condition	Condition of unequally sized pupils, sometimes due to pressure on the optic nerve as a result of trauma or lesion (Fig. 13-12).
hyphema hye FEE mah	*hypo-* under *hem/o* blood *-a* noun ending	Blood in the anterior chamber of the eye as a result of hemorrhage due to trauma.
uveitis yoo vee EYE tis	*uve/o* uvea *-itis* inflammation	Inflammation of the uvea (iris, ciliary body, and choroids).

Fig. 13-12 Anisocoria.

Terms Related to Lens Disorders

Term	Word Origin	Definition
aphakia ah FAY kee ah	*a-* no, not, without *phak/o* lens *-ia* condition	Condition of no lens, either congenital or acquired.
cataract KAT ur ackt		Progressive loss of transparency of the lens of the eye (Fig. 13-13).
glaucoma glah KOH mah	*glauc/o* gray, bluish green *-oma* mass	Group of disorders characterized by abnormal intraocular pressure (IOP) due to obstruction of the outflow of the aqueous humor. **Chronic** or **primary open-angle glaucoma** (Fig. 13-14) is characterized by an open anterior chamber angle. **Angle-closure** or **narrow-angle glaucoma** is characterized by an abnormally narrowed anterior chamber angle.

Fig. 13-13 The cloudy appearance of a lens affected by a cataract.

Fig. 13-14 Open-angle glaucoma.

Terms Related to Retina Disorders

Term	Word Origin	Definition
achromatopsia ah kroh mah TOP see ah	*a-* no, not, without *chromat/o* color *-opsia* vision condition	Impairment of color vision. Inability to distinguish between certain colors because of abnormalities of the photopigments produced in the retina. Also called **color blindness.**
age-related macular degeneration (ARMD or AMD) MACK kyoo luhr dee jen ur RAY shun		Progressive destruction of the macula lutea, resulting in a loss of central vision. This is the most common visual disorder after the age of 75 (Fig. 13-15).

Terms Related to Retina Disorders—cont'd

Term	Word Origin	Definition
diabetic retinopathy dye ah BET ick ret in OP ah thee	*retin/o* retina *-pathy* disease	Damage of the retina due to diabetes; the leading cause of blindness (Fig. 13-16). Classified according to stages from mild, nonproliferative diabetic retinopathy (NPDR) to proliferative diabetic retinopathy (PDR).
hemianopsia hem ee an NOP see ah	*hemi-* half *an-* no, not, without *-opsia* vision condition	Loss of half the visual field (VF), often as the result of a cerebrovascular accident.
nyctalopia nick tuh LOH pee ah	*nyctal/o* night *-opia* vision condition	Inability to see well in dim light. May be due to a vitamin A deficiency, retinitis pigmentosa, or chorodoretinitis.
retinal tear, retinal detachment		Separation of the retina from the choroid layer. May be due to trauma, inflammation of the interior of the eye, or aging. A hole in the retina allows fluid from the vitreous humor to leak between the two layers.
retinitis pigmentosa ret in EYE tis pig men TOH sah	*retin/o* retina *-itis* inflammation	Hereditary, degenerative disease marked by nyctalopia and a progressive loss of the VF.
scotoma skoh TOH mah	*scot/o* darkness *-oma* mass, tumor	Area of decreased vision in the VF. Commonly called a **blind spot.**

Fig. 13-15 Macular degeneration.

Fig. 13-16 Diabetic retinopathy.

⊗ **Be Careful!**

Nyctalopia *means night blindness, not night vision.*

Terms Related to Optic Nerve Disorders

Term	Word Origin	Definition
nystagmus nye STAG mus		Involuntary, back-and-forth eye movements due to a disorder of the labyrinth of the ear and/or parts of the nervous system associated with rhythmic eye movements.
optic neuritis OP tick nyoo RYE tis	*opt/o* vision *-ic* pertaining to *neur/o* nerve *-itis* inflammation	Inflammation of the optic nerve resulting in blindness; often mentioned as a predecessor to the development of multiple sclerosis.

EXERCISE 6: Disorders of the Eyeball

Match the terms with their definitions.

_____ 1. cataract   _____ 8. corneal ulcer   A. abrasion of the outer eye
                                                                B. nearsightedness
_____ 2. ARMD   _____ 9. astigmatism   C. involuntary back-and-forth movements
                                                                   of the eye
_____ 3. glaucoma   _____ 10. hyphema   D. hemorrhage within the eye
                                                                E. mal curvature of the cornea
_____ 4. anisocoria   _____ 11. scotoma   F. increased IOP
                                                                G. unequally sized pupils
_____ 5. aphakia   _____ 12. nystagmus   H. blind spot
                                                                I. loss of central vision
_____ 6. myopia (MY)   _____ 13. retinal detachment   J. loss of transparency of the lens
                                                                K. lack of a lens
_____ 7. hyperopia   L. farsightedness
                                                                M. separation of retina from choroid layer

Decode the terms.

14. nyctalopia _____

15. achromatopsia _____

16. aphakia _____

17. hemianopsia _____

18. optic neuritis _____

Build the terms.

19. inflammation of the cornea _____

20. (lack of) vision due to old age _____

21. inflammation of the uvea _____

22. disease of the retina _____

Term Related to Benign Neoplasms

Term	Word Origin	Definition
choroidal hemangioma koh ROY dul hee man jee OH mah	*choroid/o* choroid *-al* pertaining to *hemangi/o* blood vessel *-oma* tumor, mass	Tumor of the blood vessel layer under the retina (the choroid layer). May cause visual loss or retinal detachment.

Terms Related to Malignant Neoplasms

Term	Word Origin	Definition
intraocular melanoma in trah AHK yoo lur mell uh NOH mah	*intra-* within *ocul/o* eye *-ar* pertaining to *melan/o* dark, black *-oma* tumor, mass	Malignant tumor of the choroid, ciliary body, or iris that usually occurs in individuals in their 50s or 60s (Fig. 13-17).
retinoblastoma reh tih noh blas TOH mah	*retin/o* retina *blast/o* embryonic, immature *-oma* tumor, mass	An inherited condition present at birth that arises from embryonic retinal cells (Fig. 13-18).

Fig. 13-17 Intraocular melanoma.

Fig. 13-18 Retinoblastoma. White pupil is a classic sign.

EXERCISE 7: Neoplasms

Fill in the blank.

1. What is an inherited malignant condition of the eye? _____

2. What is a malignant tumor of the choroids, iris, or ciliary body? _____

3. What is a benign tumor of the vascular layer of the eye? _____

Age Matters

Pediatrics

The most prevalent disorder of the eyes is conjunctivitis, which accounts for a large number of pediatric visits. Because it is highly contagious, entire classrooms may be infected as a result of one student's infection. Routine introduction of erythromycin has severely limited the number of cases of ophthalmia neonatorum, conjunctivitis of the newborn that is usually due to gonorrhea or chlamydial infection.

Geriatrics

Age-related macular degeneration and cataracts are the most common causes of blindness in the elderly, although there are several successful procedures to treat cataracts. Currently there are no treatments to cure ARMD. Diabetic retinopathy is the most common cause of blindness, but it may also occur much earlier in life. Presbyopia is a visual disorder that usually accompanies aging, resulting in farsightedness.

DIAGNOSTIC PROCEDURES

Terms Related to Diagnostic Procedures

Term	Word Origin	Definition
Amsler grid AMZ lur		Test to assess central vision and to assist in the diagnosis of age-related macular degeneration (Fig. 13-19).
diopters DYE op turs		Level of measurement that quantifies **refraction errors,** including the amount of nearsightedness (negative numbers), farsightedness (positive numbers), and astigmatism.
fluorescein angiography FLOO reh seen an jee AH gruh fee	*angi/o* vessel *-graphy* process of recording	Procedure to confirm suspected retinal disease by injection of a fluorescein dye into the eye and use of a camera to record the vessels of the retina.
fluorescein staining FLOO reh seen		Use of a dye dropped into the eyes that allows differential staining of abnormalities of the cornea.
gonioscopy gch nee AH skuh pee	*goni/o* angle *-scopy* process of viewing	Visualization of the angle of the anterior chamber of the eye; used to diagnose glaucoma and to inspect ocular movement.
ophthalmic sonography off THALL mick	*ophthalm/o* eye *-ic* pertaining to *son/o* sound *-graphy* process of recording	Use of high-frequency sound waves to image the interior of the eye when opacities prevent other imaging techniques. May be used for diagnosing retinal detachments, inflammatory conditions, vascular malformations, and suspicious masses.
ophthalmoscopy off thal MAH skuh pee	*ophthalm/o* eye *-scopy* process of viewing	Any visual examination of the interior of the eye with an ophthalmoscope.
Schirmer tear test SHURR mur		Test to determine the amount of tear production; useful in diagnosing dry eye (xerophthalmia).

Terms Related to Diagnostic Procedures—cont'd

Term	Word Origin	Definition
slit lamp examination		Part of a routine eye examination; used to examine the various layers of the eye. Medications may be used to dilate the pupils (mydriatics), numb the eye (anesthetics), or dye the eye (fluorescein staining).
tonometry toh NAH meh tree	*ton/o* tone, tension *-metry* process of measuring	Measurement of IOP; used in the diagnosis of glaucoma. In **Goldmann applanation** tonometry, the eye is numbed and measurements are taken directly on the eye. In **air-puff tonometry,** a puff of air is blown onto the cornea.
visual acuity (VA) assessment ah KYOO ih tee		Test of the clearness or sharpness of vision; also called the **Snellen test.** Normal vision is described as being 20/20. The top figure is the number of feet the examinee is standing from the **Snellen chart** (Fig. 13-20); the bottom figure is the number of feet a normal person would be from the chart and still be able to read the smallest letters. Thus if the result is 20/40, the highest line that the individual can read is what a person with normal vision can read at 40 feet.
visual field (VF) test		Test to determine the area of physical space visible to an individual. A normal VF is 65 degrees upward, 75 degrees downward, 60 degrees inward, and 90 degrees outward.

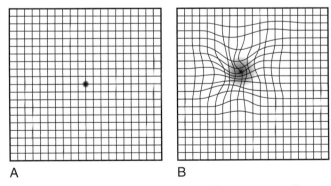

Fig. 13-19 Amsler grid. **A,** How it would appear normally. **B,** How it might appear to someone with age-related macular degeneration (ARMD).

Fig. 13-20 Snellen chart.

EXERCISE 8: Diagnostic Procedures

Matching.

_____ 1. measure of the area of physical space visible to an individual

_____ 2. exam of IOP

_____ 3. visual exam of interior of eye

_____ 4. test of sharpness of vision

_____ 5. visualization of angle of anterior chamber

_____ 6. test to measure central vision

_____ 7. test to determine amount of tear production

_____ 8. exam of abnormalities of cornea

_____ 9. part of routine eye exam of layers of the eye

_____ 10. use of injected dye to record suspected retinal disease

_____ 11. measurement units used to determine refraction errors

A. slit lamp exam
B. VA test
C. Schirmer test
D. fluorescein staining
E. VF test
F. ophthalmoscopy
G. Amsler grid
H. tonometry
I. gonioscopy
J. fluorescein angiography
K. diopters

Case Study Johanna Reynolds

Johanna Reynolds, a 62-year-old store manager, was having problems reading the reports of sales figures, and it seemed like she couldn't get enough light on her morning newspaper to read it without straining her eyes. She makes an appointment with an ophthalmologist near her and goes in on a Saturday morning. Dr. Pennswood performs a routine ophthalmic examine, then asks her to look at an Amsler grid. After the exam, he tells Johanna that she is in the early stages of ARMD. Dr. Pennswood explains that the deterioration of the macula lutea, located in the back of the eye, causes a loss of central vision. He says that drugs called *ophthalmic angiogenesis inhibitors* could be used to treat it, but there is currently no cure for the disease.

1. What does ARMD stand for? _____
_____
_____

2. The Amsler grid tests the health of one's _____ vision.
   a. central
   b. peripheral

3. The macula lutea is located in which coat of the eye?
   a. fibrous
   b. vascular
   c. nervous

4. Angiogenesis is the production of _____. (Use your knowledge of previously learned word parts.)
   a. blood vessels
   b. muscles
   c. glands
   d. blood

THERAPEUTIC INTERVENTIONS

Terms Related to Interventions of the Eyeball and Adnexa

Term	Word Origin	Definition
blepharoplasty BLEFF or uh plas tee	*blephar/o* eyelid *-plasty* surgical repair	Surgical repair of the eyelids. May be done to correct blepharoptosis or blepharochalasis (Fig. 13-21).
blepharorrhaphy BLEFF ar oh rah fee	*blephar/o* eyelid *-rrhaphy* suturing	Suture of the eyelids.
dacryocystorhinostomy dak ree oh sis toh rye NOSS tuh mee	*dacryocyst/o* lacrimal sac *rhin/o* nose *-stomy* new opening	Creation of an opening between the tear sac and the nose.
enucleation of the eye eh noo klee AY shun	*e-* out *nucle/o* nucleus *-ation* process of	Removal of the entire eyeball.
evisceration of the eye eh vis uh RAY shun	*e-* out *viscer/o* organ *-ation* process of	Removal of the contents of the eyeball, leaving the outer coat (the sclera) intact.
exenteration of the eye eck sen tur RAY shun		Removal of the entire contents of the orbit.

Fig. 13-21 Upper-lid blepharoplasty. **A,** Incision marked where skin will be removed. **B,** Prolapsed fat is snipped.

Terms Related to Scleral and Corneal Procedures

Term	Word Origin	Definition
anterior ciliary sclerotomy (ACS) sklair AH tuh mee	*scler/o* sclera *-tomy* incision	Incision in the sclera to treat presbyopia.
corneal incision procedure		Any keratotomy procedure in which the cornea is cut to change shape, thereby correcting a refractive error.
astigmatic keratotomy (AK) as tig MAT ick kair uh TAH tuh mee	*kerat/o* cornea *-tomy* incision	Corneal incision process that treats astigmatism by affecting a more rounded cornea.
photorefractive keratectomy (PRK) foh toh ree FRACK tiv kair uh TECK tuh mee	*kerat/o* cornea *-ectomy* removal	Treatment for astigmatism, hyperopia, and MY that uses an excimer laser to reshape the cornea.
corneal transplant		Transplantation of corneal tissue from a donor or the patient's own (autograft) cornea. May be either full- or partial-thickness grafts; also called **keratoplasty** (KAIR uh toh plas tee).
flap procedure		Any procedure in which a segment of the cornea is cut as a means of access to the structures below (LASIK).
laser-assisted in-situ keratomileusis (LASIK) kair uh toh mih LOO sis	*kerat/o* cornea	Flap procedure in which an excimer laser is used to remove material under the corneal flap. Corrects astigmatism, MY, and hyperopia (Fig. 13-22).

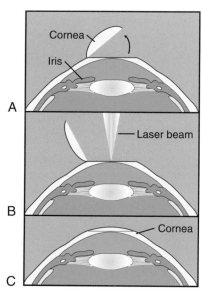

Fig. 13-22 Laser-assisted in-situ keratomileusis (LASIK) surgery. **A,** A microkeratome is used to create a hinged cap of tissue, which is lifted off the cornea. **B,** An excimer laser is used to vaporize and reshape underlying tissue. **C,** Tissue cap is replaced.

Terms Related to Lens Interventions

Term	Word Origin	Definition
cataract extraction	*ex-* out *tract/o* pull *-ion* process of	Removal of the lens to treat cataracts. May be **intracapsular cataract extraction (ICCE)**, in which the entire lens and capsule are removed, or **extracapsular cataract extraction (ECCE)**, in which the lens capsule is left in place (Fig. 13-23).
intraocular lenses (IOLs)	*intra-* within *ocul/o* eye *-ar* pertaining to	Use of an artificial lens implanted behind the iris and in front of the natural abnormal lens to treat MY and hyperopia. Also called **implantable contact lenses (ICLs)**.
phacoemulsification and aspiration of cataract fay koh ee mull sih fih KAY shun	*phac/o* lens	Vision correction accomplished through the destruction and removal of the contents of the capsule by breaking it into small pieces and removing them by suction.

EXTRACAPSULAR
CATARACT EXTRACTION

INTRACAPSULAR
CATARACT EXTRACTION

Posterior lens
capsule remains

Lens and anterior
capsule removed

Lens and entire
capsule removed

Fig. 13-23 Lens removal.

Terms Related to Iris Interventions

Term	Word Origin	Definition
coreoplasty KORE ee oh plas tee	*core/o* pupil *-plasty* surgical repair	Surgical repair to form an artificial pupil.
goniotomy goh nee AH tuh mee	*goni/o* angle *-tomy* incision	Incision of the Schlemm canal to correct glaucoma by providing an exit for the aqueous humor.
trabeculotomy tuh beck kyoo LAH tuh mee	*trabecul/o* little beam *-tomy* incision	Incision of the orbital network of the eye to promote intraocular circulation and decrease IOP.

Terms Related to Retina Interventions

Term	Word Origin	Definition
retinal photocoagulation RET in ul foh toh koh agg yoo LAY shun	*retin/o* retina *-al* pertaining to *phot/o* light *-coagulation* to clot	Destruction of retinal lesions using light rays to solidify tissue.
scleral buckling SKLAIR ul BUCK ling	*scler/o* sclera *-al* pertaining to	Reattachment of the retina with a cryoprobe and the use of a silicone sponge to push the sclera in toward the retinal scar; includes the removal of fluid from the subretinal space (Fig. 13-24).
vitrectomy vih TRECK tuh mee	*vitr/o* vitreous humor, glassy *-ectomy* removal	Removal of part or all of the vitreous humor.

Fig. 13-24 Scleral buckling procedure.

⊘ EXERCISE 9: Therapeutic Interventions

Match the interventions with their definitions.

_____ 1. suture of the eyelids

_____ 2. removal of vitreous humor

_____ 3. surgical repair of a pupil defect

_____ 4. destruction of retinal lesions with light

_____ 5. incision of the Schlemm canal to correct glaucoma

_____ 6. removal of contents of eyeball, except for outer coat

_____ 7. any keratotomy procedure to correct a refractive error

_____ 8. procedure to cut cornea to access deeper structures

_____ 9. implantable contact lenses (ICLs)

_____ 10. corneal transplant

_____ 11. removal of entire orbital contents

_____ 12. reattachment of retina

_____ 13. removal of entire eyeball

A. retinal photocoagulation
B. scleral buckling
C. enucleation of eye
D. intraocular lenses (IOLs)
E. exenteration of the eye
F. flap procedure
G. vitrectomy
H. blepharorrhaphy
I. corneal incision procedure
J. goniotomy
K. evisceration of eye
L. coreoplasty
M. keratoplasty

Decode the terms.

14. trabeculotomy _____

15. dacryocystorhinostomy _____

16. vitrectomy _____

PHARMACOLOGY

antibiotics: Medications used to treat bacterial infections. Examples include gentamicin (Garamycin) and ciprofloxacin (Ciloxan).

antiglaucoma drugs: Decrease the IOP by decreasing the amount of fluid in the eye or increasing the drainage. Examples include carbonic anhydrase (dorzolamide), cholinergics (pilocarpine), prostaglandin agonists (latanoprost), beta blockers (levobunolol) and alpha-2 agonists (brimonidine).

antihistamines: Drugs used to treat allergic conditions, such as itchy or watery eyes. Diphenhydramine (Benadryl) is a common oral over-the-counter (OTC) product used to treat allergies. Ketotifen (Zaditor) is an example of OTC eye drops.

cycloplegics: Induce paralysis of the ciliary body to allow examination of the eye. One example is atropine eye drops.

lubricants: Keep the eyes moist, mimicking natural tears.

miotics: Cause the pupils to constrict; often used to treat glaucoma.

mydriatics: Cause the pupils to dilate; used in diagnostic and refractive examination of the eye. An example is cyclopentolate (Cyclogyl).

ophthalmic angiogenesis inhibitors: Drugs that bind to vascular endothelial growth factor to prevent blood vessel growth in the eye. Administered via ophthalmic intravitreal injection. Used to treat age-related macular degeneration. Ranibizumab (Lucentis), aflibercept (Eylea), pegaptanib (Macugen), and bevacizumab (Avastin) are examples.

ophthalmics: Drugs applied directly to the eye. These may be in the form of solutions or ointments.

topical anesthetics: Temporarily anesthetize the eye for the purpose of examination.

EXERCISE 10: Pharmacology

Matching.

_____ 1. used to treat allergic conditions

_____ 2. used to constrict pupils

_____ 3. used to allow examination of eye by paralyzing ciliary body

_____ 4. used to dilate pupils

_____ 5. used to keep eyes moist

A. mydriatics
B. cycloplegics
C. antihistamines
D. lubricants
E. miotics

Case Study   Lizzie Kawa

Lizzie Kawa is a 28-year-old nurse with astigmatism and hyperopia. She is at her ophthalmologist's office to discuss the possibility of LASIK surgery to replace her contact lenses. She says that she started wearing glasses when she was 13, switched to contact lenses when she was 16, and has wanted LASIK ever since she heard that it was an option. Her optometrist tests her eyes and finds that her vision has been relatively stable for the last 2 years. He explains that patients with autoimmune disorders or chronic dry eye are probably not good candidates for LASIK. Lizzie says that she does not have either of those conditions and wants to go ahead with the procedure.

1. Malcurvature of the cornea that leads to blurred vision is called _____.
   a. hyperopia
   b. myopia
   c. astigmatism
   d. presbyopia

2. What is the common name for hyperopia?
   a. farsightedness
   b. nearsightedness
   c. cataract
   d. astigmatism

3. What is the term for dry eye?
   a. blepharoptosis
   b. keratitis
   c. hyphema
   d. xerophthalmia

4. What part of the eye is LASIK performed on?
   a. cornea
   b. retina
   c. eyelid
   d. pupil

5. The L in LASIK stands for?
   a. lacrimal gland
   b. lens
   c. lacrimal sac
   d. laser

Medical Record *Alfred Olson*

OLSON, ALFRED U - 600048 Opened by WESTGATE, ADAM MD

Task   Edit   View   Time Scale   Options   Help

As Of 09:22

| OLSON, ALFRED U | Age: 75 years | Sex: Male | Loc: WHC-SMMC |
| | DOB: 11/11/1940 | MRN: 600048 | FIN: 3506004 |

Reference Text Browser | Form Browser | Medication Profile

Orders | Last 48 Hours | ED | Lab | Radiology | Assessments | **Surgery** | Clinical Notes | Pt. Info | Pt. Schedule | Task List | I & O | MAR

Flowsheet: Surgery   Level: Operative Report   ⦿ Table   ○ Group   ○ List

Navigator

✔ Operative Report

Patient is a 75-year-old gentleman with a visually significant cataract of the right eye. He was seen preoperatively by his family physician and cleared for local anesthetic. Patient was brought into the outpatient surgical suite and underwent uncomplicated phacoemulsification and posterior lens implant of the right eye under local standby using topical anesthetic.

He was taken to the recovery room in good condition.

PROD | MAHAFC | 25 April 2015 | 09:22

⟳ EXERCISE 11: Operative Record

Using the preceding operative report, answer the following questions.

1. What is the condition that the procedure is intended to correct? _____

2. When was he seen by his family physician? _____

3. Phacoemulsification means that the lens was _____.

4. How do you know that he received a new lens? _____

5. What type of anesthetic was used during the surgery? _____

Abbreviations

Abbreviation	Meaning	Abbreviation	Meaning
Acc	accommodation	IOP	intraocular pressure
ACS	anterior ciliary sclerotomy	LASIK	laser-assisted in-situ keratomileusis
AK	astigmatic keratotomy		
ARMD, AMD	age-related macular degeneration	MY	myopia
		NPDR	nonproliferative diabetic retinopathy
Astigm, As, Ast	astigmatism		
ECCE	extracapsular cataract extraction	Ophth	ophthalmology
EM, Em	emmetropia	PDR	proliferative diabetic retinopathy
EOM	extraocular movements		
ICCE	intracapsular cataract extraction	PRK	photorefractive keratectomy
ICL	implantable contact lens	VA	visual acuity
IOL	intraocular lens	VF	visual field

EXERCISE 12: Abbreviations

Write out the following abbreviations.

1. Jonathan Sobel was diagnosed with MY in his left eye. _____

2. Marlena decided to consider the merits of LASIK and PRK before she had her prescription filled.

   _____

3. Katsuko's vision was described as 20/300 on his VA test. _____

4. The patient had ARMD. _____

5. Arielle was referred to Ophth. _____

6. The patient's IOP is described as being within normal limits. _____

7. An Amsler grid is used to test the patient's VF. _____

THE EAR

ANATOMY AND PHYSIOLOGY

The ear is regionally divided into the outer, middle, and inner **ear** (Fig. 13-25). Sound is conducted through air, bone, and fluid through these divisions. The majority of the ear is contained within the **petrous** (PEH trus) portion of the temporal bone. *Petrous* refers to the hard (*petr/o* = stone) nature of the temporal bone that protects the ear. The **mastoid process** is a hard, small projection of the temporal bone that is behind the opening of the auditory canal.

Outer (External) Ear

Sound waves are initially gathered by the flesh-covered cartilage of the outer ear called the **pinna** (PIN nuh), or **auricle** (ORE ick kul). The gathered sound is then funneled into the **external auditory canal.** Earwax, or **cerumen** (sih ROO mun), is secreted by modified sweat glands within the external auditory canal and protects the ear with its antiseptic property and its stickiness, trapping foreign debris and moving it out of the ear. The opening of the outer ear is the **external auditory meatus** (AH dih tor ee mee AY tus). The **tympanic** (tim PAN ick) **membrane (TM),** or **eardrum,** marks the end of the external ear and the beginning of the middle ear. It is a thin membrane in the middle ear that transmits sound vibrations from the external auditory canal through the middle ear and then to the inner ear.

Middle Ear

The eardrum conducts sound to three tiny bones in the middle ear called the **ossicles** (AH sick kuls), or the **ossicular chain.** These ossicles are named for their shapes: the **malleus** (MAL ee us), or hammer; the **incus** (ING kus), or anvil; and the **stapes** (STAY peez) (*pl.* stapedes), or stirrup. The ossicles transmit the sound to the **oval window** through the stapes. Within the middle ear is the opening for the **pharyngotympanic tube,** also called the *auditory tube* or *eustachian tube,* a mucous membrane–lined connection between the ears and the throat that equalizes pressure within the middle ear.

ear = ot/o, aur/o, auricul/o
mastoid process = mastoid/o
cerumen, earwax = cerumin/o
meatus = meat/o
eardrum = tympan/o, myring/o
ossicle = ossicul/o
stapes = staped/o
eustachian tube = salping/o
pharyngotympanic   pharyng/o = pharynx   tympan/o = eardrum   -ic = pertaining to

Fig. 13-25 The ear.

Be Careful! *The combining form* **salping/o** *means both fallopian tube and eustachian tube.*

 Be Careful! **Malleus** *means one of the ossicles in the ear.* **Malleolus** *means one of the processes on the distal tibia and fibula.*

Inner Ear

labyrinth, inner ear = labyrinth/o

perilymph
  peri- = surrounding
  lymph/o = lymph

endolymph
  endo- = within
  lymph/o = lymph

vestibule = vestibul/o

cochlea = cochle/o

macula = macul/o

hearing = audi/o, acous/o

 Be Careful!

Do not confuse **oral** *meaning pertaining to the mouth with* **aural** *meaning pertaining to the ear.*

Once sound is conducted to the oval window, it is transmitted to a structure called the **labyrinth** (LAB uh rinth), or the **inner ear.** The labyrinth is the organ of receptors for hearing and balance. A membranous labyrinth is enclosed within a bony labyrinth. Between the two, and surrounding the inner labyrinth, is a fluid called **perilymph** (PAIR ee limf). Within the membranous labyrinth is a fluid called **endolymph** (EN doh limf). Hair cells within the inner ear fluids act as nerve endings that function as sensory receptors for hearing and equilibrium. The outer, bony labyrinth is composed of three parts: the vestibule, the semicircular canals, and the cochlea. The **vestibule** (VES tih byool) and **semicircular canals** function to provide information about the body's sense of equilibrium, whereas the **cochlea** (KAH klee ah) is an organ of hearing.

Within the vestibule, two saclike structures called the **utricle** (YOO trick ul) and the **saccule** (SACK yool) function to determine the body's static equilibrium. A specialized patch of epithelium called the **macula** (MACK yoo lah), found in both the utricle and the saccule, provides information about the position of the head and a sense of acceleration and deceleration. The semicircular canals detect dynamic equilibrium, or a sense of sudden rotation, through the function of a structure called the **crista ampullaris** (KRIS tah am pyoo LAIR is).

The cochlea receives the vibrations from the perilymph and transmits them to the cochlear duct, which is filled with endolymph. The transmission of sound continues through the endolymph to the **organ of Corti,** where the hearing receptor cells (hairs) stimulate a branch of the eighth cranial nerve, the vestibulocochlear nerve, to transmit the information to the temporal lobe of the brain.

EXERCISE 13: Anatomy of the Ear

Match the combining forms with the correct parts of the ear. More than one answer may be correct.

_____ 1. eardrum

_____ 2. bones of the ear

_____ 3. earwax

_____ 4. inner ear

_____ 5. hearing

_____ 6. eustachian tube

_____ 7. ear

_____ 8. stirrup-shaped ear bone

A. labyrinth/o
B. ossicul/o
C. cerumin/o
D. staped/o
E. myring/o
F. salping/o
G. ot/o
H. audi/o
I. tympan/o
J. aur/o

Decode the terms.

9. preauricular _____

10. supratympanic _____

11. circumaural _____

 EXERCISE 14: Anatomy of the Ear

Label the drawing using the terms provided.

malleus
mastoid process
tympanic
  membrane (TM)
oval window
vestibule
stapes
cochlea
incus
semicircular
  canals
external auditory
  canal
pharyngotympanic
  tube
auricle

You can review the anatomy of the ear by clicking on **Body Spectrum Electronic Anatomy Coloring Book → Senses → Ear.** Choose **Hear It, Spell It** to practice spelling the anatomy and physiology terms for the ear.

Combining and Adjective Forms for the Anatomy and Physiology of the Ear

Meaning	Combining Form	Adjective Form
cerumen, earwax	cerumin/o	ceruminous
cochlea	cochle/o	cochlear
ear	ot/o, aur/o, auricul/o	otic, aural, auricular
eardrum	tympan/o, myring/o	tympanic
eustachian tube	salping/o	salpingeal
hearing	audi/o, acous/o	acoustic
labyrinth, inner ear	labyrinth/o	labyrinthine
lymph	lymph/o, lymphat/o	lymphatic
macula	macul/o	macular
mastoid process	mastoid/o	mastoidal
meatus	meat/o	meatal
ossicle	ossicul/o	ossicular
stapes	staped/o	stapedial
vestibule	vestibul/o	vestibular

Prefixes for Anatomy of the Ear

Prefix	Meaning
endo-	within
peri-	surrounding

 *Click on **Label It** to practice labeling the structures of the ear.*

PATHOLOGY

Terms Related to Symptomatic Disorders

Term	Word Origin	Definition
otalgia oh TAL juh	*ot/o* ear *-algia* pain	Earache, pain in the ear; also called **otodynia** (oh toh DIN nee ah).
otorrhea oh tuh REE ah	*ot/o* ear *-rrhea* discharge	Discharge from the auditory canal; may be serous, bloody, or purulent.
tinnitus tin EYE tis		Abnormal sound heard in one or both ears caused by trauma or disease; may be a ringing, buzzing, or jingling.
vertigo VUR tih goh		Dizziness; abnormal sensation of movement when there is none, either of one's self moving, or of objects moving around oneself. May be caused by middle ear infections or the toxic effects of alcohol, sunstroke, and certain medications.

Terms Related to Outer Ear Disorders

Term	Word Origin	Definition
impacted cerumen sur ROO mun		Blockage of the external auditory canal with cerumen.
macrotia mah KROH sha	*macro-* large *ot/o* ear *-ia* condition	Condition of abnormally large auricles.
microtia mye KROH sha	*micro-* small *ot/o* ear *-ia* condition	Condition of abnormally small auricles.
otitis externa oh TYE tis eck STER nah	*ot/o* ear *-itis* inflammation externa outer	Inflammation of the outer ear and ear canal. Also called **swimmer's ear.**

Terms Related to Middle Ear Disorders

Term	Word Origin	Definition
cholesteatoma koh less tee ah TOH mah	*chol/e* bile *steat/o* fat *-oma* tumor	Cystic mass composed of epithelial cells and cholesterol. Mass may occlude middle ear and destroy adjacent bones.
infectious myringitis meer in JYE tis	*myring/o* eardrum *-itis* inflammation	Inflammation of the eardrum due to a bacterial or viral infection.
mastoiditis mass toy DYE tis	*mastoid/o* mastoid process *-itis* inflammation	Inflammation of the mastoid process of the temporal bone (Fig. 13-26).
otitis media (OM) oh TYE tis MEE dee ah	*ot/o* ear *-itis* inflammation media middle	Inflammation of the middle ear. **Suppurative OM** is characterized by a pus-filled fluid. **Secretory OM** is characterized by clear fluid discharge (Fig. 13-27).
otosclerosis oh toh sklair ROH sis	*ot/o* ear *-sclerosis* condition of hardening	Development of bone around the oval window with resulting ankylosis of the stapes to the oval window; usually results in progressive deafness.

Fig. 13-26 Mastoiditis.

Fig. 13-27 Otitis media (OM). Tympanic membrane (TM) is erythematous, opaque, and bulging.

Terms Related to Inner Ear Disorders

Term	Word Origin	Definition
labyrinthitis lab uh rinth EYE tis	*labyrinth/o* labyrinth *-itis* inflammation	Inflammation of the inner ear that may be due to infection or trauma; symptoms may include vertigo, nausea, and nystagmus.
Meniere disease may nee UR		Chronic condition of the inner ear characterized by vertigo, hearing loss, and tinnitus. The cause is unknown.
ruptured tympanic membrane (TM)		Tear (perforation) of the eardrum due to trauma or disease process (Fig. 13-28).

Terms Related to Hearing Loss Disorders

Term	Word Origin	Definition
anacusis an uh KYOO sis	*an-* no, not, without *-acusis* hearing	General term for hearing loss or deafness.
conductive hearing loss		Hearing loss resulting from damage to or malformation of the middle or outer ear.
paracusis pair uh KYOO sis	*para-* abnormal *-cusis* hearing	Abnormality of hearing.
presbycusis prez bee KYOO sis	*presby-* old age *-cusis* hearing	Loss of hearing common in old age.
sensorineural hearing loss sen suh ree NOOR uhl		Hearing loss resulting from damage to the inner ear (cochlea) or the auditory nerve.

EXERCISE 15: Disorders of the Ear

Matching.

_____ 1. cholesteatoma

_____ 2. vertigo

_____ 3. otorrhea

_____ 4. macrotia

_____ 5. labyrinthitis

_____ 6. otitis media (OM)

_____ 7. tinnitus

_____ 8. presbycusis

_____ 9. Meniere disease

_____ 10. anacusis

_____ 11. otitis externa

_____ 12. paracusis

A. cystic mass in the middle ear composed of cholesterol
B. ringing in the ears
C. inner ear condition characterized by vertigo, hearing loss, and tinnitus
D. loss of hearing typical of aging
E. hearing loss
F. inflammation of inner ear
G. abnormally large auricles
H. abnormal sense of movement
I. middle ear infection
J. inflammation of outer ear
K. discharge from the ear
L. abnormality of hearing

Build the terms.

13. ear pain _____

14. condition of small ears _____

15. condition of hardening of the ear _____

Case Study   Carole Hancock

Carole Hancock is a 45-year-old financial advisor for a small firm. One afternoon at work she experiences hearing loss, fullness in the ear, dizziness, and ringing in the ears. The dizziness is so severe that she needs to call her daughter to give her a ride home. Her daughter urges Carole to see her doctor, because this is the third time that Carole has experienced similar symptoms. She is able to get an appointment right away, and her doctor asks her about the number and severity of her symptoms. He also performs quick audiometric tests. He suspects that Carole has Meniere disease but schedules her for imaging tests. She is prescribed meclizine (Antivert) to help manage the dizziness along with a diuretic to help alleviate the symptom of fullness in the ear.

1. What is the term that means dizziness? _____

2. What is the term that means ringing in the ears? _____

3. If you know what the combining form *audi/o* means, you'll know that audiometric tests measure _____ loss.

Terms Related to Benign Neoplasms

Term	Word Origin	Definition
acoustic neuroma ah KOO stik noo ROH mah	*acous/o* hearing *-tic* pertaining to *neur/o* nerve *-oma* tumor, mass	A benign tumor of the eighth cranial nerve (vestibulocochlear) that causes tinnitus, vertigo, and hearing loss. Also called **vestibular schwannoma** (Fig. 13-29).
ceruminoma seh roo min NOH mah	*cerumin/o* cerumen, earwax *-oma* tumor, mass	A benign adenoma of the glands that produce earwax.

Fig. 13-28 Tympanic membrane (TM) perforation.

Fig. 13-29 Computed tomography (CT) scan of acoustic neuroma. A large tumor *(arrow)* is pressing on and displacing the brainstem.

EXERCISE 16: Neoplasms

Fill in the blank.

1. What is a benign tumor of the eighth cranial nerve? _____

2. What is a benign adenoma of the glands that produce earwax? _____

 Click on **Hear It, Spell It** *to practice spelling the pathology terms that you have learned in this chapter. To review the pathology terms in this chapter, play* **Medical Millionaire.**

Medical Record *Luis Pujols*

PUJOLS, LUIS A - 645233 Opened by WASHINGTON, FELIX MD   ⊟ ⊞ ⊠

Task   Edit   View   Time Scale   Options   Help

PUJOLS, LUIS A	Age: 2 years DOB: 05/24/2013	Sex: Male MRN: 645233	Loc: WHC-SMMC FIN: 3506004

Reference Text Browser	Form Browser	Medication Profile

| Orders | Last 48 Hours | ED | Lab | Radiology | Assessments | Surgery | **Clinical Notes** | Pt. Info | Pt. Schedule | Task List | I & O | MAR |

Flowsheet: Clinical Notes ▼ ...   Level: Progress Note ▼   ⦿ Table ○ Group ○ List

Navigator ⊠
✓ Progress Note

This 2-year-old male comes in with a temperature of 101.1 F. In some pain, and mother has noted him to be lethargic. Patient has had frequent ear infections in the past. He also has history of strep throat.

PHYSICAL EXAM:	Alert male, lethargic, but responsive Not in acute respiratory distress
Temperature:	101.1, Pulse 120, BP 120/80
Neck:	No lymphadenopathy or stiffness. Full ROM
Lungs:	Clear with upper respiratory sounds, but no wheezing
Cardiac:	Regular rate and rhythm
HEENT:	Reveals dull red right TM. Oropharyngeal exam normal.
ASSESSMENT:	Right otitis media Treat with Zithromax 200 per 5. Given Auralgan suspension, 3 drops to right ear.

PROD MAHAFC   05 Jun 2015   15:20

⊘ EXERCISE 17: Progress Note

Using the preceding progress note, answer the following questions.

1. How do you know that the patient had no disease of his lymph glands? _____

2. What term tells you that the patient did not exhibit a whistling sound made during breathing?

   _____

3. The patient's right eardrum is examined and is found to be dull and red. What do you think TM

   stands for? _____

4. What area of the throat appears normal on exam? _____

5. The diagnosis is an inflammation of the middle ear. What is the term? _____

 Age Matters

Pediatrics

Although very few babies are born with a hearing loss, the Universal Newborn Hearing Screening (UNHS) test is a means to detect deafness in infancy. Once given the diagnosis, the parents can begin to plan for how to best handle the condition.

OM is the most frequently diagnosed childhood ear disease.

Geriatrics

Hearing loss that may accompany the aging process is termed *presbycusis*.

DIAGNOSTIC PROCEDURES

Terms Related to Hearing Tests

Term	Word Origin	Definition
audiometric testing ah dee oh MEH trick	*audi/o* hearing *-metric* pertaining to measurement	Measurement of hearing, usually with an instrument called an **audiometer** (ah dee AH met tur). The graphic representation of the results is called an **audiogram** (Fig. 13-30)
otoscopy oh TAH skuh pee	*ot/o* ear *-scopy* process of viewing	Visual examination of the external auditory canal and the TM using an **otoscope.**
pure tone audiometry ah dee AH meh tree	*audi/o* hearing *-metry* process of measuring	Measurement of perception of pure tones with extraneous sound screened out.
Rinne tuning fork test RIH nuh		Method of distinguishing conductive from sensorineural hearing loss.

Continued

Terms Related to Hearing Tests—cont'd

Term	Word Origin	Definition
speech audiometry	*audi/o* hearing *-metry* process of measuring	Measurement of ability to hear and understand speech.
tympanometry tim pan NAH muh tree	*tympan/o* eardrum *-metry* process of measuring	Measurement of the condition and mobility function of the eardrum. The resultant graph is called a **tympanogram.**
Universal Newborn Hearing Screening (UNHS) test		Test that uses **otoacoustic emissions (OAEs)** measured by the insertion of a probe into the baby's ear canal, and **auditory brainstem response (ABR),** which involves the placement of four electrodes on the baby's head to measure the change in electrical activity of the brain in response to sound while the baby is sleeping.
Weber tuning fork test WEB ur		Method of testing auditory acuity.

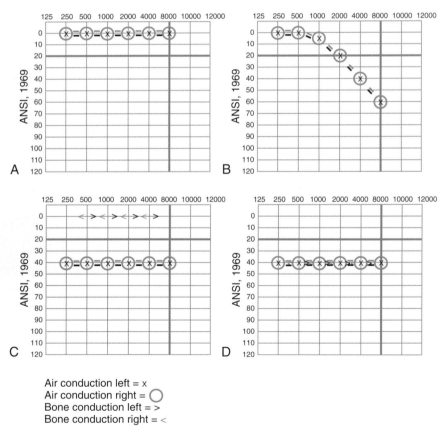

Air conduction left = x
Air conduction right = ○
Bone conduction left = >
Bone conduction right = <

Fig. 13-30 Audiograms. **A,** Normal hearing. **B,** Conductive hearing loss. **C,** High-frequency hearing loss. **D,** Sensorineural hearing loss.

EXERCISE 18: Diagnostic Procedures

Matching.

_____ 1. instrument to measure hearing

_____ 2. test of auditory acuity

_____ 3. record of function of eardrum

_____ 4. instrument to visually examine the ears

_____ 5. test to distinguish between conductive and sensorineural hearing loss

_____ 6. measurement of ability to hear and understand speech

A. otoscope
B. Rinne tuning fork test
C. speech audiometry
D. Weber tuning fork test
E. audiometer
F. tympanogram

Decode the terms.

7. otoscopy _____

8. tympanometry _____

9. audiometric _____

THERAPEUTIC INTERVENTIONS

Terms Related to Therapeutic Interventions

Term	Word Origin	Definition
cochlear implant KAH klee ur	*cochle/o* cochlea *-ar* pertaining to	Implanted device that assists those with hearing loss by electrically stimulating the cochlea (Fig. 13-31).
hearing aid		Electronic device that amplifies sound.
mastoidectomy mass toyd ECK tuh mee	*mastoid/o* mastoid process *-ectomy* removal	Removal of the mastoid process, usually to treat intractable mastoiditis.
otoplasty OH toh plas tee	*ot/o* ear *-plasty* surgical repair	Surgical or plastic repair and/or reconstruction of the external ear.
stapedectomy stay puh DECK tuh mee	*staped/o* stapes *-ectomy* removal	Removal of the third ossicle, the stapes, from the middle ear. Done to correct otosclerosis.
tympanoplasty TIM pan oh plas tee	*tympan/o* eardrum *-plasty* surgical repair	Surgical repair of the eardrum, with or without ossicular chain reconstruction. Some patients may require a prosthesis (an artificial replacement) for one or more of the ossicles.
tympanostomy tim pan AH stuh mee	*tympan/o* eardrum *-stomy* new opening	Surgical creation of an opening through the eardrum to promote drainage and/or allow the introduction of artificial tubes to maintain the opening (Fig. 13-32); also called a **myringostomy** (mir ring AH stuh mee).
tympanotomy tim pan AH tuh mee	*tympan/o* eardrum *-tomy* incision	Incision of an eardrum; also called a **myringotomy** (mir ring AH tuh mee).

Microphone
Implant
Headpiece
Electrode system
Auditory nerve
Cochlea
Sound processor

Fig. 13-31 Cochlear implant.

Fig. 13-32 Tympanostomy tube in place.

EXERCISE 19: Therapeutic Interventions

Match the interventions with their definitions.

_____ 1. incision of eardrum

_____ 2. surgical reconstruction of the external ear

_____ 3. surgical creation of a new opening through the eardrum

_____ 4. device implanted in inner ear to stimulate hearing

_____ 5. excision of ossicle that strikes the oval window

A. cochlear implant
B. otoplasty
C. tympanostomy
D. stapedectomy
E. myringotomy

Case Study   Raheem Amari

Two-year-old Raheem Amari has been fussy and says that his ear hurts. On Monday his mother takes him to his pediatrician, Dr. Kelley. Dr. Kelley examines Raheem's ears and finds that he has a middle ear infection. Raheem's mother asks whether his son will need tubes because his older sister did. Dr. Kelley says that tympanic tubes are not necessary for Raheem, but that untreated ear infections could lead to an inflammation of the mastoid process behind the ear.

1. What is the medical term for a middle ear infection?

_____

2. What instrument is used to examine the external and middle ear? _____

3. What is an inflammation of the mastoid process? ___

_____

4. What term means a surgical creation of an opening in the eardrum to promote drainage and to introduce of artificial tubes?
   a. otoplasty
   b. mastoidectomy
   c. myringotomy
   d. stapedectomy

5. What is another term for myringotomy? _____

_____

6. Removal of the mastoid process to treat intractable mastoiditis is called _____.

Click on **Hear It, Spell It** to practice spelling the diagnostic and therapeutic terms that you have learned in this chapter.

PHARMACOLOGY

antibiotics: Treat bacterial infections. A commonly used oral agent to treat ear infections is amoxicillin (Amoxil). A topical example is ciprofloxacin with hydrocortisone (Cipro HC Otic).

ceruminolytics: Soften and break down earwax. An example is triethanol-amine polypeptide oleate (Cerumenex).

decongestants: Relieve congestion associated with a cold, allergy, or sinus pressure. These drugs may be available as a nasal spray or an oral product. Examples include pseudoephedrine (Sudafed) and oxymetazoline (Afrin).

otics: Drugs applied directly to the external ear canal. These may be administered in the form of solutions, suspensions, or ointments.

 EXERCISE 20: Pharmacology

Matching.

_____ 1. otics

_____ 2. ceruminolytics

_____ 3. antibiotics

_____ 4. decongestants

A. drugs used to treat infection
B. drugs used to relieve congestion
C. drugs applied to the external ear canal
D. medications to soften and break down earwax

Case Study **Susan Zietz**

Susan Zietz, a 37-year-old truck driver, notices that she is missing parts of radio broadcasts as she drives across the country delivering loads to large box stores. After returning home from one of her deliveries, she calls and makes an appointment with her family physician. On examination, it is determined that one of her ears is clogged with impacted earwax. An attempt at irrigation and removal of the earwax is successful, but she is prescribed ear drops to prevent future buildups. Glad that she has her hearing back, she asks if there is a possibility of earwax causing a serious problem. Her physician tells her that it is rare, but a tumor of the glands that produce earwax can develop.

1. What is the medical term that means earwax? _____

   _____

2. What is the medication that breaks down earwax?

   _____

3. What is a tumor of the glands that produce earwax?

   _____

4. Earwax is a normal secretion in which part of the ear?
   a. internal
   b. external
   c. middle

Abbreviations

Abbreviation	Meaning	Abbreviation	Meaning
ABR	auditory brainstem response	oto	otology
ASL	American sign language	TM	tympanic membrane
ENT	ear, nose, throat	UNHS	Universal Newborn Hearing Screening test
OAE	otoacoustic emission		
OM	otitis media		

 EXERCISE 21: Abbreviations

Matching.

_____ 1. OM

_____ 2. ASL

_____ 3. TM

_____ 4. ENT

_____ 5. OAE

A. tympanic membrane
B. otoacoustic emission
C. American sign language
D. ear, nose, throat
E. otitis media

 Be Careful! *The abbreviations for left ear (AS), right ear (AD), and each ear (AU) have been declared "dangerous" by the Institute of Safe Medical Practice. Write out the full term instead of using an abbreviation.*

Chapter Review

Match the word parts to their definitions.

Word Part Definitions

Prefix/Suffix		Definition
an-	1. _____	surgical repair
-cusis	2. _____	outside
exo-	3. _____	inflammation
extra-	4. _____	outward
-itis	5. _____	hearing
macro-	6. _____	not
micro-	7. _____	old age
-opsia	8. _____	vision condition
-plasty	9. _____	large
presby-	10. _____	small

Combining Form		Definition
acous/o	11. _____	tears
audi/o	12. _____	cornea
auricul/o	13. _____	earwax
blephar/o	14. _____	eardrum
cerumin/o	15. _____	lacrimal sac
core/o	16. _____	ear
dacryoaden/o	17. _____	vision
dacryocyst/o	18. _____	hearing
irid/o	19. _____	eyelid
kerat/o	20. _____	inner ear
labyrinth/o	21. _____	eardrum
lacrim/o	22. _____	eye
myring/o	23. _____	pupil
ocul/o	24. _____	eye
ophthalm/o	25. _____	hearing
opt/o	26. _____	optic disk
ot/o	27. _____	eyelid
palpebr/o	28. _____	iris
papill/o	29. _____	ear
phac/o	30. _____	lens
salping/o	31. _____	eustachian tube
tympan/o	32. _____	lacrimal gland

Wordshop

Prefixes	Combining Forms	Suffixes
a-	ambul/o	-ia
acro-	anthrop/o	-ism
agora-	claustr/o	-lalia
an-	cycl/o	-logy
dys-	hedon/o	-mania
echo-	klept/o	-osis
eu-	orex/o	-phobia
para-	phren/o	-thymia
	psych/o	
	pyr/o	
	schiz/o	
	somn/o	
	till/o	
	trich/o	

Build the following terms by combining the preceding word parts. Some word parts may be used more than once. Some may not be used at all. The number in parentheses is the number of word parts needed to build the terms.

Definition	Term
1. condition of small ear (3)	_____
2. condition of no lens (3)	_____
3. discharge from the ear (2)	_____
4. (loss of) hearing due to old age (2)	_____
5. incision of the eardrum (2)	_____
6. abnormal hearing (2)	_____
7. abnormal condition of hardening of the ear (2)	_____
8. inflammation of the inner ear (2)	_____
9. condition of no color vision (3)	_____
10. process of measurement of hearing (2)	_____
11. inflammation of the tear glands (2)	_____
12. drooping of the eyelids (2)	_____
13. pertaining to the nose and tears (3)	_____
14. condition of aversion to light (2)	_____
15. process of measurement of pressure (of the eye) (2)	_____

Sort the terms into the correct categories.

Term Sorting

Anatomy and Physiology	Pathology	Diagnostic Procedures	Therapeutic Interventions

accommodation	fovea	otoplasty	slit lamp
Amsler grid	gonioscopy	otorrhea	stapedectomy
anacusis	IOLs	otosclerosis	stapes
audiometer	iridotomy	otoscopy	strabismus
cerumen	labyrinth	phacoemulsification	tinnitus
chalazion	lacrimation	pinna	tonometry
cochlea	miotics	refraction	tympanometry
coreoplasty	nyctalopia	sclera	tympanostomy
diopters	ophthalmoscopy	scleral buckling	tympanotomy
exophthalmia	otalgia	scotoma	VA

Replace the highlighted words with the correct terms.

Translations

1. Maria was complaining of **extreme sensitivity to light** and **excessive lacrimation.**

2. The pediatrician used an **instrument to view the ear** to diagnose baby Grace's **inflammation of the middle ear.**

3. The auto accident victim came to the ED with **a condition of unequally sized pupils** and **blood in the anterior chamber of the eye.**

4. During Michael's eye examination, it was discovered that he had red/green **impairment of color vision** and slight **nearsightedness.**

5. The 80-year-old patient was evaluated by **one who specializes in the study of hearing** and was found to have **loss of hearing common in old age.**

6. Rose's **disorder characterized by abnormal intraocular pressure** was tested with **measurement of intraocular pressure.**

7. Terrance had **a surgical repair of the eyelids** to correct his **drooping of the upper eyelid.**

8. The patient had **reattachment of the retina with a cryoprobe** to correct a **separation of the retina from the choroid layer.**

9. Mrs. M came to the ED complaining of **an abnormal sound heard in the ear** and **dizziness.**

10. The patient had **a creation of an opening between the tear sac and the nose** to correct a blockage in her **pertaining to tears** sac.

11. A **test to determine the amount of tear production** was used to determine the degree of the patient's **dry eye.**

12. Mary Kate's **inability to see well in dim light** was a result of **a hereditary degenerative disease marked by nyctalopiaand a progressive loss of visual field.**

13. A bilateral **surgical repair of the external ear** was performed to correct the patient's **condition of abnormally large auricles.**

14. Carl's **hearing loss** was caused by a **development of bone around the oval window.**

Medical Record Mary Ellen Wright

O'Connor Eye Associates
456 Humphrey St.
Philadelphia, PA 19117

Morgan Ophthalmology Associates   August 12, 2015
789 Henry Ave.
Philadelphia, PA 19118

Re: Mary Ellen Wright, DOB: 4/1/1977

Dear Dr. Morgan:

I have had the pleasure of treating Mary Ellen Wright for the past 11 years. She has asked me to summarize her treatment for you.

Ms. Wright had received comprehensive optometric care from her previous optometrist from 1995 to 2001. Her previous records reflected good binocular oculomotor function and good ocular health, including the absence of posterior vitreous detachment, retinal breaks, or peripheral retinal degeneration in either eye. She specifically denies any incidence of trauma, diplopia, or cephalgia. She also denies any personal or family history of glaucoma, strabismus, retinal disease, diabetes, hypertension, heart disease, or breathing problems. She is on no medications. Entrance tests, such as EOMs, pupils, color vision, confrontation fields, and cover test, appeared unchanged from previously reported exams. Refractive correction for compound myopic astigmatism contained the following parameters:

Spectacle Correction: Right eye   7.50 - 1.00 × 165 20/20   Contact Lenses: Right eye 20/15; Left eye 20/15
Left eye   7.50 - 1.00 × 180 20/20

She came for her last comprehensive examination without any visual or ocular complaints. She desired a new supply of disposable contact lenses. She reported clear and comfortable vision at distance, intermediate, and near with both her glasses and contact lenses.

Eye Health Assessment: Slit lamp examination revealed clean lids with good tonicity and apposition to the globe. The lashes and lid margins were clear of debris. There was no discharge from either eye. The corneas were clear with no fluorescein staining either eye. Pupils were equal, round, and reactive to light and accommodation without apparent defect. Intraocular pressures measured 10 mm Hg right eye, left eye at 1:30 pm with Goldmann applanation tonometry.

If any further information is needed, please feel free to contact me regarding this patient.

Sincerely,

Roland O'Connor, OD

 MEDICAL LETTER

Using the preceding medical letter, answer the following questions.

1. Mary Ellen denies diplopia and cephalgia. Explain these terms.

2. Mary Ellen has been diagnosed with myopic astigmatism. In your own words, explain this visual disorder.

3. What is the name of the test for glaucoma? _____

4. Explain the term *paralimbal*. _____

14

Endocrine System

OBJECTIVES

- Recognize and use terms related to the anatomy and physiology of the endocrine system.
- Recognize and use terms related to the pathology of the endocrine system.
- Recognize and use terms related to the diagnostic procedures for the endocrine system.
- Recognize and use terms related to the therapeutic interventions for the endocrine system.

For interactive learning go to the Shiland Evolve website, and click on:
- **Match the Word Parts** to review endocrine word parts.
- **Word Shop** to practice word building.
- **Tournament of Terminology** to test your knowledge of endocrine terms.
- **Term Sorting** to practice sorting endocrine terms into categories.

*Click on **Chapter at a Glance** to print off a list of key terms and word parts for this chapter.*

FUNCTIONS OF THE ENDOCRINE SYSTEM

The **endocrine** (EN doh krin) system assists in the function of achieving the delicate physiologic balance necessary for survival. The endocrine system uses the circulatory system and chemical messengers called **hormones** to regulate a number of body functions, including metabolism, growth, reproduction, and water and electrolyte balances.

SPECIALISTS/SPECIALTIES

Endocrinology is the study of the glands that secrete hormones within the body. An **endocrinologist** is a medical doctor who diagnoses and treats diseases and disorders of the endocrine system.

ANATOMY AND PHYSIOLOGY

The endocrine system is composed of several single and paired ductless glands that secrete hormones into the bloodstream. The hormones regulate specific body functions by acting on target cells with receptor sites for those particular hormones only. See Fig. 14-1 for an illustration of the body with the locations of the endocrine glands.

Pituitary Gland

The **pituitary** (pih TOO ih tare ree) **gland,** also known as the **hypophysis** (hye POFF ih sis), is a tiny gland located behind the optic nerve in the cranial cavity. Sometimes called the *master gland* because of its role in controlling the

endocrine
  endo- = within
  -crine = to secrete

endocrinology
  endo- = within
  crin/o = to secrete
  -logy = study of

Be Careful!

*Do not confuse **aden/o**, which means gland, with **adren/o**, which means the adrenal gland.*

pituitary gland = hypophys/o, pituitar/o

gland = aden/o

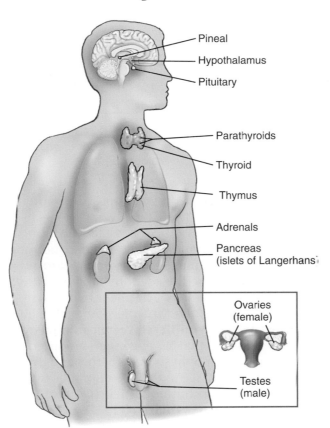

Fig. 14-1 Locations of the endocrine glands.

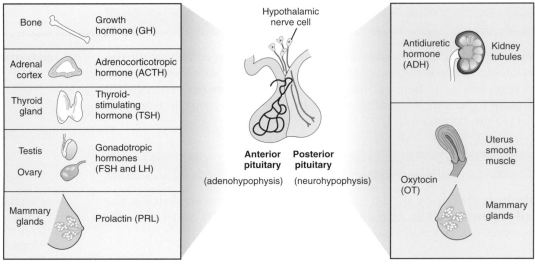

Fig. 14-2 Pituitary hormones. Principal anterior and posterior pituitary hormones and their target organs.

Adenohypophysis Hormones and Their Effects

Adenohypophysis Hormone	Effect
Adrenocorticotropic hormone (ACTH)	Stimulates the adrenal cortex to release steroids.
Gonadotropic hormones (include **follicle-stimulating hormone [FSH]**, **luteinizing hormone [LH]**, and **interstitial cell-stimulating hormone [ICSH]**)	FSH stimulates the development of gametes in the respective sexes. LH stimulates ovulation in the female and the secretion of sex hormones in both the male and the female. ICSH stimulates production of reproductive cells in the male.
Growth hormone (GH) (also called **human growth hormone [hGH]** or **somatotropin hormone [STH]**)	Stimulates growth of long bones and skeletal muscle; converts proteins to glucose.
Prolactin (PRL) (also called **lactogenic hormone**)	Stimulates milk production in the breast.
Thyrotropin (also called **thyroid-stimulating hormone [TSH]**)	Stimulates thyroid to release two other thyroid hormones.

 Be Careful!   *The combining form **trop/o** means turning, whereas **troph/o** means development or nourishment.*

lobe = lob/o

hypothalamus
  hypo- = under
  thalam/o = thalamus
  -us = structure

functions of other endocrine glands, it is composed of anterior and posterior lobes, each with its own functions.

The **anterior lobe,** or **adenohypophysis** (add uh noh hye POFF ih sis), is composed of glandular tissue and secretes myriad hormones in response to stimulation by the hypothalamus. The **hypothalamus** sends hormones through blood vessels, which cause the adenohypophysis either to release or to inhibit the release of specific hormones. The adenohypophysis has a wide range of effects on the body, as Fig. 14-2 and the preceding table illustrate.

The **posterior lobe (neurohypophysis)** of the pituitary gland is composed of nervous tissue. The hormones that it secretes are produced in the hypothalamus, transported to the neurohypophysis directly through the tissue connecting the organs, and released from storage in the posterior lobe by neural stimulation from the hypothalamus. The two hormones released by this lobe are **antidiuretic hormone (ADH)** and **oxytocin (OT).** See the following table and Fig. 14-2 for the hormones secreted by the neurohypophysis and their effects.

Neurohypophysis Hormones and Their Effects

Neurohypophysis Hormone	Effect
Antidiuretic hormone (ADH) (also called vasopressin)	Stimulates the kidneys to reabsorb water and return it to circulation; is also a vasoconstrictor, resulting in higher blood pressure.
Oxytocin (OT)	Stimulates the muscles of the uterus during the delivery of an infant and the muscles surrounding the mammary ducts to contract, releasing milk.

 Be Careful! *Oxytocin should not be confused with* **oxytocia,** *which means a rapid delivery.*

Thyroid Gland

The **thyroid gland** is a single organ located in the anterior part of the neck. It regulates the metabolism of the body and normal growth and development, and controls the amount of calcium (Ca) deposited into bone. The following table describes the hormones secreted by the thyroid and their effects.

thyroid gland = thyr/o, thyroid/o

calcium = calc/o

Thyroid Gland Hormones and Their Effects

Thyroid Gland Hormone	Effect
Calcitonin	Regulates the amount of calcium in the bloodstream.
Tetraiodothyronine (also called **thyroxine** [T_4])	Increases cell metabolism.
Triiodothyronine (T_3)	Increases cell metabolism.

 Be Careful! *Don't confuse* **calc/o** *meaning calcium with* **calic/o** *meaning calyx and* **kal/i** *meaning potassium.*

Parathyroid Glands

The **parathyroids** (pair uh THIGH royds) are four small glands located on the posterior surface of the thyroid gland in the neck. They secrete **parathyroid hormone (PTH)** in response to a low level of calcium in the blood. When low calcium is detected, the PTH increases calcium by causing it to be released from the bone, which results in calcium reabsorption by the kidneys and the digestive system. PTH is inhibited by high levels of calcium.

parathyroid gland = parathyroid/o

Adrenal Glands (Suprarenals)

The **adrenal** (uh DREE nul) **glands,** also called the **suprarenals,** are paired, one on top of each kidney. Different hormones are secreted by the two different parts of these glands: the external portion called the **adrenal cortex** (uh DREE nul KORE tecks) and an internal portion called the **adrenal medulla** (uh DREE nul muh DOO lah).

The adrenal cortex secretes three hormones that are called *steroids.*

The adrenal medulla is the inner portion of the adrenal gland. It produces sympathomimetic hormones that stimulate the fight-or-flight response to stress, similar to the action of the sympathetic nervous system.

adrenal gland = adren/o

suprarenal
  supra- = above
  ren/o = kidney
  -al = pertaining to

cortex = cortic/o

medulla = medull/o

Adrenal Cortex Hormones and Their Effects

Adrenal Cortex Hormones	Effect
Glucocorticoids (e.g., cortisol [hydrocortisone])	Respond to stress; have antiinflammatory properties.
Mineralocorticoids (e.g., aldosterone)	Regulate blood volume, blood pressure, and electrolytes.
Sex hormones (e.g., estrogen, androgen)	Responsible for secondary sex characteristics.

Adrenal Medulla Hormones and Their Effects

Adrenal Medulla Hormones (Catecholamines)	Effect
Dopamine	Dilates arteries and increases production of urine, blood pressure, and cardiac rate. Acts as a neurotransmitter in the nervous system.
Epinephrine (also called **adrenaline**)	Dilates bronchi, increases heart rate, raises blood pressure, dilates pupils, and elevates blood sugar levels.
Norepinephrine (also called **noradrenaline**)	Increases heart rate and blood pressure and elevates blood sugar levels for energy use.

pancreas = pancreat/o

exocrine
  exo- = outward
  -crine = to secrete

glucose, sugar = gluc/o, glyc/o

ketone = ket/o, keton/o

thymus gland = thym/o

Pancreas

The pancreas, located inferior and posterior to the stomach, is a gland with both exocrine and endocrine functions. The **exocrine function** is to release digestive enzymes through a duct into the small intestines. The **endocrine function,** accomplished through a variety of types of cells called **islets of Langerhans** (EYE lets of LANG gur hahnz), is to regulate the level of glucose in the blood by stimulating the liver. The two main types of islets of Langerhans cells are alpha and beta cells. Alpha cells produce the hormone glucagon that increases the level of glucose in the blood when levels are low. Beta cells secrete **insulin** (IN suh lin) that decreases the level of glucose in the blood when levels are high. Insulin is needed to transport glucose out of the bloodstream and into the cells. In the absence of glucose in the cells, proteins and fats are broken down, causing excessive fatty acids and **ketones** in the blood. Normally, these hormones regulate glucose levels through the metabolism of fats, carbohydrates, and proteins.

Thymus Gland

The **thymus** (THIGH mus) gland is located in the mediastinum above the heart. It releases a hormone called **thymosin** that is responsible for stimulating key cells in the immune response. See Chapter 9 for more details about the blood, lymphatic, and immune systems.

 Be Careful!   *Do not confuse **thyr/o**, which means thyroid, and **thym/o**, which means thymus.*

Ovaries and Testes

The **ovaries** and **testes,** the female and male **gonads,** also act as endocrine glands, which influence reproductive functions.

gonads = gonad/o

Pineal Gland

The **pineal** (PIH nee ul) gland is located in the center of the brain, functioning to secrete the hormone **melatonin,** thought to be responsible for inducing sleep.

⊘ EXERCISE 1: Endocrine Anatomy and Physiology

Fill in the blanks.

1. The pituitary gland, or the _____, is called the master gland because of its control over other endocrine glands.

2. The pituitary gland is controlled by the _____.

3. The anterior lobe of the pituitary gland is also known as the _____.

4. The thyroid gland is responsible for regulation of the body's _____ and

   controls the amount of _____ deposited into bone.

5. Adrenal glands are named for their location above the _____
   _____.

6. The inner part of the adrenal gland is the adrenal _____, whereas the

   outer part of the adrenal gland is the adrenal _____.

7. The endocrine function of the pancreas is to regulate glucose in the blood through its hormones

   _____ and _____.

8. Fatty acids and _____ are produced if glucose cannot pass out of the bloodstream and into the cells to be metabolized.

9. The thymus gland is located in the _____ above the heart and is

   responsible for stimulating key cells in the _____ response.

10. The _____ gland is located in the center of the brain, functioning to

    secrete the hormone _____, thought to be responsible for inducing _____.

Match the endocrine word parts with their definitions.

_____ 11. -al

_____ 20. ren/o

_____ 28. trop/o

_____ 12. aden/o

_____ 21. cortic/o

_____ 29. endo-

_____ 13. hypophys/o

_____ 22. medull/o

_____ 30. supra-

_____ 14. lob/o

_____ 23. pancreat/o

_____ 31. exo-

_____ 15. thalam/o

_____ 24. gluc/o

_____ 32. hypo-

_____ 16. thyr/o

_____ 25. thym/o

_____ 33. -crine

_____ 17. calc/o

_____ 26. ket/o

_____ 34. -logy

_____ 18. parathyroid/o

_____ 27. gonad/o

_____ 35. -us

_____ 19. adren/o

A. kidney
B. above
C. to secrete
D. calcium
E. outside
F. turning
G. sugar
H. structure
I. gland with exocrine and
   endocrine functions
J. reproductive organ
K. gland
L. the study of
M. medulla

N. within
O. ketone
P. gland in mediastinum
Q. pertaining to
R. master gland
S. under
T. suprarenal gland
U. cortex
V. gland regulating metabolism
W. glands regulating calcium in the blood
X. lobe
Y. thalamus

Decode the terms.

36. perithyroidal _____

37. hypoglycemic _____

38. retropancreatic _____

39. interlobar _____

 *Choose **Hear It, Spell It** to practice spelling the anatomy and physiology terms that you have learned in this chapter.*

EXERCISE 2: Endocrine Glands

Label the drawing using the terms provided.

thymus
pituitary
pancreas
ovaries
hypothalamus
pineal
parathyroids
testes
thyroid
adrenals

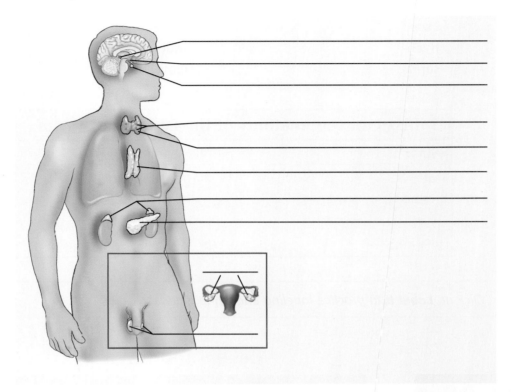

Combining and Adjective Forms for the Anatomy and Physiology of the Endocrine System

Meaning	Combining Form	Adjective Form
adrenal gland	adren/o, adrenal/o	adrenal
calcium	calc/o	
cortex	cortic/o	cortical
gland	aden/o	
glucose, sugar	gluc/o, glyc/o, glucos/o	
gonads	gonad/o	gonadal
ketone	ket/o, keton/o	
kidney	ren/o, nephr/o	renal
lobe	lob/o	lobar
medulla	medull/o	medullary
pancreas	pancreat/o	pancreatic
parathyroid gland	parathyroid/o	parathyroidal
pituitary gland	hypophys/o, pituitar/o	hypophyseal
thalamus	thalam/o	thalamic
thymus gland	thym/o	thymic
thyroid gland	thyr/o, thyroid/o	thyroidal
to secrete	crin/o	
turning	trop/o	tropic

Prefixes for the Anatomy of the Endocrine System

Prefix	Meaning
endo-	within
exo-	outward
hypo-	under
supra-	above

Suffixes for the Anatomy of the Endocrine System

Suffix	Meaning
-al	pertaining to
-crine	to secrete
-logy	study of
-us, -is	structure

 *Click on **Label It** to practice labeling endocrine glands.*

Fig. 14-3 Exophthalmia.

PATHOLOGY

Most of the pathology of the endocrine system is the result of either *hyper-* (too much) or *hypo-* (too little) hormonal secretion. Developmental issues also play a role in determining when the malfunction occurs and what the results will be.

Terms Related to Signs and Symptoms of Endocrine Disorders

Term	Word Origin	Definition
anorexia an oh RECK see ah	*an-* without *orex/o* appetite *-ia* condition	Lack of **appetite.** Anorexia nervosa is an eating disorder.
exophthalmia eck soff THAL mee ah	*ex-* out *ophthalm/o* eye *-ia* condition	Protrusion of eyeballs from their orbits (Fig. 14-3).
glucosuria gloo koh SOOR ee ah	*glucos/o* sugar, glucose *-uria* urinary condition	Presence of glucose in the urine. May indicate diabetes mellitus (DM). Also called **glycosuria.**
goiter GOY tur		Enlargement of the thyroid gland, not due to a tumor (Fig. 14-4).
hirsutism HUR soo tiz um		Abnormal hairiness, especially in women (Fig. 14-5). Also called **hypertrichosis.**

Terms Related to Signs and Symptoms of Endocrine Disorders—cont'd

Term	Word Origin	Definition
hypocalcemia hye poh kal SEE mee ah	*hypo-* deficient *calc/o* calcium *-emia* blood condition	Condition of deficient calcium (Ca) in the blood. The opposite is **hypercalcemia**—excessive calcium in the blood.
hypoglycemia hye poh gly SEE mee ah	*hypo-* deficient *glyc/o* sugar, glucose *-emia* blood condition	Condition of deficient sugar in the blood. The opposite is **hyperglycemia**—excessive sugar in the blood.
hypokalemia hye poh kuh LEE mee ah	*hypo-* deficient *kal/i* potassium *-emia* blood condition	Condition of deficient potassium (K) in the blood. The opposite is **hyperkalemia**—excessive potassium in the blood.
hyponatremia hye poh nuh TREE mee ah	*hypo-* deficient *natr/o* sodium *-emia* blood condition	Condition of deficient sodium (Na) in the blood. The opposite is **hypernatremia**—excessive sodium in the blood.
ketoacidosis kee toh ass ih DOH sis	*ket/o* ketone *acid/o* acid *-osis* abnormal condition	Excessive number of ketone acids in the bloodstream.
ketonuria kee toh NOOR ee ah	*keton/o* ketone *-uria* urinary condition	Presence of ketones in urine.
paresthesia pair uh STHEE zsa	*par-* abnormal *esthesi/o* feeling *-ia* condition	Abnormal sensation, such as prickling.
polydipsia pah lee DIP see ah	*poly-* excessive *-dipsia* condition of thirst	Condition of excessive thirst.
polyphagia pah lee FAY jee ah	*poly-* excessive *phag/o* to eat, swallow *-ia* condition	Condition of excessive appetite.
polyuria pah lee YOO ree ah	*poly-* excessive *ur/o* urine *-ia* condition	Condition of excessive urination.
tetany TET uh nee		Continuous muscle spasms.

Fig. 14-4 Goiter.

Fig. 14-5 Hirsutism.

EXERCISE 3: Signs and Symptoms

_____ 1. goiter

_____ 2. hirsutism

_____ 3. tetany

_____ 4. polydipsia

_____ 5. exophthalmia

_____ 6. anorexia

_____ 7. polyphagia

_____ 8. polyuria

_____ 9. ketonuria

_____ 10. ketoacidosis

A. condition of excessive appetite
B. presence of ketones in urine
C. condition of excessive urination
D. enlargement of thyroid gland
E. abnormal hairiness
F. condition of excessive thirst
G. lack of appetite
H. protrusion of eyeballs from orbits
I. excessive quantity of ketone acids in blood
J. continuous muscle spasms

Decode the terms.

11. hypoglycemia _____

12. paresthesia _____

13. hypercalcemia _____

Build the terms.

14. condition of deficient sodium in the blood _____

15. condition of excessive potassium in the blood _____

16. condition of glucose in the urine _____

Terms Related to Pituitary Gland Disorders

Term	Word Origin	Definition
acromegaly ack roh MEG uh lee	*acro-* extremities *-megaly* enlargement	Hypersecretion of somatotropin from the adenohypophysis during adulthood; leads to an enlargement of the extremities (hands and feet), jaw, nose, and forehead (Fig. 14-6). Usually caused by an adenoma of the pituitary gland.
diabetes insipidus (DI) dye ah BEE teez in SIP ih dus		Deficiency of ADH, which causes the patient to excrete large quantities of urine (**polyuria**) and exhibit excessive thirst (**polydipsia**).

Fig. 14-6 The progression of acromegaly.

Terms Related to Pituitary Gland Disorders—cont'd

Term	Word Origin	Definition
gigantism jye GAN tiz um		Hypersecretion of somatotropin from adenohypophysis during childhood, leading to excessive growth (Fig. 14-7).
growth hormone deficiency (GHD)		Somatotropin deficiency due to dysfunction of adenohypophysis during childhood results in **dwarfism** (Fig. 14-8). If the deficiency occurs during adulthood, patients may develop obesity and may experience weakness and cardiac difficulties.
panhypopituitarism pan hye poh pih TOO ih tur iz um	*pan-* all *hypo-* deficient *pituitar/o* pituitary *-ism* condition	Deficiency or lack of all pituitary hormones causing hypotension, weight loss, weakness, and loss of libido; also called **Simmonds disease.**
syndrome of inappropriate antidiuretic hormone (SIADH)		Oversecretion of ADH from the neurohypophysis leading to severe hyponatremia and the inability to excrete diluted urine.

Fig. 14-7 A case of gigantism.

Fig. 14-8 The normal 3½ year-old boy is in the 50th percentile for height. The short, 3-year-old girl exhibits the characteristic "kewpie doll" appearance, suggesting a diagnosis of growth hormone deficiency (GHD).

Case Study   *Chakor Patel*

Chakor Patel, a 25-year-old chemical engineer, has been more thirsty than normal, but thinks it might be due to the hot, dry weather. Although he could store a supply of water at his desk, he has had to deal with an expected increase in trips to the men's room. One day he decides that he can't put up with it anymore and makes an appointment with his physician. He is diagnosed with diabetes insipidus (DI). He is treated with desmopressin to replace his ADH, and he is able to cut down on his trips to the men's room.

1. Diabetes insipidus is a disorder of the _____ _____ gland.

2. Which lobe of the gland is affected?
   a. neurohypophysis
   b. adenohypophysis

3. What does ADH stand for? _____ _____

4. What is the medical term that means excessive thirst? _____

5. What is the medical term that means excessive urination? _____

Terms Related to Thyroid Disorders

Term	Word Origin	Definition
hyperthyroidism hye pur THIGH roy diz um	*hyper-* excessive *thyroid/o* thyroid gland *-ism* condition	Excessive thyroid hormone production; also called **thyrotoxicosis,** the most common form of which is **Graves disease,** which may be accompanied by exophthalmia. Ketonuria is a diagnostic sign.
hypothyroidism hye poh THIGH roy diz um	*hypo-* deficient *thyroid/o* thyroid gland *-ism* condition	Deficient thyroid hormone production. If it occurs during childhood, it causes a condition called **cretinism,** which results in stunted mental and physical growth. The extreme adult form is called **myxedema** (mick suh DEE mah), which is characterized by facial and orbital edema.

Terms Related to Parathyroid Disorders

Term	Word Origin	Definition
hyperparathyroidism hye pur pair uh THIGH roy diz um	*hyper-* excessive *parathyroid/o* parathyroid gland *-ism* condition	Overproduction of PTH; symptoms include polyuria, hypercalcemia, hypertension, and kidney stones.
hypoparathyroidism hye poh pair uh THIGH roy diz um	*hypo-* deficient *parathyroid/o* parathyroid gland *-ism* condition	Deficient PTH production results in tetany, hypocalcemia, irritability, and muscle cramps.

Terms Related to Adrenal Gland Disorders

Term	Word Origin	Definition
Addison disease ADD ih sun		Insufficient secretion of acrenal cortisol from the adrenal cortex is manifested by gastric complaints, hypotension, fatigue, and hyperpigmentation of skin and mucous membranes (Fig. 14-9).
Cushing disease CUSH ing		Excessive secretion of cortisol by the adrenal cortex causes symptoms of obesity, leukocytosis, hirsutism, hypokalemia, hyperglycemia, and muscle wasting (Fig. 14-10).

Fig. 14-9 Pigmentation of buccal membranes caused by Addison disease.

Fig. 14-10 Cushing disease. **A,** First diagnosed with Cushing disease. **B,** Four months later after treatment.

Terms Related to Pancreas (Islets of Langerhans) Disorders

Term	Word Origin	Definition
diabetes mellitus (DM)		DM is a group of metabolic disorders characterized by high glucose levels that result from inadequate amounts of insulin, resistance to insulin, or a combination of both.
type 1 diabetes		Total lack of insulin production resulting in glycosuria, polydipsia, polyphagia, polyuria, blurred vision, fatigue, and frequent infections. Thought to be an autoimmune disorder. Previously called **insulin-dependent diabetes mellitus (IDDM).**
type 2 diabetes		Deficient insulin production with symptoms similar to type 1 diabetes. Cause unknown but associated with obesity and family history; previously called **non–insulin-dependent diabetes mellitus (NIDDM).**
gestational diabetes		Insulin resistance acquired during pregnancy. Usually resolves after birth, although some women develop type 2 diabetes later in life.
hyperinsulinism hye pur IN suh lin iz um	*hyper-* excessive *insulin/o* insulin *-ism* condition	Oversecretion of insulin; seen in some newborns of diabetic mothers. Causes severe hypoglycemia.
prediabetes		A condition in which an individual's blood glucose level is higher than normal, but not high enough for a diagnosis of type 2 diabetes.

Nutritional Recommendations for Persons with Diabetes

Recommendation	Description
Calories	Sufficient to achieve and maintain reasonable weight.
Carbohydrates	May be up to 45% to 55% of total calories. Emphasis is on unrefined carbohydrates with fiber; modest amounts of sucrose and other refined sugars may be acceptable contingent on diabetes control and body weight.
Protein	Usual intake is double the amount needed; exact ideal percentage of total calories is unknown; usually, intake is 10% to 20%.
Fat	Ideally, less than 30% of total calories; must be individualized because 30% may be too low for some individuals. • Polyunsaturated fats: 6% to 8% • Saturated fats: < 10% • Monounsaturated fats: Remaining percentage
Fiber	Up to 40 g/day; 25 g/1000 cal for low-calorie diet.
Alternative sweeteners	Use of various nutritive and nonnutritive sweeteners is acceptable.
Sodium	1000 mg/1000 cal, not to exceed 3000 mg/day; modified for those with special medical conditions.
Vitamins/minerals	No evidence that diabetes influences vitamin/mineral needs.

EXERCISE 4: Diseases and Disorders of the Endocrine System

Fill in the blanks with the following choices.

type 2 diabetes, pituitary, cortex, SIADH, hypoparathyroidism, thyroid, hormones, cretinism, myxedema, type 1 diabetes

1. Most endocrine disorders are the result of an abnormal secretion of _____.

2. Graves disease is a disorder of the _____ gland.

3. Addison and Cushing diseases are endocrine disorders of the adrenal _____.

4. DI is a disorder of the _____.

5. _____ is characterized by tetany.

6. Hypothyroidism in childhood results in _____ and _____ in adults.

7. _____ is the result of oversecretion of ADH.

8. Lack of insulin leads to _____. Deficient insulin production leads to _____.

Decode the terms.

9. hyperinsulinism _____

10. hypothyroidism _____

11. acromegaly _____

Case Study   Enya Sanza

Enya Sanza, a 25-year-old graphic artist, is being treated for hypoparathyroidism. Four months ago, she experienced muscle cramps that progressed to continuous spasms. She also noticed that she felt tingling in her fingers and toes along with headaches that wouldn't seem to go away. It was the continuous spasms along with the fatigue that brought her in to see her doctor. Lab tests shows that she is deficient in calcium, and hormone tests show abnormally low PTH. Treatment includes calcium and vitamin D supplementation.

1. Hypocalcemia means that Enya has deficient _____ in her blood.

2. The term that means continuous muscle spasms is _____.

3. PTH stands for _____ _____.

4. There are a total of _____ parathyroid glands.

Terms Related to Benign Neoplasms

Term	Word Origin	Definition
pheochromocytoma fee oh kroh mah sye TOH mah	**phe/o** dark **chrom/o** color **cyt/o** cell **-oma** tumor, mass	Usually benign tumor of the adrenal medulla.
prolactinoma pro lack tih NOH mah	**prolactin/o** prolactin **-oma** tumor, mass	Most common type of pituitary tumor (Fig. 14-11). Causes the pituitary to oversecrete PRL.
thymoma thigh MOH mah	**thym/o** thymus **-oma** tumor, mass	Noncancerous tumor of epithelial origin that is often associated with myasthenia gravis.

Terms Related to Malignant Neoplasms

Term	Word Origin	Definition
islet cell carcinoma EYE let	*carcin/o* epithelial cancer *-oma* tumor, mass	Also called **pancreatic cancer;** fourth leading cause of cancer death in the United States. Treated with a Whipple procedure (pancreatoduodenectomy).
malignant thymoma thigh MOH mah	*thym/o* thymus gland *-oma* tumor, mass	Rare cancer of the thymus gland.
thyroid carcinoma kar sih NOH mah	*carcin/o* epithelial cancer *-oma* tumor, mass	The most common types of thyroid carcinoma are follicular and papillary (Fig. 14-12). Both have high 5-year survival rates.

Fig. 14-11 Pituitary tumor (prolactinoma).

Fig. 14-12 Carcinoma of the thyroid entirely replacing the gland and extending into the surrounding skeletal muscle.

EXERCISE 5: Neoplasms

Match the neoplasms with their definitions.

_____ 1. malignant thymoma

_____ 2. islet cell carcinoma

_____ 3. pheochromocytoma

_____ 4. thyroid carcinoma

_____ 5. thymoma

_____ 6. prolactinoma

A. most common type of pituitary tumor
B. rare cancer of the thymus gland
C. most common thyroid cancer
D. benign tumor of adrenal medulla
E. benign thymus tumor
F. pancreatic cancer

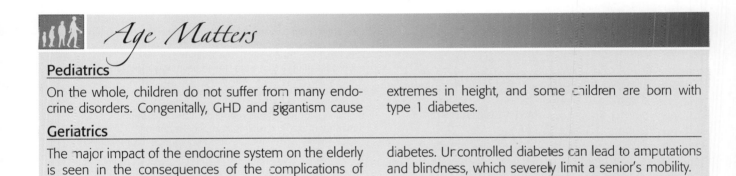

Age Matters

Pediatrics

On the whole, children do not suffer from many endocrine disorders. Congenitally, GHD and gigantism cause extremes in height, and some children are born with type 1 diabetes.

Geriatrics

The major impact of the endocrine system on the elderly is seen in the consequences of the complications of diabetes. Uncontrolled diabetes can lead to amputations and blindness, which severely limit a senior's mobility.

*Click on **Hear It, Spell It** to practice spelling the pathology terms you have learned in this chapter. To review the pathology terms in this chapter, play **Medical Millionaire**.*

⟳ EXERCISE 6: Admission History and Physical

Using the preceding form, answer the following questions.

1. Which type (number) of diabetes does this patient have? _____

2. What is the term for the eye disease that the patient has in her past history? _____

3. What particular complication of DM is this patient being seen for? _____

4. What does the term *afebrile* tell you about the patient's temperature? _____

DIAGNOSTIC PROCEDURES

Terms Related to Laboratory Tests

Term	Word Origin	Definition
A1c		Measure of average blood glucose during a 3-month time span. Used to monitor response to diabetes treatment. Also called **glycosylated hemoglobin** or **HbA1c**.
fasting plasma glucose (FPG)		After a period of fasting, blood is drawn. The amount of glucose present is used to measure the body's ability to break down and use glucose. 100 to 125 mg/dL = prediabetes; more than 126 = diabetes. Previously called **fasting blood sugar (FBS)**.
glucometer gloo KAH muh tur	*gluc/o* sugar, glucose *-meter* instrument to measure	An instrument for measurement of blood sugar.
hormone tests		Measure the amount of ADH, cortisol, GH, or PTH in the blood.
oral glucose tolerance test (OGTT)		Blood test to measure the body's response to a concentrated glucose solution. May be used to diagnose DM or gestational diabetes.
radioimmunoassay (RIA) studies ray dee oh ih myoo noh ASS say		Nuclear medicine tests used to tag and detect hormones in the blood through the use of radionuclides.
thyroid function tests (TFTs)		Blood tests done to assess T_3, T_4, and calcitonin. May be used to evaluate abnormalities of thyroid function.
total calcium		Measures the amount of calcium in the blood. Results may be used to assess parathyroid function, calcium metabolism, or cancerous conditions.
urinalysis (UA) yoor in AL ih sis	*urin/o* urine *-lysis* breaking down	Physical, chemical, and microscopic examination of urine.
urine glucose		Used as a screen for or to monitor DM; a urine specimen is tested for the presence of glucose.
urine ketones KEE tones		Test to detect presence of ketones in a urine specimen; may indicate DM or hyperthyroidism.

Terms Related to Imaging

Term	Word Origin	Definition
computed tomography (CT) scan	*tom/o* slice *-graphy* process of recording	May be used to test for bone density in hypoparathyroidism and the size of the adrenal glands in Addison disease.
magnetic resonance imaging (MRI)		May be used to examine changes in the size of soft tissues (for example, the pituitary, pancreas, or hypothalamus).
radioactive iodine uptake (RAIU) scan		May be used to test thyroid function by measuring the gland's ability to concentrate and retain iodine. Useful to test for hyperthyroidism (Fig. 14-13).
radiography	*radi/o* ray *-graphy* process of recording	X-rays are done to examine suspected endocrine changes that affect the density or thickness of bone; also may reveal underlying causes of an endocrine disorder.
sonography	*son/o* sound *-graphy* process of recording	Aside from visualizing the pancreas (Fig. 14-14), sonography may be used to guide biopsies of the thyroid gland to discern the differences between solid and fluid-filled cysts.

Fig. 14-13 Radioactive iodine uptake (RAIU) scan demonstrating hyperthyroidism. The thyroid gland absorbed 65% of the iodine.

Fig. 14-14 Transverse scan over the epigastric region of the abdomen, demonstrating a normal pancreas *(cross marks)*. AO, Aorta; *IVC,* inferior vena cava; *L,* left lobe of the liver; *SMV,* superior mesenteric vein; *arrow,* superior mesenteric artery.

EXERCISE 7: Diagnostic Procedures

Fill in the blank.

1. High-frequency sound waves may be used to image the pancreas, adrenals, or thyroid in a procedure called a/n _____.

2. Detailed images of soft tissues (such as, the pituitary, pancreas, or hypothalamus) may be acquired through a technique called _____.

3. A test used to monitor a patient's response to diabetes treatment is _____.

4. Parathyroid dysfunction may be detected through a blood test for PTH or a test for

   _____.

5. Which type of test can be used to screen for DM? _____

6. Blood sugar can be measured using a/n _____.

Case Study Evonne Wright

Evonne Wright, a 52-year-old healthcare administrator, noticed that her clothes were fitting more loosely. Although she was not dieting, a quick check on her dusty bathroom scale showed that she had lost almost ten pounds from the last time she had weighed herself. The weight loss, along with a sense that her eyes seemed to be protruding a bit, sent her to her doctor's office. A quick history and physical and clinical observation led to testing that revealed an overactive thyroid gland. Evonne is diagnosed with Graves disease and is treated with radioactive iodine.

1. The general term for an overactive thyroid gland is _____.

2. The term for the condition where eyes protrude from their sockets is _____.

3. A test that measures the thyroid gland's ability to concentrate and retain iodine is called a _____ _____.

4. The abbreviation for the lab tests for measuring the function of the thyroid gland is _____ _____.

5. The medical term for the extreme form of excessive thyroid hormone production is _____ _____.

THERAPEUTIC INTERVENTIONS

Most of the therapeutic interventions for endocrine system disorders are excisions. Unlike the case with other body systems, incisions, repairs, or new openings are not as helpful as the removal of part, or all, of the malfunctioning gland.

Terms Related to Excisions

Term	Word Origin	Definition
adrenalectomy uh dree nuh LECK tuh mee	*adrenal/o* adrenal gland *-ectomy* excision	Bilateral removal of the adrenal glands to reduce excess hormone secretion.
hypophysectomy hye poff uh SECK tuh mee	*hypophys/o* pituitary gland *-ectomy* excision	Excision of the pituitary gland; usually done to remove a pituitary tumor (Fig. 14-15).
pancreatectomy pan kree uh TECK tuh mee	*pancreat/o* pancreas *-ectomy* excision	Excision of all or part of the pancreas to remove a tumor or to treat an intractable inflammation of the pancreas.
pancreatoduodenectomy pan kree ah toh doo ah den ECK tuh mee	*pancreat/o* pancreas *duoden/o* duodenum *-ectomy* excision	Excision of the head of the pancreas together with the duodenum; used to treat pancreatic cancer. Also called **Whipple procedure.**
parathyroidectomy pair uh thigh roy DECK tuh mee	*parathyroid/o* parathyroid gland *-ectomy* excision	Removal of the parathyroid gland, usually to treat hyperparathyroidism.
thyroidectomy thigh roy DECK tuh mee	*thyroid/o* thyroid gland *-ectomy* excision	Removal of part or all of the thyroid gland to treat goiter, tumor, or hyperthyroidism that does not respond to medication. Removal of most, but not all, of this gland results in a regrowth of the gland with normal function. If cancer is detected a total thyroidectomy is performed.

Fig. 14-15 Hypophysectomy.

EXERCISE 8: Therapeutic Interventions

Build the terms.

1. excision of the pancreas _____

2. excision of the adrenal gland _____

3. excision of the pituitary gland _____

4. excision of the parathyroid gland _____

5. excision of the thyroid gland _____

PHARMACOLOGY

Most of the pharmacologic interventions for endocrine disorders are provided to correct imbalances, either inhibiting or replacing abnormal hormone levels.

antidiabetics: Manage glucose levels in the body when the pancreas or insulin receptors are no longer functioning properly. These drugs are also known as *hypoglycemic agents* and encompass various oral agents and replacement insulin. Type 1 diabetes typically requires insulin therapy. Management of type 2 diabetes begins with antidiabetics, such as metformin (Glucophage), glipizide (Glucotrol), or albiglutide (Tanzeum). Insulin is typically used as a last resort. See Figs. 14-16 and 14-17 for sites of insulin injection and an insulin pump.

antithyroid agents: Treat hyperthyroidism. Examples include methimazole (Tapazole) and propylthiouracil (PTU).

corticosteroids: Mimic or replace the body's steroids normally produced by the adrenal glands. Underfunctioning adrenal cortices (Addison disease) may be treated with prednisone (Deltasone). Corticosteroids are classified as glucosteroids and mineralocorticoids, depending on structure and function.

growth hormones: Treat various disease-causing growth inhibitions. Human growth hormone (hGH) is available as the prescription somatropin (Genotropin, Nutropin).

posterior pituitary hormones: Vasopressin and desmopressin acetate are used to treat diabetes insipidus.

thyroid hormones: Treat hypothyroidism. Examples include natural thyroid hormones (Armour Thyroid) and levothyroxine (Levoxyl, Synthroid).

Fig. 14-16 Sites for insulin injection.

Indwelling subcutaneous needle

Insulin pump

Subcutaneous tissue

Fig. 14-17 Insulin pump. The device is worn externally and is connected to an indwelling subcutaneous needle, which is usually inserted into the abdomen.

 EXERCISE 9: Pharmacology

Match the pharmacologic agent with the correct disease or disorder.

_____ 1. insulin

_____ 2. prednisone

_____ 3. vasopressin

_____ 4. Synthroid

    A. Addison disease
    B. hypothyroidism
    C. diabetes mellitus (DM)
    D. diabetes insipidus (DI)

Case Study   Roma Steen

Roma Steen wears purple in honor of her Uncle Ted who died of pancreatic cancer last year. He had been having problems with abdominal pain, bloating, and nausea last Thanksgiving. The cancer was diagnosed after testing that included ultrasound of the pancreas. When he was diagnosed, his cancer had not yet spread beyond the pancreas, but despite chemotherapy and a pancreatoduodenectomy, he died in early spring. Roma hopes that someday soon, there will be a way to diagnose pancreatic cancer earlier so that it can be treated more effectively.

1. The pancreas functions as an exocrine as well as a/n _____ gland.

2. Another name for a pancreatoduodenectomy is a/n _____ procedure.

3. The imaging procedure that uses ultrasound to detect abnormal growths within the body is _____.

4. Another term for pancreatic cancer is _____ _____.

5. *Duoden/o* in the term pancreatoduodenectomy refers to the first part of the _____ _____.

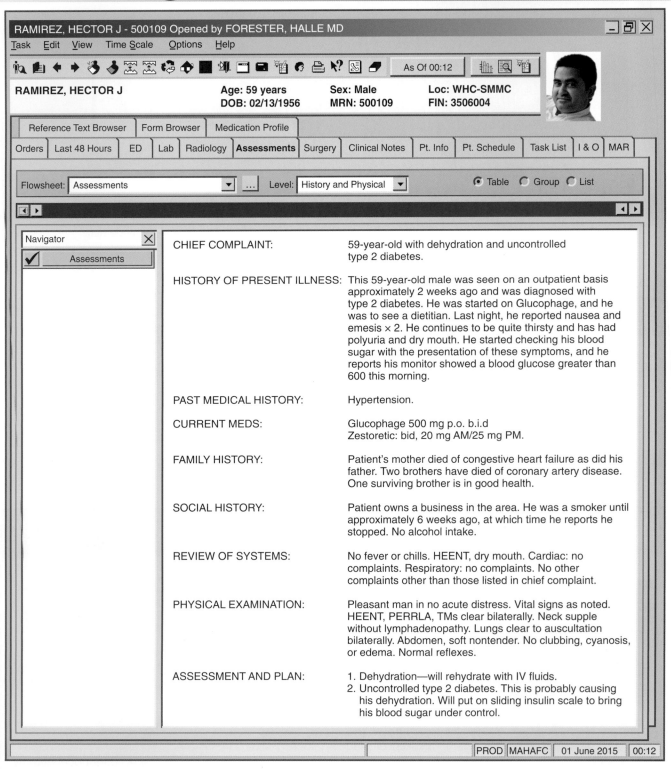

Medical Record — Hector Ramirez

RAMIREZ, HECTOR J - 500109 Opened by FORESTER, HALLE MD

Task   Edit   View   Time Scale   Options   Help

As Of 00:12

RAMIREZ, HECTOR J   Age: 59 years   Sex: Male   Loc: WHC-SMMC
DOB: 02/13/1956   MRN: 500109   FIN: 3506004

Reference Text Browser | Form Browser | Medication Profile

Orders | Last 48 Hours | ED | Lab | Radiology | **Assessments** | Surgery | Clinical Notes | Pt. Info | Pt. Schedule | Task List | I & O | MAR

Flowsheet: Assessments   Level: History and Physical   ⦿ Table ○ Group ○ List

Navigator
✓ Assessments

CHIEF COMPLAINT:	59-year-old with dehydration and uncontrolled type 2 diabetes.
HISTORY OF PRESENT ILLNESS:	This 59-year-old male was seen on an outpatient basis approximately 2 weeks ago and was diagnosed with type 2 diabetes. He was started on Glucophage, and he was to see a dietitian. Last night, he reported nausea and emesis × 2. He continues to be quite thirsty and has had polyuria and dry mouth. He started checking his blood sugar with the presentation of these symptoms, and he reports his monitor showed a blood glucose greater than 600 this morning.
PAST MEDICAL HISTORY:	Hypertension.
CURRENT MEDS:	Glucophage 500 mg p.o. b.i.d Zestoretic: bid, 20 mg AM/25 mg PM.
FAMILY HISTORY:	Patient's mother died of congestive heart failure as did his father. Two brothers have died of coronary artery disease. One surviving brother is in good health.
SOCIAL HISTORY:	Patient owns a business in the area. He was a smoker until approximately 6 weeks ago, at which time he reports he stopped. No alcohol intake.
REVIEW OF SYSTEMS:	No fever or chills. HEENT, dry mouth. Cardiac: no complaints. Respiratory: no complaints. No other complaints other than those listed in chief complaint.
PHYSICAL EXAMINATION:	Pleasant man in no acute distress. Vital signs as noted. HEENT, PERRLA, TMs clear bilaterally. Neck supple without lymphadenopathy. Lungs clear to auscultation bilaterally. Abdomen, soft nontender. No clubbing, cyanosis, or edema. Normal reflexes.
ASSESSMENT AND PLAN:	1. Dehydration—will rehydrate with IV fluids. 2. Uncontrolled type 2 diabetes. This is probably causing his dehydration. Will put on sliding insulin scale to bring his blood sugar under control.

PROD | MAHAFC | 01 June 2015 | 00:12

---

*Click on **Hear It, Spell It** to practice spelling the diagnostic and therapeutic terms that you have learned in this chapter.*

EXERCISE 10: Admission History and Physical

Using the preceding form, answer the following questions.

1. What type of diabetes does this patient have? _____

2. What is the complication that he has? _____

3. What medication is he taking for his diabetes? _____

4. What treatment is being performed for his complication? _____

Abbreviations

Abbreviation	Meaning
A1c	average glucose level
ACTH	adrenocorticotropic hormone
ADH	antidiuretic hormone
Ca	calcium
Dl	diabetes insipidus
FBS	fasting blood sugar
FPG	fasting plasma glucose
FSH	follicle-stimulating hormone
GH	growth hormone
GHD	growth hormone deficiency
hGH	human growth hormone
ICSH	interstitial cell-stimulating hormone
IDDM	insulin-dependent diabetes mellitus
K	potassium
LH	luteinizing hormone
Na	sodium

Abbreviation	Meaning
NIDDM	non–insulin-dependent diabetes mellitus
OGTT	oral glucose tolerance test
OT	oxytocin
PGH	pituitary growth hormone
PRL	prolactin
PTH	parathyroid hormone
RAIU	radioactive iodine uptake (scan)
RIA	radioimmunoassay
SIADH	syndrome of inappropriate antidiuretic hormone
STH	somatotropic hormone
T_3	triiodothyronine
T_4	thyroxine
TFT	thyroid function test
TSH	thyroid-stimulating hormone
UA	urinalysis

EXERCISE 11: Abbreviations

Match the abbreviations with their definitions.

_____ 1. Ca   _____ 5. DI

_____ 2. K   _____ 6. OGTT

_____ 3. Na   _____ 7. ADH

_____ 4. OT

A. diabetes insipidus
B. oxytocin
C. potassium
D. oral glucose tolerance test
E. calcium
F. sodium
G. antidiuretic hormone

Match the word parts to their definitions.

Word Part Definitions

Prefix/Suffix

acro-
-crine
-ectomy
-emia
endo-
exo-
-graphy
hyper-
hypo-
pan-
poly-
supra-

Definition

1. _____ process of recording
2. _____ all
3. _____ within
4. _____ excessive
5. _____ above
6. _____ deficient
7. _____ blood condition
8. _____ outward
9. _____ to secrete
10. _____ extremities
11. _____ excessive
12. _____ excision

Combining Form

aden/o
adren/o
calc/o
crin/o
chrom/o
cyt/o
gluc/o
glyc/o
gonad/o
hypophys/o
kal/i
natr/o
pancreat/o
parathyroid/o
phe/o
pituitar/o
thalam/o
thym/o
thyr/o
trop/o

Definition

13. _____ potassium
14. _____ pituitary gland
15. _____ color
16. _____ sodium
17. _____ glucose, sugar
18. _____ gonads
19. _____ parathyroid gland
20. _____ turning
21. _____ gland
22. _____ thymus gland
23. _____ sugar, glucose
24. _____ dark
25. _____ to secrete
26. _____ thyroid gland
27. _____ thalamus
28. _____ adrenal gland
29. _____ calcium
30. _____ pancreas
31. _____ cell
32. _____ pituitary gland

Wordshop

Prefixes	Combining Forms	Suffixes
a-	blephar/o	-opia
an-	phak/o	-ia
par-	chromat/o	-opsia
para-	dacryoaden/o	-rrhea
presby-	dacryocyst/o	-ptosis
micro-	nas/o	-ectomy
	rhin/o	-cusis
	lacrim/o	-tomy
	phot/o	-sclerosis
	ton/o	-itis
	labyrinth/o	-metry
	ot/o	-stomy
	audi/o	-al
	tympan/o	-phobia

Build the following terms by combining the preceding word parts. Some word parts may be used more than once. Some may not be used at all. The number in parentheses is the number of word parts needed to build the terms.

Definition	Term
1. condition of excessive sodium in the blood (3)	_____
2. enlargement of the extremities (2)	_____
3. condition of sugar in the urine (2)	_____
4. condition of an eye (that protrudes) outward (3)	_____
5. instrument to measure (blood) sugar (2)	_____
6. condition of excessive urination (2)	_____
7. condition of ketones in the urine (2)	_____
8. abnormal condition of acidity due to ketones (3)	_____
9. condition of excessive eating (3)	_____
10. condition of abnormal sensation (2)	_____
11. removal of the parathyroid gland (2)	_____
12. condition of excessive thirst (2)	_____
13. study of the glands that secrete within (3)	_____
14. condition of excessive blood sugar (3)	_____
15. condition of deficient potassium in the blood (3)	_____

Sort the terms into the correct categories.

Term Sorting

Anatomy and Physiology	Pathology	Diagnostic Procedures	Therapeutic Interventions

A1c	GH	MRI	RAIU
ACTH	GHD	OGTT	RIA
adrenalectomy	gigantism	orchiectomy	SIADH
anorexia	glucagon	OT	sonography
antidiabetics	glucometer	pancreas	TFT
cortex	goiter	pancreatectomy	thymectomy
DI	hirsutism	pancreatoduodenectomy	thymoma
endocrine	hyperinsulinism	parathyroidectomy	thyroidectomy
epinephrine	hypophysectomy	polydipsia	UA
FPG	hypophysis	prednisone	vasopressin

Replace the highlighted words with the correct terms.

Translations

1. After experiencing **condition of excessive thirst** and **condition of excessive urination,** Tilda was diagnosed with diabetes insipidus.

2. Victor's **protrusion of eyeballs from their orbits** was caused by **condition of excessive thyroid production.**

3. Moira went to the endocrinologist with symptoms of **condition of deficient calcium production** and **continuous muscle spasms.** She was diagnosed with **condition of deficient parathyroid hormone production.**

4. The child suffered from **deficient thyroid hormone production that occurs in childhood.** Her aunt suffered from the **extreme adult form of deficient hormone production.**

5. Soo Lin had **abnormal hairiness,** easy bruising, **condition of excessive sugar in the blood** and **condition of deficient potassium in the blood,** which led to a diagnosis of Cushing disease.

6. The patient's **condition of oversecretion of insulin** caused a **severe condition of deficient sugar in the blood.**

7. Franco had **a pancreatic cancer,** which was treated with an **excision of the head of the pancreas and the duodenum.**

8. The patient with **total lack of insulin production** was instructed to purchase **an instrument for measurement of blood sugar.**

9. A **partial removal of the thyroid gland** was performed to treat thepatient's **enlargement of the thyroid gland not due to a tumor.**

10. Severe **condition of deficient sodium in the blood** and the inability to excrete diluted urine were two symptoms of **oversecretion of ADH from the neurohypophysis.**

11. Kyonia's **insulin resistance acquired during pregnancy** developed into **deficient insulin production** when she was in her forties.

12. After undergoing **a blood test done after fasting,** Mrs. Brown was diagnosed with a **condition in which an individual's blood glucose level is higher than normal, but not high enough for type 2 diabetes.**

13. When she was an adult, Martha developed **enlargement of the extremities** due to hypersecretion of somatotropin from the **anterior part of her pituitary gland.**

14. Maria suffered from **lack of appetite** and **abnormal sensation of prickling.**

Medical Record Darren Williams

WILLIAMS, DARREN D - 492891 Opened by BURNS, CHRISTOPHER MD

Task   Edit   View   Time Scale   Options   Help

As Of 10:23

| WILLIAMS, DARREN D | Age: 57 years | Sex: Male | Loc: WHC-SMMC |
| | DOB: 08/13/1957 | MRN: 492891 | FIN: 3506004 |

Reference Text Browser | Form Browser | Medication Profile

Orders | Last 48 Hours | ED | Lab | Radiology | Assessments | Surgery | **Clinical Notes** | Pt. Info | Pt. Schedule | Task List | I & O | MAR

Flowsheet: Clinical Notes   ...   Level: Office Visit   ⦿ Table   ○ Group   ○ List

Navigator
✓ Office Visit

HISTORY OF PRESENT ILLNESS: This is a return visit to the office for the patient with history of hypothyroidism. He is 57 years old. His last visit was about 6 months ago. Since that time, the patient states his health has remained unchanged. Currently, primary complaint is one of fatigue that he feels throughout the day. Patient states that he is not having signs or symptoms of thyroid excess or hypothyroidism. His weight has been stable. He is not reporting proximal muscle weakness.

CURRENT MEDICATIONS:
Levothyroxine 125 micrograms p.o. once daily; Glucotrol; Avandamet; Synthroid; Byetta injected twice daily.

PHYSICAL EXAMINATION:
GENERAL: Patient is an overweight, very peasant man, in no acute distress. VITAL SIGNS: Temperature 96.9, pulse 85, respirations not counted, blood pressure 135/65, and weight 85.7 kg. NECK: Reveals well healed surgical scar in the anteroinferior aspect of the neck. There is no palpable thyroid tissue noted on this examination today. There is no lymphadeno-pathy. THORAX: Reveals lungs that are clear, PA and lateral, without adventitous sounds. CARDIOVASCULAR: Demonstrated regular rate and rhythm. S1 and S2 without murmur. No S3, no S4 is auscultated. EXTREMITIES: Deep tendon reflexes 2+/4 without a delayed relaxation phase. No fine resting tremor of the outstretched upper extremity. SKIN, HAIR, AND NAILS: All are unremarkable.

LABORATORY DATABASE: Lab data on 08/18/14 showed the following: Thyroglobulin quantitative less than 0.5 and thyroglobulin antibody less than 20, free T4 1.35, and TSH suppressed at 0.121.

ASSESSMENT AND PLAN:
1. Acquired hypothyroidism, status post total thyroidectomy for papillary carcinoma in 2012.
2. Plan to continue following thyroglobulin levels.
3. Plan to obtain a free T4, TSH, and thyroglobulin levels today.
4. Have the patient call the clinic next week for followup and continued management of his hypothyroid state.
5. Plan today is to repeat his thyroid function studies. This case was discussed with Dr. Xavier and his recommendation is for us to taper his medication to get his TSH somewhere between 0.41 or less. Therefore, labs have been drawn. We plan to see the patient back in approximately 6 months.

PROD | MAHAFC | 18 Aug 2014 | 10:23

OFFICE VISIT SUMMARY

Using the preceding office visit summary, answer the following questions.

1. Mr. Williams has hypothyroidism. Does he have excessive or deficient thyroid production?

   _____

2. What is the extreme form of hypothyroidism called? _____

3. The childhood form of hypothyroidism is called _____.

4. A T$_4$ assessment is a type of TFT or _____.

5. TSH stands for _____.

6. TSH is also known as _____.

15 Mental and Behavioral Health

OBJECTIVES

- Understand the role of DSM-5 and definitions of mental and behavioral health.
- Recognize and use terms related to the pathology of mental and behavioral health.

- Recognize and use terms related to the diagnostic procedures for mental and behavioral health.
- Recognize and use terms related to the therapeutic interventions for mental and behavioral health.

For interactive learning go to the Shiland Evolve website, and click on:
- **Match the Word Parts** to review mental and behavioral health word parts.
- **Word Shop** to practice word building.
- **Tournament of Terminology** to test your knowledge of mental and behavioral health terms.
- **Term Sorting** to practice sorting mental and behavioral health terms into categories.

*Click on **Chapter at a Glance** to print off a list of key terms and word parts for this chapter.*

INTRODUCTION TO MENTAL AND BEHAVIORAL HEALTH

Many body system disorders are described by their abnormal laboratory, physical, or clinical findings, but mental and behavioral disorders are not as easily defined. In the United States, the American Psychiatric Association (APA) publishes the official listing of diagnosable mental and behavioral disorders called the *Diagnostic and Statistical Manual of Mental Disorders*. This manual is now in its fifth edition (DSM-5). This revision will eventually result in a closer alignment to the International Classification of Diseases, 10th revision (ICD-10) and its single axis format.

Consider the following:

- One of every four American adults and children has been diagnosed with a mental condition.
- More than 30% of the 20 top-selling medications are for psychiatric disorders.
- The fourth most common diagnostic category for inpatient admissions is substance-related mental disorders.
- Approximately 40 million Americans are diagnosed with anxiety.
- The number of discharges for patients with substance-related mental health disorders has sharply escalated from 20,000 in 1998 to 110,000 in 2008.
- Approximately 7.5 million Americans are classified as mentally retarded.*

Given these statistics, the terminology related to mental and behavioral disorders is content that cannot be ignored.

Mental health may be defined as a relative state of mind in which a person who is healthy is able to cope with and adjust to the recurrent stresses of everyday living in a culturally acceptable way. Thus mental illness may be generally defined as a functional impairment that substantially interferes with or limits one or more major life activities for a significant duration.

The term *behavioral health* reflects an integration of the outdated concept of the separate nature of the body (physical health/illness) and the mind (mental health/illness). Advances in research continually acknowledge the roles of culture, environment, and spirituality in influencing physical and behavioral health. The use of the term *behavior* refers to observable, measurable activities that may be used to evaluate the progress of treatment.

Similar to previous chapters, this chapter examines disorders that result when an individual has a maladaptive response to his or her environment (internal or external). (See Chapter 12 for an explanation of the anatomy and physiology of the brain and nervous system.) However, even though some mental illnesses have organic causes in which neurotransmitters and other known brain functions play a role, there is no mental "anatomy" per se. Instead, behavioral health is a complex interaction among an individual's emotional, physical, mental, and behavioral processes in an environment that includes cultural and spiritual influences.

SPECIALTIES/SPECIALISTS

Psychologists work with the diagnosis and treatment of mental health disorders. Most psychologists will have a doctoral degree (PhD or PsyD). Their specialty is psychology. **Psychiatrists** are medical doctors who specialize in the treatment of mental health disorders. Their discipline is **psychiatry.**

mind = psych/o, thym/o, phren/o

treatment = iatr/o

 Be Careful!

Don't confuse **psychiatry,** *the treatment of mental disorders,* with **physiatry,** *the treatment of physical disorders*

psychologist
  psych/o = mind
  -logist = one who specializes in the study of

psychiatrist
  psych/o = mind
  -iatrist = one who specializes in treatment

---

*It should be noted that mental retardation (MR) is not an illness; it is a condition characterized by developmental delays and difficulty with learning and social situations.

Combining and Adjective Forms for Mental Health

Meaning	Combining Form	Adjective Form
attraction	phil/o	
mind	psych/o, thym/o, phren/o	psychic, thymic
treatment	iatr/o	

Suffixes for Mental Health

Suffix	Meaning
-ia, -ism	condition
-iatrist	one who specializes in treatment
-mania	condition of madness
-phobia	condition of fear

PATHOLOGY

Terms Related to General Symptoms

Term	Word Origin	Definition
akathisia ack uh THEE zsa	*a-* lack of *kathis/o* sitting *-ia* condition	Inability to remain calm, still, and free of anxiety.
amnesia am NEE zsa		Inability to remember either isolated parts of the past or one's entire past; may be caused by brain damage or severe emotional trauma.
anhedonia an hee DOH nee ah	*an-* without *hedon/o* pleasure *-ia* condition	Absence of the ability to experience either pleasure or joy, even in the face of causative events.
catatonia kat tah TOH nee ah	*cata-* down *ton/o* tension *-ia* condition	Paralysis or immobility from psychological or emotional rather than physical causes.
confabulation kon fab byoo LAY shun		Effort to conceal a gap in memory by fabricating detailed, often believable stories. Associated with alcohol abuse.
defense mechanism		Unconscious mechanism for psychological coping, adjustment, or self-preservation in the face of stress or a threat. Examples include **denial** of an unpleasant situation or condition and **projection** of intolerable aspects onto another individual.

Terms Related to General Symptoms—cont'd

Term	Word Origin	Definition
delirium dih LEER ree um		Condition of confused, unfocused, irrational agitation. In mental disorders, agitation and confusion may also be accompanied by a more intense disorientation, incoherence, or fear, and illusions, hallucinations, and delusions.
delusion dih LOO zhun		Persistent belief in a demonstrable untruth or a provable inaccurate perception despite clear evidence to the contrary.
dementia dih MEN shah		Mental disorder in which the individual experiences a progressive loss of memory, personality alterations, confusion, loss of touch with reality, and **stupor** (seeming unawareness of, and disconnection with, one's surroundings).
echolalia eh koh LAYL yuh	*echo-* reverberation *-lalia* condition of babbling	Repetition of words or phrases spoken by others.
hallucination hah loo sih NAY shun		Any unreal sensory perception that occurs with no external cause.
illusion ill LOO zhun		Inaccurate sensory perception based on a real stimulus; examples include mirages and interpreting music or wind as voices.
libido lih BEE doh		Normal psychological impulse drive associated with sensuality, expressions of desire, or creativity. Abnormality occurs only when such drives are excessively heightened or depressed.
psychosis sye KOH sis	*psych/o* mind *-osis* abnormal condition	Disassociation with or impaired perception of reality; may be accompanied by hallucinations, delusions, incoherence, akathisia, and/or disorganized behavior.
somnambulism som NAM byoo liz um	*somn/o* sleep *ambul/o* walking *-ism* condition	Sleepwalking.

 Be Careful! *Don't confuse* **delusion**, *a persistent belief in an untruth, with* **illusion**, *an inaccurate sensory perception based on a real stimulus.*

Affects

Affects are observable demonstrations of emotion that can be described in terms of quality, range, and appropriateness. The following list defines the most significant affects encountered in behavioral health:

blunted: Moderately reduced range of affect.
flat: The diminishment or loss of emotional expression sometimes observed in schizophrenia, MR, and some depressive disorders.
labile: Multiple, abrupt changes in affect seen in certain types of schizophrenia and bipolar disorder (BD).
full/wide range of affect: Generally appropriate emotional response.

Terms Related to Moods

Term	Word Origin	Definition
anxiety		Anticipation of impending danger and dread accompanied by restlessness, tension, tachycardia, and breathing difficulty not associated with an apparent stimulus.
dysphoria dis FOR ree ah	*dys-* abnormal *phor/o* to carry, to bear *-ia* condition	Generalized negative mood characterized by depression.
euphoria yoo FOR ree ah	*eu-* good, well *phor/o* to carry, to bear *-ia* condition	Exaggerated sense of physical and emotional well-being not based on reality, disproportionate to the cause, or inappropriate to the situation.
euthymia yoo THIGH mee ah	*eu-* good, well *-thymia* condition of the mind	Normal range of moods and emotions.

⊗ **Be Careful!** *The suffix* **-thymia** *means a condition of the mind, but* **thym/o** *refers to the thymus gland or to the mind.*

 EXERCISE 1: Symptoms, Affects, and Moods of Mental Illness

Matching.

_____ 1. delusion

_____ 2. hallucination

_____ 3. dementia

_____ 4. dysphoria

_____ 5. amnesia

_____ 6. akathisia

_____ 7. confabulation

_____ 8. delirium

_____ 9. catatonia

_____ 10. illusion

_____ 11. libido

A. paralysis from psychological causes
B. lack of memory
C. restlessness, inability to sit still
D. normal drive of sensuality, creativity, desire
E. mental condition characterized by confusion and agitation
F. inaccurate sensory perception based on a real stimulus
G. belief in a falsehood
H. negative mood characterized by depression
I. making up stories to conceal lack of memory
J. unreal sensory perception
K. condition characterized by loss of memory, personality changes, confusion, and loss of touch with reality

Circle the correct answer.

12. Anger, anxiety, and dysphoria are examples of a patient's *(affect, mood)*.

13. Individuals whose emotions change rapidly are said to have a *(labile, blunted)* affect.

14. Patients who subconsciously blame another person for their own problems are using a defense mechanism called *(denial, projection)*.

Build the term.

15. abnormal condition of the mind _____

16. condition of sleep walking _____

17. condition of well mind _____

18. condition of no pleasure _____

Terms Related to Disorders Usually First Diagnosed in Childhood

Term	Word Origin	Definition
attention-deficit/ hyperactivity disorder (ADHD)		Series of syndromes that includes impulsiveness, inability to concentrate, and short attention span.
conduct disorder		Any of a number of disorders characterized by patterns of persistent aggressive and defiant behaviors. **Oppositional defiant disorder (ODD),** an example of a conduct disorder, is characterized by hostile, disobedient behavior.
mental retardation (MR)		Condition of subaverage intellectual ability, with impairments in social and educational functioning. The intelligence quotient (IQ) is a measure of an individual's intellectual functioning compared with the general population. DSM-5 refers to this condition as **intellectual disability,** but the renaming has caused debate. **Mild MR:** IQ range of 50 to 69; learning difficulties result. **Moderate MR:** IQ range of 35 to 49; support needed to function in society. **Severe MR:** IQ of 20 to 34; continuous need for support to live in society. **Profound MR:** IQ less than 20; severe self-care limitations.
autism spectrum disorder (ASD)		A group of developmental delay disorders characterized by impairment of communication skills and social interactions.
autistic disorder ah TISS tick	*auto-* self *-istic* pertaining to	Condition of abnormal development of social interaction, impaired communication (including delayed language acquisition), and repetitive behaviors.
Asperger disorder AS pur gur		Disorder characterized by impairment of social interaction and repetitive patterns of inappropriate behavior without the delays of language acquisition and cognitive functions of autistic disorder.

EXERCISE 2: Disorders Usually First Diagnosed in Childhood

Choose the correct answer from the following list.

ADHD, mild MR, severe MR, autistic disorder, Asperger disorder, conduct disorder, ODD, moderate MR

1. Type of MR in which the IQ range is 20 to 34. _____

2. Disorder characterized by impairment of social interaction caused by repetitive patterns of inappropriate behavior without language delay. _____

3. Group of disorders characterized by persistent aggressive and defiant behaviors. _____

4. IQ range of 50 to 69. Most prevalent form of MR, which manifests itself in learning difficulties. _____

5. IQ range of 35 to 49. Adults will need support to live in society. _____

6. A series of syndromes that include impulsiveness, inability to concentrate, and a short attention span. _____

7. Condition of pathologic social withdrawal, impairment of communication, and repetitive behaviors, along with language delay. _____

8. Persistent negative behavior characterized by hostile, disobedient behavior. _____

Substance-Related Disorders

The most rapidly increasing group of disorders is substance-related disorders. These include abuse of a number of substances, including alcohol, opioids, cannabinoids, sedatives or hypnotics, cocaine, stimulants (including caffeine), hallucinogens, tobacco, and volatile solvents (inhalants). Classifications for substance abuse include psychotic, amnesiac, and late-onset disorders. It is important to be aware that addiction is not a character flaw. Rather, addiction has a neurologic basis; the effects of specific drugs are localized to equally specific areas of the brain.

An individual is considered an "abuser" if he or she uses substances in ways that threaten health or impair social or economic functioning. Levels of abuse vary.

Terms Related to Substance Abuse

Term	Word Origin	Definition
acute intoxication	*in-* in *toxic/o* poison *-ation* process of	Episode of behavioral disturbance following ingestion of alcohol or psychotropic drugs.
delirium tremens (DTs) deh LEER ee um TREM uns		Acute and sometimes fatal delirium induced by the cessation of ingesting excessive amounts of alcohol over a long period of time.
dependence syndrome		Difficulty in controlling use of a drug.
harmful use		Pattern of drug use that causes damage to health.
tolerance		State in which the body becomes accustomed to the substances ingested; hence the user requires greater amounts to create the desired effect.
withdrawal state		Group of symptoms that occur during cessation of the use of a regularly taken drug.

Case Study Curtis Rossner

Curtis Rossner developed a drinking problem when he was a college student. He drank on weekends to celebrate the end of grueling study sessions during the week, but later he started to drink during the week also. He continued to drink after getting a job in finance because the hours were grueling. Twice he remembers blacking out from drinking shots, and he realizes that he has a problem when he wakes up one morning sitting in his car on the side of the road with no idea of how he got there. His friends encourage him to make an appointment with an addiction counselor, who can help him deal with his issues with alcohol.

1. What is the term for a state in which the body becomes accustomed to the substances it ingests, causing the user to require greater amounts to achieve the desired effect?
   a. acute intoxication
   b. dependence syndrome
   c. harmful use
   d. tolerance

2. What is the term for a pattern of substance use that causes damage to health?
   a. acute intoxication
   b. dependence syndrome
   c. harmful use
   d. tolerance

3. Difficulty in controlling use of a substance is called _____ syndrome?
   a. acute intoxication
   b. dependence
   c. harmful use
   d. tolerance

4. An episode of behavioral disturbance following ingestion of alcohol or a psychotropic drug is called acute _____.

5. A _____ state is a group of symptoms that occur during cessation of the use of a regularly taken drug.
   a. acute intoxication
   b. dependence syndrome
   c. harmful use
   d. withdrawal

Fig. 15-1 A, Drawing by a delusional patient with schizophrenia. **B,** This drawing by a patient with schizophrenia demonstrates thought disorder.

Terms Related to Schizophrenia and Delusional Disorders

Term	Word Origin	Definition
acute and transient psychotic disorders		Group of disorders characterized by the acute onset (2 weeks or less) of psychotic symptoms (such as, delusions, hallucinations, and perceptual disturbances) and by the severe disruption of ordinary behavior. Condition is not severe enough to justify a diagnosis of delirium. May be associated with acute stress.
persistent delusional disorders		Variety of disorders in which long-standing delusions constitute the only clinical characteristic.
schizophrenia	*schiz/o* split *-phrenia* condition of mind	Disorders characterized by fundamental distortions of thinking and perception, coupled with affects that are inappropriate or blunted (Fig. 15-1).

⊗ Be Careful! *The combining form* **phren/o** *can mean mind or diaphragm.*

 EXERCISE 3: Substance Abuse and Schizophrenic Disorders

Fill in the blanks with the following terms.

schizophrenia, persistent delusional, alcohol, inhalants, controlling substance use

1. A patient with the DTs is showing withdrawal symptoms from _____.

2. Volatile solvents are included under the category of _____.

3. Dependence syndrome is a condition in which the patient has difficulty _____.

4. Auditory hallucinations, delusions, and thought disturbances are characteristic of _____.

5. The only, or most conspicuous, clinical characteristic of patients with _____ disorders is the presence of long-standing aberrant beliefs or perceptions.

Case Study   Mirasol Bebanco

Mirasol Bebanco is a 19-year-old student who is being seen for treatment for schizophrenia. She started hearing voices when she turned 18, and the condition worsened until one day the voices told her to attack shoppers in her local supermarket. Aside from the voices and feelings of persecution, her family said that Mirasol seemed to have no emotion and just didn't seem herself. Now that she is in therapy and on medication, she is able to talk to her family about the disorder and is able to express her emotions more fully.

1. An unreal sensory perception that occurs without an external cause is a/n _____.
   a. illusion   b. delusion
   c. hallucination   d. phobia

2. A persistent belief in a demonstrable untruth is a/n _____.
   a. illusion   b. delusion
   c. hallucination   d. phobia

3. What does the combining form *phren/o* mean?
   _____

4. The term for the condition characterized by fundamental distortions of thinking and perception is____
   _____.

5. What kind of affect is one that means the patient shows no emotion?
   a. flat   b. labile
   c. full   d. blunted

Mood Disorders

Patients with mood disorders, also called *affective disorders,* show a disturbance of affect ranging from depression (with or without associated anxiety) to elation. The mood change is usually accompanied by a change in the overall level of activity; most of the other symptoms are either secondary to, or easily understood in the context of, the change in mood and activity. Most of these disorders tend to be recurrent, and the onset of individual episodes can often be related to stressful events or situations.

Terms Related to Mood Disorders

Term	Word Origin	Definition
bipolar disorder (BD), BP bye POH lur	*bi-* two *pol/o* pole *-ar* pertaining to	Disorder characterized by swings between an elevation of mood, increased energy and activity (hypomania and mania), and a lowering of mood and decreased energy and activity (depression).
cyclothymia sye kloh THIGH mee ah	*cycl/o* recurring *-thymia* condition of the mind	Disorder characterized by recurring episodes of mild elation and depression that are not severe enough to warrant a diagnosis of BD.

Continued

Terms Related to Mood Disorders—cont'd

Term	Word Origin	Definition
depressive disorder		Depression typically characterized by its degree (minimal, moderate, or severe) or number of occurrences (single or recurrent, persistent). Patient exhibits dysphoria, reduction of energy, and decrease in activity. Symptoms include anhedonia, lack of ability to concentrate, and fatigue. Patient may experience **parasomnias** (abnormal sleep patterns), diminished appetite, and loss of self-esteem.
dysthymia dis THIGH mee ah	*dys-* difficult *-thymia* condition of the mind	Mild, chronic depression of mood that lasts for years but is not severe enough to justify a diagnosis of depression.
hypomania hye poh MAY nee ah	*hypo-* decreased *-mania* condition of madness	Disorder characterized by an inappropriate elevation of mood that may include positive and negative aspects. Patient may report increased feelings of well-being, energy, and activity but may also report irritability and conceit.
persistent mood disorders		Group of long-term, cyclic mood disorders in which the majority of the individual episodes are not sufficiently severe to warrant being described as hypomanic or mild depressive episodes.
seasonal affective disorder (SAD)		Weather-induced depression resulting from decreased exposure to sunlight in autumn and winter.

Terms Related to Anxiety Disorders

Term	Word Origin	Definition
acrophobia ack roh FOH bee ah	*acro-* heights, extremities *-phobia* condition of fear	Fear of heights.
agoraphobia ah gore uh FOH bee ah	*agora-* marketplace *-phobia* condition of fear	Fear of leaving home and entering crowded places.
anthropophobia an throh poh FOH bee ah	*anthrop/o* man *-phobia* condition of fear	Fear of scrutiny by other people; also called **social phobia.**
claustrophobia klos troh FOH bee ah	*claustr/o* a closing *-phobia* condition of fear	Fear of enclosed spaces.
generalized anxiety disorder (GAD)		One of the most common diagnoses assigned but not specific to any particular situation or circumstance. Symptoms may include persistent nervousness, trembling, muscular tensions, sweating, lightheadedness, palpitations, dizziness, and epigastric discomfort.
obsessive-compulsive disorder (OCD)		Characterized by recurrent, distressing, and unavoidable preoccupations or irresistible drives to perform specific rituals (e.g., constantly checking locks, excessive hand washing) that the patient feels will prevent some harmful event.

Terms Related to Anxiety Disorders—cont'd

Term	Word Origin	Definition
panic disorder (PD)		Recurrent, unpredictable attacks of severe anxiety (panic) that are not restricted to any particular situation. Symptoms may include vertigo, chest pain, and heart palpitations.
posttraumatic stress disorder (PTSD)		Extended emotional response to a traumatic event. Symptoms may include flashbacks, recurring nightmares, anhedonia, insomnia, hypervigilance, anxiety, depression, suicidal thoughts, and emotional blunting.

Terms Related to Adjustment Disorder, Dissociative Identity Disorder, and Somatoform Disorder

Term	Word Origin	Definition
adjustment disorder		Disorder that tends to manifest during periods of stressful life changes (e.g., divorce, death, relocation, job loss). Symptoms include anxiety, impaired coping mechanisms, social dysfunction, and a reduced ability to perform normal daily activities.
dissociative identity disorder		Maladaptive coping with severe stress by developing one or more separate personalities. A less severe form, **dissociative disorder** or **dissociative reaction,** results in identity confusion accompanied by amnesia, a dreamlike state, and somnambulism.
somatoform disorder soh MAT toh form	*somat/o* body	Any disorder that has unfounded physical complaints by the patient, despite medical assurance that no physiologic problem exists. One type of somatoform disorder is **illness anxiety disorder,** which is the preoccupation with the possibility of having one or more serious and progressive physical disorders.

Terms Related to Eating Disorders

Term	Word Origin	Definition
anorexia nervosa an oh RECKS see ah nur VOH sah	*an-* without *orex/o* appetite *-ia* condition	Prolonged refusal to eat adequate amounts of food and an altered perception of what constitutes a normal minimum body weight caused by an intense fear of becoming obese. Primarily affects adolescent females; emaciation and amenorrhea result (Fig. 15-2).
bulimia nervosa boo LIM ee ah nur VOH sah		Eating disorder in which the individual eats large quantities of food and then purges the body through self-induced vomiting or inappropriate use of laxatives.

Fig. 15-2 The perception of body shape and size can be evaluated with the use of special computer drawing programs that allow a subject to distort (increase or decrease) the width of an actual picture of a person's body by as much as 20%. Subjects with anorexia consistently adjusted their own body picture to a size 20% larger than its true form, which suggests that they have a major problem with the perception of self-image.

Actual size   Constricted image   Expanded image
(−20%)   (+20%)

Term Related to Sleep Disorders

Term	Word Origin	Definition
parasomnia pair ah SAHM nee ah	*para-* abnormal *somn/o* sleep *-ia* condition	Abnormal activation of physiologic functions during the sleep cycle. Examples include **sleep terrors,** in which repeated episodes of sudden awakening are accompanied by intense anxiety, agitation, amnesia, and somnambulism.

Terms Related to Sexual Dysfunction

Term	Word Origin	Definition
hypoactive sexual disorder		Indifference or unresponsiveness to sexual stimuli; inability to achieve orgasm during intercourse. Formerly called **frigidity.**
nymphomania nim foh MAY nee ah	*nymph/o* woman *-mania* condition of madness	Relentless drive to achieve sexual orgasm in the female. In the male, the condition is called **satyriasis** (sat tih RYE ah sis).
sexual anhedonia an hee DOH nee ah	*an-* without *hedon/o* pleasure *-ia* condition	Inability to enjoy sexual pleasure.

Personality Disorders

Personality disorders have several common characteristics, including long-standing, inflexible, dysfunctional behavior patterns and personality traits that result in an inability to function successfully in society. These characteristics are not caused by stress, and affected patients have very little to no insight into their disorder.

Terms Related to Personality Disorders

Term	Word Origin	Definition
borderline personality disorder		Disorder characterized by impulsive, unpredictable mood and self-image, resulting in unstable interpersonal relationships and a tendency to see and respond to others as unwaveringly good or evil.
dissocial personality disorder		Disorder in which the patient shows a complete lack of interest in social obligations to the extreme of showing antipathy for other individuals. Patients frustrate easily, are quick to display aggression, show a tendency to blame others, and do not change their behavior even after punishment. Also called **dyssocial personality disorder.**
paranoid personality disorder		State in which the individual exhibits inappropriately suspicious thinking, self-importance, a lack of ability to forgive perceived insults, and an extreme sense of personal rights.
schizoid personality disorder		Condition in which the patient withdraws into a fantasy world with little need for social interaction. Most patients have a limited capacity to experience pleasure or to express their feelings.

Terms Related to Habit and Impulse Disorders

Term	Word Origin	Definition
kleptomania klep toh MAY nee ah	*klept/o* steal *-mania* condition of madness	Uncontrollable impulse to steal.
pyromania pye roh MAY nee ah	*pyr/o* fire *-mania* condition of madness	Uncontrollable impulse to set fires.
trichotillomania trick oh till oh MAY nee ah	*trich/o* hair *till/o* pulling *-mania* condition of madness	Uncontrollable impulse to pull one's hair out by the roots.

Terms Related to Paraphilias (Sexual Perversion) or Disorders of Sexual Preference

Term	Word Origin	Definition
exhibitionism eck sih BISH uh niz um		Condition in which the patient derives sexual arousal from the exposure of his or her genitals to strangers.
fetishism FET ish iz um		Reliance on an object as a stimulus for sexual arousal and pleasure.
pedophilia ped oh FILL ee ah	*ped/o* child *phil/o* attraction *-ia* condition	Sexual preference, either in fantasy or actuality, for children as a means of achieving sexual excitement and gratification.
sadomasochism say doh MASS oh kiz um		Preference for sexual activity that involves inflicting or receiving pain and/or humiliation.
voyeurism VOY yur iz um		Condition in which an individual derives sexual pleasure and gratification from surreptitiously looking at individuals engaged in intimate behavior.

EXERCISE 4: Miscellaneous Behavioral Disorders

Fill in the blanks with the following terms.

acrophobia, PTSD, anorexia nervosa, hypomania, satyriasis, somnambulism, sadomasochism, dysthymia, BD, OCD, social phobia, cyclothymia, PD, paranoid personality disorder, pyromania, depressive disorder, illness anxiety disorder, dissociative identity disorder, GAD, claustrophobia

1.   An alternative name for anthropophobia is _____.

2.   Fear of enclosed spaces is called _____.

3.   Patients who experience symptoms of persistent nervousness, trembling, muscular tension, sweating, lightheadedness, palpitations, dizziness, and epigastric discomfort may be given the diagnosis of

   _____.

4.   Patients who are compelled to have repetitive thoughts or to repeat specific rituals may have a

   diagnosis of _____.

5.   Extreme trauma that may result in flashbacks, nightmares, hypervigilance, or reliving the trauma is

   called _____.

6.   Patients who develop separate personalities as a result of a severely stressful situation are given the

   diagnosis of what disorder? _____.

7.   Patients who continually express physical complaints that have no real basis have a type of

   _____.

8.   Episodes of mood change from depression to mania are called _____.

9.   Patients who have a loss of energy, of pleasure, and of interest in life may be experiencing

   _____.

10.   An inappropriate, persistent elevation of mood that may include irritability is called

   _____.

11.   Recurring episodes of mild elation and depression not severe enough to warrant diagnosis of

   BD is called _____.

12.   A chronic depression that lasts for years but does not warrant a diagnosis of depression may be

   termed _____.

13. What is the healthcare term for walking in one's sleep? _____

14. What is the term for an insatiable sexual desire in men? _____

15. What are recurrent unpredictable attacks of severe anxiety? _____

16. What is the disorder in which patients refuse to maintain a body weight that is a minimum weight

for height? _____

17. What is the healthcare term for the pathologic impulse to set fires? _____

18. What is the healthcare term for a severe, enduring personality disorder with paranoid tendencies?

_____

19. A preference for sexual activity that involves pain and humiliation is called _____.

20. Fear of heights is called _____.

Decode the term.

21. pedophilia _____

22. parasomnia _____

23. kleptomania _____

24. agoraphobia _____

25. trichotillomania _____

 *Click on **Hear It, Spell It** to practice spelling the pathology terms that you have learned in this chapter. To review the pathology terms in this chapter, play **Medical Millionaire.***

Age Matters

Pediatrics

Aside from the disorders first diagnosed in childhood—Asperger disorder, ADHD, autistic disorder, conduct disorders and mental retardation—children are being diagnosed in increasing numbers for depressive disorders, substance abuse, and eating disorders.

Geriatrics

Seniors are seen with disorders associated with depression and anxiety, along with those caused by dementia.

DIAGNOSTIC PROCEDURES

Behavioral diagnoses must take into account underlying healthcare abnormalities that may cause or influence a patient's mental health. Some of the common laboratory and imaging procedures are mentioned here, along with procedures that are traditionally considered to be psychological.

Mental Status Examination

A diagnostic procedure to determine a patient's current mental state. It includes assessment of the patient's appearance, affect, thought processes, cognitive function, insight, and judgment.

Laboratory Tests

Patients may have blood counts (complete blood cell count [CBC] with differential), blood chemistry, thyroid function panels, screening tests for syphilis (rapid plasma reagin [RPR] or microhemagglutination assay-*Treponema pallidum* [MHA-TP]), urinalyses with drug screen, urine pregnancy checks for females with childbearing potential, blood alcohol levels, serum levels of medications, and human immunodeficiency virus (HIV) tests in high-risk patients.

Imaging

Imaging is most helpful in ruling out neurologic disorders and in research; it is less helpful in diagnosing or treating psychiatric problems. Computed tomography (CT) scans and magnetic resonance imaging (MRI) can be used to screen for brain lesions. Positron emission tomography (PET) scans can be used to examine and map the metabolic activity of the brain (Fig. 15-3).

Fig. 15-3 Positron emission tomography (PET) scans of the same depressed individual's brain when depressed *(left)* and after recovery through treatment with medication *(right)*. Several brain areas, particularly the prefrontal cortex *(at top)*, show diminished activity *(darker colors)* during depression.

Psychological Testing

Bender Gestalt Test: A test of visuomotor and spatial abilities; useful for children and adults.

Draw-a-Person (DAP) Test: Analysis of patient's drawings of male and female individuals. Used to assess personality.

Minnesota Multiphasic Personality Inventory (MMPI): Assessment of personality characteristics through a battery of forced-choice questions.

Rorschach inkblot test: A projective test using inkblots to determine the patient's ability to integrate intellectual and emotional factors into his or her perception of the environment (Fig. 15-4).

Thematic Apperception Test (TAT): Test in which patients are asked to make up stories about the pictures they are shown. This test may provide information about a patient's interpersonal relationships, fantasies, needs, conflicts, and defenses.

Wechsler Adult Intelligence Scale (WAIS): Measure of verbal IQ, performance IQ, and full-scale IQ.

Fig. 15-4 Rorschach inkblot test.

EXERCISE 5: Diagnostic Procedures

Match the diagnostic procedures with their definitions.

_____ 1. WAIS

_____ 2. TAT

_____ 3. PET scan

_____ 4. MMPI

_____ 5. Rorschach

_____ 6. Bender Gestalt

A. provides information about needs, fantasies, and interpersonal relationships
B. measures personality characteristics
C. IQ test
D. test of visuomotor and spatial skills
E. imaging of metabolic activity (in brain)
F. examines integration of emotional and intellectual factors

Medical Record Leah Wellor

WELLOR, LEAH H - 818077 Opened by JEZIK, LATISHA

Task   Edit   View   Time Scale   Options   Help

WELLOR, LEAH H   Age: 26 years   Sex: Female   Loc: WHC-SMMC
                        DOB: 12/18/1988   MRN: 818077   FIN: 3506004

Reference Text Browser | Form Browser | Medication Profile

Orders | Last 48 Hours | ED | Lab | Radiology | Assessments | Surgery | Clinical Notes | Pt. Info | Pt. Schedule | Task List | I & O | MAR

Flowsheet: Assessment   Level: Mental Health Exam   ○ Table   ○ Group   ○ List

Navigator
☑ Mental Health Exam

Patient was a pleasant, alert, well-groomed woman who showed no evidence of distractibility. Orientation was intact for person, time, and place. Eye contact was appropriate. There were no abnormalities of gait, posture, or demeanor. Vocabulary and grammar skills were suggestive of intellectual functioning within the high average range.

The patient's attitude was warm, open, and cooperative. Her mood was euthymic. She had full affect range. Memory functions were grossly intact with respect to immediate and remote recall of events and factual information. Her thought processes were intact, goal oriented, and well organized. Thought content revealed no evidence of delusions, paranoia, or suicidal/homicidal ideation. There was no evidence of perceptual disorder. Her level of personal insight appeared to be very good, as evidenced by her ability to state her current diagnosis of PTSD and to identify events that contributed to its exacerbations. Social judgment appeared good, as evidenced by appropriate interactions with other patients in the waiting room.

PROD MAHAFC   03 Nov 2015   14:41

EXERCISE 6: Mental Status Record

Using the preceding mental status report, answer the following questions.

1. What term indicates that the patient exhibited a normal range of emotions?

2. What term indicates that the patient exhibited a variety of moods that were appropriate to the conversation?

3. How do you know that the patient did not exhibit any persistent beliefs in things that are untrue?

4. What is her current diagnosis?

THERAPEUTIC INTERVENTIONS

Terms Related to Psychotherapy

Term	Word Origin	Definition
behavioral therapy		Therapeutic attempt to alter an undesired behavior by substituting a new response or set of responses to a given stimulus.
cognitive therapy		Wide variety of treatment techniques that attempt to help the individual alter inaccurate or unhealthy perceptions and patterns of thinking.
psychoanalysis sye koh uh NAL ih sis	*psych/o* mind *ana-* up, apart *-lysis* breakdown	Behavioral treatment developed initially by Sigmund Freud to analyze and treat any dysfunctional effects of unconscious factors on a patient's mental state. This therapy uses techniques that include analysis of defense mechanisms and dream interpretation.

Terms Related to Other Therapeutic Methods

Term	Word Origin	Definition
detoxification dee tock sih fih KAY shun	*de-* lack of, removal *toxic/o* poison *-ation* process of	Removal of a chemical substance (drug or alcohol) as an initial step in treatment of a chemically dependent individual.
electroconvulsive therapy (ECT) ee leck troh kun VUHL siv		Method of inducing convulsions to treat affective disorders in patients who have been resistant or unresponsive to drug therapy.
hypnosis hip NOH sis	*hypn/o* sleep *-sis* state	The induction of an altered state of consciousness to change an unwanted behavior or emotional response.
light therapy		Exposure of the body to light waves to treat patients with depression due to seasonal fluctuations (Fig. 15-5).
narcosynthesis nar koh SIN thih sis	*narc/o* sleep, stupor *-synthesis* bring together	The use of intravenous barbiturates to elicit repressed memories or thoughts.
pharmacotherapy far mah koh THAIR uh pee	*pharmac/o* drugs *-therapy* treatment	The use of medication to affect behavior and/or emotions.

Fig. 15-5 Broad-spectrum, fluorescent lamps, such as this one, are used in daily therapy sessions from autumn into spring for individuals with seasonal affective disorder (SAD). Patients report that they feel less depressed within 3 to 7 days. (Courtesy of Apollo Light Systems.)

Case Study Elena Georgio

Recently Elena Georgio discovered that her grandmother had been hospitalized for depression and anhedonia when she was in her 40s. Elena was very interested in hearing the reason why, so she asked her mother, Martina. Martina says that there is a family history of depression and that she has had her own issues with dysthymia. Martina says that Elena's grandmother's depression was so severe that she was given multiple treatments of ECT. After the seventh treatment, she remembered her mother feeling much better, and although she still sees her psychologist on an "as needed" basis, she has never had to go back for treatment again.

1. ECT stands for _____ _____.

2. The term for a mild, chronic depression that lasts for years but is not severe enough to warrant a diagnosis of depression is _____ _____.

3. Another name for a mood disorder is a/n _____ _____ disorder.

4. A diagnostic procedure to determine a patient's current mental state that includes an assessment of the patient's appearance, affect, thought processes, cognitive function, insight, and judgment is a _____.
   a. MMPI
   b. Bender Gestalt test
   c. Rorschach inkblot test
   d. mental status exam

5. The absence of ability to experience pleasure is called _____.

EXERCISE 7: Therapeutic Interventions

Fill in the blanks with the following terms.

hypnosis, cognitive therapy, ECT, behavioral, pharmacotherapy, light therapy, psychoanalysis, narcosynthesis

1. Patients are treated with _____ therapy when an attempt is made to replace maladjusted patterns with a new response to a given stimulus.

2. What type of therapy uses exposure of the body to light waves to treat patients with depression caused by seasonal fluctuations?

   _____

3. What is a method of inducing convulsions to treat affective disorders in patients who have been resistant or unresponsive to drug therapy?

   _____

4. What therapy is used to analyze and treat any dysfunctional effects of unconscious factors on a patient's mental state?

   _____

5. What are any of the various methods of treating mental and emotional disorders that help a person change attitudes, perceptions, and patterns of thinking?

   _____

6. What therapy induces an altered state of unconsciousness to change an unwanted behavior or emotional response? _____

7. The use of intravenous barbiturates to elicit repressed memories or thoughts.

_____

8. The use of medication to affect behavior and/or emotions. _____

PHARMACOLOGY

A major part of treatment for behavioral disorders is the use of drug therapy. Various neurotransmitters may be out of balance in the brain, causing mental disorders. Many drugs have been developed to improve this balance and minimize symptoms of these disorders. The psychiatric medications described appear in the top 100 prescribed medications in the United States. Medications are continually being developed and reevaluated and are closely regulated by the Food and Drug Administration. Examples include the following:

antialcoholics: Discourage use of alcohol. Naltrexone (ReVia) can be used for alcohol and narcotic withdrawal. Disulfiram (Antabuse) is used to deter alcohol consumption.

antidepressants: Relieve symptoms of depressed mood. Many drug classes are available, including selective serotonin reuptake inhibitors (SSRIs), tricyclic antidepressants (TCAs), monoamine oxidase inhibitors (MAOIs), and some newer unclassified agents. Examples include fluoxetine (Prozac), sertraline (Zoloft), mirtazapine (Remeron), bupropion (Wellbutrin), and venlafaxine (Effexor).

antipsychotics or neuroleptics: Control psychotic symptoms, such as hallucinations and delusions. Haloperidol (Haldol) and chlorpromazine (Thorazine) are examples of typical antipsychotics; olanzapine (Zyprexa) and risperidone (Risperdal) are examples of the newer atypical antipsychotics.

anxiolytics: Relieve symptoms of anxiety. These drugs are often used as sedatives or sedative-hypnotics as well. Examples are lorazepam (Ativan), buspirone (BuSpar), and alprazolam (Xanax).

mood stabilizers: Balance neurotransmitters in the brain to reduce or prevent acute mood swings (mania or depression). Lithium (Lithobid) is the most well-known mood stabilizer. Some anticonvulsants such as valproic acid (Depakene) and lamotrigine (Lamictal) are also considered mood stabilizers.

NMDA receptor antagonists: Preserve cognitive function in patients suffering from progressive memory loss by blocking glutamate activity. Memantine (Namenda) is the only drug of this class currently used for this purpose.

sedatives and sedative-hypnotics: Exert a calming effect with or without inducing sleep. The most commonly used agents are benzodiazepines and barbiturates.

stimulants: Generally increase synaptic activity of targeted neurons to increase alertness. Examples include methylphenidate (Ritalin) and caffeine.

EXERCISE 8: Pharmacology

Match the drug class with the drug action.

_____ 1. mood stabilizer   _____ 4. anxiolytic

_____ 2. antidepressant   _____ 5. stimulant

_____ 3. sedative   _____ 6. antialcoholic

A. discourages use of alcohol
B. increases synaptic activity to
   increase alertness
C. relieves symptoms of depression
D. reduces anxiety
E. prevents acute mood swings
F. calms and relaxes

Case Study **Jermaine Wolston**

Jermaine Wolston, a 37-year-old artist, is being seen today because he is having trouble sleeping, and he has started sleepwalking. He says that the problems started shortly after his return from a tour of duty in Afghanistan. He said that in the army, he was counseled to seek therapy to deal with his recurrent flashbacks, but he didn't think he needed it. After talking to his physician about his options, he was given a prescription for an anxiolytic and a referral to a psychologist to discuss a possible diagnosis of PTSD.

1. What is the medical term for sleepwalking? _____
   _____

2. What is a medication to treat anxiety? _____
   _____

3. What is the term for an anticipation of impending danger and dread not associated with an apparent stimulus? _____

4. Which type of therapy alters an undesired behavior by substituting a new response or set of responses to a given stimulus?
   a. behavioral
   b. psychoanalysis
   c. cognitive therapy

5. What does PTSD stand for? _____
   _____

Medical Record *Sherry Prichet*

PRICHET, SHERILYN B - 620018 Opened by REXFORD, CHRISTIANA MD

Task   Edit   View   Time Scale   Options   Help

PRICHET, SHERILYN B   Age: 54 years   Sex: Female   Loc: WHC-SMMC
                                  DOB: 05/07/1960   MRN: 620018   FIN: 3506004

| Reference Text Browser | Form Browser | Medication Profile |

| Orders | Last 48 Hours | ED | Lab | Radiology | Assessments | Surgery | **Clinical Notes** | Pt. Info | Pt. Schedule | Task List | I & O | MAR |

Flowsheet: Clinical Notes   Level: Progress Note   ◉ Table ○ Group ○ List

Navigator
✓ Progress Note

54-year-old female says she is anxious, can't sleep, and has recurring panic attacks.

Issues circle around behavior of her autistic son and excessive workload at her job. Past history includes molestation. Suffers from somnambulism. Is having nightmares of being robbed. She just can't take it anymore and would like a sleeping pill.

IMPRESSION: Insomnia associated with nightmares, anxiety and panic disorder.

PLAN: Issued trazodone 25 mg to take 1-2 hours before bed for the next several nights. She is to schedule visit with a psychologist to begin to resolve these issues on a more prolonged basis.

PROD   MA-AFC   08 May 2015   11:52

EXERCISE 9: Progress Note

Using the preceding progress note, answer the following questions.

1. The impression notes that the patient has "insomnia." What is the meaning of the term?

   _____

2. What healthcare professional is she scheduled to visit? _____

3. What class of drug do you expect trazodone to be in? _____

4. She is diagnosed with a disorder in which the mood may be described as an "anticipation of impending danger and dread accompanied by restlessness, tension, tachycardia, and breathing

   difficulty not associated with the general stimulus." What is it? _____

Click on **Hear It, Spell It** to practice spelling the diagnostic and therapeutic terms that you have learned in this chapter.

Abbreviations

Abbreviation	Definition	Abbreviation	Definition
ADHD	attention-deficit/hyperactivity disorder	IQ	intelligence quotient
APA	American Psychiatric Association	MMPI	Minnesota Multiphasic Personality Inventory
ASD	autism spectrum disorder	MR	mental retardation
BD, BP	bipolar disorder	OCD	obsessive-compulsive disorder
DAP	Draw-a-Person (Test)	ODD	oppositional defiant disorder
DSM	Diagnostic and Statistical Manual of Mental Disorders	PD	panic disorder
		PTSD	posttraumatic stress disorder
DTs	delirium tremens	SAD	seasonal affective disorder
ECT	electroconvulsive therapy	SSRI	selective serotonin reuptake inhibitor
GAD	generalized anxiety disorder		
ICD	International Classification of Diseases	TAT	Thematic Apperception Test
		WAIS	Wechsler Adult Intelligence Scale

EXERCISE 10: Abbreviations

Write out the abbreviations in the following sentences.

1. Michele was being treated with light therapy for her SAD. _____

2. John was diagnosed with GAD after exhibiting symptoms of difficulty concentrating, excessive worry, and disturbed sleep over the last year. _____

3. The patient had a diagnosis of mild MR, with an IQ of 55, as determined by the WAIS.

   _____

4. Roger was referred to the school psychologist by his teacher to be evaluated for the possibility of an ADHD diagnosis after many behavioral problems at school and at home.

   _____

5. The patient was diagnosed with PTSD after she was assaulted. _____

Match the word parts to their definitions.

Word Part Definitions

Prefix/Suffix		Definition
acro-	1. _____	babbling
agora-	2. _____	condition of madness
an-	3. _____	without
bi-	4. _____	condition of fear
dys-	5. _____	condition of mind
eu-	6. _____	marketplace
-ia	7. _____	good, well
-iatrist	8. _____	one who specializes in the study of
-lalia	9. _____	two
-logist	10. _____	condition
-mania	11. _____	heights
-phobia	12. _____	one who specializes in treatment
-thymia	13. _____	difficult

Combining Form		Definition
anthrop/o	14. _____	pleasure
claustr/o	15. _____	recurring
cycl/o	16. _____	appetite
hedon/o	17. _____	mind
iatr/o	18. _____	body
kathis/o	19. _____	man
klept/o	20. _____	woman
nymph/o	21. _____	sitting
orex/o	22. _____	pole
ped/o	23. _____	mind
phil/o	24. _____	steal
phor/o	25. _____	child
phren/o	26. _____	treatment
pol/o	27. _____	sleep
psych/o	28. _____	mind
pyr/o	29. _____	attraction
somat/o	30. _____	fire
somn/o	31. _____	a closing
thym/o	32. _____	to carry, bear

Wordshop

Prefixes	Combining Forms	Suffixes
aero-	acid/a	-dipsia
an-	erin/o	-eetomy
endo-	esthesi/o	-emia
ex-	glue/a	-ia
hyper-	glueos/o	-logy
hypo-	glye/o	-megaly
par-	kal/i	-meter
para-	ket/o	-osis
poly-	keton/o	-tomy
	natr/o	-uria
	ophthalmia	
	parathyroid/a	
	phag/o	

Build the following terms by combining the preceding word parts. Some word parts may be used more than once. Some may not be used at all. The number in parentheses is the number of word parts needed to build the terms.

Definition	Term
1. condition of no pleasure (3)	_____
2. study of the mind (2)	_____
3. fear of men (people) (2)	_____
4. abnormal condition of the mind (2)	_____
5. condition of compulsion (to set) fires (2)	_____
6. fear of closed spaces (2)	_____
7. condition of a healthy state of mind (2)	_____
8. fear of heights (2)	_____
9. condition of split mind (3)	_____
10. condition of sleep walking (3)	_____
11. condition of compulsion to pull (one's own) hair (3)	_____
12. condition of abnormal sleep (3)	_____
13. fear of the marketplace (2)	_____
14. condition of babbling repetition of words spoken by others (2)	_____
15. condition of no appetite (3)	_____

Sort the terms into the correct categories.

Term Sorting

Pathology	Pathology	Diagnostic Procedures	Therapeutic Interventions

acrophobia	confabulation	GAF	PTSD
ADHD	cyclothymia	hallucination	pyromania
akathisia	DAP	hypomania	Rorschach
anhedonia	delusion	hypnosis	schizophrenia
antidepressants	detoxification	MMPI	sedative
anxiety	DSM-5	OCD	somnambulism
anxiolytics	DTs	PD	stimulants
Bender Gestalt	ECT	psychoanalysis	TAT
catatonia	GAD	psychosis	WAIS

Replace the highlighted words with the correct terms.

Translations

1. The patient had a **moderately reduced range of affect** and **mild, chronic depression of mood.**

2. Amy was admitted with a diagnosis of **prolonged refusal to eat adequate amounts of food** and **fear of leaving home and entering crowded places.**

3. The patient was referred to a sleep therapist for **abnormal activation of physiologic functions during the sleep cycle** and **sleepwalking.**

4. Marielle was diagnosed with **a weather-induced depression** after telling her doctor that she had a loss of **normal psychological impulse drive associated with sensuality or creativity** and **absence of the ability to experience pleasure or joy.**

5. Because Mr. Ballestero was experiencing **generalized negative mood characterized by depression** and **an exaggerated sense of well-being not based on reality,** he was diagnosed with **a disordercharacterized by elevation and lowering of mood.**

6. After Andrew McKlin returned home from Iraq, he suffered from **anticipation of impending danger and dread** and **extended emotional response to a traumatic event.**

7. Cho Ling told her **one who specializes in the study of the mind** that she thought she had **fear of heights** and **fear of enclosed spaces.**

8. Adam was washing his hands 40 times a day and his **one who specializes in treatment of the mind** diagnosed **recurrent, distressing, and unavoidable preoccupation to perform specific rituals.**

9. The patient's **impaired perception of reality** was accompanied by **unreal sensory perceptions that occur with no external cause.**

10. Tiffany showed signs of **a syndrome that includes impulsiveness, inability to concentrate and short attention span.**

11. Sixteen-year-old Ray Huggins was diagnosed with **a conduct disorder characterized by hostile, disobedient behavior** and **an uncontrollable impulse to set fires.**

12. By the time Brooke was 20 years old, she had no eyelashes because she had suffered from **an uncontrollable impulse to pull one's hair out by the roots** since she was 8 years old.

13. Dr. Linder used **the use of medication to affect behavior and/or emotions** to treat Sylvia's depression.

Medical Record Walter Hu

Hu, Walter W - 733382 Opened by McGuire, Patrick MD

Task   Edit   View   Time Scale   Options   Help

Hu, Walter W | Age: 76 years | Sex: Male | Loc: WHC-SMMC
| DOB: 03/08/1939 | MRN: 733382 | FIN: 3526641

Reference Text Browser | Form Browser | Medication Profile

Orders | Last 48 Hours | ED | Lab | Radiology | Assessments | Surgery | **Clinical Notes** | Pt. nfo | Pt. Schedule | Task List | I & O | MAR

Flowsheet: Clinical Notes   Level: SOAP Note   ● Table ○ Group ○ List

Navigator
✓ Progress Note

S: This 76-year-old Asian male was brought here today by his daughter. He has a history of hypertension, GERD, and constipation. His daughter states, "Dad has been eating very poorly and seems uninterested in life since my mom's death." The patient says that he has come only because his daughter insisted and admits that he has not been eating or sleeping well. He has been using Correctol for his constipation, but says that it causes runny stools.

O: General: The patient is an older Asian male who appears to be fatigued and somewhat sad and tearful. HEENT: Tympanic membranes were clear bilaterally. Nose had some pale mucosa, otherwise clear. Throat was clear. Neck was supple. Lungs: Clear to auscultation. Cardiovascular: Regular rate and rhythm without murmur. Abdomen: Soft and diffusely tender to mild degree. Bowel sounds were active.

A: (1) Depression. (2) Hypertension. (3) GERD. (4) Contipation.

P: (1) He will be referred to a psychotherapist for cognitive therapy. If he does not seem improved within the month, a prescription for Zoloft or Prozac will be considered. (2) His hypertension has been controlled through diet and is within normal limits today. (3) His GERD is being treated with Tagamet. (4) For his constipation, I recommended Citrucel or some similar type of fiber, increasing his fluid intake, and closely monitoring his diet for additional roughage.

PROD | MAHAFC | 08 March 2015 | 11:52

SOAP NOTE

1. What is the diagnosis of the patient's mental state? _____

2. What is the meaning of GERD? _____

3. Zoloft and Prozac are what types of medications? _____

4. What type of therapy uses medication to affect behavior and emotions? _____

5. What type of therapy has been suggested for Mr. Hu? _____

16

Oncology

CHAPTER OUTLINE

Specialties/Specialists
Carcinogenesis
Naming Malignant Tumors
Staging and Grading
  Case Study: Mark Samson
Pathology

Diagnostic Procedures
  Medical Record: Terrence McAffee
Therapeutic Interventions
  Case Study: Tamara Ramos
  Case Study: Akiyo Kato

Pharmacology
  Medical Record: Stella Yates
Chapter Review
  Medical Record: Clifford Walker

OBJECTIVES

- Recognize and use terms related to the physiology of neoplasms.
- Recognize and use terms related to neoplasm pathology.

- Recognize and use terms related to the diagnostic procedures for detecting neoplasms.
- Recognize and use terms related to the therapeutic interventions for treating neoplasms.

For interactive learning, go to the Shiland Evolve website, and click on:
- **Match the Word Parts** to review oncology word parts.
- **Word Shop** to practice word building.
- **Tournament of Terminology** to test your knowledge of oncology terms.
- **Term Sorting** to practice sorting oncology terms into categories.

*Click on **Chapter at a Glance** to print off a list of key terms and word parts for this chapter.*

Where there is life, there is cancer. Although the types of cancer and their incidence (the number of new types diagnosed each year) may vary by geography, sex, race, age, and ethnicity, cancer exists in every population and has since ancient times. Archeologists have found evidence of cancer in dinosaur bones and human mummies. Written descriptions of cancer treatment have been discovered dating back to 1600 BC. The name itself comes from the Greek word for crab, used by Hippocrates to describe the appearance of the most common type of cancer, carcinoma.

SPECIALTIES/SPECIALISTS

Oncology is the study of tumors, both benign (noncancerous) and malignant (cancerous). An **oncologist** is a specialist in the diagnosis, treatment, and prevention of tumors.

Certified cancer registrars (CTRs) (also called **tumor registrars**) are specialists in cancer data management. Their primary responsibility is to report and track patients with cancer who are diagnosed and/or treated at the registrar's healthcare facility.

CARCINOGENESIS

Cancer is not *one* disease but a group of hundreds of diseases with similar characteristics. The shared characteristics are uncontrolled cell growth and a spread of altered cells. Different types of cancers have different occurrence rates and different causes.

Current research suggests that there is no single cause of cancer. Radiation, bacteria, viruses, genetics, diet, smoking (or exposure to tobacco smoke), alcohol, and other factors all contribute to the development of cancer termed **carcinogenesis.** Each of these factors is instrumental in disrupting the normal balance of cell growth and destruction within the body by causing a mutation in the deoxyribonucleic acid (DNA) of cells (Fig. 16-1). Once this **mutation** takes place, a process of uncontrolled cell growth may begin. It is important to note that the cancer cells that replace normal cells no longer function to keep the body working. The only mission of cancer cells is to reproduce. Fig. 16-2 illustrates the process of **apoptosis** (a pop TOH sis), the body's normal restraining function to keep cell growth in check. Fig. 16-3 shows the progression from normally functioning skin tissue to **hyperplasia,** to **dysplasia,** and finally to carcinoma in situ (CIS). Cancer is a continuum—from tissue made up of

cancer = carcin/o

oncologist
onc/o = tumor
-logist = one who studies

carcinogenesis
carcin/o = cancer
-genesis = production, origin

mutation
mut/a = change
-tion = process of

apoptosis
apo- = away from
-ptosis = falling

hyperplasia
hyper- = excessive
-plasia = condition of formation

dysplasia
dys- = abnormal
-plasia = condition of formation

Normal cell division	Cancer due to activation of oncogenes	Cancer due to action of mutated tumor suppressor genes
Regulated by tumor suppressor genes		Loss or mutation of tumor suppressor genes
Proto-oncogenes	Proto-oncogenes	Proto-oncogenes
stimulate	activate	
	Oncogenes	
Cell growth and proliferation	Increased rate of cell growth and proliferation	Cell growth and proliferation
	Malignant transformation	Malignant transformation

Fig. 16-1 Normal cell growth versus oncogenesis.

Fig. 16-2 Apoptosis.

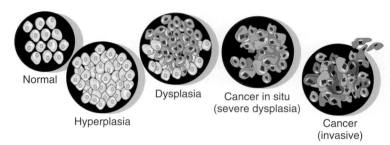

Fig. 16-3 Progression of skin cancer from hyperplasia to cancer.

Fig. 16-4 Metastasis.

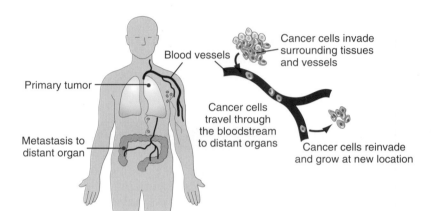

normally functioning cells fulfilling their role to keep the body healthy, to tissue replaced by cancerous cells that no longer perform the work of the tissue and now perform only the function of reproducing themselves. Cancers are capable of destroying not only the tissue in which they originate (the primary site), but also other tissues, through the process of **metastasis,** the spread of cancer. Metastasis can occur by direct extension to contiguous organs and tissues or to distant sites through blood (Fig. 16-4) or lymphatic involvement.

NAMING MALIGNANT TUMORS

All cancers are **neoplasms** (new growths), but not all neoplasms are cancerous. Cancerous **tumors** are termed *malignant*, whereas noncancerous tumors are termed *benign*.

Although the hundreds of known types of malignant tumors commonly share the characteristics listed previously, the names that they are given reflect their differences. All tissues (and hence organs) are derived from the progression of three embryonic germ layers that differentiate into specific tissues and organs. Tumors are generally divided into two broad categories and a varying number of other categories, based on their **embryonic** origin. Fig. 16-5 illustrates the different types of cancers and where they occur.

- **Carcinomas:** Approximately 80% to 90% of malignant tumors are derived from the outer **(ectodermal)** and inner **(endodermal)** layers of the embryo that develop into epithelial tissue that either covers or lines the surfaces of the body. This category of cancer is divided into two main types. If derived from an organ or gland, it is an adenocarcinoma; if derived from squamous

---

metastasis
 meta- = beyond, change
 -stasis = controlling,
 stopping

tumor = onc/o, -oma

neoplasm
 neo- = new
 -plasm = formation

embryonic = blast/o, -blast

carcinoma
 carcin/o = cancer
 -oma = tumor, mass

ectodermal
 ecto- = outer
 derm/o = skin
 -al = pertaining to

endodermal
 endo- = within
 derm/o = skin
 -al = pertaining to

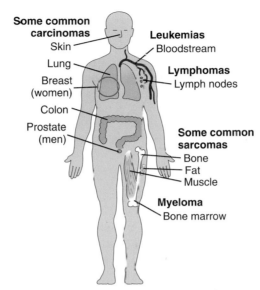

Fig. 16-5 Common cancers and where they occur.

epithelium, it is a squamous cell carcinoma. Examples include gastric adeno-carcinoma and squamous cell carcinoma of the lung.

- **Sarcomas** are derived from the middle **(mesodermal)** layer, which becomes connective tissue (bones, muscle, cartilage, blood vessels, and fat). Most end in the suffix *-sarcoma.* Examples include osteosarcoma, chondrosarcoma, hemangiosarcoma, mesothelioma, and glioma.
- **Lymphomas** develop in lymphatic tissue (vessels, nodes, and organs, including the spleen, tonsils, and thymus gland). Lymphomas are solid cancers and may also appear outside of the sites of lymphatic organs in the stomach, breast, or brain; these are called **extranodal lymphomas.** All lymphomas may be divided into two categories: Hodgkin lymphoma and non-Hodgkin lymphoma.
- **Leukemia** is cancer of the bone marrow. An example is acute myelocytic leukemia.
- **Myelomas** arise from the plasma cells in the bone marrow. An example is multiple myeloma.
- **Mixed tumors** are a combination of cells from within one category or between two cancer categories. Examples are **teratocarcinoma** and **carcinosarcoma.**

STAGING AND GRADING

To treat cancer, the treating physician must determine the severity of the cancer, the grade, and its stage, or size and spread. Cancers at different grades and stages react differently to various treatments.

Grading (G) is the first means of affixing a value to a clinical opinion of the degree of **dedifferentiation (anaplasia)** of cancer cells, or how much the cells appear different from their original form. Healthy cells are well differentiated; cancer cells are poorly differentiated. The pathologist determines this difference and assigns a grade ranging from 1 to 4. The higher the grade, the more cancerous, or dedifferentiated, is the tissue sample. Grading is a measure of the cancer's *severity.*

The other means of determining the *size and spread* of the cancer from its original site, which is called **staging.** A number of systems are used to describe staging. Some are specific to the type of cancer; others are general systems. If staging is determined by various diagnostic techniques, it is referred to as **clinical staging.** If it is determined by the pathologist's report, it is called

---

mesodermal
  meso- = middle
  derm/o = skin
  -al = pertaining to

connective tissue cancer
  = sarc/o, -sarcoma

extranodal
  extra- = outside
  nod/o = node
  -al = pertaining to

myeloma
  myel/o = bone marrow, spinal cord
  -oma = tumor, mass

teratocarcinoma
  terat/o = deformity
  -carcinoma = cancer of epithelial origin

carcinosarcoma
  carcin/o = cancer
  -sarcoma = connective tissue cancer

anaplasia
  ana- = up, apart
  -plasia = condition of formation

pathologic
  path/o = disease
  -logic = pertaining to studying

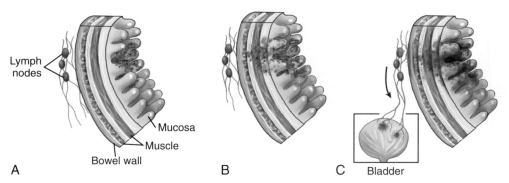

Fig. 16-6 Staging of colon cancer. **A,** Stage I; **B,** stage II; **C,** stage III.

Be Careful!

Don't confuse **sarc/o** *meaning flesh with* **sacr/o** *meaning sacrum.*

pathologic staging. An example is TNM staging. In this system, **T** stands for the size of the **tumor**, **N** stands for the number of lymph **nodes** positive for cancer, and **M** stands for the presence of distant **metastasis** (meh TAS tuh sis). Summary staging puts together the TNM to give one number as a stage. Again, this helps the clinician to determine the type of treatment that is most effective. Fig. 16-6 illustrates a staging system. If the cancer cells appear only at the original site and have not invaded the organ of origin, it is called **carcinoma in situ (CIS).**

Cancer that begins in an organ is referred to as a *primary tumor.* When a cancer spreads to another site in the body from that primary tumor, the new tumor is referred to as *secondary,* or **metastatic.** The cells in the metastatic tumor are composed of the same tissue as the cancer at the original site. For example, a patient can have a primary liver cancer that begins in the liver, or a metastatic brain tumor that is composed of cells from a primary liver cancer that has spread. The abbreviation **mets** stands for **metatases,** the resultant secondary tumors that have traveled from the original site.

EXERCISE 1: General Oncology Terms

Match the word part with its correct meaning.

_____ 1. -stasis   _____ 6. -carcinoma

_____ 2. -oma   _____ 7. ana-

_____ 3. -plasia   _____ 8. hyper-

_____ 4. meta-   _____ 9. neo-

_____ 5. dys-   _____ 10. sarcoma

A. up, apart
B. abnormal
C. connective tissue tumor
D. new
E. cancer of epithelial tissue origin
F. stopping, controlling
G. beyond, change
H. tumor
I. excessive
J. formation

Circle the correct answer.

11. Tumors that are cancerous are considered to be *(benign, malignant).*

12. The most common type of malignant cancer is *(carcinoma, sarcoma, leukemia, lymphoma, myeloma, mixed cell cancer).*

13. Cancer composed of connective tissue is classified as *(carcinoma, sarcoma, leukemia, lymphoma, myeloma, mixed cell cancer).*

14. Cancer cells that derive from plasma cells in the bone marrow are classified as *(carcinoma, sarcoma, leukemia, lymphoma, myeloma, mixed cell cancer).*

15. Healthy cells are *(well, poorly)* differentiated.

16. A determination of the degree of dedifferentiation of cancer cells is called *(grading, staging)*.

17. A system of determining how far a cancer has spread from its original site is called *(grading, staging)*.

18. The site where the cancer originates is referred to as the *(primary, metastatic)* site.

Case Study Mark Samson

Mark Samson is spending part of his Friday at a city hospital to see if a career in cancer registry is something he would like to do. He asks one of the registrars, Betsy Hanson, how she got interested in the field. Betsy says that during one of her anatomy and physiology classes, the professor had lectured on carcinogenesis and the many different toxic substances and exposures that can lead to the formation of a malignant neoplasm. Betsy says that she wrote a paper on cancer that helped her understand the difference between grading and staging and why they are important in cancer treatment.

1. Carcinogenesis means producing or causing _____ _____.

2. The term for assigning a clinical value to a malignant tumor's degree of anaplasia is _____.
   a. grading   b. staging

3. Noncancerous tumors are described as being benign, whereas cancerous tumors are _____.

4. The term that means "new formation" is _____.
   a. tumor   b. sarcoma
   c. cancer   d. neoplasm

5. A system that describes the size and spread of a tumor is____.
   a. staging   b. grading

 *Choose **Hear It, Spell It** to practice spelling the staging and grading terms that you have learned in this chapter.*

Combining and Adjective Forms for Oncology

Meaning	Combining Form	Adjective Form
change	mut/a	
disease	path/o	
embryo	blast/o	embryonic
node	nod/o	nodal
tumor	onc/o	

Prefixes for Oncology

Prefix	Meaning	Prefix	Meaning
ana-	up, apart	extra-	outside
apo-	away from	hyper-	excessive
dys-	abnormal	meso-	middle
ecto-	outer	meta-	beyond, change
endo-	within	neo-	new

Suffixes for Oncology

Suffix	Meaning
-carcinoma	cancer of epithelial origin
-genesis	production, origin
-oma	tumor, mass
-plasia	condition of formation
-plasm	formation
-ptosis	falling
-sarcoma	connective tissue cancer
-stasis	controlling, stopping

PATHOLOGY

Signs and Symptoms

The signs and symptoms of cancer are manifestations of how cancer cells replace the functions of healthy tissue. Some examples include anorexia (lack of appetite), bruising, leukocytosis (slight increase of white blood cells), fatigue, cachexia (wasting), and thrombocytopenia (deficiency of clotting cells).

Neoplasia by Body System

The following tables summarize characteristics of benign and malignant tumors by body system. Note that a particular system does not always have all one type of cancer because organs are composed of a variety of tissues with different embryonic origins. The integumentary system has both carcinomas and sarcomas.

Comparison of Benign and Malignant Neoplasms

Characteristics	Benign	Malignant
Mode of growth	Relatively slow growth by expansion; encapsulated; cells adhere to each other	Rapid growth; invades surrounding tissue by infiltration
Cells under microscopic examination	Resemble tissue of origin; well differentiated; appear normal	Do not resemble tissue of origin; vary in size and shape; abnormal appearance and function
Spread	Remains isolated	Metastasis; cancer cells carried by blood and lymphatics to one or more other locations; secondary tumors occur
Other properties	No tissue destruction; not prone to hemorrhage; may be smooth and freely movable	Ulceration and/or necrosis; prone to hemorrhage, irregular and less movable
Recurrence	Rare after excision	A common characteristic
Pathogenesis	Symptoms related to location with obstruction and/or compression of surrounding tissue or organs; usually not life threatening unless inaccessible	Cachexia; pain; fatal if not controlled

From Frazier MS, Drzymkowski JW: *Essentials of human diseases and conditions,* ed 5, Philadelphia, 2012, Saunders.

Examples of Neoplasms by Body System*

Body System	Organ	Benign Neoplasms	Malignant Neoplasms

Musculoskeletal (MS)	bone
	cartilage
	muscle
		osteoma
		chondroma
		rhabdomyoma,
		    leiomyoma
			Ewing sarcoma, osteosarcoma
			chondrosarcoma
			rhabdomyosarcoma,
			    leiomyosarcoma

Integumentary	skin	dermatofibroma	basal cell carcinoma, squamous
			    cell carcinoma, malignant
			    melanoma, Kaposi sarcoma

Gastrointestinal (GI)	esophagus
	
	stomach
	pancreas
	colon/rectum
		leiomyoma
		
		polyp
		gastric adenoma
			adenocarcinoma of the
			    esophagus, stomach, pancreas,
			    colon, and/or rectum

Urinary	kidney
	
	bladder
		nephroma	hypernephroma/renal cell
			    carcinoma, Wilms tumor/
			    nephroblastoma
			transitional cell carcinoma
			    (bladder cancer)

Male reproductive	testis prostate	benign prostatic hyperplasia	seminoma, teratoma adenocarcinoma of the prostate

Female reproductive	breast
	
	uterus
	ovaries
	cervix
		fibrocystic changes in
		    the breast
		fibroids
		ovarian cyst
		cervical dysplasia
			infiltrating ductal adenocarcinoma
			    of the breast
			stromal endometrial carcinoma
			epithelial ovarian carcinoma
			squamous cell carcinoma of the
			    cervix

Blood/ lymphatic/ immune	blood lymph vessels thymus gland	 thymoma	leukemia non-Hodgkin lymphoma, Hodgkin lymphoma malignant thymoma
Cardiovascular	blood vessels heart	hemangioma myxoma	hemangiosarcoma myxosarcoma

Respiratory	epithelial tissue of respiratory
	    tract, lung, bronchus
		papilloma of lung	adenocarcinoma of the lung, small
			    cell carcinoma, mesothelioma,
			    bronchogenic carcinoma

Nervous	Central nervous system (CNS;
	    brain, spinal cord, meninges)
	Peripheral nervous system (PNS)
		neuroma, neurofibroma,
		    meningioma
			glioblastoma multiforme

Endocrine	pituitary thyroid adrenal medulla	benign pituitary tumor pheochromocytoma	 thyroid carcinoma
Eyes and ears	retina choroid acoustic nerve	 choroidal hemangioma acoustic neuroma	retinoblastoma

*See also neoplasm tables in Chapters 3 to 14.

Click on **Hear It, Spell It** to practice spelling the pathology terms that you have learned in this chapter. To hear how well you pronounce the pathology terms in this chapter, click on **Hear It, Say It.** To review the pathology terms in this chapter, play **Medical Millionaire.**

Age Matters

Pediatrics

Childhood cancer is such a rarity that incidence rates are routinely expressed as the number of cases per million, instead of per 100,000 as with adult cancers. Still, certain cancers have a childhood form. Wilms tumor (children's kidney cancer), acute lymphocytic leukemia, retinoblastoma, and Ewing sarcoma are examples of cancers that seldom occur outside of childhood.

Geriatrics

The cumulative exposure to a lifetime of carcinogens reveals itself in cancer statistics that show cancer rates to increase as age increases. Lung, prostate, breast, colon, and skin cancers are common in elderly patients. Researchers estimate that 97% of men who have the prostate cancer gene will develop prostate cancer by the time they are 85.

DIAGNOSTIC PROCEDURES

Patient History

Along with the various clinical techniques described, the patient's history is especially important, including information regarding family history (for genetic information) and social history, such as tobacco and alcohol use, diet, and sexual history. A patient's smoking history is described in terms of "pack years." Pack years equals the average number of packs smoked per day multiplied by the number of years of smoking. For example: 1 pack/day × 25 years of smoking represents 25 pack years. A patient's current or former occupation may also shed light on the type of cancer. For example, exposure to asbestos, through an occupation of ship building or working with brake repair, may lead to a rare type of lung cancer—mesothelioma.

Tumor Markers

Tumor marker tests measure the levels of a variety of biochemical substances detected in the blood, urine, or body tissues that often appear in higher than normal amounts in individuals with certain neoplasms. Because other factors may influence the amount of the tumor marker present, they are not intended to be used as a sole means of diagnosis. Examples include the following:

alpha fetoprotein (AFP) test: Increased levels may indicate liver or testicular cancer.

beta-2 microglobulin (B2M): Levels are elevated in multiple myeloma and chronic lymphocytic leukemia.

bladder tumor antigen (BTA): Present in the urine of patients with bladder cancer.

CA125: Used for ovarian cancer detection and management.

CA15-3: Levels are measured to determine the stage of breast cancer.

CA19-9: Levels are elevated in stomach, colorectal and pancreatic cancers.

CA27-29: Used to monitor breast cancer; especially useful in testing for recurrences.

carcinoembryonic antigen (CEA): Monitors colorectal cancer when the disease has spread or after treatment to measure the patient's response.

human chorionic gonadotropin (hCG): Used as a screen for choriocarcinoma and testicular and ovarian cancers.

neuron-specific enolase (NSE): Used to measure the stage and/or patient's response to treatment of small cell cancer and neuroblastoma.

prostate-specific antigen (PSA): Increased levels may be due to benign prostatic hyperplasia/hypertrophy (BPH) or prostate cancer.

TA-90: Used to detect the spread of malignant melanoma.

Other lab tests include **fecal occult blood test (FOBT)** to test for colon cancer and **Papanicolaou test (Pap)** to test for cervical and vaginal cancer.

Biopsy (Bx)

See Chapter 4 for additional information on types of biopsies.

Imaging

computed tomography (CT) scans: CT scans provide information about a tumor's shape, size, and location, along with the source of its blood supply. They are useful in detecting, evaluating, and monitoring cancer, especially liver, pancreatic, bone, lung, and adrenal gland cancers. CT scans are also useful in staging cancer and guiding needles for aspiration biopsy (bx) (Fig. 16-7).

magnetic resonance imaging (MRI): Areas of the body that are often difficult to image are possible to see with MRI because of its three-dimensional (3D) capabilities. MRI is useful in detecting cancer in the CNS and the MS system. It is also used to stage breast and endometrial cancer before surgery and to detect metastatic spread of cancer to the liver.

nuclear scans: Nuclear scans are useful in locating and staging cancer of the thyroid and the bone. A **positron emission tomography (PET) scan** provides information about the metabolism of an internal structure, along with its size and shape. It is primarily used for images of the brain, neck, colon, rectum, ovary, and lung. It may also help to identify more aggressive tumors (Fig. 16-8). **Single-photon emission computed tomography (SPECT)** uses a rotating camera to create 3D images with the use of radioactive substances. It is useful in identifying metastases to the bone. *Monoclonal antibodies* are used to evaluate cancer of the prostate, colon, breast, and ovaries and melanoma.

Fig. 16-7 Computed tomography (CT) scan of needle biopsy (bx) of the liver clearly shows the needle in the liver on the left. (Courtesy of Riverside Methodist Hospitals, Columbus, OH.)

Fig. 16-8 High resolution positron emission tomography (PET) scan showing neck cancer *(arrow)*.

radiography: Because tumors are usually denser than the tissue surrounding them, they may appear as a lighter shade of gray (blocking more radiation). Abdominal x-rays may reveal tumors of the stomach, liver, kidneys, and so on, whereas chest x-rays are useful in detecting lung cancer. If a contrast medium is used, as in an upper or lower GI series or intravenous urogram (IVU), tumors of the esophagus, rectum, colon, or kidneys may be detected. Another special type of x-ray is a **mammogram,** which is useful in the early detection of breast cancer. **Stereotactic (3D) mammography** may be used for an image-guided biopsy (bx).

Self-Detection

Self-detection remains the most important method of discovering cancer. The American Cancer Society (ACS) has developed a series of reminders and rules to help individuals become aware of cancer signs and symptoms. For general detection of cancer, they have developed the following CAUTION criteria:

CAUTION Criteria
Change in bowel or bladder habits **A** sore that does not heal **U**nusual bleeding or discharge **T**hickening or lump in the breast, testicles, or elsewhere **I**ndigestion or difficulty swallowing **O**bvious change in the size, shape, color, or thickness of a wart, mole, or mouth sore **N**agging cough or hoarseness

For discovering skin cancer, the ACS has come up with the following ABCDE rule (Fig. 16-9):

ABCDE Rule
A for **asymmetry:** A mole that, when divided in half, does not look the same on both sides. **B** for **border:** A mole with blurry or jagged edges. **C** for **color:** Changes in the color of a mole, including darkening, spread of color, loss of color, or the appearance of multiple colors, such as blue, red, white, pink, purple, or gray. **D** for **diameter:** A mole larger than $\frac{1}{4}$ inch in diameter. **E** for **elevation:** A mole that is raised above the skin and has an uneven surface. (E can also stand for **evolution,** describing how a mole evolves or changes over time.)

The ACS also has criteria for breast self-examination (BSE) and testicular self-examination (TSE).

Fig. 16-9 Malignant melanomas. Note the presence of the ABCDE characteristics (**a**symmetry, **b**order, **c**olor, **d**iameter, and **e**levation)

EXERCISE 2: Diagnostic Procedures

Fill in the blank.

1. A patient's history of smoking may be described as pack years, which is the number of

    _____ smoked per day × the number of years of smoking.

2. Information regarding previous diet, alcohol use, and family members with cancer may be found in

    the _____ section of a patient's medical record.

3. Levels of biochemical substances present in the blood that may indicate neoplastic activity are

    referred to as _____.

4. Removal of a sample of tissue to be examined for signs of cancer is a _____.

5. Mammography may be done to test for cancer of the _____.

Medical Record   *Terrence McAffee*

McAFFEE, TERRENCE C - 599999 Opened by CLINTON, ANNALIESE MD

Task   Edit   View   Time Scale   Options   Help

| McAFFEE, TERRENCE C | Age: 68 years | Sex: Male | Loc: WHC-SMMC |
| | DOB: 01/27/1947 | MRN: 599999 | FIN: 3506004 |

Reference Text Browser   Form Browser   Medication Profile

Orders | Last 48 Hours | ED | Lab | Radiology | Assessments | **Surgery** | Clinical Notes | Pt. Info | Pt. Schedule | Task List | I & O | MAR

Flowsheet: Surgery   Level: Operative Report   ⊙ Table   ○ Group   ○ List

Navigator
✓   Operative Report

Preoperative diagnosis:	History of colon cancer, multiple colon polyps
Postoperative diagnosis:	History of colon cancer, multiple colon polyps
Surgery:	Colonoscopy with polypectomy ×5

This 68-year-old male has colon polyps and a previous history of colon carcinoma. Patient was taken to the endoscopy suite and in the left lateral position, the long colonoscope was inserted without difficulty. The perirectal area was normal. Rectal ampulla was normal. The left colon showed a few diverticula. The right colon had multiple polyps, five of which were removed with hot forceps. The patient tolerated the procedure well and went to the recovery room in stable condition.

PROD MAHAFC   26 April 2015   08:27

⟳ EXERCISE 3: Operative Report

Using the preceding operative report, fill in the blanks.

1. What are "polyps," and why do you think they were removed? _____

2. What is the medical term for colon cancer? _____

3. Give example of procedures done in an endoscopy suite. _____

4. What is a colonoscope? _____

5. Explain the meaning of the procedure "colonoscopy with polypectomy ×5."

_____

THERAPEUTIC INTERVENTIONS

Surgery

The primary treatment for cancer has always been, and remains, removal of the tumor. When the tumor is relatively small and is present only in the organ that is removed, surgery is most effective.

The amount of tissue removed varies with the stage and grade of the cancer. In breast cancer surgery, for example, the types of surgery are as follows:

en bloc resection: Removal of the cancerous tumor and the lymph nodes.

lumpectomy: Removal of the tumor only.

lymph node dissection: The removal of clinically involved lymph nodes. **Lymph node mapping** determines a pattern of spread from the primary tumor site through the lymph nodes. The **sentinel node** is the first node in which lymphatic drainage occurs in a particular area. If this node is negative for cancer upon dissection, then the lymph system is free of cancer, and no other nodes need to be excised.

radical mastectomy: Removal of the breast containing the cancer, along with the lymph nodes and the muscle under the breast. When the surgical report discusses **margins,** it refers to the borders of normal tissue surrounding the cancer. A **wide margin resection** means that the cancer is removed with a significant amount of tissue around the tumor to ensure that all cancer cells are removed. If the margins are reported as negative, no cancer cells are seen. If the margins are reported as positive, cancer cells have been detected by the pathologist.

simple mastectomy: Removal of the breast containing the cancer.

Radiotherapy

Approximately half of all cancer patients receive radiation. The goal of radiation therapy is to destroy the nucleus of the cancer cells, thereby destroying their ability to reproduce and spread.

Although radiation is usually started after removal of the tumor, sometimes it is done before removal to shrink the tumor. Some cancers may be treated solely with radiation.

three-dimensional conformal radiation therapy (3DCRT): Targeted radiation therapy that uses digital diagnostic imaging and specialized software to treat tumors without damaging surrounding tissue (Fig. 16-10).

brachytherapy (bray kee THAIR uh pee): The use of radiation placed directly on or within the cancer through the use of needles or beads containing radioactive gold, cobalt, or radium (Fig. 16-11).

gamma knife surgery: A noninvasive type of surgery that uses gamma radiation to destroy a brain tumor.

intensity-modulated radiation therapy (IMRT): High-dosage radiation delivered via a beam that changes its dosage and shape.

Systemic Therapy

bone marrow transplant (BMT): Patients who are incapable of producing healthy blood cells are given bone marrow from a matching donor to stimulate normal blood cell growth. Patients with specific types of leukemia may receive BMTs after chemotherapy has effectively destroyed the functioning of their own bone marrow.

chemotherapy
chem/o = drug, chemical
-therapy = treatment

Fig. 16-10 Dosimetry plan showing nine different radiation fields used to treat a pancreatic tumor.

Fig. 16-11 Prostate brachytherapy. Radioactive seeds are implanted with a needle guided by sonography and a template grid.

chemotherapy: Chemotherapy is the circulation of cancer-destroying medicine throughout the body. Chemotherapy may also be used as an adjuvant (aid) to other forms of treatment to relieve symptoms or slow down the spread of cancer. Combination chemotherapy is the use of two or more anticancer drugs at one time. See the Pharmacology section for more details on chemotherapy drugs.

complementary and alternative medicine (CAM) techniques: Prayer, massage, diet, exercise, and mind-body techniques constitute the majority of CAM methods used in cancer treatment. The US government has established the National Center for Complementary and Alternative Medicine, which reports on results of research studies on the use of CAM techniques for various disorders (http://www.nccam.nih.gov).

immunotherapy: Immunotherapy is the use of the body's own defense system to attack cancer cells. See the description of interleukins in the Pharmacology section.

brachytherapy
brachy- = short
-therapy = treatment

Preventive Measures

vaccines: Two vaccines are currently in use to prevent specific cancers. The hepatitis B vaccine prevents hepatitis B with its sequelae of liver cancer and cirrhosis. The cervical cancer vaccine protects a woman against strains 16 and 18 of the human papillomavirus (HPV).

EXERCISE 4: Therapeutic Interventions

Fill in the blank.

1. Treatment with radioactive beads near or inside the cancer is called _____.

2. A determination of the spread of the primary tumor through the lymph nodes is referred to as lymph node _____.

3. The first node in which lymphatic drainage occurs is the _____ node.

4. Removal of the tumor and lymph nodes is called_____.

5. The borders of normal tissue surrounding the cancer are called _____.

6. Use of the body's own defense system to attack cancer cells is called _____.

7. Prayer, massage, exercise, and mind-body techniques are examples of _____.

8. Three-dimensional targeted radiation treatment to treat tumors without damaging surrounding tissue is _____.

Case Study   Tamara Ramos

Tamara Ramos' cousin, Virginia, is currently undergoing treatment for metastatic breast cancer and has started a blog to keep family and friends informed on her progress. Because Virginia's and Tamara's mothers are sisters in a large family, Virginia has posted a family history. One of the grandmothers had breast cancer when she was in her 70s, but it went into remission for a decade. She had been diagnosed through a routine mammography and treated with a mastectomy and chemotherapy. Her sister, one of the great aunts, posted that she had been diagnosed with cervical dysplasia at age 44.

1. The combining forms in the terms mammography and mastectomy both refer to the _____.

2. Chemotherapy refers to treatment with what?
   a. drugs
   b. x-rays
   c. surgery

3. The term *metastatic* means that the cancer has _____.
   a. been cured
   b. spread
   c. been contained

4. The term *complete remission* means that the cancer has____.
   a. reoccurred
   b. spread
   c. disappeared

5. Dysplasia refers to a/n _____ formation.
   a. abnormal
   b. normal

Case Study   Akiyo Kato

After a high PSA level triggered further testing, Akiyo Kato was diagnosed with prostate cancer last year. Although his urologist initially had hoped that Akiyo might have hyperplasia, the diagnosis was adenocarcinoma of the prostate, stage III. After unsuccessful treatment with a transurethral resection of the prostate (TURP) and brachytherapy, he s now receiving palliative therapy in hospice.

1. PSA stands for _____ specific antigen.
   a. prostatic
   b. permanent
   c. patient

2. Hyperplasia refers to a/n _____ condition of formation.
   a. lack of
   b. excessive

3. The prefix *brachy-* in brachytherapy refers to the _____ distance the radiation needs to travel to destroy the tumor.
   a. long
   b. short

4. An adenocarcinoma is a _____ tumor.
   a. benign
   b. malignant

5. What is the purpose of palliative treatment?
   a. to make the patient comfortable
   b. to cure the patient
   c. to treat the tumor

PHARMACOLOGY

Chemotherapy works by disrupting the cycle of cell replication. All cells go through a cycle of reproducing themselves, but, unlike cancer cells, they have a built-in mechanism that limits their growth. The side effects of cancer therapy (such as, hair loss or nausea) are due to the inability of chemotherapeutic agents to differentiate between normal and cancerous cells. Thus cells that reproduce rapidly (such as, hair cells or those that line the stomach) are also affected. It should also be noted that two or more chemotherapeutic agents usually are used together to effectively attack the cancer at various stages. This is referred to as a *drug protocol* or *plan*.

Most of the pharmaceuticals prescribed to treat cancer are referred to as *antineoplastic agents*. They accomplish the goal of slowing or stopping the progression of cancer in different ways:

alkylating agents: Interfere with DNA replication to lead to cancer cell death or dysfunction. Examples include cisplatin (Platinol AQ), nitrosoureas like carmustine (Gliadel), and nitrogen mustards like cyclophosphamide (Cytoxan).

antimetabolites: Replace compounds that cancer cells need to grow and/or replicate. Examples are methotrexate and fluorouracil (5-FU).

antineoplastic antibiotics: Prevent or delay cell replication. Examples include doxorubicin (Rubex, Adriamycin) and dactinomycin (Cosmegen).

antineoplastic hormones: Interfere with receptors for growth-stimulating proteins. Examples include flutamide (Eulexin) and tamoxifen (Nolvadex).

interleukins: Stimulate cells of the immune system to boost attacks on cancer cells. An example is aldesleukin (Proleukin).

mitotic inhibitors: Prevent cell division. An example is paclitaxel (Taxol).

vinca alkaloids: Prevent formation of chromosome spindles necessary for cell duplication. Examples include vincristine (Oncovin) and vinblastine (Velban).

EXERCISE 5: Pharmacology

Circle the correct answer.

1. Patients who are prescribed chemotherapy receive a drug *(protocol, adjuvant)*.

2. Side effects of chemotherapy frequently occur because the drugs used to kill cancer cells often *(stimulate, kill)* normal cells.

3. Most chemotherapeutic agents work by disrupting the cycle of cell *(replication, movement)*.

4. Drugs that interfere with receptors for growth-stimulating proteins are *(antineoplastic hormones, antimetabolites)*.

5. Drugs that interfere with DNA replication are called *(antineoplastic, antibiotics, alkylating agents)*.

6. Drugs that replace compounds that cancer cells need to grow or replicate are *(interleukins, antimetabolites)*.

7. Cell division is prevented by *(vinca alkaloids, miotic inhibitors)*.

 *Click on **Hear It, Spell It** to practice spelling the diagnostic and therapeutic terms that you have learned in this chapter.*

Medical Record — Stella Yates

YATES, STELLA M - 618022 Opened by SINGH, SHEPHALI

Task   Edit   View   Time Scale   Options   Help

YATES, STELLA M

Age: 40 years
DOB: 03/02/1975

Sex: Female
MRN: 618022

Loc: WHC-SMMC
FIN: 3506004

As Of 20:25

Reference Text Browser | Form Browser | Medication Profile

Orders | Last 48 Hours | ED | Lab | Radiology | Assessments | Surgery | **Clinical Notes** | Pt. Info | Pt. Schedule | Task List | I & O | MAR

Flowsheet: Clinical Notes   Level: Discharge Summary   ○ Table ○ Group ○ List

Navigator

✓ Discharge Summary

Final Diagnosis: 1. Metastatic breast cancer

2. Dehydration with confusion

SUMMARY: This is a 40-year-old woman who developed breast cancer approximately 1 year ago. She had surgery and chemotherapy, seemed to be doing well, but this fall developed recurrence. This was present in the neck and liver. She underwent cycles of chemotherapy. Although the nodes in her neck subsided, she has had advancing cancer in the liver and does not seem to be responding to chemotherapy, and in fact, the chemotherapy is making her quite ill. This has been discussed with her family, and because this therapy is not going to cure her and is making her ill, she has decided to forego any more chemotherapy at this time, which seems appropriate.

She has had some right flank pain, I presume from the liver metastases. She has had a very poor appetite and poor oral intake, and has become quite dehydrated and confused. She came to the hospital in an extremely weak and confused condition. She was noted to have hyponatremia with sodium down to 125, extremely dry mucous membranes. White count was elevated to 16.5. Hemoglobin has been right around 10. Initial labs also suggested a urinary tract infection, although the culture did not grow anything.

She was admitted and treated with IV fluids and nausea medication, and started on Cipro for presumed UTI. Her condition improved so that she became mentally clear. She continues to have poor oral intake and needs a lot of encouragement, but is discharged home to be followed by hospice. Her long-term prognosis is poor, probably in the range of months.

Discharge medications include Cipro 500 mg for an additional 7 days. Compazine 10 mg po every 6 hr for nausea, Ultram 1 to 2 tablets t.i.d. for pain, and Senokot 1 to 2 tablets p.r.n. for constipation. Plan of care was discussed with her and her family, and hospice will be following her.

PROD MAHAFC 04/07/2015 20:25

⊘ EXERCISE 6: Discharge Summary

Using the preceding discharge summary, fill in the blanks.

1. This patient has metastatic breast cancer. What does this mean? _____

2. Where has the cancer spread to? _____

3. What type of treatment has she received? _____

4. The patient is dehydrated and hyponatremia is noted. What is hyponatremia? _____

5. Explain what "her long-term prognosis is poor, probably in the range of months" means.

_____

Abbreviations

Abbreviations	Meaning	Abbreviations	Meaning
3DCRT	three-dimensional conformal radiation therapy	FOBT	fecal occult blood test
		G	grade
ACS	American Cancer Society	GI	gastrointestinal
AFP	alpha fetoprotein (test)	hCG	human chorionic gonadotropin
B2M	beta-2 microglobulin	IMRT	intensity-modulated radiation therapy
BMT	bone marrow transplant		
BSE	breast self-examination	IVU	intravenous urogram
BTA	bladder tumor antigen	mets	metastases
Bx	biopsy	MS	musculoskeletal
CA	cancer	NSE	neuron-specific enolase
CA125	tumor marker primarily for ovarian cancer	Pap	Papanicolaou test for cervical/vaginal cancer
CA15-3	tumor marker to monitor breast cancer	PET	positron emission tomography
CA19-9	tumor marker for pancreatic, stomach, and bile duct cancer	PSA	prostate-specific antigen
CA27-29	tumor marker to check for recurrence of breast cancer	SPECT	single-photon emission computed tomography
		TA-90	tumor marker for spread of malignant melanoma
CAM	complementary and alternative medicine	TNM	tumor-nodes-metastases (staging)
CEA	carcinoembryonic antigen		
CIS	carcinoma in situ	TSE	testicular self-examination
CTR	certified tumor registrar		

EXERCISE 7: Abbreviations

Write the meaning of the following abbreviations.

1. The patient appeared for a Bx of a suspicious mole.

   _____

2. The prognosis was poor for the lung cancer patient with a G IV finding on his pathology report.

   _____

3. The 50-year-old woman made an appointment for a colonoscopy to check for CA after she had a positive finding on a home FOBT.

   _____

4. The CTR at Montgomery Memorial recorded the TNM stage for the patient's abstract.

   _____

5. SPECT was used to detect bone mets in the patient with advanced breast cancer.

   _____

Chapter Review

Match the word parts to their definitions.

Word Part Definitions

Prefix/Suffix
ana-
apo-
-blast
-carcinoma
dys-
ecto-
-genesis
hyper-
meta-
neo-
-oma
-plasia
-plasm
-ptosis
-sarcoma
-stasis

Definition

1. _____ new
2. _____ condition of formation
3. _____ tumor
4. _____ away from
5. _____ abnormal
6. _____ production, origin
7. _____ up, apart
8. _____ embryonic
9. _____ cancer of epithelial origin
10. _____ outer
11. _____ controlling, stopping
12. _____ connective tissue cancer
13. _____ beyond, change
14. _____ formation
15. _____ excessive
16. _____ falling

Combining Form
blast/o
carcin/o
derm/o
mut/a
nod/o
onc/o
path/o
sarc/o

Definition

17. _____ change
18. _____ embryonic
19. _____ connective tissue cancer
20. _____ tumor
21. _____ disease
22. _____ node
23. _____ skin
24. _____ cancer

Wordshop

Prefixes	Combining Forms	Suffixes
ana-	aden/o	-oma
apo-	astr/o	-plasia
brachy-	blast/o	-ptosis
	chrom/o	-sarcoma
	cyt/o	-therapy
	hemangi/o	-tion
	meningi/o	
	mut/a	
	nephr/o	
	neur/o	
	oste/o	
	phe/o	
	retin/o	

Build the following terms by combining the preceding word parts. Some word parts will be used more than once. Some may not be used at all. The number in parentheses indicates the number of word parts needed to build the terms.

Definition	Term
1. tumor of a nerve (2)	_____
2. tumor of a blood vessel (2)	_____
3. malignant tumor of bone (2)	_____
4. tumor of a gland (2)	_____
5. tumor of embryonic retinal (cells) (3)	_____
6. treatment using short distance (radiation) (2)	_____
7. condition of formation apart (dedifferentiation) (2)	_____
8. falling away (cell suicide) (2)	_____
9. process of change (2)	_____
10. tumor of the meninges (2)	_____
11. star cell tumor (3)	_____
12. kidney tumor (2)	_____
13. dark color cell tumor (4)	_____

Sort the terms into the correct categories.

Term Sorting

Benign Neoplasms	Malignant Neoplasms	Diagnostic Procedures	Therapeutic Interventions

3DCRT	chemotherapy	IMRT	osteoma
acoustic neuroma	CT scan	Kaposi sarcoma	PET
adenocarcinoma	dermatofibroma	leiomyoma	pheochromocytoma
AFP	Ewing sarcoma	leukemia	PSA
biopsy (bx)	fibroids	lumpectomy	radiotherapy
BMT	gamma knife surgery	mammogram	retinoblastoma
BPH	hcG	mastectomy	seminoma
brachytherapy	hemangiosarcoma	meningioma	SPECT
BTA	hypernephroma	myxosarcoma	thymoma
CA125	immunotherapy	neuroma	Wilms tumor

Replace the highlighted words with the correct terms.

Translations

1. The cancer registry student had four cases to abstract: one **testicular cancer,** one **cancer of the bone marrow,** and **two glandular cancers of the lung.**

2. The pathologist described the cancer as **appearing to have cells that retain most of their intended function.**

3. The patient was diagnosed with **spreading beyond control** of breast cancer.

4. The **test for vaginal and cervical cancer** revealed severe **abnormal condition of formation** of the cervical cells.

5. As a result of a breast self-examination, Bonita's Stage I breast cancer was treated with **a removal of the tumor only, treatment with x-rays** and **circulation of cancer-destroying medicine throughout the body.**

6. Allen's prostate cancer was treated with the use of **radioactive beads directly in the tumor.**

7. Ellen was diagnosed with **cancer of white blood cells** and was treated with **cancer-destroying medicine throughout the body** and **bone marrow from a matching donor.**

DISCHARGE SUMMARY

Using the discharge summary above, answer the following questions.

1. What was the patient's diagnosis?

   _____

2. How was his cancer diagnosed?

   _____

3. What procedures were done?

   _____

4. How do we know that there was no cancer in the lymph nodes?

   _____

Appendix A

Word Parts and Definitions

Word Part	Meaning	Word Part	Meaning
-a	noun ending	amyl/o	starch
a-	no, not, without	-an	pertaining to
ab-	away from	an-	no, not, without
abdomin/o	abdomen	an/o	anus
-ablation	removal	ana-	up, apart, away
-abrasion	scraping of	andr/o	male
-ac	pertaining to	angi/o	vessel
acid/o	acid	ankyl/o	stiffening
acous/o	hearing	ante-	forward, in front of, before
acro-	heights, extremities	anter/o	front
acromi/o	acromion	anthrop/o	man
acu-	sharp	anti-	against
-acusis	hearing	antr/o	antrum, cavity
-ad	toward	aort/o	aorta (largest artery)
ad-	toward	-apheresis	removal
aden/o	gland	aphth/o	ulceration
adenoid/o	adenoid (pharyngeal tonsil)	apic/o	pointed extremity, apex
adip/o	fat	apo-	separate, away from
adnex/o	accessory	append/o	vermiform appendix, that which is added
adren/o	adrenal gland		
aer/o	air	appendic/o	vermiform appendix, that which is added
af-	toward		
agglutin/o	clumping	-ar	pertaining to
agora-	marketplace	-arche	beginning
-al	pertaining to	arteri/o	artery
albin/o	white	arteriol/o	arteriole (small artery)
albumin/o	protein	arthr/o	articulation (joint)
-algia	pain	articul/o	articulation (joint)
aliment/o	nutrition	-ary	pertaining to
allo-	other, different	-ase	enzyme
alveol/o	alveolus	astr/o	star
ambly/o	dull, dim	ather/o	fatty plaque
ambul/o	walking	-atic	pertaining to
amni/o	amnion	-ation	process of
-amnios	amnion, inner fetal sac	atri/o	atrium
amphi-	both	audi/o	hearing

Word Parts and Definitions—cont'd

Word Part	Meaning	Word Part	Meaning
aur/o	ear	cardi/o	heart
auricul/o	ear	-cardia	condition of the heart
auto-	self	carp/o	carpus (wrist)
axill/o	axilla (armpit)	cartilag/o	cartilage
az/o	nitrogen	cata-	down
azot/o	nitrogen	caud/o	tail
bacteri/o	bacteria	cauter/i	burning
balan/o	glans penis	cec/o	cecum (first part of large intestine)
bar/o	pressure, weight		
bartholin/o	Bartholin gland	-cele	herniation, protrusion
bas/o	base, bottom	celi/o	abdomen
bi-	two	cellul/o	cell
bi/o	life, living	-centesis	surgical puncture
bil/i	bile	cephal/o	head
bin-	two	cerebell/o	cerebellum
-blast	embryonic, immature	cerebr/o	cerebrum
blast/o	embryonic, immature	cerumin/o	cerumen (earwax)
blephar/o	eyelid	cervic/o	neck, cervix
bol/o	to throw, throwing	-chalasia	condition of relaxation, slackening
brachi/o	arm		
brachy-	short	-chalasis	relaxation, slackening
brady-	slow	cheil/o	lips
bronch/o	bronchus	chem/o	drug, chemical
bronchi/o	bronchus	-chezia	condition of stools
bronchiol/o	bronchiole	chol/e	bile, gall
bucc/o	cheek	cholangi/o	bile vessel
bunion/o	bunion	cholecyst/o	gallbladder
burs/o	bursa	choledoch/o	common bile duct
calc/o, calc/i	calcium	cholesterol/o	cholesterol
calcane/o	calcaneus (heel bone)	chondr/o	cartilage
calcul/o	stone, calculus	chord/o	cord, spinal cord
cali/o	calyx, calix	chori/o	chorion (outer fetal sac)
calic/o	calyx, calix	chorion/o	chorion (outer fetal sac)
calyc/o	calyx, calix	choroid/o	choroid, vascular membrane
cancer/o	cancer, malignancy	chrom/o	color
canth/o	canthus (corner of eye)	chromat/o	color
capit/o	head	chym/o	juice
capn/o	carbon dioxide	circum-	around
carcin/o	cancer	cirrh/o	orange-yellow
-carcinoma	cancer of epithelial origin	-cision	process of cutting

Word Parts and Definitions—cont'd

Word Part	Meaning	Word Part	Meaning
-clasis	intentional breaking	-cusis	hearing
-clast	breaking down	cut/o	skin
claustr/o	closing	cutane/o	skin
clavicul/o	clavicle (collarbone)	cyan/o	blue
cleid/o	clavicle (collarbone)	cycl/o	ciliary body, recurring, round
clitorid/o	clitoris	-cyesis	pregnancy, gestation
-coagulation	process of clotting	cyst/o	bladder, sac
coccyg/o	coccyx (tailbone)	cyt/o	cell
cochle/o	cochlea	-cyte	cell
col/o	colon (large intestine)	-cytosis	abnormal increase in cells
coll/o	neck	dacry/o	tear
colon/o	colon (large intestine)	dacryoaden/o	lacrimal gland
colp/o	vagina	dacryocyst/o	lacrimal sac
commissur/o	connection	dactyl/o	digitus (finger or toe)
con-	together	de-	down, lack of
con/o	cone	dendr/o	dendrite, tree
condyl/o	condyle, knob	dent/i	teeth
coni/o	dust	derm/o	skin
conjunctiv/o	conjunctiva	dermat/o	skin
contra-	opposite, against	-desis	binding
cor/o	pupil	dextr/o	right
cord/o	cord, spinal cord	di-	two, both
cordi/o	heart	dia-	through, complete
core/o	pupil	diaphragm/o	diaphragm
corne/o	cornea	diaphragmat/o	diaphragm
coron/o	crown, heart	digit/o	finger or toe
corpor/o	body	dipl/o	double
cortic/o	cortex (outer portion)	dips/o	thirst
cost/o	costa (rib)	-dipsia	condition of thirst
cox/o	coxa (hip)	dis-	bad, abnormal, apart
crani/o	cranium (skull)	dist/o	far
crin/o	to secrete, secreting	diverticul/o	diverticulum, pouch
-crine	to secrete, secreting	dors/o	back
-crit	to separate, separating	-drome	to run, running
crur/o	leg	duct/o	to carry, carrying
cry/o	extreme cold	duoden/o	duodenum
crypt-	hidden	dur/o	dura mater, hard
cubit/o	elbow, forearm	-dynia	pain
culd/o	cul-de-sac (rectouterine pouch)	dys-	bad, difficult, painful, abnormal

Word Parts and Definitions—cont'd

Word Part	Meaning	Word Part	Meaning
-e	noun ending	ethmoid/o	ethmoid bone
e-	outward, out	eu-	healthy, normal
-eal	pertaining to	ex-	out
ec-	out, outward	exanthemat/o	rash
echo-	sound, reverberation	-exia	condition
-ectasia	condition of expansion, dilation	exo-	outside
-ectasis	expansion, dilation	extra-	outside
ecto-	outward, outer	faci/o	face
-ectomy	removal, excision	fallopi/o	fallopian tube
-edema	swelling	fasci/o	fascia
ef-	away from	fec/a	feces, stool
electr/o	electricity	femor/o	femur (thigh bone)
-emesis	vomiting, vomit	fer/o	to bear, carry
-emia	blood condition	-ferous	pertaining to carrying
-emic	pertaining to blood condition	ferr/o	iron
en-	in	fet/o	fetus
encephal/o	brain	fibr/o	fiber
end-	within	fibrin/o	fibrous substance
endo-	within	fibul/o	fibula (lower lateral leg bone)
endocardi/o	inner lining of the heart	-fida	to split, splitting
endometri/o	endometrium	flex/o	to bend, bending
enter/o	small intestines, intestines	fluor/o	to flow, flowing
eosin/o	rosy-colored	-flux	to flow, flowing
epi-	above, upon	follicul/o	follicle, small sac
epicardi/o	epicardium	foramin/o	hole, foramen
epicondyl/o	epicondyle	fornic/o	arched structure, fornix
epididym/o	epididymis	foss/o	hollow, depression
epiglott/o	epiglottis	front/o	front, forehead
episi/o	vulva (external female genitalia)	fund/o	fundus (base, bottom)
epitheli/o	epithelium	fung/i	fungus
erg/o	work	-fusion	process of pouring
erythr/o	red	galact/o	milk
erythrocyt/o	red blood cell	gastr/o	stomach
eschar/o	scab	-gen	producing, produced by
-esis	state of	gen/o	origin, originate
eso-	inward	-genesis	production, origin
esophag/o	esophagus	-genic	pertaining to produced by
esthesi/o	feeling, sensation	-genous	pertaining to originating from
		ger/o	old age

Word Parts and Definitions—cont'd

Word Part	Meaning	Word Part	Meaning
geus/o	taste	hil/o	hilum
gingiv/o	gums	hist/o	tissue
glauc/o	gray, bluish green	home/o	same
-glia	glia cell, glue	homo-	same
-globin	protein substance	humer/o	humerus (upper arm bone)
-globulin	protein substance	humor/o	liquid
glomerul/o	glomerulus	hydr/o	water, fluid
gloss/o	tongue	hymen/o	hymen
gluc/o	sugar, glucose	hyper-	excessive, above
glute/o	gluteus (buttocks)	hypo-	deficient, below, under
glyc/o	sugar, glucose	hypophys/o	hypophysis, pituitary
glycos/o	sugar, glucose	hyster/o	uterus
gnath/o	jaw, entire	-i	noun ending
gnos/o	knowledge	-ia	condition, state of
gon/o	seed	-iac	pertaining to
gonad/o	gonad, sex organ	-iasis	condition, presence of
goni/o	angle	iatr/o	treatment
-gram	record, recording	-iatric	pertaining to treatment
granul/o	little grain	-iatrician	one who specializes in treatment
-graph	instrument to record	-iatrist	one who specializes in treatment
graph/o	to write, writing		
-graphy	process of recording	-iatry	process of treatment
gravid/o	pregnancy, gestation	-ic	pertaining to
-gravida	pregnancy, gestation	ichthy/o	fishlike
gynec/o	female, woman	-ician	one who studies
halit/o	breath	-icle	small, tiny
hal/o	to breathe, breathing	-id	pertaining to
hedon/o	pleasure	idi/o	unique, unknown
hem/o	blood	-ile	pertaining to
hemangi/o	blood vessel	ile/o	ileum (third part small intestines)
hemat/o	blood		
hemi-	half	ili/o	ilium (superior, widest pelvic bone)
hemorrhoid/o	hemorrhoid		
hepat/o	liver	immun/o	safety, protection
herni/o	hernia	-in	substance
heter/o	different	in-	in, not
hiat/o	an opening	-ine	pertaining to
hidr/o	sweat	infer/o	downward
hidraden/o	sudoriferous gland (sweat gland)	infra-	down

Word Parts and Definitions—cont'd

Word Part	Meaning	Word Part	Meaning
inguin/o	groin	-lalia	condition of babbling
insulin/o	insulin	lamin/o	lamina, thin plate
inter-	between	lapar/o	abdomen
interstit/o	space between	-lapse	falling, dropping, prolapse
intestin/o	intestine	laryng/o	larynx (voice box)
intra-	within	later/o	side
-ion	process of	lei/o	smooth
-ior	pertaining to	leiomy/o	smooth muscle
ipsi-	same	-lepsy	seizure
ir/o	iris	leuk/o	white
irid/o	iris	leukocyt/o	white blood cell
-is	structure, thing, noun ending	levo-	left
is/o	equal	lex/o	word, speech
isch/o	hold back, suppress	ligament/o	ligament
ischi/o	ischium (lower part of pelvic bone)	ligat/o	to tie, tying
		lingu/o	tongue
-ism	condition, state of	lip/o	fat
-ist	one who specializes	lipid/o	lipid, fat
-itis	inflammation	-listhesis	slipping
-itic	pertaining to	lith/o	stone, calculus
-ium	structure, membrane	-lithotomy	removal of a stone
-ive	pertaining to	lob/o	lobe, section
-ization	process of	lobul/o	small lobe
jejun/o	second part of small intestine jejunum	log/o	study
		-logist	one who specializes in the study of
kal/i	potassium	-logy	study of
kary/o	nucleus	long/o	long
kathis/o	sitting	lord/o	swayback
kerat/o	hard, horny, cornea	lumb/o	lower back
ket/o	ketone	lumin/o	lumen (space within vessel)
keton/o	ketone	lymph/o	lymph
-kine	movement	lymphaden/o	lymph gland (lymph node)
kinesi/o	movement	lymphangi/o	lymph vessel
-kinin	movement substance	lymphat/o	lymph
klept/o	to steal, stealing	lys/o	break down, dissolve
kyph/o	round back	-lysis	breaking down, dissolving, loosening, freeing from adhesions
labi/o	lips, labia		
labyrinth/o	labyrinth (inner ear)		
lacrim/o	tear	-lytic	pertaining to breaking down
lact/o	milk		

Word Parts and Definitions—cont'd

Word Part	Meaning	Word Part	Meaning
macro-	large	mitochondri/o	mitochondria
macul/o	macula, macule, macula lutea, spot	mono-	one
		morph/o	shape, form
mal-	bad, poor	muc/o	mucus
-malacia	condition of softening	multi-	many
malle/o	malleus, hammer	muscul/o	muscle
malleol/o	distal process lower leg, little malleolus	mut/a	change
		my/o	muscle, to shut
mamm/o	breast	myc/o	fungus
man/o	scanty pressure	myel/o	bone marrow, spinal cord
mandibul/o	lower jaw	myocardi/o	myocardium (heart muscle)
-mania	condition of madness	myos/o	muscle
man/u	hand	myring/o	eardrum
mast/o	breast	myx/o	mucus
mastoid/o	mastoid process	narc/o	sleep, stupor
maxill/o	maxilla (upper jaw bone)	nas/o	nose
meat/o	meatus (opening)	nat/o	birth, born
medi/o	middle	natr/o	sodium
mediastin/o	mediastinum (space between lungs)	necr/o	death, dead
		neo-	new
medull/o	medulla, inner portion	nephr/o	kidney
-megaly	enlargement	neur/o	nerve
melan/o	black, dark	neutr/o	neutral
men/o	menstruation, menses	nev/o	nevus, birthmark
mening/o	meninges	nid/o	nest
meningi/o	meninges	noct/i	night
menisc/o	meniscus, crescent	nod/o	node, knot
menstru/o	menstruation	-noia	condition of mind
ment/o	mind, chin	non-	not
meso-	middle	nuch/o	neck
meta-	beyond, change	nucle/o	nucleus
metacarp/o	metacarpal (hand bone)	nulli-	none
metatars/o	metatarsal (foot bone)	nyctal/o	night
-meter	instrument to measure	nymph/o	woman, female
metr/o	uterus	o/o	ovum, egg, female sex cell
metri/o	uterus	occipit/o	occiput, back of head
-metry	process of measurement	occlus/o	to close, closing, a blockage
micro-	small	-occlusion	condition of closure
mid-	middle	-occult	secret, hidden
-mission	to send, sending		

Word Parts and Definitions—cont'd

Word Part	Meaning	Word Part	Meaning
ocul/o	eye	oxy-	rapid
odont/o	teeth	palat/o	palate, roof of mouth, palatine bone
-oid	resembling, like		
olecran/o	elbow	palm/o	palm
olig/o	scanty, few	palpebr/o	eyelid
-oma	tumor, mass	pan-	all
omphal/o	umbilicus (navel)	pancreat/o	pancreas
onc/o	tumor	papill/o	papilla, nipple, optic disk
-on	structure	papul/o	papule, pimple
-one	hormone, substance that forms	par-	beside, near
		-para	delivery, parturition
onych/o	nail	para-	near, beside, abnormal
oophor/o	ovary (female gonad)	parathyroid/o	parathyroid
ophthalm/o	eye	parenchym/o	parenchyma
-opia	vision condition	-paresis	slight paralysis
-opsia	vision condition	pariet/o	wall, partition
-opsy	process of viewing	part/o	parturition (delivery)
opt/o	vision	-partum	parturition (delivery)
optic/o	vision	patell/o, patell/a	patella (kneecap)
or/o	mouth, oral cavity		
orbit/o	orbit	path/o	disease
orch/o	testis, testicle (male gonad)	-pathy	disease process
orchi/o	testis, testicle (male gonad)	-pause	stop, cease
orchid/o	testis, testicle (male gonad)	pector/o	chest
orex/o	appetite	ped/o	foot, child
organ/o	organ, viscus	pedicul/o	lice
orth/o	straight, upright	pelv/i, pelv/o	pelvis
-ose	pertaining to, full of	pen/i	penis
-osis	abnormal condition	-penia	deficiency condition
osm/o	sense of smell	-pepsia	digestion condition
oss/i	bone	per-	through
osse/o	bone	peri-	surrounding, around
ossicul/o	ossicle (tiny bone)	pericardi/o	sac surrounding the heart
oste/o	bone	perine/o	perineum
ot/o	ear	peritone/o, periton/o	peritoneum
-ous	pertaining to		
ov/o	ovum (egg)	perone/o	lower, lateral leg bone, fibula
ovari/o	ovary (female gonad)	-pexy	fixation, suspension
ovul/o	ovum (female sex cell)	phac/o	lens
ox/i, ox/o	oxygen	phag/o	to eat, swallow

Word Parts and Definitions—cont'd

Word Part	Meaning	Word Part	Meaning
phak/o	lens	pne/o	to breathe, breathing
phalang/o	phalanx (finger/toe bones)	pneum/o	lung, air
phall/o	penis	pneumon/o	lung
pharyng/o	pharynx (throat)	-poiesis	formation, production
phas/o	speech	-poietin	forming substance
phe/o	dark	pol/o	pole
-pheresis	removal	poly-	many, much, excessive, frequent
-phil	attraction		
phil/o	attraction	polyp/o	polyp
-philia	condition of attraction, increase	poplite/o	back of knee
		por/o	passage
phleb/o	vein	post-	behind, after
-phobia	condition of fear, extreme sensitivity	poster/o	back
		potass/o	potassium
phon/o	sound, voice	prax/o	purposeful movement
phor/o	to carry, to bear	pre-	before, in front of
phot/o	light	preputi/o	prepuce (foreskin)
phren/o	diaphragm, mind	presby-	old age
-phylaxis	protection	press/o	pressure
physi/o	growth, nature	primi-	first
-physis	growth, nature	pro-	forward, in front of, in favor of
phyt/o	growth, nature		
pil/o	hair	proct/o	rectum and anus
pituitar/o	pituitary	prolactin/o	prolactin
placent/o	placenta	prostat/o	prostate
-plakia	condition of patches	prosth/o, prosthes/o	addition
plant/o	sole of foot		
plas/o	formation	proxim/o	near
-plasia	condition of formation, development	psych/o	mind
		-ptosis	drooping, prolapse, falling
-plasm	formation	-ptysis	spitting
plasm/o	plasma	pub/o	pubis, anterior pelvic bone
plast/o	formation	pulmon/o	lung
-plastin	forming substance	pupill/o	pupil
-plasty	surgical repair	puerper/o	childbirth, puerperium
-plegia	paralysis	purpur/o	purple
pleur/o	pleura, membrane surrounding lungs	pustul/o	pustule
		py/o	pus
plethysm/o	volume	pyel/o	renal pelvis
plic/o	fold, plica	pylor/o	pylorus
-pnea	breathing		

Word Parts and Definitions—cont'd

Word Part	Meaning	Word Part	Meaning
pyr/o	fever, fire	scoli/o	curvature
pyret/o	fever, fire	-scope	instrument to view
quadri-	four	-scopic	pertaining to viewing
rachi/o	spinal column, backbone	-scopy	process of viewing
radi/o	radius (lower lateral arm bone)	scot/o	dark
		scrot/o	scrotum (sac holding testes)
radi/o	rays	sebac/o	sebum, oil
radicul/o	nerve root, spinal nerve root	seb/o	sebum, oil
re-	back, backward, again	semin/i	semen
rect/o	rectum, straight	seps/o	infection
ren/o	kidney	-sepsis	infection
reticul/o	network	sept/o	septum, wall, partition
retin/o	retina	septic/o	infection
retro-	backward	ser/o	serum
rhabd/o	striated	sial/o	saliva
rhabdomy/o	striated (skeletal) muscle	sialaden/o	salivary gland
rheumat/o	watery flow	sider/o	iron
rhin/o	nose	-siderin	iron substance
rhiz/o	spinal nerve root, nerve root	sigmoid/o	sigmoid colon
rhythm/o	rhythm	sin/o	sinus, cavity
rhytid/o	wrinkle	sinistr/o	left
rib/o	ribose	sinus/o	sinus, cavity
rot/o	wheel	-sis	state of, condition
-rrhagia, -rrhage	bursting forth	skelet/o	skeleton
		somat/o	body
-rrhaphy	suture, repair	somn/o	sleep
-rrhea	discharge, flow	son/o	sound
-rrheic	pertaining to discharge	-spadias	a rent or tear
-rrhexis	rupture	-spasm	spasm, sudden, involuntary contraction
rug/o	rugae, ridge		
sacr/o	sacrum	sperm/o	spermatozoon (male sex cell)
sagitt/o	arrow, separating the sides	spermat/o	spermatozoon (male sex cell)
salping/o	tube, fallopian or eustachian	sphenoid/o	sphenoid
-salpinx	fallopian, tube	spin/o	spine
sarc/o	flesh	spir/o	to breathe, breathing
-sarcoma	connective tissue cancer	splen/o	spleen
scapul/o	scapula (shoulder blade)	spondyl/o	vertebra, backbone, spine
schiz/o	split	squam/o	scaly
scler/o	sclera, hard	-stalsis	contraction
-sclerosis	abnormal condition of hardening	staped/o	stapes (third ossicle in ear)

Word Parts and Definitions—cont'd

Word Part	Meaning	Word Part	Meaning
-stasis	controlling, stopping	testicul/o	testis, testicle (male gonad)
steat/o	fat	tetra-	four
-stenosis	abnormal condition of narrowing	thalam/o	thalamus
		thalass/o	sea
ster/o	steroid	thel/e	nipple
stere/o	three-dimensional	-therapy	treatment
stern/o	sternum (breastbone)	therm/o	heat, temperature
steth/o	chest	thorac/o	thorax (chest)
sthen/o	strength	-thorax	chest (pleural cavity)
-sthenia	condition of strength	thromb/o	clotting, clot
stom/o	an opening, a mouth	-thrombin	clotting substance
stomat/o	mouth, oral cavity	thrombocyt/o	clotting cell
-stomy	new opening	thym/o	thymus gland, mind
strom/o	stroma (supportive tissue)	-thymia	condition/state of mind
sub-	under, below	thyr/o	thyroid gland, shield
sudor/i	sweat	thyroid/o	thyroid gland
sulc/o	sulcus, groove	tibi/o	tibia (shinbone)
super/o	upward	-tic	pertaining to
supra-	upward, above	-tion	process of
sur/o	calf	toc/o	labor, delivery
sympath/o	to feel with	-tocia	condition of labor, delivery
syn-	together, joined	tom/o	section, cutting
syndesm/o	ligament (structure connecting bone)	-tome	instrument to cut
		-tomy	incision, cutting
synovi/o	synovium	ton/o	tension, tone
tachy-	fast, rapid	tonsill/o	tonsil
tars/o	tarsal bone (ankle bone)	top/o	place, location
tax/o	order, coordination	tox/o	poison
tel/e	end, far, complete	toxic/o	poison
tele/o	end, far, complete	trabecul/o	little beam
tempor/o	temporal bone	trache/o	trachea (windpipe)
ten/o	tendon (structure connecting muscles to bones)	tract/o	to pull, pulling
tend/o	tendon (structure connecting muscles to bones)	trans-	through, across
		-tresia	condition of an opening
tendin/o	tendon (structure connecting muscles to bones)	tri-	three
		trich/o	hair
tens/o	stretching	trigon/o	trigone
-tension	process of stretching, pressure	-tripsy	process of crushing
terat/o	deformity	-tripter	machine to crush
test/o	testis, testicle (male gonad)	-trite	instrument to crush

Word Parts and Definitions—cont'd

Word Part	Meaning	Word Part	Meaning
trochanter/o	trochanter	vas/o	vessel, ductus deferens, vas deferens
trop/o	to turn, turning	vascul/o	vessel
troph/o	development, nourishment	ven/o	vein
-trophy	process of nourishment, development	ventr/o	belly side
tub/o	tube, pipe	ventricul/o	ventricle
tubercul/o	tubercle, a swelling	venul/o	venule, small vein
tympan/o	eardrum, drum	-verse	to turn
-ule	small	vers/o	to turn
uln/o	ulna (lower medial arm bone)	-version	process of turning
ultra-	beyond	vertebr/o	vertebra, spine
-um	structure, thing, membrane	vesic/o	bladder
umbilic/o	umbilicus (navel)	vesicul/o	small sac, seminal vesicle, blister
ungu/o	nail	vestibul/o	vestibule (small space at entrance to canal)
uni-	one	vill/o	villus
ur/o	urine, urinary system	vir/o	virus
ureter/o	ureter	viscer/o	viscera, organ
urethr/o	urethra	vitre/o	vitreous humor, glassy
-uria	urinary condition	vol/o	volume
urin/o	urine, urinary system	vomer/o	vomer
-us	structure, thing, noun ending	vulgar/o	common
uter/o	uterus	vulv/o	vulva (external female genitalia)
uve/o	uvea	xen/o	foreign
uvul/o	uvula	xer/o	dry
vag/o	vagus nerve	xiph/i	xiphoid process, sword
vagin/o	vagina	-y	process of; condition
valv/o	valve	zo/o	animal
valvul/o	valve	zygom/o	zygoma (cheekbone)
varic/o	varices	zygomat/o	zygoma (cheekbone)

Appendix B

Definitions and Word Parts

Meaning	Word Part	Meaning	Word Part
abdomen	abdomin/o, celi/o, lapar/o	arrow, separating the sides	sagitt/o
abnormal	para-, dys-	arteriole (small artery)	arteriol/o
abnormal condition	-osis	artery	arteri/o
abnormal condition of hardening	-sclerosis	atrium	atri/o
		attraction	phil/o, -phil
abnormal condition of narrowing	-stenosis	away from	ab-, ef-, apo-
		back	dors/o, poster/o
abnormal increase in cells	-cytosis	backbone	rachi/o
above, upon	epi-	back of knee	poplite/o
accessory	adnex/o	back, again	re-
acid	acid/o	backward	retro-, re-
acromion	-acromion	bacteria	bacteri/o
addition	prosth/o, prosthes/o	bad, abnormal, apart	dis-
adenoid (pharyngeal tonsil)	adenoid/o	bad, difficult, painful, abnormal	dys-
adrenal gland	adren/o	bad, poor	mal-
again	re-	Bartholin gland	bartholin/o
against	anti-	base, bottom	bas/o
air	aer/o, pneum/o	bear, carry	fer/o, phor/o, duct/o
all	pan-	before, in front of	pre-
alveolus	alveol/o	beginning	-arche
amnion	amni/o	behind, after	post-
amnion (inner fetal sac)	-amnios	belly side	ventr/o
angle	goni/o	below	hypo-
animal	zo/o	bend, bending	flex/o
ankle bone (tarsal bone)	tars/o	beside, near	par-
antrum, cavity	antr/o	between	inter-
anus	an/o	beyond	ultra-
aorta (largest artery)	aort/o	beyond, change	meta-
appendix, vermiform	append/o, appendic/o	bile, gall	bil/i, chol/e
appetite	orex/o	bile vessel	cholangi/o
arm	brachi/o	binding	-desis
		birth, born	nat/o
armpit (axilla)	axill/o	black, dark	melan/o
around	circum-	bladder	vesic/o
		bladder, sac	cyst/o

629

Definitions and Word Parts—cont'd

Meaning	Word Part	Meaning	Word Part
blister	vesicul/o	cartilage	cartilag/o, chondr/o
blood	hem/o, hemat/o	cecum (first part of large intestine)	cec/o
blood condition	-emia		
blood vessel	hemangi/o	cell	cellul/o, cyt/o, cyte
blue	cyan/o	cerebellum	cerebell/o
bluish green	glauc/o	cerebrum	cerebr/o
body	corpor/o, somat/o, som/o	cervix	cervic/o
		change	mut/a
bone	oss/i, osse/o, oste/o	cheek	bucc/o
bone marrow, spinal cord	myel/o	cheekbone (zygoma)	zygom/o, zygomat/o
		chest (thorax)	pector/o, steth/o, thorac/o
both	amphi-		
brain	encephal/o	chest (pleural cavity)	-thorax
break down, dissolve	lys/o	child, foot	ped/o
break down, freeing from adhesions, dissolving, loosening	-lysis	childbirth, puerperium	puerper/o
		chin	ment/o
		cholesterol	cholesterol/o
breaking down	-clast	choroid	choroid/o
breast	mamm/o, mast/o	chorion (outer fetal sac)	chori/o, chorion/o
breastbone (sternum)	stern/o		
breath	halit/o	ciliary body	cycl/o
breathe, breathing	pne/o	clitoris	clitorid/o
breathing, to breathe	-pnea, spir/o, hal/o	close, closing, a blockage	occlus/o
bronchiole	bronchiol/o		
bronchus	bronch/o, bronchi/o	closing	claustr/o
bunion	bunion/o	clotting cell	thrombocyt/o
burning	cauter/i	clotting substance	-thrombin
bursa	burs/o	clotting, clot	thromb/o
bursting forth	-rrhagia, -rrhage	clumping	agglutin/o
buttocks	glute/o	cochlea	cochle/o
calcium	calc/o, calc/i	collarbone (clavicle)	cleid/o, clavicul/o
calf	sur/o	color	chrom/o, chromat/o
calyx, calix	cali/o, calic/o, calyc/o	common	vulgar/o
cancer	carcin/o	common bile duct	choledoch/o
cancer of epithelial origin	-carcinoma	condition of an opening	-tresia
cancer, malignancy	cancer/o	condition of attraction; increase	-philia
canthus (corner of eye)	canth/o		
carbon dioxide	capn/o	condition of babbling	-lalia
carry, carrying	duct/o	condition of closure	-occlusion
carry, to bear	phor/o	condition of expansion, dilation	-ectasia

Definitions and Word Parts—cont'd

Meaning	Word Part	Meaning	Word Part
condition of fear, extreme sensitivity	-phobia	diaphragm	diaphragm/o, diaphragmat/o
condition of formation, development	-plasia	diaphragm, mind	phren/o
		different	heter/o
condition of labor, delivery	-tocia	digestion condition	-pepsia
		discharge, flow	-rrhea
condition of madness	-mania	disease	path/o
condition of patches	-plakia	disease process	-pathy
condition of relaxation, slackening	-chalasia	distal process lower leg, little malleolus	malleol/o
condition of softening	-malacia	diverticulum, pouch	diverticul/o
condition of stools	-chezia	double	dipl/o
condition of strength	-sthenia	down	cata- infra-
condition of the heart	-cardia	down, lack of	de-
condition of thirst	-dipsia	downward	infer/o
condition, presence of	-iasis	drooping, prolapse	-ptosis
condition, state of	-exia, -ia, -ism, -y	drug, chemical	chem/o
condition/state of mind	-thymia, -noia	dry	xer/o
condyle, knob	condyl/o	dull, dim	ambly/o
cone	con/o	duodenum	duoden/o
conjunctiva	conjunctiv/o	dust	coni/o
connection	commissur/o	ear	aur/o, auricul/o, ot/o
connective tissue cancer	-sarcoma	earwax, cerumen	cerumin/o
		eardrum, drum	myring/o, tympan/o
contraction	-stalsis	eat, swallow	phag/o
controlling, stopping	-stasis	elbow	olecran/o
cord, spinal cord	chord/o	elbow (forearm)	cubit/o
cornea	corne/o, kerat/o	electricity	electr/o
cortex (outer portion)	cortic/o	embryonic, immature	-blast, blast/o
crown	coron/o	end, far, complete	tel/e, tele/o
curvature	scoli/o	endocardium (inner lining of the heart)	endocardi/o
dark	phe/o, scot/o	endometrium	endometri/o
death, dead	necr/o	enlargement	-megaly
deficiency condition	-penia	enzyme	-ase
deficient, below, under	hypo-	epicardium	epicardi/o
deformity	terat/o	epicondyle	epicondyl/o
delivery, parturition	-para	epididymis	epididym/o
dendrite, tree	dendr/o	epiglottis	epiglott/o
development	troph/o	epithelium	epitheli/o

Definitions and Word Parts—cont'd

Meaning	Word Part	Meaning	Word Part
equal	is/o	formation, production	plas/o, plast/o, -poiesis, -plasm
esophagus	esophag/o	forming substance	-plastin, -poietin
ethmoid bone	ethmoid/o	fornix	fornic/o
excessive, above	hyper-	forward, in front of	ante-, pro-
expansion, dilation	-ectasis	four	quadri-, tetra-
extreme cold	cry/o	frequent	poly-
eye	ocul/o, ophthalm/o	front, forehead	anter/o, front/o
eyelid	blephar/o, palpebr/o	fungus	myc/o, fung/i
face	faci/o	fundus (base, bottom)	fund/o
falling, drooping, prolapse	-lapse, -ptosis	gallbladder	cholecyst/o
		gland	aden/o
fallopian tube	fallopi/o, salping/o, -salpinx	glans penis	balan/o
		glomerulus	glomerul/o
far	tel/e, tele/o	glue, glia cell	-glia
fascia	fasci/o	gonad, sex organ	gonad/o
fast, rapid	tachy-	groin	inguin/o
fat	adip/o, lip/o, steat/o	growth, nature	physi/o, -physis, phyt/o
fatty plaque	ather/o	gums	gingiv/o
feces, stool	fec/a	hair	pil/o, trich/o
feel with	sympath/o	half	hemi-
feeling, sensation	esthesi/o	hand	man/u
female, woman	gynec/o, nymph/o	hard (dura mater)	dur/o
femur (thighbone)	femor/o	hard, horny, cornea	kerat/o
fetus	fet/o	head	capit/o, cephal/o
fever, fire	pyr/o, pyret/o	healthy, normal	eu-
fiber	fibr/o	hearing	acous/o, audi/o, -acusis
fibrous substance	fibrin/o	heart	cardi/o, cordi/o, coron/o
fibula	fibul/o, perone/o		
finger or toe (digitus)	dactyl/o, digit/o	heat, temperature	therm/o
finger/toe bones (phalanx)	phalang/o	heel bone (calcaneus)	calcane/o
first	primi-	heights, extremes, extremities	acro-
fishlike	ichthy/o		
fixation, suspension	-pexy	hemorrhoid	hemorrhoid/o
flesh	sarc/o	hernia	herni/o
flow, flowing	fluor/o	herniation, protrusion	-cele
fold, plica	plic/o	hidden	crypt-
follicle, small sac	follicul/o	hilum	hil/o
foot, child	ped/o	hip (coxa)	cox/o
foreign	xen/o	hold back, suppress	isch/o
foreskin (prepuce)	preputi/o	hole, foramen	foramin/o

Definitions and Word Parts—cont'd

Meaning	Word Part	Meaning	Word Part
hollow, depression	foss/o	large intestine (colon)	col/o, colon/o
hormone, substance that forms	-one	left	levo-, sinistr/o
		leg	crur/o
humerus (upper arm bone)	humer/o	lens	phac/o, phak/o
		lice	pedicul/i
hymen	hymen/o	life, living	bi/o
ileum	ile/o	ligament	ligament/o, syndesm/o
ilium (superior, widest pelvic bone)	ili/o	light	phot/o
		lipid, fat	lipid/o
in	en-, in-	lips	cheil/o
in favor of	pro-	lips (labia)	labi/o
incision, cutting	-tomy	liquid	humor/o
infection	seps/o, -sepsis, septic/o	little beam	trabecul/o
inflammation	-itis	little grain	granul/o
inner ear (labyrinth)	labyrinth/o	liver	hepat/o
instrument to crush	-trite	lobe, section	lob/o
instrument to cut	-tome	long	long/o
instrument to measure	-meter	lower back	lumb/o
instrument to record	-graph	lower jaw	mandibul/o
instrument to view	-scope	lumen (space within vessel)	lumin/o
insulin	insulin/o		
intentional breaking	-clasis	lung	pneumon/o, pulmon/o, pneum/o
intestine	intestin/o, enter/o		
inward	eso-	lymph	lymph/o, lymphat/o
iris	ir/o, irid/o	lymph gland (lymph node)	lymphaden/o
iron	ferr/o, sider/o		
iron substance	-siderin	lymph vessel	lymphangi/o
ischium	ischi/o	machine to crush	-tripter
jaw, entire	gnath/o	male	andr/o
jejunum	jejun/o	male sex cell, spermatozoon	spermat/o
joint (articulation)	arthr/o, articul/o		
juice	chym/o	malleus, hammer	malle/o
ketone	ket/o, keton/o	man	anthrop/o
kidney	nephr/o, ren/o	many	multi-
kneecap (patella)	patell/o, patell/a	many, much, excessive	poly-
knowledge	gnos/o	marketplace	agora-
labor, delivery	toc/o	mass	-oma
lacrimal gland	dacryoaden/o	mastoid process	mastoid/o
lacrimal sac	dacrocyst/o	meatus (opening)	meat/o
lamina, thin plate	lamin/o	mediastinum	mediastin/o
large	macro-	medulla	medull/o

Definitions and Word Parts—cont'd

Meaning	Word Part
meninges	mening/o, meningi/o
meniscus	menisc/o
menstruation, menses	menstru/o, men/o
metacarpal (hand bone)	metacarp/o
metatarsal (foot bone)	metatars/o
middle	medi/o, meso-, mid-
milk	galact/o, lact/o
mind	ment/o, phren/o, psych/o
mitochondria	mitochondri/o
mouth, oral cavity	or/o, stomat/o
movement	-kine, kinesi/o
movement substance	-kinin
mucus	muc/o, myx/o
muscle	muscul/o, my/o, myos/o
myocardium (heart muscle)	myocardi/o, cardiomy/o
nail	onych/o, ungu/o
near	proxim/o
near, beside, abnormal	para-, par-
neck	nuch/o, coll/o
neck, cervix	cervic/o
nerve	neur/o
nerve root	radicul/o, rhiz/o
nest	nid/o
network	reticul/o
neutral	neutr/o
nevus, birthmark	nev/o
new	neo-
new opening	-stomy
night	noct/i, nyctal/o
nipple	thel/e
nipple	papill/o
nitrogen	az/o, azot/o
no, not, without	a-, an-, in-, non-
node, knot	nod/o
none	nulli-
nose	nas/o, rhin/o

Meaning	Word Part
nourishment	troph/o
noun ending	-a, -e, -i, -is, -um, -on, -ium, -us
nucleus	kary/o, nucle/o
nutrition	aliment/o
occiput, back of head	occipit/o
old age	ger/o, presby-
one	mono-, uni-
one who specializes	-ist
one who specializes in the study of	-logist
one who specializes in treatment	-iatrician, -iatrist
optic disk	papill/o
one who studies	-ician
opening	hiat/o
opening, a mouth	stom/o
opposite, against	contra-
optic disk	papill/o
orange-yellow	cirrh/o
order, coordination	tax/o
organ, viscera	organ/o, viscer/o
origin, originate	gen/o
ossicle	ossicul/o
other, different	allo-
out, outward	ec-, ex-
outside	exo-, extra-
outward	e-, ecto-
ovary	oophor/o, ovari/o
ovum, egg	o/o, ovul/o, ov/o
oxygen	ox/i, ox/o
pain	-algia, -dynia
palate, roof of mouth, palatine bone	palat/o
palm	palm/o
pancreas	pancreat/o
papilla	papill/o
papule	papul/o
paralysis	-plegia
paralysis, slight	-paresis

Definitions and Word Parts—cont'd

Meaning	Word Part	Meaning	Word Part
parathyroid	parathyroid/o	pregnancy, gestation	-cyesis, gravid/o, gravida
parenchyma	parenchym/o	pressure	press/o
parturition, delivery	part/o, -partum	pressure, weight	bar/o
passage	por/o	process of viewing	-opsy
pelvis	pelv/i, pelv/o	process of	-ation, -ion, -ization, -tion, -y
penis	pen/i, phall/o	process of clotting	-coagulation
perineum	perine/o	process of crushing	-tripsy
peritoneum	peritone/o, periton/o	process of cutting	-cision
peroneum	perone/o	process of measurement	-metry
pertaining to	-ac, -al, -an, -ar, -ary, -atic, -eal, -iac, -ac, -ic, -id, -ile, -ine, -ior, -itic, -ive, -ous, -tic	process of nourishment, development	-trophy
pertaining to blood condition	-emic	process of pouring	-fusion
pertaining to breaking down	-lytic	process of recording	-graphy
pertaining to carrying	-ferous	process of stretching, pressure	-tension
pertaining to discharge	-rrheic	process of treatment	-iatry
pertaining to originating from	-genous	process of turning	-version
pertaining to produced by	-genic	process of viewing	-scopy
pertaining to treatment	-iatric	producing, produced by	-gen
pertaining to viewing	-scopic	production	-genesis
pertaining to, full of	-ose	prolactin	prolact/o
pimple	papul/o	prolapse	-ptosis
pituitary, hypophysis	hypophys/o, pituitar/o	prostate	prostat/o
place, location	top/o	protection	-phylaxis
placenta	placent/o	protein	albumin/o
plasma	plasm/a	protein substance	-globin, -globulin
pleasure	hedon/o	pubis, anterior pelvic bone	pub/o
pleura (membrane surrounding lungs)	pleur/o	pull, pulling	tract/o
pointed extremity, apex	apic/o	pupil	cor/o, core/o, pupill/o
poison	tox/o, toxic/o	purple	purpur/o
pole	pol/o	purposeful movement	prax/o
polyp	polyp/o	pus	py/o
potassium	kal/i, potass/o	pustule	pustul/o
pouch, diverticulum	diverticul/o	pylorus	pylor/o
		radius	radi/o

Definitions and Word Parts—cont'd

Meaning	Word Part	Meaning	Word Part
rapid, fast	oxy-, tachy-	sclera, hard	scler/o
rash	exanthemat/o	scraping of	-abrasion
rays	radi/o	scrotum	scrot/o
record, recording	-gram	sea	thalass/o
rectouterine pouch (cul-de-sac)	culd/o	sebum, oil	seb/o, sebac/o
rectum and anus	proct/o	secret, hidden	-occult
rectum, straight	rect/o	secrete, secreting	crin/o, -crine
recurring, round	cycl/o	section, cutting	tom/o
red	erythr/o	seed	gon/o
red blood cell	erythrocyt/o	seizure	-lepsy
relaxation, slackening	-chalasis	self	auto-
removal of a stone	-lithotomy	semen	semin/i
removal, excision	-ablation, -apheresis, -pheresis, -ectomy	send, sending	-mission
renal pelvis	pyel/o	sense of smell	osm/o
rent or tear	-spadias	separate, separating	-crit
repair	-rrhaphy	separate, away	apo-
resembling, like	-oid	septum	sept/o
retina	retin/o	serum	ser/o
rhythm	rhythm/o	shape, form	morph/o
rib (costa)	cost/o	sharp	acu-
ribose	rib/o	shinbone (tibia)	tibi/o
right	dextr/o	short	brachy-
rosy-colored	eosin/o	shoulder blade (scapula)	scapul/o
round back	kyph/o	side	later/o
rugae, ridge	rug/o	sigmoid colon	sigmoid/o
run, running	-drome	sinus, cavity	sin/o, sinus/o
rupture	-rrhexis	sitting	kathis/o
sac surrounding the heart	pericardi/o	skeleton	skelet/o
sacrum	sacr/o	skin	cut/o, cutane/o, derm/o, dermat/o
safety, protection	immun/o	skull (cranium)	crani/o
saliva	sial/o	sleep, stupor	narc/o, somn/o
salivary gland	sialaden/o	slight paralysis	-paresis
same	home/o, homo-, ipsi-	slipping	-listhesis
scab	eschar/o	slow	brady-
scaly	squam/o	small	micro-, -ule
scanty, few	olig/o	small intestines, intestines	enter/o
scanty, pressure	man/o	small lobe	lobul/o

Definitions and Word Parts—cont'd

Meaning	Word Part
small sac, seminal vesicle	vesicul/o
smooth	lei/o
smooth muscle	leiomy/o
sodium	natr/o
softening	-malacia
sole of foot	plant/o
sound	echo-, son/o
sound, voice	phon/o
space between	interstit/o
spasm	-spasm
speech	phas/o
spermatozoon	sperm/o
sphenoid	sphenoid/o
spinal column	rachi/o
spinal cord	cord/o, myel/o
spinal nerve root	rhiz/o, radicul/o
spine	spin/o, vertebr/o
spitting	-ptysis
spleen	splen/o
split	schiz/o, -fida
split, splitting	-fida
spot, macula lutea, macule	macul/o
stapes	staped/o
star	astr/o
starch	amyl/o
state of	-esis, -sis
state of relaxation	-chalasis
steal, stealing	klept/o
steroid	ster/o
stiffening	ankyl/o
stomach	gastr/o
stone (calculus)	calcul/o, lith/o
stop, cease	-pause
straight, upright	orth/o
strength	sthen/o
stretching	tens/o
striated	rhabd/o

Meaning	Word Part
striated (skeletal) muscle	rhabdomy/o
stroma (supportive tissue)	strom/o
structure, membrane, thing	-um, -ium
structure, thing, noun ending	-us, -on, -is
study	log/o
study of	-logy
substance	-in
sugar, glucose	glycos/o, gluc/o, glyc/o
sulcus, groove	sulc/o
surgical puncture	-centesis
surgical repair	-plasty
surrounding, around	peri-
suture	-rrhaphy
swallow, eat	phag/o
swayback	lord/o
sweat	hidr/o, sudor/i
sweat gland (sudoriferous gland)	hidraden/o
swelling	-edema, tubercul/o
synovium	synovi/o
tail	caud/o
tailbone (coccyx)	coccyg/o
taste	geus/o
tear	dacry/o, lacrim/o
teeth	dent/i, odont/o
temporal bone	tempor/o
tendon	ten/o, tend/o, tendin/o
tension, tone	ton/o
testis, testicle	orch/o, orchi/o, orchid/o, test/o, testicul/o
thalamus	thalam/o
thirst	dips/o
three	tri-
three-dimensional	stere/o
throat (pharynx)	pharyng/o

Definitions and Word Parts—cont'd

Meaning	Word Part
through	per-
through, across	trans-
through, complete	dia-
thymus gland, mind	thym/o
thyroid gland	thyroid/o
thyroid gland, shield	thyr/o
tissue	hist/o
throw, throwing	bol/o
tie, tying	ligat/o
to flow, flowing	fluor/o
together	con-
together, joined	syn-
tongue	gloss/o, lingu/o
tonsil	tonsill/o
to shut	my/o
toward	ad-, -ad, af-
treatment	iatr/o, -therapy
tree	dendr/o
trochanter	trochanter/o
trigone	trigon/o
tube, fallopian	-salpinx
tube, fallopian or eustachian	salping/o
tube, pipe	tub/o
tumor	onc/o
tumor, mass	-oma
tubercle	tubercul/o
turn, turning	trop/o, vers/o, -verse
twisting	tors/o
two	bi-, bin-
two (both)	di-
ulceration	aphth/o
ulna	uln/o
umbilicus (navel)	omphal/o, umbilic/o
under, below	sub-, hypo-
unique, unknown	idi/o
up, apart, away	ana-
upper jaw bone (maxilla)	maxill/o
upward	super/o, supra-

Meaning	Word Part
ureter	ureter/o
urethra	urethr/o
urinary condition	-uria
urine, urinary system	ur/o, urin/o
uterus	hyster/o, metr/o, metri/o, uter/o
uvea	uve/o
uvula	uvul/o
vagina	colp/o, vagin/o
vagus nerve	vag/o
valve	valv/o, valvul/o
varices	varic/o
vas deferens	vas/o
vein	phleb/o, ven/o
ventricle	ventricul/o
venule (small vein)	venul/o
vertebra, spine	spondyl/o, vertebr/o
vessel	angi/o, vascul/o, vas/o
vessel, ductus deferens, vas deferens	vas/o
villus	vill/o
vestibule	vestibul/o
virus	vir/o
vision	opt/o, optic/o
vision condition	-opia, -opsia
vitreous humor, glassy	vitre/o
voice box (larynx)	laryng/o
volume	plethysm/o, vol/o
vomer	vomer/o
vomiting	-emesis
vulva	episi/o, vulv/o
walking	ambul/o
wall, partition, septum	pariet/o, sept/o
water, fluid	hydr/o
watery flow	rheumat/o
wheel	rot/o
white	albin/o, leuk/o
white blood cell	leukocyt/o
windpipe (trachea)	trache/o

Word Parts and Definitions—cont'd

Meaning	Word Part	Meaning	Word Part
within	end, endo-, intra-	wrinkle	rhytid/o
woman, female	nymph/o	wrist (carpus)	carp/o
word, speech	lex/o	write, writing	graph/o
work	erg/o	xiphoid process	xiph/i

Appendix C

Abbreviations

Abbreviation	Meaning	Abbreviation	Meaning
#	fracture	ANS	autonomic nervous system
3DCRT	three-dimensional conformal radiation therapy	AP	anteroposterior
		APA	American Psychiatric Association
A	action	ARF	acute renal failure; acute respiratory failure
A&P	auscultation and percussion		
A, B, AB, O	blood types	ARMD, AMD	age-related macular degeneration
A1c	average glucose level	AS	aortic stenosis
ABG	arterial blood gas	ASD	atrial septal defect; autism spectrum disorder
ABR	auditory brainstem response		
Acc	accommodation	ASHD	arteriosclerotic heart disease
ACE	angiotensin-converting enzyme	ASL	American sign language
ACS	anterior ciliary sclerotomy; American Cancer Society	Astig, As, Ast	astigmatism
		AV	atrioventricular
ACTH	adrenocorticotropic hormone	B2M	beta-2 microglobulin
AD	Alzheimer disease	BaS	barium swallow
ADH	antidiuretic hormone	basos	basophils
ADHD	attention-deficit hyperactivity disorder	BBB	blood-brain barrier; bundle branch block
ADLs	activities of daily living	BCC	basal cell carcinoma
AEB	atrial ectopic beat	BCP	birth control pill
AF	atrial fibrillation	BD	bipolar disorder
AFP	alpha fetoprotein	BE	barium enema
AHIMA	American Health Information Management Association	BM	bowel movement
		BMP	basic metabolic panel
AI	artificial insemination	BMT	bone marrow transplant
AICD	automatic implantable cardioverter-defibrillator	BP	blood pressure
		BPH	benign prostatic hyperplasia, benign prostatic hypertrophy
AIDS	acquired immunodeficiency syndrome		
		bpm	beats per minute
AK	astigmatic keratotomy	BSE	breast self-examination
ALL	acute lymphocytic leukemia	BTA	bladder tumor antigen
ALS	amyotrophic lateral sclerosis	BUN	blood urea nitrogen
AMA	American Medical Association	Bx	biopsy
AMI	acute myocardial infarction	C1-C7	first cervical through seventh cervical vertebrae
AML	acute myelogenous leukemia		
ANA	antinuclear antibody	C1-C8	cervical nerves

Abbreviations—cont'd

Abbreviation	Meaning	Abbreviation	Meaning
Ca	calcium	CPT	Current Procedural Terminology
CA	cancer	CR	closed reduction
CA125	tumor marker primarily for ovarian cancer	CREF	closed reduction, external fixation
CA15-3	tumor marker used to monitor breast cancer	CRP	C-reactive protein
CA19-9	tumor marker for pancreatic, stomach, and bile duct cancer	CS, C-section	cesarean section
CA27-29	tumor marker used to check for recurrence of breast cancer	CSF	cerebrospinal fluid; colony-stimulating factor
CABG	coronary artery bypass graft	CST	contraction stress test
CAD	coronary artery disease	CT scan	computed tomography scan
CAM	complementary and alternative medicine	CTA	clear to auscultation
CAPD	continuous ambulatory peritoneal dialysis	CTR	certified tumor registrar
CAT	computed axial tomography	CTS	carpal tunnel syndrome
Cath	(cardiac) catheterization	CV	cardiovascular
CBC	complete blood cell (count)	CVA	cerebrovascular accident
CCB	calcium channel blocker(s)	CVS	chorionic villus sampling
CCPD	continuous cycling peritoneal dialysis	CWP	coal workers' pneumoconiosis
CEA	carcinoembryonic antigen	Cx	cervix
CF	cystic fibrosis	CXR	chest x-ray
CHF	congestive heart failure	D&C	dilation and curettage
CIN	cervical intraepithelial neoplasia	D1-D12	first dorsal through twelfth dorsal vertebrae
CIS	carcinoma in situ	DAP Test	Draw-a-Person Test
CKD	chronic kidney disease	decub	decubitus ulcer
Cl	chloride	DEXA, DXA	dual-energy x-ray absorptiometry
CLL	chronic lymphocytic leukemia	DI	diabetes insipidus
CML	chronic myelogenous leukemia	diff	differential (WBC count)
CMP	comprehensive metabolic panel	DIP	distal interphalangeal joint
CNS	central nervous system	DJD	degenerative joint disease
CO_2	carbon dioxide	DLE	disseminated lupus erythematosus
COPD	chronic obstructive pulmonary disease	DM	diabetes mellitus
COX-2	cyclooxygenase-2	DMARD	disease-modifying antirheumatic drug
CP	cerebral palsy	DNA	deoxyribonucleic acid
CPAP	continuous positive airway pressure	DOE	dyspnea on exertion
		DRE	digital rectal exam
CPK	creatine phosphokinase	DSA	digital subtraction angiography
CPR	cardiopulmonary resuscitation	DSM	Diagnostic and Statistical Manual of Mental Disorders
		DSM-5	Diagnostic and Statistical Manual of Mental Disorders, fifth edition

Abbreviations—cont'd

Abbreviation	Meaning
DT	delirium tremens
DTR	deep tendon reflex
DUB	dysfunctional uterine bleeding
DVT	deep vein thrombosis
EBV	Epstein-Barr virus
ECC	extracorporeal circulation
ECCE	extracapsular cataract extraction
ECG, EKG	electrocardiography, electrocardiogram
ECHO	echocardiography
ECP	emergency contraceptive pill
ECT	electroconvulsive therapy
ED	emergency department; erectile dysfunction
EDD	estimated delivery date
EEG	electroencephalography, electroencephalogram
EF	external fixation
EGD	esophagogastroduodenoscopy
ELISA	enzyme-linked immunosorbent assay
EM, Em	emmetropia
EMG	electromyography
ENT	ears, nose, and throat
EOC	epithelial ovarian cancer
EOM	extraocular movements
eosins	eosinophils
EP	evoked potential
ERCP	endoscopic retrograde cholangiopancreatography
ERT	estrogen replacement therapy
ESR	erythrocyte sedimentation rate
ESRD	end-stage renal disease
EST	exercise stress test
ESWL	extracorporeal shock wave lithotripsy
EVLT	endovenous laser ablation
FB	foreign body
FBS	fasting blood sugar
FEV	forced expiratory volume
FOBT	fecal occult blood test

Abbreviation	Meaning
FPG	fasting plasma glucose
FRC	forced residual capacity
FSH	follicle-stimulating hormone
FTA-ABS	fluorescent treponemal antibody absorption
FVC	forced vital capacity
Fx	fracture
G	grade, pregnancy
GAD	generalized anxiety disorder
GARS	gait assessment rating scale
GB	gallbladder
Gc	gonococcus
G-CSF	granulocyte colony-stimulating factor
GCT	germ cell tumor
GERD	gastroesophageal reflux disease
GFR	glomerular filtration rate
GGT	gamma-glutamyl transferase
GH	growth hormone
GHD	growth hormone deficiency
GI	gastrointestinal
GIFT	gamete intrafallopian transfer
GM-CSF	granulocyte-macrophage colony-stimulating factor
GN	glomerulonephritis
GPA	gravida, para, abortion
GRH	gonadotropin-releasing hormone
GU	genitourinary
H	hypodermic
H2RA	histamine-2 receptor antagonist
HAV	hepatitis A virus
Hb	hemoglobin
HBV	hepatitis B virus
hCG	human chorionic gonadotropin
Hct	hematocrit
HD	hemodialysis
HDL	high-density lipoprotein
HDN	hemolytic disease of the newborn
HF	heart failure
Hg	millimeters of mercury

Abbreviations—cont'd

Abbreviation	Meaning	Abbreviation	Meaning
Hgb	hemoglobin	IQ	intelligence quotient
hGH	human growth hormone	IUD	intrauterine device
HHN	hand-held nebulizer	IV	intravenous
HIM	health information management	IVF	in vitro fertilization
HIV	human immunodeficiency virus	IVP	intravenous pyelography
HIVD	herniated intervertebral disk	IVU	intravenous urography; intravenous urogram
hMG	human menopausal gonadotropin	K	potassium
HPV	human papillomavirus	KS	Kaposi sarcoma
HRT	hormone replacement therapy	KUB	kidney, ureter, and bladder
HSG	hysterosalpingography	L1-L5	lumbar vertebrae, first through fifth; lumbar nerves
HSV	herpes simplex virus	LA	left atrium
HSV-1	herpes simplex virus-1	Lap	laparoscopy
HSV-2	herpes simplex virus-2; herpes genitalis	LASIK	laser-assisted in-situ keratomileusis
HTN	hypertension	lat	lateral
I&D	incision and drainage	LCA	left circumflex artery; left coronary artery
IBD	inflammatory bowel disease	LDH	lactate dehydrogenase
IBS	irritable bowel syndrome	LDL	low-density lipoprotein
IC	inspiratory capacity	LEEP	loop electrocautery excision procedure
ICCE	intracapsular cataract extraction	LES	lower esophageal sphincter
ICD	International Classification of Diseases	LFT	liver function test
ICD-10	International Classification of Diseases, 10th revision	LGA	light for gestational age
ICD-10-CM	International Classification of Diseases, 10th revision, Clinical Modification	LH	luteinizing hormone
		LLL	left lower lobe
ICL	implantable contact lens	LLQ	lower left quadrant
ICP	intracranial pressure	LMP	last menstrual period
ICSH	interstitial cell-stimulating hormone	LP	lumbar puncture
ICSI	intracytoplasmic sperm injection	LRQ	lower right quadrant
ID	intradermal	LUL	left upper lobe
IDC	infiltrating ductal carcinoma	LUQ	left upper quadrant
IDDM	insulin-dependent diabetes mellitus	LV	left ventricle
IF	internal fixation	LVAD	left ventricular assist device
Ig	immunoglobulin	lymphs	lymphocytes
IMRT	intensity-modulated radiation therapy	MAOI	monoamine oxidase inhibitor
		MCH	mean corpuscular hemoglobin
IOL	intraocular lens	MCHC	mean corpuscular hemoglobin concentration
IOP	intraocular pressure		

Abbreviations—cont'd

Abbreviation	Meaning	Abbreviation	Meaning
MD	muscular dystrophy; medical doctor	O	origin
MDI	metered dose inhaler	O_2	oxygen
MDRTB	multidrug-resistant tuberculosis	OA	osteoarthritis
mets	metastases	OAE	otoacoustic emission
MHA-TP	microhemagglutination assay-*Treponema pallidum*	OCD	obsessive-compulsive disorder
		OCP	oral contraceptive pill
MI	myocardial infarction	ODD	oppositional defiant disorder
MIDCAB	minimally invasive direct coronary artery bypass	OGTT	oral glucose tolerance test
MMPI	Minnesota Multiphasic Personality Inventory	OM	otitis media
		Ophth	ophthalmology
MR	mental retardation; mitral regurgitation	OR	open reduction
		ORIF	open reduction, internal fixation
MRA	magnetic resonance angiography	OSA	obstructive sleep apnea
MRI	magnetic resonance imaging	OT	oxytocin
MS	multiple sclerosis; mitral stenosis; musculoskeletal	OTC	over the counter
		Oto	otology
MSH	melanocyte-stimulating hormone	PA	physician's assistant; posteroanterior; pulmonary artery
MSLT	multiple sleep latency test		
MUGA	multigated (radionuclide) angiogram	PAC	premature atrial contraction
		PACAB	port-access coronary artery bypass
MV	mitral valve	Pap	Papanicolaou (test for cervical/vaginal cancer)
MVP	mitral valve prolapse		
MY	myopia	PCOS	polycystic ovary syndrome
N&V	nausea and vomiting	PCV	packed-cell volume
Na	sodium	PD	panic disorder; Parkinson disease
neuts	neutrophils	PDA	patent ductus arteriosus
NGU	nongonococcal urethritis	PDD	pervasive developmental disorders
NIDDM	non–insulin-dependent diabetes mellitus (type 2 diabetes)	PDR	proliferative diabetic retinopathy
		PEG	percutaneous endoscopic gastrostomy
NIH	National Institutes of Health		
NK	natural killer (cell)	PET scan	positron emission tomography scan
NPDR	nonproliferative diabetic retinopathy		
		PFT	pulmonary function test
NSAID	nonsteroidal antiinflammatory drug	PGH	pituitary growth hormone
		pH	acidity/alkalinity
NSCLC	non–small cell lung cancer	PICC	peripherally inserted central catheter
NSE	neuron-specific enolase		
NSR	normal sinus rhythm	PID	pelvic inflammatory disease
NST	nonstress test	PIP	proximal interphalangeal joint
NTG	nitroglycerin	PK	penetrating keratoplasty (corneal transplant)

Abbreviations—cont'd

Abbreviation	Meaning	Abbreviation	Meaning
PKD	polycystic kidney disease	RIA	radioimmunoassay
PKU	phenylketonuria	RLL	right lower lobe (of the lung)
plats	platelets; thrombocytes	RLQ	right lower quadrant
PMB	postmenopausal bleeding	RML	right middle lobe (of the lung)
PMDD	premenstrual dysphoric disorder	RNA	ribonucleic acid
PMN	polymorphonucleocyte	ROM	range of motion
PMNs, polys	polymorphonucleocytes	RPR	rapid plasma reagin
PMS	premenstrual syndrome	RSV	respiratory syncytial virus
PNS	peripheral nervous system	RUL	right upper lobe (of the lung)
pos	posterior	RUQ	right upper quadrant
PPB	positive-pressure breathing	RV	right ventricle
PPD	purified protein derivative	Rx	prescribed
PRK	photorefractive keratectomy	S1-S5	sacral vertebrae, first through fifth; sacral nerves
PRL	prolactin		
PSA	prostate-specific antigen	SA	sinoatrial
PSG	polysomnography	SAD	seasonal affective disorder
PT	prothrombin time	SARS	severe acute respiratory syndrome
PTA	prothrombin activator		
PTC/PTCA	percutaneous transhepatic cholangiography	SCC	squamous cell carcinoma
		SCLC	small cell lung cancer
PTCA	percutaneous transluminal coronary angioplasty	SG	skin graft; specific gravity
		SIADH	syndrome of inappropriate antidiuretic hormone
PTH	parathyroid hormone		
PTSD	posttraumatic stress disorder	SIRS	systemic inflammatory response syndrome
PTT	partial thromboplastin time		
PTU	propylthiouracil	SLE	systemic lupus erythematosus
PUD	peptic ulcer disease	SNS	somatic nervous system
PUVA	psoralen plus ultraviolet A	SOB	shortness of breath
PV	pulmonary vein	SPECT	single-photon emission computed tomography
PVC	premature ventricular contraction		
PVD	peripheral vascular disease	SPF	sun protection factor
QFT	QuantiFERON-TB	SSRI	selective serotonin reuptake inhibitor
RA	rheumatoid arthritis; right atrium		
RAD	reactive airway disease	SSS	sick sinus syndrome
RAIU	radioactive iodine uptake	STD	sexually transmitted disease
RBC	red blood cell (count)	STH	somatotropic hormone
RCA	right coronary artery	STI	sexually transmitted infection
RF	rheumatoid factor	STSG	split-thickness skin graft
RFCA	radiofrequency catheter ablation	sup	superior
		SVT	superficial vein thrombosis
Rh	Rhesus (factor)	sx	symptoms

Abbreviations—cont'd

Abbreviation	Meaning	Abbreviation	Meaning
T	tumor	TUR	transurethral resection (of the prostate)
T1-T12	thoracic vertebrae, first through twelfth; thoracic nerves	TURP	transurethral resection of the prostate
T_3	triiodothyronine	TV	tidal volume; tricuspid valve
T_4	thyroxine	UA	urinalysis
TA-90	tumor marker for spread of malignant melanoma	UAE	uterine artery embolization
TAH-BSO	total abdominal hysterectomy with a bilateral salpingo-oophorectomy	UCL	ulnar collateral ligament
		uE3	unconjugated estradiol
		ULQ	upper left quadrant
TAT	Thematic Apperception Test	UNHS	Universal Newborn Hearing Screening
TB	tuberculosis		
TCA	tricyclic antidepressant	URI	upper respiratory infection
TCC	transitional cell carcinoma	URQ	upper right quadrant
TEA	thromboendarterectomy	UTI	urinary tract infection
TEE	transesophageal echocardiography	UV	ultraviolet
TENS	transcutaneous electrical nerve stimulation	VA	visual acuity
		VBAC	vaginal birth after cesarean section
TFT	thyroid function test		
THR	total hip replacement	VCUG	voiding cystourethrography
TIA	transient ischemic attack	VD	venereal disease
TKR	total knee replacement	VDRL	Venereal Disease Research Laboratory
TLC	total lung capacity		
TM	tympanic membrane	VEB	ventricular ectopic beat
TMJ	temporomandibular joint disorder	VF	visual field
TMR	transmyocardial revascularization	VHD	valvular heart disease
TNM	tumor-node-metastases (staging)	VMA	urine vanillylmandelic acid
tPA	tissue plasminogen activator	VP	vasopressin
TS	tricuspid stenosis	VSD	ventricular septal defect
TSE	testicular self-examination	WAIS	Wechsler Adult Intelligence Scale
TSH	thyroid-stimulating hormone	WBC	white blood cell (count)
TTS	transdermal therapeutic system	WHO	World Health Organization
TUIP	transurethral incision of the prostate	ZIFT	zygote intrafallopian transfer

Institute for Safe Medication Practices

ISMP's List of *Error-Prone Abbreviations, Symbols,* and *Dose Designations*

The abbreviations, symbols, and dose designations found in this table have been reported to ISMP through the ISMP National Medication Errors Reporting Program (ISMP MERP) as being frequently misinterpreted and involved in harmful medication errors. They should **NEVER** be used when communicating medical information. This includes internal communications, telephone/verbal prescriptions, computer-generated labels, labels for drug storage bins, medication administration records, as well as pharmacy and prescriber computer order entry screens.

Abbreviations	Intended Meaning	Misinterpretation	Correction
μg	Microgram	Mistaken as "mg"	Use "mcg"
AD, AS, AU	Right ear, left ear, each ear	Mistaken as OD, OS, OU (right eye, left eye, each eye)	Use "right ear," "left ear," or "each ear"
OD, OS, OU	Right eye, left eye, each eye	Mistaken as AD, AS, AU (right ear, left ear, each ear)	Use "right eye," "left eye," or "each eye"
BT	Bedtime	Mistaken as "BID" (twice daily)	Use "bedtime"
cc	Cubic centimeters	Mistaken as "u" (units)	Use "mL"
D/C	Discharge or discontinue	Premature discontinuation of medications if D/C (intended to mean "discharge") has been misinterpreted as "discontinued" when followed by a list of discharge medications	Use "discharge" and "discontinue"
IJ	Injection	Mistaken as "IV" or "intrajugular"	Use "injection"
IN	Intranasal	Mistaken as "IM" or "IV"	Use "intranasal" or "NAS"
HS	Half-strength	Mistaken as bedtime	Use "half-strength" or "bedtime"
hs	At bedtime, hours of sleep	Mistaken as half-strength	
IU**	International unit	Mistaken as IV (intravenous) or 10 (ten)	Use "units"
o.d. or OD	Once daily	Mistaken as "right eye" (OD-oculus dexter), leading to oral liquid medications administered in the eye	Use "daily"
OJ	Orange juice	Mistaken as OD or OS (right or left eye); drugs meant to be diluted in orange juice may be given in the eye	Use "orange juice"
Per os	By mouth, orally	The "os" can be mistaken as "left eye" (OS-oculus sinister)	Use "PO," "by mouth," or "orally"
q.d. or QD**	Every day	Mistaken as q.i.d., especially if the period after the "q" or the tail of the "q" is misunderstood as an "i"	Use "daily"
qhs	Nightly at bedtime	Mistaken as "qhr" or every hour	Use "nightly"
qn	Nightly or at bedtime	Mistaken as "qh" (every hour)	Use "nightly" or "at bedtime"
q.o.d. or QOD**	Every other day	Mistaken as "q.d." (daily) or "q.i.d. (four times daily) if the "o" is poorly written	Use "every other day"
q1d	Daily	Mistaken as q.i.d. (four times daily)	Use "daily"
q6PM, etc.	Every evening at 6 PM	Mistaken as every 6 hours	Use "daily at 6 PM" or "6 PM daily"
SC, SQ, sub q	Subcutaneous	SC mistaken as SL (sublingual); SQ mistaken as "5 every;" the "q" in "sub q" has been mistaken as "every" (e.g., a heparin dose ordered "sub q 2 hours before surgery" misunderstood as every 2 hours before surgery)	Use "subcut" or "subcutaneously"
ss	Sliding scale (insulin) or ½ (apothecary)	Mistaken as "55"	Spell out "sliding scale;" use "one-half" or "½"
SSRI	Sliding scale regular insulin	Mistaken as selective-serotonin reuptake inhibitor	Spell out "sliding scale (insulin)"
SSI	Sliding scale insulin	Mistaken as Strong Solution of Iodine (Lugol's)	
i/d	One daily	Mistaken as "tid"	Use "1 daily"
TIW or tiw	3 times a week	Mistaken as "3 times a day" or "twice in a week"	Use "3 times weekly"
U or u**	Unit	Mistaken as the number 0 or 4, causing a 10-fold overdose or greater (e.g., 4U seen as "40" or 4u seen as "44"); mistaken as "cc" so dose given in volume instead of units (e.g., 4u seen as 4cc)	Use "unit"
UD	As directed ("ut dictum")	Mistaken as unit dose (e.g., diltiazem 125 mg IV infusion "UD" misinterpreted as meaning to give the entire infusion as a unit [bolus] dose)	Use "as directed"

Dose Designations and Other Information	Intended Meaning	Misinterpretation	Correction
Trailing zero after decimal point (e.g., 1.0 mg)**	1 mg	Mistaken as 10 mg if the decimal point is not seen	Do not use trailing zeros for doses expressed in whole numbers
"Naked" decimal point (e.g., .5 mg)**	0.5 mg	Mistaken as 5 mg if the decimal point is not seen	Use zero before a decimal point when the dose is less than a whole unit
Abbreviations such as mg. or mL. with a period following the abbreviation	mg mL	The period is unnecessary and could be mistaken as the number 1 if written poorly	Use mg, mL, etc. without a terminal period

Institute for Safe Medication Practices

ISMP's List of *Error-Prone Abbreviations, Symbols,* and *Dose Designations* (continued)

Dose Designations and Other Information	Intended Meaning	Misinterpretation	Correction
Drug name and dose run together (especially problematic for drug names that end in "l" such as Inderal40 mg; Tegretol300 mg)	Inderal 40 mg Tegretol 300 mg	Mistaken as Inderal 140 mg Mistaken as Tegretol 1300 mg	Place adequate space between the drug name, dose, and unit of measure
Numerical dose and unit of measure run together (e.g., 10mg, 100mL)	10 mg 100 mL	The "m" is sometimes mistaken as a zero or two zeros, risking a 10- to 100-fold overdose	Place adequate space between the dose and unit of measure
Large doses without properly placed commas (e.g., 100000 units; 1000000 units)	100,000 units 1,000,000 units	100000 has been mistaken as 10,000 or 1,000,000; 1000000 has been mistaken as 100,000	Use commas for dosing units at or above 1,000, or use words such as 100 "thousand" or 1 "million" to improve readability

Drug Name Abbreviations	Intended Meaning	Misinterpretation	Correction
To avoid confusion, do not abbreviate drug names when communicating medical information. Examples of drug name abbreviations involved in medication errors include:			
APAP	acetaminophen	Not recognized as acetaminophen	Use complete drug name
ARA A	vidarabine	Mistaken as cytarabine (ARA C)	Use complete drug name
AZT	zidovudine (Retrovir)	Mistaken as azathioprine or aztreonam	Use complete drug name
CPZ	Compazine (prochlorperazine)	Mistaken as chlorpromazine	Use complete drug name
DPT	Demerol-Phenergan-Thorazine	Mistaken as diphtheria-pertussis-tetanus (vaccine)	Use complete drug name
DTO	Diluted tincture of opium, or deodorized tincture of opium (Paregoric)	Mistaken as tincture of opium	Use complete drug name
HCl	hydrochloric acid or hydrochloride	Mistaken as potassium chloride (The "H" is misinterpreted as "K")	Use complete drug name unless expressed as a salt of a drug
HCT	hydrocortisone	Mistaken as hydrochlorothiazide	Use complete drug name
HCTZ	hydrochlorothiazide	Mistaken as hydrocortisone (seen as HCT250 mg)	Use complete drug name
MgSO4**	magnesium sulfate	Mistaken as morphine sulfate	Use complete drug name
MS, MSO4**	morphine sulfate	Mistaken as magnesium sulfate	Use complete drug name
MTX	methotrexate	Mistaken as mitoxantrone	Use complete drug name
PCA	procainamide	Mistaken as patient controlled analgesia	Use complete drug name
PTU	propylthiouracil	Mistaken as mercaptopurine	Use complete drug name
T3	Tylenol with codeine No. 3	Mistaken as liothyronine	Use complete drug name
TAC	triamcinolone	Mistaken as tetracaine, Adrenalin, cocaine	Use complete drug name
TNK	TNKase	Mistaken as "TPA"	Use complete drug name
ZnSO4	zinc sulfate	Mistaken as morphine sulfate	Use complete drug name

Stemmed Drug Names	Intended Meaning	Misinterpretation	Correction
"Nitro" drip	nitroglycerin infusion	Mistaken as sodium nitroprusside infusion	Use complete drug name
"Norflox"	norfloxacin	Mistaken as Norflex	Use complete drug name
"IV Vanc"	intravenous vancomycin	Mistaken as Invanz	Use complete drug name

Symbols	Intended Meaning	Misinterpretation	Correction
ℨ ♏	Dram Minim	Symbol for dram mistaken as "3" Symbol for minim mistaken as "mL"	Use the metric system
x3d	For three days	Mistaken as "3 doses"	Use "for three days"
> and <	Greater than and less than	Mistaken as opposite of intended; mistakenly use incorrect symbol; "< 10" mistaken as "40"	Use "greater than" or "less than"
/ (slash mark)	Separates two doses or indicates "per"	Mistaken as the number 1 (e.g., "25 units/10 units" misread as "25 units and 110" units)	Use "per" rather than a slash mark to separate doses
@	At	Mistaken as "2"	Use "at"
&	And	Mistaken as "2"	Use "and"
+	Plus or and	Mistaken as "4"	Use "and"
°	Hour	Mistaken as a zero (e.g., q2° seen as q 20)	Use "hr," "h," or "hour"
Φ or ⌀	zero, null sign	Mistaken as numerals 4, 6, 8, and 9	Use 0 or zero, or describe intent using whole words

**These abbreviations are included on The Joint Commission's "minimum list" of dangerous abbreviations, acronyms, and symbols that must be included on an organization's "Do Not Use" list, effective January 1, 2004. Visit www.jointcommission.org for more information about this Joint Commission requirement.

ISMP
INSTITUTE FOR SAFE MEDICATION PRACTICES
www.ismp.org

Appendix D

English-to-Spanish Translation Guide: Key Medical Questions

The following is a guide to help you complete the history and examination of Spanish-speaking patients. Initial questions presented are general ones used at the beginning of the examination. Questions for pain assessment follow. The remainder of the translations are arranged in order of the body systems. Each system's section contains basic vocabulary, questions used for history taking, and instructions that would facilitate examination. The intent of this guide is to offer an array of questions and phrases from which the examiner can choose as appropriate for assessment.

Hints for Pronunciation of Spanish Words

1. *h* is silent.
2. *j* is pronounced as *h*.
3. *ll* is pronounced as a *y* sound.
4. *r* is pronounced with a trilled sound, and *rr* is trilled even more.
5. *v* is pronounced with a *b* sound.
6. A *y* by itself is pronounced with a long *e* sound.
7. Accent marks over the vowel indicate the syllable that is to be stressed.

Introductory	
I am _____.	Soy _____.
What is your name?	¿Cómo se llama usted?
I would like to examine you now.	Quisiera examinarlo(a) ahora.

General	
How do you feel?	¿Cómo se siente?
Good	Bien
Bad	Mal
Do you feel better today?	¿Se siente mejor hoy?
Where do you work?	¿Dónde trabaja? (Cuál es su profesión o trabajo?) (¿Qué hace usted?)
Are you allergic to anything?	¿Tiene usted alérgias?
Medications, foods, insect bites?	¿Medicinas, alimentos, picaduras de insectos?
Do you take any medications?	¿Toma usted alguna medicina?
Do you have any drug allergies?	¿Es usted alérgico(a) a algún medicamento?
Do you have a history of	¿Padece usted:
Heart disease?	de alguna enfermedad del corazón?
Diabetes?	del diabetes?
Epilepsy?	la epilépsia?
Bronchitis?	de bronquitis?
Emphysema?	de enfisema?
Asthma?	de asma?

From Seidel HM: *Mosby's guide to physical examination,* ed 5, St Louis, 2003, Mosby.

Pain

Have you any pain?	¿Tiene dolor?
Where is the pain?	¿Dónde está el dolor?
Do you have any pain here?	¿Tiene usted dolor aquí?

How severe is the pain?
   Mild, moderate, sharp, or severe?
	¿Qué tan fuerte es el dolor?
	   ¿Ligero, moderado, agudo, o severo?

What were you doing when the pain started?	¿Qué hacía usted cuando le comenzóel dolor?
Have you ever had this pain before?	¿Ha tenido este dolor antes?
	(¿Ha sido siempre así?)
Do you have a pain in your side?	¿Tiene usted dolor en el costado?
Is it worse now?	¿Está peor ahora?
Does it still pain you?	¿Le duele todavía?

Did you feel much pain at the time?
   Show me where.
	¿Sintió mucho dolor entonces?
	   Muéstreme dónde.

Does it hurt when I press here?	¿Le duele cuando aprieto aquí?

Head

Vocabulary

Head	La cabeza
Face	La cara

History

How does your head feel?	¿Cómo siente la cabeza?
Have you any pain in the head?	¿Le duele la cabeza?
Do you have headaches?	¿Tiene usted dolores de cabeza?
Do you have migraines?	¿Tiene usted migrañas?
What causes the headaches?	¿Qué le causa los dolores de cabeza?

Examination

Lift up your head.	Levante la cabeza.

Eyes

Vocabulary

Eye	El ojo

History

Have you had pain in your eyes?	¿Ha tenido dolor en los ojos?
Do you wear glasses?	¿Usa usted anteojos/gafas/lentes/espejuelos?
Do you wear contact lenses?	¿Usa usted lentes de contacto?

Can you see clearly?
   Better at a distance?
	¿Puede ver claramente?
	   ¿Mejor a cierta distancia?

Do you sometimes see things double?	¿Ve las cosas doble algunas veces?
Do you see things through a mist?	¿Ve las cosas nubladas?
Were you exposed to anything that could have injured your eye?	¿Fue expuesto(a) a cualquier cosa que pudiera haberle dañado el ojo?
Do your eyes water much?	¿Le lagrimean mucho los ojos?

Examination

Look up.	Mire para arriba.
Look down.	Mire para abajo.

Look toward your nose.	Mírese la nariz.
Look at me.	Míreme.
Tell me what number it is.	Dígame qué número es éste.
Tell me what letter it is.	Dígame qué letra es ésta.

Ears/Nose/Throat

Vocabulary

Ears	Los oídos
Eardrum	El tímpano
Laryngitis	La laringitis
Lip	El labio
Mouth	La boca
Nose	La naríz
Tongue	La lengua

History

Do you have any hearing problems?	¿Tiene usted problemas al oir?
Do you use a hearing aid?	¿Usa usted un audífono?
Do you have ringing in the ears?	¿Le zumban los oídos?
Do you have allergies?	¿Tiene alérgias?
Do you use dentures?	¿Usa usted dentadura postiza?
Do you have any loose teeth, removable bridges, or any prosthesis?	¿Tiene dientes flojos, dientes postizos, o cualiquier prótesis?
Do you have a cold?	¿Tiene usted un resfriado/resfrío?
Do you have a sore throat frequently?	¿Le duele la garganta con frecuencia?
Have you ever had a strep throat?	¿Ha tenido alguna vez infección de la garganta?

Examination

Open your mouth.	Abra la boca.
I want to take a throat culture. This will not hurt.	Quiero hacer un cultivo de la garganta. Esto no le va a doler.

Cardiovascular

Vocabulary

Heart	El corazón
Heart attack	El ataque al corazón
Heart disease	La enfermedad del corazón
Heart murmur	El soplo del corazón
High blood pressure	Alta presión

History

Have you ever had any chest pain? Where?	¿Ha tenido alguna vez dolor de pecho? ¿Dónde?
Do you notice any irregularity of heartbeat or any palpitations?	¿Nota cualquier latido o palpitación irregular?
Do you get short of breath? When?	¿Tiene usted problemas con la respiración? ¿Cuándo?
Do you take medicine for your heart? How often?	¿Toma medicina para el corazón? ¿Con qué frecuencia?

Do you know if you have high blood pressure?	¿Sabe usted si tiene la presión alta?
Is there a history of hypertension in your family?	¿En su familia se encuentran varias personas con alta presión?
Are any of your limbs swollen? Hands, feet, legs?	¿Están hinchados algunos de sus miembros? ¿Manos, pies, piernas?
How long have they been swollen like this?	¿Desde cuándo están hinchados así? (¿Qué tanto tiempo tiene usted con esta hinchazón?)

Examination

Let me feel your pulse.	Déjeme tomarle el pulso.
I am going to take your blood pressure now.	Le voy a tomar la presión ahora.

Respiratory

Vocabulary

Chest	El pecho
Lungs	Los pulmones

History

Do you smoke? How many packs a day?	¿Fuma usted? ¿Cuántos paquetes al día?
Have you any difficulty in breathing?	¿Tiene dificultad al respirar?
How long have you been coughing?	¿Desde cuándo tiene tos?
Do you cough up phlegm?	¿Al toser, escupe usted flema(s)?
What is the color of your expectorations?	¿Cuándo usted escupe, qué color es?
Do you cough up blood?	¿Al toser, arroja usted sangre?
Do you wheeze?	¿Le silba a usted el pecho?

Examination

Take a deep breath.	Respìre profundo.
Breathe normally.	Respìre normalmente.
Cough.	Tosa.
Cough again.	Tosa otra vez.

Gastrointestinal

Vocabulary

Abdomen	El abdomen
Intestines/bowels	Los intestinos/las entrañas
Liver	El hígado
Nausea	Náusea
Gastric ulcer	La úlcera gástrica
Stomach	El estómago, la panza, la barriga
Stomachache	El dolor de estómago

History

What foods disagree with you?	¿Qué alimentos le caen mal?
Do you get heartburn?	¿Suele tener ardor en el pecho?
Do you have indigestion often?	¿Tiene indigestion con frecuencia?
Are you going to vomit?	¿Va a vomitar (arrojar)?
Do you have blood in your vomit?	¿Tiene usted vómitos con sangre?

Do you have abdominal pain?	¿Tiene dolor en el abdomen?
How are your stools?	¿Cómo son sus defecaciones?
Are they regular?	¿Son regulares?
Have you noticed their color?	¿Se ha fijado en el color?
Are you constipated?	¿Está estreñido?
Do you have diarrhea?	¿Tiene diarrea?

Genitourinary
Vocabulary

Genitals	Los genitales
Kidney	El riñón
Penis	El pene, el miembro
Urine	La orina

History

Have you any difficulty passing water?	¿Tiene dificultad en orinar?
Do you pass water involuntarily?	¿Orina sin querer?
Do you have a urethral discharge?	¿Tiene desecho de la uretra?
Do you have burning with urination?	¿Tiene ardor al orinar?

Musculoskeletal
Vocabulary

Ankle	El tobillo
Arm	El brazo
Back	La espalda
Bones	Los huesos
Elbow	El codo
Finger	El dedo
Foot	El pie
Fracture	La fractura
Hand	La mano
Hip	La cadera
Knee	La rodilla
Leg	La pierna
Muscles	Los músculos
Rib	La costilla
Shoulder	El hombro
Thigh	El muslo

History

Did you fall, and how did you fall?	¿Se cayó, y cómo se cayó?
How did this happen?	¿Cómo sucedió esto?
How long ago?	¿Hace cuanto tiempo?

Examination

Raise your arm.	Levante el brazo.
Raise it more.	Más alto.
Now the other.	Ahora el otro.
Stand up and walk.	Parese y camine.

Straighten your leg.	Enderece la pierna.
Bend your knee.	Doble la rodilla.
Push	Empuje
Pull	Jale
Up	Arriba
Down	Abajo
In/out	Adentro/afuera
Rest	Descanse
Kneel	Arrodíllese

Neurologic

Vocabulary

Brain	El cerebro
Dizziness	El vertigo, el mareo
Epilepsy	La epilépsia
Fainting spell	El desmayo

History

Have you ever had a head injury?	¿Ha tenido alguna vez daño en la cabeza?
Do you have convulsions?	¿Tiene convulsiones?
Do you have tingling sensations?	¿Tiene hormigueos?
Do you have numbness in your hands, arms, or feet?	¿Siente entumecidos las manos, los brazos, o los pies?
Have you ever lost consciousness? For how long?	¿Perdió alguna vez el sentido? (inconsiente) ¿Por cuánto tiempo?
How often does this happen?	¿Con qué frecuencia ocurre esto?

Examination

Squeeze my hand.	Apriete mi mano.
Can you not do it better than that?	¿No puede hacerlo más fuerte?
Turn on your left/right side.	Voltéese al lado izquierdo/al lado derecho.
Roll over and sit up over the edge of the bed.	Voltéese y siéntese sobre el borde de la cama.
Stand up slowly. Put your weight only on your right/left foot.	Párese despacio. Ponga peso solo en la pierna derecha/izquierda.
Take a step to the side.	Dé un paso al lado.
Turn to your left/right.	Doble a la izquierda/derecha.
Is this hot or cold?	¿Está frío o caliente esto?
Am I sticking you with the point or the head of the pin?	¿Le estoy pinchando con el punto o la cabeza del alfiler?

Endocrine/Reproductive

Vocabulary

Uterus	El útero, la matríz
Vagina	La vagina

History

Have you had any problems with your thyroid?	¿Ha tenido alguna vez problemas con tiroides?
Have you noticed any significant weight gain or loss?	¿Ha notado pérdida o aumento de peso?

What is your usual weight?	¿Cuál es su peso usual?
How is your appetite?	¿Qué tal su apetito?

Women

How old were you when your periods started?	¿Cuántos años tenía cuando tuvo la primera regla?
How many days between periods?	¿Cuántos dias entre las reglas?
When was your last menstrual period?	¿Cuándo fue su última regla?
Have you ever been pregnant?	¿Ha estado embarazada?
How many children do you have?	¿Cuántos hijos tiene?
When was your last Pap smear?	¿Cuándo fue su última prueba de Papanicolau?
Would you like information on birth control methods?	¿Quiere usted información sobre los métodos del control de la natalidad?
Do you have a vaginal discharge?	¿Tiene desecho vaginal?

Illustration Credits

Adam A, Dixon AK: *Grainger & Allison's diagnostic radiology,* ed 5, Oxford, 2008, Churchill Livingstone (Fig. 12-25).

Albert D: *Albert & Jakobiec's principles and practice of ophthalmology,* ed 3, London, 2008, Saunders/Elsevier (Fig. 13-12).

Beare PG, Myers JL: *Adult health nursing,* ed 3, St Louis, 1998, Mosby/Elsevier (Fig. 11-20, *D*).

Bird D, Robinson D: *Torres and Ehrlich modern dental assisting,* ed 8, Philadelphia, 2005, Saunders/Elsevier (Fig. 5-10, *E*).

Black JM, Hawks JH, Keene A: *Medical surgical nursing: clinical management for positive outcomes,* ed 8, Philadelphia, 2009, Saunders/Elsevier (Figs. 5-12; 6-22; 8-17; 9-12; 11-16, *A*; 12-18, *B*; 12-22, *B*; 13-13; 13-30; 14-17).

Blumgart L: *Surgery of the liver, biliary tract, and pancreas,* ed 4, St Louis, 2007, Saunders/Elsevier (Fig. 5-24).

Bolognia JL: *Dermatology,* ed 2, St Louis, 2008, Mosby/Elsevier (Figs. 5-8, 9-11).

Bonewit-West K: *Clinical procedures for medical assistants,* ed 7, Philadelphia, 2008, Saunders/Elsevier (Figs. 6-11, 6-12, 9-20).

Bontrager KL: *Textbook of radiographic positioning and related anatomy,* ed 7, St Louis, 2009, Mosby/Elsevier (Fig. 6-15).

Bork K, Brauninger W: *Skin disease in clinical practice,* ed 2, Philadelphia, 1999, Saunders/Elsevier (Fig. 4-16).

Brody HJ: *Chemical peeling,* ed 2, St Louis, 1997, Mosby/Elsevier (Fig. 4-38).

Callen JP, Greer KE, Saller AS, et al: *Color atlas of dermatology,* ed 3, Philadelphia, 2003, Saunders/Elsevier (Figs. 4-6, 4-13, 4-15, 4-19 to 4-22).

The Centers for Disease Control (Fig. 4-30).

Christian PE: *Nuclear Medicine and PET/CT: technology and techniques,* ed 7, 2012, Mosby/Elsevier (Fig. 16-8).

Christensen BL: *Foundations and adult health nursing,* ed 6, St Louis, 2010, Mosby/Elsevier (Fig. 11-20, *D*).

Cotran RS, Kumar V, Collins: *Robbins' pathologic basis of disease,* ed 6, Philadelphia, 1999, Saunders/Elsevier (Fig. 10-18, *B*).

de la Maza LM, Pezzlo MT, Baron EJ: *Color atlas of diagnostic microbiology,* St Louis, 1997, Mosby/Elsevier (Fig. 7-15).

Damjanov I: *Anderson's pathology,* ed 10, St Louis, 2000, Mosby/Elsevier (Figs. 3-20, 4-26, 5-29, 6-10, 7-12, 8-13, 9-15, 10-20, 13-18, 14-11).

Damjanov I: *Pathology: a color atlas,* St Louis, 2000, Mosby/Elsevier (Figs. 5-13; 5-15, *A*; 5-17; 5-18, *B*; 10-16; 10-17, *B-C*; 11-7; 11-11; 12-11).

Early PJ, Sodee DB: *Nuclear medicine: principles and practice,* ed 2, St Louis, 1994, Mosby/Elsevier (Fig. 11-17).

Eisen D, Lynch DP: *The mouth: diagnosis and treatment,* St Louis, 1998, Mosby/Elsevier (Fig. 5-11).

Eisenberg RL, Johnson N: *Comprehensive radiographic pathology,* ed 4, St Louis, 2007, Mosby/Elsevier (Fig. 11-16, *B*).

Elkin MK, Perry AG, Potter PA: *Nursing intervention and clinical skills,* ed 4, St Louis, 2008, Mosby/Elsevier (Figs. 4-17, 6-14).

Epstein E: *Common skin disorders,* ed 5, Philadelphia, 2001, Saunders/Elsevier (Fig. 4-8).

Feldman M, Friedman LS, Brandt LJ: *Sleisenger and Fordtran's gastrointestinal and liver disease,* ed 8, Philadelphia, 2006, Saunders/Elsevier (Fig. 1-1).

Fenichel G: *Clinical pediatric neurology,* ed 5, Philadelphia, 2005, Saunders/Elsevier (Fig. 13-29).

Fletcher CD: *Diagnostic histopathology of tumors,* ed 3, London, 2008, Churchill Livingstone (Figs. 8-11, *B*; 10-19).

Fortinash KM: *Psychiatric mental health nursing,* ed 4, St Louis, 2008, Mosby/Elsevier (Fig. 15-3).

Frank ED, Long BW, Smith BJ: *Merrill's atlas of radiographic positions and radiologic procedures,* ed 12, St Louis, 2012, Mosby/Elsevier (Figs. 2-3; 2-4; 3-11; 3-14, *B*; 3-22; 5-25; 5-26; 5-27; 6-8; 6-13; 8-11, *A*; 8-14; 9-17; 10-21; 10-23; 10-24, *A*; 10-27; 14-14; 16-11).

Frazier MS, Drzymkowski JW: *Essentials of human diseases and conditions,* ed 4, Philadelphia, 2008, Saunders/Elsevier (Figs. 4-14, 5-19, 6-16, *B*).

Frowen P, et al: *Neale's disorders of the foot,* ed 8, Oxford, 2010, Churchill Livingstone (Fig. 11-5).

Fuller JK: *Surgical technology,* ed 4, Philadelphia, 2006, Saunders/Elsevier (Figs. 1-9; 3-21, *B*; 5-31, *B*; 13-21).

Garrels M: *Laboratory testing for ambulatory settings,* ed 2, St Louis, 2011, Saunders/Elsevier (Fig. 4-5).

Goldberg JG, Falcone T: *Atlas of endoscopic techniques in gynecology,* Philadelphia, 2000, Saunders/Elsevier (Fig. 8-21).

Habif TP: *Clinical dermatology,* ed 5, St Louis, 2010, Mosby/Elsevier (Figs. 4-11, 4-24, 4-36, 9-19).

Hagen-Ansert SL: *Textbook of diagnostic sonography,* ed 7, St Louis, 2012, Mosby/Elsevier (Figs. 8-10; 8-15, *B*; 8-16; 10-24, *B*).

Herlihy B, Maebius NK: *The human body in health and illness,* ed 4, Philadelphia, 2011, Saunders/Elsevier (Figs. 9-6, 9-9, 13-1, 13-11).

Hill MJ: *Skin disorders,* St Louis, 1994, Mosby/Elsevier (Figs. 4-12, 4-14).

Ignatavicius DD, Workman ML: *Medical-surgical nursing: critical thinking for collaborative care,* ed 6, Philadelphia, 2011, Saunders/Elsevier (Figs. 4-34; 6-7; 6-21, *A-B*; 11-22; 13-20; 13-23; 13-24; 14-6; 14-15).

Kanski J, Bowling B: *Clinical ophthalmology,* ed 7, London, 2011, Saunders/Elsevier (Fig. 13-10).

Kliegman R, Stanton BF, St. Geme JW, et al: *Nelson textbook of pediatrics,* ed 19, St Louis, 2011, Saunders/Elsevier (Figs. 5-9, 12-9).

Kowalczyk N: *Radiographic pathology for technologists,* ed 5, St Louis, 2009, Mosby/Elsevier (Figs. 3-25, *A*; 16-7).

Kumar P, Clark ML: *Kumar and Clarks's clinical medicine,* ed 7, Philadelphia, 2009, Saunders/Elsevier (Figs. 6-9, 7-11, 9-10, 12-18).

Kumar V, Abbas AK, Fausto N: *Basic pathology,* ed 7, Philadelphia, 2003, Saunders/Elsevier (Fig. 12-20).

Kumar V, et al: *Robbins basic pathology,* ed 8, Philadelphia, 2007, Saunders/Elsevier (Fig. 11-14).

LaTrenta G: *Atlas of aesthetic face and neck surgery,* Philadelphia, 2004, Saunders/Elsevier (Fig. 4-37).

Lewis SM: *Medical-surgical nursing: assessment and management of clinical problems,* ed 8, St Louis, 2011, Mosby/Elsevier (Figs. 3-12; 3-21, *A*; 6-5; 6-14; 10-9, *B-C*; 10-18; 12-30).

Liu G, Volpe N, Galetta S: *Neuro-ophthalmology,* ed 2, London, 2010, Saunders/Elsevier (Fig. 13-9).

Lowdermilk DL, Perry SE, Bobak IM: *Maternity and women's health care,* ed 10, St Louis, 2012, Mosby/Elsevier (Figs. 8-12, 8-27).

Mahan LK, Escott-Stump S: *Krause's food and nutrition therapy,* ed 12, Philadelphia, 2008, Saunders/Elsevier (Fig. 5-18, *A*).

Marks JG Jr, Miller JJ: *Lookingbill & Marks' principles of dermatology,* ed 4, London, 2006, Saunders/Elsevier (Fig. 4-10).

Marx J, Hockberger R, Walls R: *Rosen's emergency medicine,* ed 7, Philadelphia, 2010, Saunders/Elsevier (Fig. 13-7).

McCance KL, Huether SE: *Pathophysiology: the biologic basis for disease in adults and children,* ed 6, St Louis, 2010, Mosby/Elsevier (Figs. 4-27, 4-32).

Miller RG, Ashar B, Sisson SD: *The Johns Hopkins internal medicine board review 2010-2011,* ed 3, Philadelphia, 2010, Mosby/Elsevier (Fig. 13-19).

Mosby's medical nursing and allied health dictionary, ed 8, St Louis, 2009, Mosby/Elsevier (Figs. 7-9, 7-10, 14-5).

Murray SS: *Foundations of maternal newborn & women's health nursing,* ed 5, Philadelphia, 2010, Saunders/Elsevier (Fig. 8-24).

Nguyen Q, Rodrigues EB, Farah ME, et al: *Retinal pharmacotherapy,* London, 2010, Saunders/Elsevier (Fig. 13-17).

Potter PA, Perry AG: *Fundamentals of nursing,* ed 7, St Louis, 2011, Mosby/Elsevier (Figs. 5-29, *B;* 11-20, *A-C*).

Rosai J: *Rosai and Ackerman's surgical pathology,* ed 10, Edinburgh, 2011, Mosby/Elsevier (Fig. 14-12).

Rothrock J: *Alexander's care of the patient in surgery,* ed 14, St Louis, 2011, Mosby/Elsevier (Fig. 16-9).

Sainani GS, Joshi VR, Sainani RG: *Manual of clinical & practical medicine,* New Delhi, 2010, Elsevier India (Fig. 14-7).

Salvo SG: *Massage therapy,* ed 3, St Louis, 2007, Saunders/Elsevier (Fig. 8-4).

Salvo SG: *Mosby's pathology for massage therapists,* ed 2, St Louis, 2009, Mosby/Elsevier (Fig. 5-18).

Seidel HM, Ball JW, Dains JE, et al: *Mosby's guide to physical examination,* ed 7, St Louis, 2011, Mosby/Elsevier (Figs. 4-9; 4-31; 7-6; 7-7; 12-2, *A;* 13-3; 13-6).

Shiland B: *Medical terminology & anatomy for ICD-10 coding,* St Louis, 2012, Mosby/Elsevier (Figs. 3-35, 3-39, 8-20, 8-12, 12-29, 13-9, 15-3).

Sorrentino SA: *Textbook for long-term care nursing assistants,* ed 6, St Louis, 2011, Mosby/Elsevier (Fig. 11-19).

Sorrentino SA: *Assisting with patient care,* ed 2, St Louis, 2004, Mosby/Elsevier (Fig. 13-4).

Stone DR, Gorbach SL: *Atlas of infectious diseases,* Philadelphia, 2000, Saunders/Elsevier (Fig. 13-26).

Stuart GW, Laraia MT: *Principles and practice of psychiatric nursing,* ed 9, St Louis, 2009, Mosby/Elsevier (Figs. 15-1, 15-2, 15-3).

Thibodeau GA, Patton KT: *Anatomy and physiology,* ed 7, St Louis, 2010, Mosby/Elsevier (Figs. 9-13, 10-18, *B*).

Thibodeau GA, Patton KT: *The human body in health and disease,* ed 5, St Louis, 2010, Mosby/Elsevier (Figs. 12-5, 12-17, 14-4, 14-9).

White S, Pharoah M: *Oral radiology,* ed 6, St Louis, 2009, Mosby/Elsevier (Fig. 5-21).

Wilson SF, Giddens JF: *Health assessment for nursing practice,* ed 4, St Louis, 2012, Mosby/Elsevier (Figs. 3-14, *A;* 3-23; 4-7).

Young AP, Proctor DB: *Kinn's the medical assistant,* ed 11, Philadelphia, 2011, Saunders/Elsevier (Figs. 10-25, 11-18).

Ziessman HA: *Nuclear medicine, the requisites,* ed 3, St Louis, 2011, Mosby/Elsevier (Fig. 14-13).

Zitelli BJ, Davis HW: *Atlas of pediatric physical diagnosis,* ed 5, St Louis, 2007, Mosby/Elsevier (Figs. 3-9, 3-10, 5-6, 5-14, 5-20, 7-3, 11-4, 11-6, 12-10, 13-5, 13-27, 13-28, 13-32, 14-8).

Answers to Exercises and Review Questions

Chapter 1

Exercise 1
1. C 2. D 3. E 4. B 5. F
6. A

Exercise 2
1. C 2. D 3. A 4. E 5. B

Exercise 3
1. B 2. D 3. E 4. A 5. C

Exercise 4
1. ophthalm/o (eye) + -logy (study of)
   Def: study of the eye
2. ot/o (ear) + -plasty (surgical repair)
   Def: surgical repair of the ear
3. gastr/o (stomach) + -algia (pain)
   Def: pain in the stomach
4. arthr/o (joint) + -scope (instrument to view)
   Def: instrument to view a joint
5. rhin/o (nose) + -tomy (incision)
   Def: incision of the nose

Exercise 5
1. E 2. G 3. J 4. I 5. H
6. A 7. C 8. D 9. F 10. B
11. cardi/o (heart) + -megaly (enlargement)
    Def: enlargement of the heart
12. oste/o (bone) + -malacia (softening)
    Def: softening of the bone
13. valvul/o (valve) + -itis (inflammation)
    Def: inflammation of a valve
14. cephal/o (head) + -ic (pertaining to)
    Def: pertaining to the head
15. gastr/o (stomach) + -ptosis (prolapse)
    Def: prolapse of the stomach

Exercise 6
1. E 2. I 3. H 4. F 5. J
6. C 7. D 8. A 9. G 10. B
11. oste/o (bone) + -logist (one who specializes in the study of)
    Def: one who specializes in the study of bones
12. spir/o (breathing) + -meter (instrument to measure)
    Def: instrument to measure breathing
13. hyster/o (uterus) + -scopy (process of viewing)
    Def: process of viewing the uterus

14. cyst/o (bladder, sac) + -scope (instrument to view)
    Def: instrument to view the bladder
15. splen/o (spleen) + -ectomy (removal)
    Def: removal of the spleen

Case Study: Debbie Halloran
1. b
2. a
3. c
4. b
5. d

Exercise 7
1. C 2. H 3. F 4. I 5. B
6. D 7. E 8. J 9. A 10. G
11. sub- (under) + hepat/o (liver) + -ic (pertaining to)
    Def: pertaining to under the liver
12. peri- (around) + cardi/o (heart) + -um (structure)
    Def: structure around the heart
13. dys- (difficult) + pne/o (breathing) + -ic (pertaining to)
    Def: pertaining to difficult breathing
14. per- (through) + cutane/o (skin) + -ous (pertaining to)
    Def: pertaining to through the skin
15. hypo- (deficient) + glyc/o (sugar) + -emia (blood condition)
    Def: blood condition of deficient sugar

Case Study: Kate Martin
1. a
2. b
3. a
4. d
5. a

Exercise 8
1. esophagi
2. larynges
3. fornices
4. pleurae
5. diagnoses
6. myocardia
7. cardiomyopathies
8. hepatitides

Exercise 9
x, ph, pn, eu, pt, ps

Case Study: Harry Chu
1. bladder
2. eye
3. ear
4. bone
5. d

Case Study: Medical Terminology Class
1. arthritis
2. cardiology
3. endoscopy
4. epigastric
5. paranasal

Chapter 1 Review

Word Part Definitions
1. inter-
2. per-
3. par-
4. intra-
5. anti-
6. a-
7. peri-
8. para-
9. pre-
10. poly-
11. sub-
12. dys-
13. –dynia
14. –rrhea
15. –stenosis
16. –oma
17. –tripter
18. –itis
19. –rrhage
20. –scopy
21. –logy
22. –tomy
23. –plasty
24. –ectomy
25. –graphy
26. –meter
27. –rrhaphy
28. –stomy
29. –osis
30. –pathy
31. –ar
32. –ia

Wordshop
1. condition (-ia) without (an-) eye (ophthalm/o)
   Term: anophthalmia
2. pertaining to (-id) near (par-) ear (ot/o)
   Term: parotid

3. pertaining to (-ic) under (sub-) liver (hepat/o)
   Term: subhepatic
4. inflammation (-itis) stomach (gastr/o) small intestines (enter/o)
   Term: gastroenteritis
5. instrument to view (-scope) ear (ot/o)
   Term: otoscope
6. structure (-um) surrounding (peri-) heart (cardi/o)
   Term: pericardium
7. new opening (-stomy) colon (col/o)
   Term: colostomy
8. process of recording (-graphy) artery (arteri/o)
   Term: arteriography
9. process of viewing (-scopy) within (endo-)
   Term: endoscopy
10. removal (-ectomy) uterus (hyster/o)
    Term: hysterectomy
11. study of (-logy) many (poly-) sleep (somn/o)
    Term: polysomnology
12. pertaining to (-al) before (pre-) birth (nat/o)
    Term: prenatal
13. pain (-algia) head (cephal/o)
    Term: cephalalgia
14. pertaining to (-ic) above (epi-) stomach (gastr/o)
    Term: epigastric
15. enlargement (-megaly) spleen (splen/o)
    Term: splenomegaly

Chapter 2

Exercise 1
1. D 2. E 3. A 4. C 5. B

Exercise 2
1. C 2. A 3. D 4. B

Exercise 3
1. D 2. F 3. A 4. B 5. H
6. C 7. E 8. G

Exercise 4
1. pertaining to within the lumen
2. pertaining to the hilum
3. pertaining to around the apex
4. pertaining to the antrum
5. pertaining to the nucleus
6. pertaining to the cytoplasm
7. pertaining to outside the body
8. pertaining to the vestibule
9. pertaining to the fundus
10. lumen
11. hilum
12. apex
13. body, corporis
14. sinuses

Case Study: Samantha Weil
1. fundus
2. sinus or antrum
3. apex
4. body or corporis
5. vestibule

Exercise 5
1. F 2. H 3. C, I 4. A
5. G 6. E 7. J 8. B
9. L 10. D 11. K

Exercise 6
1. J 2. G 3. A 4. I 5. D
6. E 7. H 8. B 9. C 10. F

Exercise 7
1. the study of cells
2. one who specializes in the study of disease
3. process of viewing dead (tissue)
4. one who specializes in the study of tissue
5. process of viewing living (tissue)

Exercise 8
1. G 2. M 3. J 4. K
5. R 6. A 7. P 8. D
9. T 10. B 11. F 12. I
13. Q 14. C 15. S 16. N
17. E 18. O 19. H 20. L

Exercise 9
See Fig. 2-2.

Exercise 10
1. I 2. P 3. N 4. L
5. M 6. J 7. R 8. B
9. K 10. F 11. D 12. O
13. G 14. A 15. Q 16. E
17. C 18. H

Exercise 11
1. C 2. A 3. F 4. K
5. I 6. J 7. L 8. E
9. D 10. H 11. G 12. B

Exercise 12
1. esophagus
2. esophagus and stomach
3. the beginning and middle portions of the esophagus were normal
4. distal esophagus

Exercise 13
1. D 2. C 3. B 4. A 5. E

Exercise 14
1. epigastric
2. lumbar
3. hypogastric
4. iliac or inguinal
5. hypochondriac

Exercise 15
See Fig. 2-7.

Exercise 16
1. transverse
2. midsagittal
3. frontal or coronal

Exercise 17
1. closer to the toes
2. inner surface
3. during
4. front to back

Exercise 18
1. posterior
2. superior
3. anterior
4. lateral
5. inferior

Case Study: Elena Novoyenko
1. epigastric
2. hypogastric
3. b
4. a
5. b
6. a

Chapter 2 Review

Word Part Definitions
1. epi-
2. meta-
3. uni-
4. endo-
5. bi-
6. af-
7. ipsi-
8. contra-
9. ef-
10. viscer/o
11. infer/o
12. anter/o
13. dist/o
14. medi/o
15. axill/o
16. super/o
17. proxim/o
18. sinistr/o
19. brachi/o
20. caud/o
21. lapar/o
22. later/o
23. dextr/o
24. poster/o
25. hist/o
26. corpor/o
27. cephal/o
28. crani/o
29. cyt/o
30. inguin/o

31. cervic/o
32. thorac/o

Wordshop

1. pertaining to (-al) middle (mid-) sagittal plane (sagitt/o)
   Term: midsagittal
2. pertaining to (-al) two (bi-) side (later/o)
   Term: bilateral
3. toward (-ad) right (dextr/o)
   Term: dextrad
4. pertaining to (-ior) back (poster/o) front (anter/o)
   Term: posteroanterior
5. pertaining to (-ic) chest (thorac/o)
   Term: thoracic
6. pertaining to (-ic) abdomen (abdomin/o) pelvis (pelv/o)
   Term: abdominopelvic
7. pertaining to (-ar) low back (lumb/o)
   Term: lumbar
8. pertaining to (-al) opposite (contra-) side (later/o)
   Term: contralateral
9. formation (-plasm) cell (cyt/o)
   Term: cytoplasm
10. pertaining to (-ior) upward (super/o)
    Term: superior
11. pertaining to (-ic) above (supra-) chest (thorac/o)
    Term: suprathoracic
12. study of (-logy) tissues (hist/o)
    Term: histology
13. pertaining to (-ic) under (hypo-) stomach (gastr/o)
    Term: hypogastric
14. pertaining to (-al) same (ipsi-) side (later/o)
    Term: ipsilateral
15. pertaining to (-al) within (intra-) skull (crani/o)
    Term: intracranial

Term Sorting

Organization of the body: apex, cytoplasm, hilum, lumen, nucleus, organ, sinus, system, vestibule, viscera
Positional and Directional Terms: afferent, anterior, distal, efferent, lateral, posterior, prone superior, supine, ventral
Body Cavities and Planes: coronal, cranial, midsagittal, pleural, sagittal, spinal, thoracic, transverse
Abdominal Regions and Quadrants: epigastric, hypochondriac, hypogastric, iliac inguinal, lumbar, umbilical

Translations

1. plantar, palmar
2. antecubital
3. bilateral
4. buccal
5. biopsy
6. lumen
7. thoracic
8. distal
9. mediastinum
10. contralateral
11. supine
12. inguinal or iliac
13. thoracic, coxal
14. epigastric

Radiology Report

1. distal end, the end closest to the wrist
2. backward
3. joint
4. pertaining to the back
5. posteroanterior, back to front

Chapter 3

Exercise 1

1. E, J   2. C, D   3. I
4. G, L   5. H, K   6. A
7. F   8. B
9. articul/o (joint) + -ar (pertaining to)
   Def: pertaining to a joint
10. tendin/o (tendon) + -ous (pertaining to)
    Def: pertaining to a tendon
11. muscul/o (muscle) + -ar (pertaining to)
    Def: pertaining to a muscle
12. syndesm/o (ligament) + -al (pertaining to)
    Def: pertaining to a ligament
13. chondr/o (cartilage) + -al (pertaining to)
    Def: pertaining to the cartilage
14. osse/o (bone) + -ous (pertaining to)
    Def: pertaining to a bone

Exercise 2

1. E   2. J   3. F   4. L
5. H   6. N   7. B   8. O
9. G   10. C   11. K   12. M
13. A   14. D   15. I
16. build, break down
17. diaphysis, epiphyses
18. periosteum, endosteum
19. depressions, processes
20. antrum

Exercise 3

See Fig. 3-2.

Exercise 4

1. I   2. K   3. F   4. G
5. N   6. J   7. M   8. B
9. E   10. D   11. A   12. O
13. C   14. H   15. L   16. P
17. sub- (under, below) + mandibul/o (mandible) + -ar (pertaining to)
    Def: pertaining to under the mandible
18. cost/o (rib) + chondr/o (cartilage) + -al (pertaining to)
    Def: pertaining to ribs and cartilage
19. lumb/o (lower back) + sacr/o (sacrum) + -al (pertaining to)
    Def: pertaining to lower back and sacrum
20. thorac/o (chest) + -ic (pertaining to)
    Def: pertaining to the chest
21. sub- (under, below) + stern/o (breastbone) + -al (pertaining to)
    Def: pertaining to under the breastbone

Exercise 5

See Fig. 3-3, *A*.

Exercise 6

See Fig. 3-4, *A*.

Exercise 7

See Fig. 3-4, *C*.

Exercise 8

See Fig. 3-4, *B*.

Exercise 9

1. F   2. I   3. G   4. H
5. A   6. J   7. C   8. D
9. E   10. B   11. P   12. N
13. K   14. O   15. Q   16. R
17. T   18. L   19. U   20. S
21. M   22. V
23. inter- (between) + phalang/o (finger or toe bones) + -eal (pertaining to)
    Def: pertaining to between the finger or toe bones
24. humer/o (upper arm bone) + uln/o (lower medial arm bone) + -ar (pertaining to)
    Def: pertaining to the upper arm bone and the lower medial arm bone
25. infra- (below) + patell/o (kneecap) + -ar (pertaining to)
    Def: pertaining to below the kneecap
26. femor/o (thigh bone) + -al (pertaining to)
    Def: pertaining to the thigh bone

15. removal (-ectomy) meniscus (menisc/o)
    Term: meniscectomy
16. surgical repair (-plasty) ligament (syndesm/o)
    Term: syndesmoplasty

Exercise 25
1. bisphosphonates
2. disease-modifying antirheumatic drugs
3. inflammation and pain
4. muscle relaxants

Case Study: Consuela Esteban
1. crepitus
2. closed fracture
3. reduction
4. pain

Case Study: Pia Romana
1. pain
2. cervical (neck)
3. between
4. myelogram
5. b

Case Study: Barbara Eversole
1. osteoarthritis
2. rheumatoid arthritis
3. range of motion
4. total knee replacement
5. antiinflammatory

Exercise 26
1. fracture of the fifth lumbar vertebra, dual energy x-ray absorptiometry
2. degenerative joint disease
3. electromyelography, muscular dystrophy
4. CTS (carpal tunnel syndrome)

Chapter 3 Review

Word Part Definitions
1. –desis
2. –plasia
3. –centesis
4. syn-
5. –malacia
6. –listhesis
7. peri-
8. –clasis
9. –physis
10. –osis
11. cleid/o
12. oste/o
13. gnath/o
14. rhabdomy/o
15. humer/o
16. carp/o
17. zygomat/o
18. femor/o
19. cervic/o

20. spondyl/o
21. chondr/o
22. myel/o
23. dactyl/o
24. phalang/o
25. cost/o
26. my/o
27. olecran/o
28. coccyg/o
29. patell/a
30. arthr/o
31. mandibul/o
32. scapul/o

Wordshop
1. structure (-um) surrounding (peri-) bone (oste/o)
   Term: periosteum
2. inflammation (-itis) many (poly-) muscle (myos/o)
   Term: polymyositis
3. inflammation (-itis) surrounding (peri-) joint (arthr/o)
   Term: periarthritis
4. softening (-malacia) cartilage (chondr/o)
   Term: chondromalacia
5. condition (-y) many (poly-) fingers or toes (dactyl/o)
   Term: polydactyly
6. destruction (-lysis) skeletal muscle (rhabdomy/o)
   Term: rhabdomyolysis
7. abnormal condition (-osis) bone (oste/o) growth (phyt/o)
   Term: osteophytosis
8. binding (-desis) joint (arthr/o)
   Term: arthrodesis
9. suture (-rrhaphy) muscle (my/o)
   Term: myorrhaphy
10. condition (-y) joined, together (syn-) fingers or toes (dactyl/o)
    Term: syndactyly
11. tumor (-oma) cartilage (chondr/o)
    Term: chondroma
12. binding (-desis) joined, together (syn-) vertebrae (spondyl/o)
    Term: spondylosyndesis
13. surgical repair (-plasty) ligament (syndesm/o)
    Term: syndesmoplasty
14. formation (-plasia) no, without (a-) cartilage (chondr/o)
    Term: achondroplasia
15. surgical repair (-plasty) tendon (ten/o) muscle (my/o)
    Term: tenomyoplasty

Term Sorting
Anatomy an... ...ysiology: articulation... costa, diaph... ...lage, humerus, liga... ...gitus, sternum, ulna ...adius,
Pathology: arthro... bursitis, CTS, ost... osteoporosis, oste... ...n, spondylolisthesis, s... tendinitis
Diagnostic Procedures: arthrography, arthrosc... DEXA, EMG, goniomet... myelogram, Phalen test, ... serum calcium
Therapeutic Interventions: arthrocentesis, arthrodesis, laminectomy, meniscectomy, myorrhaphy, osteoclasis, osteoplasty, prosthesis, tenomyoplasty, TKR

Translations
1. chondromalacia, Baker cyst
2. amputation, prosthesis
3. myorrhaphy
4. arthrocentesis, hemarthrosis
5. reduction, clavicle
6. Phalen test, carpal tunnel syndrome (CTS)
7. osteophytosis, interphalangeal joints
8. kyphosis, osteoporosis
9. osteomyelitis, radius
10. plantar fasciitis, tendinitis
11. electromyography (EMG), muscular dystrophy
12. greenstick, humerus
13. polydactyly, syndactyly
14. bunionectomy, bunion

Operative Report
1. osteoarthritis
2. the front of the knee
3. kneecap
4. near the patella
5. incision of a joint
6. turned out, away from the midline
7. an instrument to cut bone
8. increasing the angle of the joint beyond normal range

Chapter 4

Exercise 1
1. B   2. H   3. F   4. A   5. D
6. E   7. G   8. I   9. C 10. J
11. (without) + vascul/o (vessel) + -ar (pertaining to)
    Def: pertaining to without vessels

12. sub- (under, below) + ungu/o
    (nail) + -al (pertaining to)
    **Def: pertaining to under
    the nail**
13. hypo- (below) + derm/o (skin)
    + -ic (pertaining to)
    **Def: pertaining to below
    the skin**

Exercise 2
See Fig. 4-1.

Exercise 3
1. the nail bed is the tissue under
   the nail and the nail plate is the
   actual nail
2. palm
3. an instrument for compression
   of blood vessels to control blood
   flow to and from the fingertip
4. the nail root

Exercise 4
1. E   2. F   3. C   4. A
5. B   6. D   7. C   8. D
9. A   10. E   11. B   12. D
13. E 14. C   15. A   16. B

Exercise 5
1. eczema
2. atopic dermatitis
3. contact dermatitis
4. seborrheic dermatitis
5. impetigo
6. furuncle
7. pilonidal cyst
8. inflammation (-itis) of follicles
   (follicul/o)
   Term: folliculitis
9. inflammation (-itis) of cells
   (cellul/o)
   Term: cellulitis

Case Study: Devin Doughtery
1. vesicles
2. pustules
3. pruritus
4. impetigo
5. c

Exercise 6
1. D   2. C   3. F   4. B   5. H
6. A   7. G   8. E
9. abnormal condition (-osis) of
   lice (pedicul/o)
   Term: pediculosis
10. abnormal condition (-osis)
    of fungus (my/o) of the skin
    (dermat/o)
    Term: dermatomycosis

Case Study: Zander Woo
1. candidiasis
2. moniliasis
3. b
4. dermatomycosis

Exercise 7
1. psoriasis
2. hypertrichosis
3. alopecia
4. keratinous cyst
5. acne vulgaris
6. clavus
7. pressure sore, decubitus ulcer
8. milia
9. xeroderma

Case Study: Keisha Landerson
1. psoriasis
2. epithelial
3. stratum corneum
4. b

Exercise 8
1. abnormal condition (-osis)
   excessive (hyper-) sweat (hidr/o)
   Term: hyperhidrosis
2. abnormal (dys-) color (chrom/o)
   condition (-ia)
   Term: dyschromia
3. inflammation (-itis) sweat
   (hidr/o) gland (aden/o)
   Term: hidradenitis
4. abnormal condition (-osis) no
   (an-) sweat (hidr/o)
   Term: anhidrosis
5. vitiligo
6. albinism
7. miliaria

Exercise 9
1. C   2. D   3. B   4. E   5. A
6. softening (-malacia) nail
   (onych/o)
   Term: onychomalacia
7. abnormal condition (-osis)
   fungus (myc/o) nail (onych/o)
   Term: onychomycosis
8. abnormal condition (-osis)
   hidden (crypt/o) nail (onych/o)
   Term: onychocryptosis
9. separation (-lysis) nail (onych/o)
   Term: onycholysis

Case Study: Angela Trova
1. onychocryptosis
2. hidden
3. redness
4. nail plate

Exercise 10
1. C   2. A   3. D   4. B

Exercise 11
1. D   2. A   3. B   4. C   5. E
6. dermat/o (skin) + fibr/o (fiber) +
   -oma (mass, tumor)
   Def: mass of fibrous skin
7. angi/o (vessel) + -oma
   (mass, tumor)
   Def: mass of vessels

8. seb/o (sebum) + -rrheic
   (pertaining to discharge)
   kerat/o (hard, horny) + -osis
   (abnormal condition)
   **Def: abnormal horny condition
   pertaining to discharge of
   sebum**

Exercise 12
1. C   2. D   3. A   4. B

Exercise 13
1. excisional
2. needle aspiration
3. incisional
4. exfoliation
5. punch
6. F
7. C
8. E
9. B
10. G
11. A
12. D

Exercise 14
1. pruritic means pertaining to
   itching
2. no previous history of dermatitis
3. elevated and contained fluid
4. rash

Exercise 15
1. A. skin graft from self
   B. skin graft from another
      human
   C. skin graft from another
      species
2. full-thickness graft
3. dermatome
4. laser therapy
5. débridement
6. cauterization
7. cryosurgery
8. curettage
9. incision and drainage
10. shaving
11. occlusive therapy
12. Mohs surgery
13. removal (-ectomy) wrinkle
    (rhytid/o)
    Term: rhytidectomy
14. removal (-ectomy) fat
    (lip/o)
    Term: lipectomy
15. surgical repair (-plasty) eyelid
    (blephar/o)
    Term: blepharoplasty
16. scraping of (-abrasion) skin
    (derm/o)
    Term: dermabrasion
17. surgical repair (-plasty) skin
    (dermat/o)
    Term: dermatoplasty

Case Study: Anthony Xavier
1. superficial, first-degree
2. partial thickness, second-degree
3. autograft
4. allograft
5. débridement
6. escharotomy

Exercise 16
1. intradermal
2. topical
3. hypodermic
4. transdermal therapeutic system
5. anesthetic agent
6. keratolytics
7. antifungals
8. antibacterial
9. scabicide
10. antiinflammatory
11. D
12. C
13. A
14. B
15. E
16. G
17. F

Case Study: Helena Freeman
1. macule
2. papule
3. excoriations
4. pediculosis
5. pediculicide

Exercise 17
1. ID
2. UV
3. SG
4. Decub
5. FB
6. I&D
7. Bx
8. PPD
9. TTS
10. TB

Chapter 4 Review

Word Part Definitions
1. hyper-
2. –osis
3. trans-
4. intra-
5. –cide
6. sub-
7. crypt-
8. –itis
9. par-
10. –lytic
11. hidr/o
12. melan/o
13. onych/o
14. chrom/o
15. rhytid/o
16. follicul/o
17. vascul/o
18. papul/o
19. macul/o
20. hemat/o
21. xen/o
22. exanthemat/o
23. kerat/o
24. hidraden/o
25. cutane/o
26. pedicul/o
27. seb/o
28. eschar/o
29. squam/o
30. pil/o
31. adip/o
32. myc/o

Wordshop
1. abnormal condition (-osis) excessive (hyper-) hair (trich/o)
   Term: hypertrichosis
2. condition (-y) no (a-) development (troph/o)
   Term: atrophy
3. removal (-ectomy) wrinkle (rhytid/o)
   Term: rhytidectomy
4. pertaining to discharge (-rrheic) oil (seb/o)
   Term: seborrheic
5. condition (-ia) near (par-) nail (onych/o)
   Term: paronychia
6. abnormal condition (-osis) no (an-) sweat (hidr/o)
   Term: anhidrosis
7. surgical repair (-plasty) eyelid (blephar/o)
   Term: blepharoplasty
8. softening (-malacia) nail (onych/o)
   Term: onychomalacia
9. inflammation (-itis) follicle (follicul/o)
   Term: folliculitis
10. condition (-ia) abnormal (dys-) color (chrom/o)
    Term: dyschromia
11. pertaining to (-ous) under (sub-) skin (cutane/o)
    Term: subcutaneous
12. abnormal condition (-osis) fungus (myc/o) skin (dermat/o)
    Term: dermatomycosis
13. tumor (-oma) fiber (fibr/o) skin (dermat/o)
    Term: dermatofibroma
14. destruction/loosening (-lysis) nail (onych/o)
    Term: onycholysis
15. abnormal condition (-osis) hidden (crypt-) nail (onych/o)
    Term: onychocryptosis

Term Sorting
Anatomy and Physiology: epidermis, eponychium, follicle, lunula, melanocyte, papilla, perspiration, sebaceous gland, sebum, strata
Pathology: alopecia, dermatomycosis, ecchymosis, eczema, hyperhidrosis, onychomycosis, plaque, tinea pedis, verruca, vesicle
Diagnostic Procedures: bacterial analysis, excisional Bx, Mantoux test, punch biopsy, Tzanck test, Wood's light
Therapeutic Interventions: allograft, blepharoplasty, cauterization, curettage, débridement, dermabrasion, dermatoplasty, escharotomy, rhytidectomy, xenograft

Translations
1. tinea pedis
2. pruritus, scabies
3. hyperhidrosis
4. onychocryptosis, paronychia
5. keloid
6. impetigo, papules, vesicles
7. pediculosis, pediculicide
8. acne vulgaris, retinoid
9. emollient, xeroderma
10. verruca (wart), cryosurgery
11. escharotomy, allograft
12. rhytidectomy (face-lift), blepharoplasty
13. decubitus ulcer

ED Record
1. B
2. mottled (indicates redness), pain, and blisters are signs of second degree burns
3. circumscribed, ½ cm elevated lesion containing fluid

Chapter 5

Exercise 1
1. M   2. H   3. F   4. E, I
5. D, K   6. C, G   7. B   8. N
9. J   10. L   11. A
12. peri- (surrounding, around) + or/o (mouth) + -al (pertaining to)
    Def: pertaining to around the mouth
13. gingiv/o (gums) + -al (pertaining to)
    Def: pertaining to the gums

14. peri- (around) + odont/o (teeth) + -al (pertaining to)
    Def: pertaining to around the teeth
15. sub- (under, below) + mandibul/o (mandible) + -ar (pertaining to)
    Def: pertaining to under the mandible
16. nas/o (nose) + pharyng/o (pharynx) + -eal (pertaining to)
    Def: pertaining to the nose and pharynx

Exercise 2
See Fig. 5-2.

Exercise 3
1. H 2. I 3. M 4. G
5. N 6. L 7. O 8. J
9. F 10. B 11. P 12. E
13. D 14. K 15. A 16. C
17. peri- (around, surrounding) + rect/o (rectum) + -al (pertaining to)
    Def: pertaining to around the rectum
18. intra- (within) + lumin/o (lumen) + -al (pertaining to)
    Def: pertaining to within the lumen
19. epi- (above) + gastr/o (stomach) + -ic (pertaining to)
    Def: pertaining to above the stomach

Exercise 4
See Figs. 5-3 and 5-4.

Exercise 5
1. G 2. D 3. A 4. C
5. B 6. E 7. F
8. pancreat/o (pancreas) + -ic (pertaining to)
   Def: pertaining to the pancreas
9. bil/i (bile) + -ary (pertaining to)
   Def: pertaining to bile
10. sub- (under, below) + hepat/o (liver) + -ic (pertaining to)
    Def: pertaining to below the liver

Exercise 6
See Fig. 5-5.

Exercise 7
1. upper GI tract—pharynx, esophagus, stomach, duodenum
2. close to
3. fundus
4. gastroesophageal sphincter, cardiac sphincter

Exercise 8
1. G 2. H 3. D 4. F
5. A 6. I 7. B 8. C
9. E 10. D 11. B 12. E
13. C 14. A
15. condition of stools (-chezia) blood (hemat/o)
    Term: hematochezia
16. vomiting (-emesis) blood (hemat/o)
    Term: hematemesis
17. abnormal (dys-) condition of digestion (-pepsia)
    Term: dyspepsia

Exercise 9
1. esophageal atresia
2. cleft palate
3. Hirschsprung disease
4. congenital megacolon
5. pyloric stenosis

Exercise 10
1. A 2. F 3. D 4. E
5. G 6. C 7. B
8. inflammation (-itis) gums (gingiv/o)
   Term: gingivitis
9. discharge (-rrhea) pus (py/o)
   Term: pyorrhea
10. condition of patches (-plakia) white (leuk/o)
    Term: leukoplakia

Case Study: Robert Mifflin
1. dysphagia
2. cold sores, fever blisters
3. mouth
4. aphthous stomatitis, canker sores

Exercise 11
1. F 2. D, E 3. C 4. A, H, I
5. B 6. G

Exercise 12
1. G 2. I 3. L 4. B
5. O 6. M 7. C 8. F
9. J 10. E 11. D 12. K
13. P 14. H 15. N 16. A
17. inflammation (-itis) appendix (appendic/o)
    Term: appendicitis
18. abnormal condition (-osis) diverticulum (diverticul/o)
    Term: diverticulosis
19. inflammation (-itis) rectum and anus (proct/o)
    Term: proctitis

Case Study: Elizabeth Frankfort
1. flatulence
2. constipation
3. diverticulum
4. abnormal condition
5. inflammation

Exercise 13
1. cirrhosis
2. cholelithiasis
3. cholangitis
4. choledocholithiasis
5. pancreatitis
6. hepatitis
7. cholecystitis
8. jaundice

Case Study: Andrew Stockhausen
1. nausea and vomiting
2. jaundice
3. liver
4. a

Exercise 14
1. A 2. B 3. F 4. C 5. D
6. E

Exercise 15
1. polyp
2. hepatocellular carcinoma, hepatoma
3. adenocarcinoma
4. odontogenic tumor

Case Study: Bill Worth
1. needles
2. alcohol
3. upper right quadrant
4. enlargement
5. malignant

Exercise 16
1. sonography
2. barium swallow
3. computed tomography (CT) scan
4. barium enema
5. manometry
6. stool culture
7. guaiac, hemoccult
8. biopsy
9. total bilirubin
10. gamma-glutamyl transferase (GGT)
11. transhepatic cholangiography
12. cholecyst/o (gallbladder) + -graphy (process of recording)
    Def: process of recording the gallbladder
13. proct/o (rectum and anus) + -scopy (process of viewing)
    Def: process of viewing the rectum and anus
14. cholangi/o (bile vessels) + -graphy (process of recording)
    Def: process of recording the bile vessels
15. colon/o (colon) + -scopy (process of viewing)
    Def: process of viewing the colon

Case Study: Mai Tang
1. inflammation
2. yellow
3. recording
4. gallbladder (GB)

Exercise 17
1. colonoscopy
2. colonoscope
3. diverticula
4. pertaining to surrounding the rectum

Exercise 18
1. B   2. E   3. A   4. F
5. H   6. N   7. J   8. M
9. G   10. L   11. D   12. I
13. K   14. C   15. O
16. pylor/o (pylorus) + my/o (muscle) + -tomy (incision)
    Def: incision of the pylorus
17. col/o (colon) + -stomy (new opening)
    Def: new opening into the colon
18. herni/o (hernia) + -rrhaphy (suture)
    Def: suture of a hernia
19. gastr/o (stomach) + -ectomy (removal)
    Def: removal of the stomach
20. polyp/o (polyp) + -ectomy (removal)
    Def: removal of a polyp

Exercise 19
1. E   2. C   3. D   4. F   5. A
6. B

Case Study: Emmaline Jones
1. nasal
2. opening
3. stomach
4. cleft
5. palatoplasty

Case Study: Andre Jordon
1. b
2. a
3. d
4. inflammatory bowel disease (IBD)

Exercise 20
1. bowel movement
2. gallbladder
3. nausea and vomiting
4. gastroesophageal reflux disease
5. irritable bowel syndrome

Chapter 5 Review

Word Part Definitions
1. –rrhea
2. –scopy
3. –tresia
4. –stomy
5. –rrhaphy
6. –emesis
7. –chezia
8. –phagia
9. –stalsis
10. –pepsia
11. lingu/o
12. gingiv/o
13. inguin/o
14. phren/o
15. esophag/o
16. sial/o
17. cholangi/o
18. choledoch/o
19. stomat/o
20. py/o
21. gastr/o
22. proct/o
23. labi/o
24. hepat/o
25. bucc/o
26. odont/o
27. an/o
28. cholecyst/o
29. pharyng/o
30. lumin/o
31. col/o
32. enter/o

Wordshop
1. pertaining to (-eal) stomach (gastr/o) esophagus (esophag/o)
    Term: gastroesophageal
2. condition of an opening (-tresia) no (a-)
    Term: atresia
3. pertaining to (-al) surrounding (peri-) teeth (odont/o)
    Term: periodontal
4. pertaining to (-ic) nose (nas/o) stomach (gastr/o)
    Term: nasogastric
5. new opening (-stomy) colon (col/o)
    Term: colostomy
6. inflammation (-itis) gallbladder (cholecyst/o)
    Term: cholecystitis
7. new opening (-stomy) esophagus (esophag/o) stomach (gastr/o)
    Term: esophagogastrostomy
8. removal (-ectomy) gallbladder (cholecyst/o)
    Term: cholecystectomy
9. discharge (-rrhea) pus (py/o)
    Term: pyorrhea
10. condition of swallowing (-phagia) difficult, painful (dys-)
    Term: dysphagia
11. condition of digestion (-pepsia) difficult, bad (dys-)
    Term: dyspepsia
12. condition (-iasis) stone (lith/o) bile (chol/e)
    Term: cholelithiasis
13. condition (-iasis) stone (lith/o) common bile duct (choledoch/o)
    Term: choledocholithiasis
14. incision (-tomy) abdomen (lapar/o)
    Term: laparotomy
15. surgical repair (-plasty) mouth (stomat/o)
    Term: stomatoplasty

Term Sorting
Anatomy and Physiology: cholecystokinin, deglutition, esophagus, jejunum, LES, lipid, mastication, oropharynx, peristalsis, rugae
Pathology: achalasia, cheilitis, cystoadenoma, dyspepsia, halitosis, hematemesis, hematochezia, jaundice, leukoplakia, pyrosis
Diagnostic Procedures: barium enema, BaS, cholecystography, CT scan, ERCP, GGT, manometry, PTC, stool guaiac, total bilirubin
Therapeutic Interventions: anastomosis, cholecystectomy, colostomy, gastric gavage, herniorrhaphy, laparotomy, ligation, paracentesis, PEG, stomatoplasty

Translations
1. colonoscopy, polypectomy
2. hepatitis, jaundice
3. inguinal hernia, herniorrhaphy
4. achalasia, manometry
5. stool guaiac or hemoccult test
6. ligation, cholecystectomy
7. colostomy, Crohn disease
8. laxative, constipation
9. flatus, diarrhea
10. appendicitis, peritonitis
11. gingivitis, malocclusion
12. cleft palate, Hirschsprung disease
13. regurgitation, esophageal atresia
14. hematochezia, hemorrhoids

Operative Report
1. diagnosis of cholelithiasis
2. cholecystitis
3. laparoscopic cholecystectomy
4. back
5. to tie it off

Chapter 6

Exercise 1

1. C   2. F   3. D   4. A
5. E   6. G   7. B   8. L
9. J   10. H   11. M   12. I
13. K

14. trans- (through) + urethr/o (urethra) + -al (pertaining to)
    Def: pertaining to through the urethra
15. para- (near) + nephr/o (kidney) + -ic (pertaining to)
    Def: pertaining to near the kidney
16. retro- (backward) + peritone/o (peritoneum) + -al (pertaining to)
    Def: pertaining to the back of the peritoneum
17. supra- (above) + ren/o (kidney) + -al (pertaining to)
    Def: pertaining to above the kidney
18. peri- (surrounding) + vesic/o (bladder) + -al (pertaining to)
    Def: pertaining to surrounding the bladder

Exercise 2

See Figs. 6-1 and 6-3.

Exercise 3

1. retention
2. edema
3. abscess
4. azotemia or uremia
5. enuresis
6. diuresis
7. urgency
8. incontinence
9. urinary condition (-uria) pus (py/o)
   Term: pyuria
10. excessive (poly-) thirst (-dipsia)
    Term: polydipsia
11. urinary condition (-uria) painful (dys-)
    Term: dysuria
12. glycos/o (sugar) + -uria (urinary condition)
    Def: condition of sugar in the urine
13. hemat/o (blood) + -uria (urinary condition)
    Def: condition of blood in the urine
14. an- (without) + -uria (urinary condition)
    Def: condition of no urine

Exercise 4

1. C   2. F   3. D   4. E   5. G
6. A   7. B

8. condition, presence of (-iasis) stones (lith/o) kidney (nephr/o)
   Term: nephrolithiasis
9. condition, presence of (-iasis) stones (lith/o) ureter (ureter/o)
   Term: ureterolithiasis
10. condition, presence of (-iasis) stones (lith/o) bladder (cyst/o)
    Term: cystolithiasis
11. condition, presence of (-iasis) stones (lith/o) urethra (urethr/o)
    Term: urethrolithiasis

Case Study: Victor Molina

1. polycystic kidney disease
2. pertaining to sacs
3. hematuria
4. nocturia

Exercise 5

1. L   2. I   3. D   4. G
5. J   6. C   7. H   8. A
9. F   10. B   11. K   12. E

13. hydr/o (water) + nephr/o (kidney) + -osis (abnormal condition)
    Def: abnormal condition of water in the kidney
14. cyst/o (urinary bladder) + -cele (herniation)
    Def: herniation of the urinary bladder
15. nephr/o (kidney) + lith/o (stones) + -iasis (presence of)
    Def: presence of stones in the kidney
16. ren/o (kidney) + -al (pertaining to) + sclerosis (a hardening)
    Def: pertaining to hardening of the kidney

Case Study: Paulina Abernathy

1. oliguria
2. edema
3. albuminuria
4. nephrosis

Exercise 6

1. E   2. C   3. F   4. B   5. A
6. D

Exercise 7

1. inability to hold urine (incontinence)
2. herniation of the bladder (cystocele)
3. barium enema and CT scan

Exercise 8

1. F   2. G   3. E   4. H   5. D
6. C   7. B   8. A

9. machine that crushes (-tripter) stone (lith/o)
   Term: lithotripter

10. instrument to view (-scope) kidney (nephr/o)
    Term: nephroscope
11. instrument to measure (-meter) urine (urin/o)
    Term: urinometer

Case Study: Maria Alonsa Cortez

1. urethral stricture
2. urinary tract infection
3. bladder
4. urethra
5. cystoscopy

Exercise 9

1. tube that remains in the body to drain urine
2. post-
3. urinalysis and culture

Exercise 10

1. C   2. E   3. B   4. F   5. D
6. A
7. destruction of adhesions (-lysis) urethra (urethr/o)
   Term: urethrolysis
8. process of crushing (-tripsy) stone (lith/o)
   Term: lithotripsy
9. incision (-tomy) bladder (vesic/o)
   Term: vesicotomy

Exercise 11

1. D   2. E   3. A   4. F   5. C
6. B

Case Study: Henry Walker

1. glomerular filtration rate
2. chronic kidney disease
3. end-stage renal disease (ESRD)
4. hemodialysis
5. renal transplant

Exercise 12

1. diabetes mellitus
2. chronic kidney disease, hemodialysis
3. urinalysis, specific gravity, diabetes insipidus
4. urinary tract infection
5. voiding cystourethrography

Chapter 6 Review

Word Part Definitions

1. –lithotomy
2. –cele
3. –lysis
4. –tripter
5. –dipsia
6. –scopy
7. –pexy
8. –ptosis

9. –uria
10. –esis
11. glycos/o
12. cyst/o or vesic/o
13. ureter/o
14. kal/i
15. noct/i
16. trigon/o
17. natr/o
18. ur/o
19. lith/o
20. meat/o
21. nephr/o or ren/o
22. olig/o
23. glomerul/o
24. ren/o or nephr/o
25. calic/o
26. pyel/o
27. urethr/o
28. vesic/o or cyst/o
29. albumin/o
30. azot/o
31. cortic/o

Wordshop

1. pertaining to (-al) surrounding (peri-) bladder (vesic/o)
   Term: perivesical
2. process of recording (-graphy) section (tom/o) kidney (nephr/o)
   Term: nephrotomography
3. instrument to visually examine (-scope) kidney (nephr/o)
   Term: nephroscope
4. herniation (-cele) ureter (ureter/o)
   Term: ureterocele
5. urinary condition (-uria) difficult or painful (dys-)
   Term: dysuria
6. urinary condition (-uria) blood (hemat/o)
   Term: hematuria
7. inflammation (-itis) glomerulus (glomerul/o) kidney (nephr/o)
   Term: glomerulonephritis
8. condition of (-iasis) stone (lith/o) urinary system (ur/o)
   Term: urolithiasis
9. urinary condition (-uria) no, not, without (an-)
   Term: anuria
10. process of crushing (-tripsy) stone (lith/o)
    Term: lithotripsy
11. blood condition (-emia) urea nitrogen (azot/o)
    Term: azotemia
12. freeing from adhesions (-lysis) urethra (urethr/o)
    Term: urethrolysis

13. urinary condition (-uria) excessive (poly-)
    Term: polyuria
14. inflammation (-itis) renal pelvis (pyel/o) kidney (nephr/o)
    Term: pyelonephritis
15. condition of thirst (-dipsia) excessive (poly-)
    Term: polydipsia

Term Sorting

Anatomy and Physiology: cortex, glomeruli, hilum, medulla, micturition, renal medulla, trigone, urea, urethra, urinary meatus

Pathology: albuminuria, DM, enuresis, nephritis, nephroptosis, pyuria, renal adenoma, renal colic, urethral stenosis, UTI

Diagnostic Procedures: BUN, cystoscopy, cystourethroscopy, GFR, IVU, KUB, nephrotomography, UA, urinometer, VCUG

Therapeutic Interventions: CAPD, HD, lithotripsy, meatotomy, nephrolithotomy, nephropexy, nephrostomy, renal dialysis, ureterolysis, vesicotomy

Translations

1. edema, hypertension
2. BUN, creatinine clearance test
3. renal colic, urolithiasis
4. nephrolithiasis, lithotripsy
5. urinary tract infection (UTI), enuresis
6. cystoscope, cystocele
7. oligouria, azotemia
8. nephroptosis, nephropexy
9. nephrotomography, renal oncocytoma
10. polyuria, polydipsia
11. diabetes mellitus, diabetes insipidus
12. pyelonephritis
13. renal hypertension, renal failure
14. renal dialysis, renal transplant

Operative Report

1. a stone in the left ureter
2. acute
3. yes; hydronephrosis is a backup of fluid in the kidney caused by obstruction of the flow of urine
4. CT scan, cystoscopy, abdominal x-ray, renal ultrasound, ureteroscopy, retrograde pyelogram
5. atraumatically

Chapter 7

Exercise 1
1. D 2. K 3. A 4. G 5. B
6. I 7. J 8. L 9. H 10. F
11. E 12. C
13. uni- (one) + testicul/o (testicle) + -ar (pertaining to)
    Def: pertaining to one testicle
14. preputi/o (prepuce) + -al (pertaining to)
    Def: pertaining to the prepuce
15. vesicul/o (seminal vesicle) + -ar (pertaining to)
    Def: pertaining to the seminal vesicle
16. peri- (around) + prostat/o (prostate) + -ic (pertaining to)
    Def: pertaining to around the prostate
17. intra- (within) + scrot/o (scrotum) + -al (pertaining to)
    Def: pertaining to within the scrotum

Exercise 2
See Fig. 7-1.

Exercise 3
1. G 2. A 3. E 4. F 5. H
6. D 7. C 8. B
9. inflammation (-itis) glans penis (balan/o)
   Term: balanitis
10. condition (-ia) no (a-) living (zo/o) sperm (sperm/o)
    Term: azoospermia
11. inflammation (-itis) prostate (prostat/o)
    Term: prostatitis
12. excessive (hyper-) formation (-plasia) pertaining to (-ic) prostate (prostat/o)
    Term: prostatic hyperplasia
13. orch/o (testis) + -itis (inflammation)
    Def: inflammation of the testis
14. olig/o (scanty) + sperm/o (sperm) + -ia (pertaining to)
    Def: pertaining to scanty sperm
15. vesicul/o seminal vesicle + -itis = inflammation
    Def: inflammation of the seminal vesicle

Case Study: Mario Polanco
1. urethra
2. epispadias
3. above
4. a
5. chordee

Exercise 4
1. condylomata
2. syphilis
3. nongonococcal urethritis
4. gonorrhea
5. chancres
6. asymptomatic
7. human papillomavirus (HPV)
8. herpes simplex virus-2 (HSV-2)

Exercise 5
1. C 2. E 3. D 4. B 5. A
6. tumor (-oma) semen (semin/i)
   Term: seminoma
7. cancerous tumor of epithelial tissue (-carcinoma) gland (aden/o)
   Term: adenocarcinoma

Case Study: Roger Bradford
1. chancre
2. purulent
3. sexually transmitted infection
4. VD, STD

Exercise 6
1. E 2. F 3. G 4. D 5. C
6. A 7. B
8. plethys/o (volume) + -graphy (process of recording)
   Def: process of recording volume
9. epididym/o (epididymis) + vesicul/o (vesicle) + -graphy (process of recording)
   Def: process of recoding the epididymis and seminal vesicle

Case Study: Daniel Grey
1. benign prostatic hypertrophy/ hyperplasia
2. prostate, prostate gland
3. prostate-specific antigen
4. digital rectal examination

Exercise 7
1. F 2. B 3. C 4. A 5. G
6. D 7. E
8. vas/o (vas deferens) + vas/o (vas deferens) + -stomy (new opening)
   Def: new opening between the vas deferens
9. trans- (through) + urethr/o (urethra) + -al (pertaining to)
   Def: pertaining to through the urethra
10. prostat/o (prostate) + -ectomy (resection)
    Def: resection of the prostate

Exercise 8
1. through the rectum
2. increased chance of BPH
3. contribute to seminal fluid

Exercise 9
1. D 2. A 3. B 4. E 5. C

Case Study: Vithy Gupta
1. cryptorchidism
2. hidden
3. orchiopexy
4. fixation, suspension
5. orchid/o, orch/o, test/o, testicul/o

Exercise 10
1. BPH
2. STI or VD
3. syphilis
4. digital rectal examination, diagnose BPH
5. HPV
6. genitourinary

Chapter 7 Review

Word Part Definitions
1. hypo-
2. hyper-
3. –oma
4. trans-
5. –itis
6. circum-
7. –graphy
8. –cele
9. a-
10. crypt-
11. –ectomy
12. –genesis
13. –cision
14. –spadias
15. –plasia
16. andr/o
17. semin/i
18. balan/o
19. sperm/o
20. epididym/o
21. orchid/o
22. preputi/o
23. vesicul/o
24. pen/i or phall/o
25. scrot/o
26. vas/o
27. olig/o
28. prostat/o
29. plethysm/o
30. hydr/o
31. zo/o
32. phall/o or pen/i

Wordshop
1. condition of (-ia) scanty (olig/o) sperm (sperm/o)
   Term: oligospermia
2. inflammation (-itis) seminal vesicle (vesicul/o)
   Term: vesiculitis
3. fixation (-pexy) testicle (orchi/o)
   Term: orchiopexy
4. surgical repair (-plasty) glans penis (balan/o)
   Term: balanoplasty
5. removal (-ectomy) prostate (prostat/o)
   Term: prostatectomy
6. inflammation (-itis) glans penis (balan/o)
   Term: balanitis
7. study of (-logy) male (andr/o)
   Term: andrology
8. production (-genesis) sperm (spermat/o)
   Term: spermatogenesis
9. condition of (-ia) no (a-) animals (zo/o) sperm (sperm/o)
   Term: azoospermia
10. process of cutting (-cision) around (circum-)
    Term: circumcision
11. condition of (-ism) hidden (crypt-) testicle (orchid/o)
    Term: cryptorchidism
12. inflammation (-itis) epididymis (epididym/o)
    Term: epididymitis
13. removal (-ectomy) epididymis (epididym/o)
    Term: epididymectomy
14. condition of (-ism) no (an-) testicle (orch/o)
    Term: anorchism
15. removal (-ectomy) testicle (orchid/o)
    Term: orchidectomy

Term Sorting
Anatomy and Physiology: corpora cavernosa, ductus deferens, epididymis, gametes, genitalia, glans penis, prepuce, semen, spermatogenesis, tunica vaginalis
Pathology: anorchism, balanitis, BPH, ED, epididymitis, gonorrhea, hydrocele, oligospermia, phimosis, seminoma
Diagnostic Procedures: FTA-ABS, DRE, epididymovesiculography, PSA, Gram stain, plethysmography, sonography, sperm analysis, TSE, VDRL
Therapeutic Interventions: ablation, castration, circumcision, orchidectomy, orchiopexy, prostatectomy, sterilization, TUIP, TURP, vasectomy

Translations
1. sperm analysis, oligospermia (or azoospermia)

2. benign prostatic hyperplasia/hypertrophy (BPH), transurethral incision of the prostate (TUIP)
3. epididymitis
4. circumcision, phimosis
5. chancre, syphilis
6. Gram stain, gonorrhea
7. vasectomy, vasovasostomy
8. orchidectomy, cryptorchidism
9. erectile dysfunction (ED), plethysmography
10. condylomata, herpes genitalis (herpes simplex virus-2, HSV-2)
11. seminoma
12. urologist, varicocele
13. gynecomastia
14. azoospermia (or oligospermia), sterilization

Operative Report
1. abnormal enlargement of the prostate gland surrounding the urethra, leading to difficulty with urination
2. A. painful urination
   B. inability to hold urine
   C. sensation of the need to urinate immediately
   D. urinating more often than normally
   E. condition of blood in the urine
3. two
4. transurethral resection of the prostate; removal of the prostate through the urethra
5. surrounding the prostate

Chapter 8

Exercise 1
1. E 2. F 3. A 4. A 5. B
6. G 7. C 8. D 9. F 10. A
11. B 12. H
13. supra- (above) + cervic/o (cervix) + -al (pertaining to)
    Def: pertaining to above the cervix
14. intra- (within) + uter/o (uterus) + -ine (pertaining to)
    Def: pertaining to within the uterus
15. pre- (before) + menstru/o (menstruation) + -al (pertaining to)
    Def: pertaining to before menstruation
16. trans- (across, through) + vagin/o (vagina) + -al (pertaining to)
    Def: pertaining to through the vagina

Exercise 2
See Fig. 8-1.

Exercise 3
1. B, J 2. D, F 3. G 4. A, I
5. L 6. E, K 7. H 8. C
9. M
10. inter- (between) + labi/o (labia) + -al (pertaining to)
    Def: pertaining to between the labia
11. intra- (within) + mamm/o (breast) + -ary (pertaining to)
    Def: pertaining to within the breast

Exercise 4
1. C, I, K 2. B, E 3. A, H
4. M 5. D 6. F, J
7. L 8. G
9. ante- (before) + nat/o (birth) + -al (pertaining to)
   Def: pertaining to before birth
10. peri- (surrounding) + umbilic/o (umbilicus) + -al (pertaining to)
    Def: pertaining to surrounding the umbilicus

Exercise 5
See Fig. 8-5.

Exercise 6
1. pyosalpinx
2. adhesions
3. salpingitis
4. hydrosalpinx
5. polycystic ovary syndrome
6. oophar/o (ovary) + -itis (inflammation)
   Def: inflammation of the ovary
7. an- (without) + ovul/o (ovum) + -ation (process of)
   Def: process of without (release of) an ovum
8. hemat/o (blood) + -salpinx (fallopian tubes)
   Def: blood in the fallopian tubes

Case Study: Magda Petersen
1. palping/o
2. salpingitis
3. pregnancy and delivery
4. oviduct, uterine tube

Exercise 7
1. leukorrhea
2. retroflexion of the uterus
3. endometriosis
4. endometri/o (endometrium) + -itis (inflammation)
   Def: inflammation of the endometrium

5. hyster/o (uterus) + -ptosis (drooping)
   Def: drooping of the uterus
6. cervic/o (cervix) + -itis (inflammation)
   Def: inflammation of the cervix

Exercise 8
1. vaginal prolapse
2. vulvitis
3. vulvodynia
4. thelitis
5. mastitis
6. vulvovaginitis
7. galact/o (milk) + -rrhea (flow, discharge)
   Def: abnormal discharge of milk
8. mast/o (breast) + -ptosis (drooping)
   Def: drooping of the breast
9. vagin/o (vagina) + -itis (inflammation)
   Def: inflammation of the vagina

Exercise 9
1. menorrhagia
2. metrorrhagia
3. premenstrual syndrome
4. menometrorrhagia
5. premenstrual dysphoric disorder
6. dysfunctional uterine bleeding
7. dys- (painful) + men/o (menses) + -rrhea (discharge)
   Def: painful menstrual discharge
8. (without) + men/o (menses) + -rrhea (discharge)
   Def: without menstrual discharge
9. poly- (many) + men/o (menses) + -rrhea (discharge)
   Def: many (frequent) menstrual discharge
10. olig/o (scanty) + men/o (menses) + -rrhea (discharge)
    Def: scanty menstrual discharge

Case Study: Antoinette Song
1. oligomenorrhea
2. amenorrhea
3. inflammation
4. bladder
5. dysmenorrhea

Exercise 10
1. meconium
2. nuchal cord
3. abruptio placentae
4. cephalopelvic disproportion

5. ectopic pregnancy
6. abortion
7. preeclampsia
8. placenta previa
9. eclampsia
10. erythroblastosis fetalis
11. condition (-ia) without (a-) milk (galact/o)
    Term: agalactia
12. excessive (poly-) amnion (-amnios) fluid (hydr/o)
    Term: polyhydramnios
13. scanty (olig/o) amnion (-amnios) fluid (hydr/o)
    Term: oligohydramnios

Exercise 11
1. E   2. F   3. D   4. C
5. B   6. G   7. A   8. A
9. C   10. G   11. F   12. E
13. D   14. B

Exercise 12
1. one pregnancy, one delivery
2. pelvic inflammatory disease
3. dysmenorrhea
4. blood test

Exercise 13
1. hysterosalpingography
2. pelvimetry
3. cervicography
4. hysteroscopy
5. sonohysterography
6. laparoscopy
7. hormone levels
8. Pap smear
9. culd/o (cul-de-sac) + -centesis (removal of fluid)
    Def: removal of fluid from the cul-de-sac
10. mamm/o (breast) + -graphy (process of recording)
    Def: process of recording the breast
11. culd/o (cul-de-sac) + -scopy (visual examination)
    Def: process of viewing the cul-de-sac
12. colp/o (vagina) + -scopy (visual examination)
    Def: process of viewing the vagina

Case Study: Marina Santiago
1. endometriosis
2. menstruation, menses
3. menorrhagia
4. hysterectomy
5. uterus, fallopian tubes

Exercise 14
1. human chorionic gonadotropin
2. Apgar score

3. contraction stress test
4. nonstress test
5. alpha fetoprotein
6. congenital hypothyroidism
7. chorionic villus sampling
8. removal of fluid for diagnostic purposes (-centesis) amnion (amni/o)
    Term: amniocentesis

Exercise 15
1. hysteropexy
2. salpingolysis
3. bilateral oophorectomy
4. TAH-BSO
5. lumpectomy
6. pelvic exenteration
7. uterine artery embolization
8. dilation and curettage
9. colpoplasty
10. mastopexy
11. clitorid/o (clitoris) + -ectomy (removal)
    Def: removal of the clitoris
12. culd/o (cul-de-sac) + -plasty (surgical repair)
    Def: surgical repair of the cul-de-sac
13. hymen/o (hymen) + -tomy (incision)
    Def: incision of the hymen
14. removal (-ectomy) ovary (oophor/o) cyst (cyst/o)
    Term: oophorocystectomy
15. surgical repair (-plasty) nipple (thel/e)
    Term: theleplasty

Case Study: Phoebe Gilliam
1. metrorrhagia
2. human chorionic gonadotropin (hCG)
3. a
4. ectopic
5. fallopian tube

Exercise 16
1. tubal ligation
2. VBAC
3. eutocia
4. cephalic version
5. C-section
6. sterilization
7. cerclage
8. A
9. C
10. B
11. D
12. E
13. episi/o (vulva) + -tomy (incision)
    Def: incision of the vulva
14. oxy- (rapid) + -tocia (labor)
    Def: rapid labor

15. salping/o (fallopian tube) + salping/o (fallopian tube) + -stomy (new opening)
    Def: new opening between the fallopian tubes

Case Study: Elizabeth Dardenne
1. multiple
2. hypertension
3. turning
4. cesarean section

Exercise 17
1. sterilization = surgical procedure that renders a person incapable of producing children; multiparity = multiple (two or more) deliveries
2. multiparous = many (two or more) deliveries; multigravida = many (two or more) pregnancies
3. laparoscopic
4. tie off
5. infraumbilical (below the navel)

Exercise 18
1. OCP
2. barrier methods
3. condoms
4. IUDs
5. abortifacient
6. rhythm method
7. abstinence
8. spermicides
9. ECP

Exercise 19
1. increase
2. hormone replacement therapy
3. soy beans
4. induce
5. tocolytics

Case Study: Sharifa Khan
1. one pregnancy, zero deliveries, zero abortions
2. menometrorrhagia
3. endometrial
4. uterus
5. uterine artery embolization

Exercise 20
1. H   2. D   3. F   4. B   5. G
6. E   7. C   8. A

Chapter 8 Review

Word Part Definitions
1. neo-
2. primi-
3. –gravida
4. –para
5. –salpinx
6. multi-
7. nulli-
8. –ptosis

9. –rrhea
10. –tocia
11. cervic/o
12. gravid/o
13. lact/o
14. mast/o or mamm/o
15. nat/o
16. papill/o or thel/e
17. mast/o or mamm/o
18. amni/o
19. thel/e or papill/o
20. gynec/o
21. o/o
22. olig/o
23. hyster/o or metr/o
24. men/o
25. part/o
26. chori/o
27. colp/o
28. hyster/o or metr/o
29. culd/o
30. salping/o
31. oophor/o
32. episi/o

Wordshop
1. no (a-) menstruation (men/o) flow (-rrhea)
   Term: amenorrhea
2. process of recording (-graphy) uterus (hyster/o) fallopian tube (salping/o)
   Term: hysterosalpingography
3. frequent (poly-) menstruation (men/o) flow (-rrhea)
   Term: polymenorrhea
4. no (nulli-) pregnancy (-gravida)
   Term: nulligravida
5. after (post-) delivery (-partum)
   Term: postpartum
6. many (multi-) deliveries (-para)
   Term: multipara
7. painful (dys-) menstruation (men/o) flow (-rrhea)
   Term: dysmenorrhea
8. removal (-ectomy) uterus (hyster/o)
   Term: hysterectomy
9. freeing from adhesions (-lysis) fallopian tube (salping/o)
   Term: salpingolysis
10. fixation (-pexy) breast (mast/o)
    Term: mastopexy
11. pus (py/o) fallopian tube (-salpinx)
    Term: pyosalpinx
12. condition (-ia) without (a-) milk (galact/o)
    Term: agalactia
13. incision (-tomy) perineum (episi/o)
    Term: episiotomy

14. condition of labor, delivery (-tocia) healthy, normal (eu-)
    Term: eutocia
15. surgical repair (-plasty) nipple (thel/e)
    Term: theleplasty

Term Sorting
Anatomy and Physiology: areola, cervix, endometrium, fimbriae, gestation, hCG, menopause, parturition, progesterone, puerperium
Pathology: anovulation, eclampsia, hematosalpinx, hysteroptosis, leiomyoma, menorrhagia, oophoritis, polyhydramnios, pyosalpinx, vulvodynia
Diagnostic Procedures: AFP, amniocentesis, Apgar, colposcopy, CST, culdocentesis, CVS, Pap smear, pelvimetry, PKU
Therapeutic Interventions: cerclage, cervicectomy, colpopexy, D&C, LEEP, mastopexy, oophorectomy, salpingolysis, theleplasty, tubal ligation

Translations
1. gynecologist, dysmenorrhea
2. obstetrician, amniocentesis
3. neonate, nuchal cord
4. leukorrhea, cervicitis
5. fallopian adhesions, salpingolysis
6. ectopic pregnancy, tubal ligation
7. primigravida, nonstress test (NST)
8. mastectomy, infiltrating ductal carcinoma (IDC)
9. Pap smear, colposcopy
10. mastitis, thelitis (or acromastitis)
11. hysterosalpingography, salpingitis
12. hysterectomy, leiomyosarcoma
13. oxytocia, episiotomy
14. cephalopelvic disproportion, cesarean section

Operative Report
1. premature
2. first feces of the newborn
3. umbilical cord wrapped around the neck of the neonate
4. physical health of the infant at 1 and 5 minutes after birth
5. the health of the fetus

Chapter 9

Exercise 1
1. I   2. J   3. E   4. A
5. M   6. K   7. L   8. F
9. D   10. C   11. H   12. G
13. B   14. N   15. J   16. A
17. E   18. H   19. I   20. B
21. G   22. D   23. C   24. F
25. poly- (many) + nucle/o (nucleus) + -ar (pertaining to)
   Def: pertaining to many nuclei
26. (without) + granul/o (little grain) + cyt/o (cell) + -ic (pertaining to)
   Def: pertaining to cells without little grains
27. lymphat/o (lymph) + -ic (pertaining to)
   Def: pertaining to the lymph
28. (without) + nucle/o (nucleus) + -ar (pertaining to)
   Def: pertaining to without a nucleus
29. poly- (many) + morph/o (shape) + -ic (pertaining to)
   Def: pertaining to many shapes

Exercise 2
1. A, B, AB, O
2. antigens
3. A, AB
4. universal donor, universal recipient
5. Rh

Exercise 3
1. D   2. A   3. H   4. J   5. E
6. C   7. G   8. F   9. B   10. I
11. pertaining to (-ary) armpit (axill/o)
    Term: axillary
12. pertaining to (-al) groin (inguin/o)
    Term: inguinal
13. pertaining to (-al) neck (cervic/o)
    Term: cervical

Exercise 4
See Fig. 9-7.

Exercise 5
1. Nonspecific immunity is a general defense against pathogens. Specific immunity involves recognition of a given pathogen and a reaction against it.
2. mechanical (skin, mucus), physical (sneezing, coughing, vomiting, diarrhea), chemical (saliva, tears, perspiration)

3. phagocytosis, inflammation, fever, protective proteins
4. active artificial
5. passive natural
6. passive artificial
7. active natural
8. B
9. F
10. D
11. E
12. C
13. A
14. G
15. H
16. I
17. J

Exercise 6

1. sickle-cell anemia
2. autoimmune acquired hemolytic anemia
3. thalassemia
4. aplastic anemia
5. pancytopenia
6. pernicious anemia
7. acute posthemorrhagic anemia
8. hypo- (deficient) + vol/o (volume) + -emia (blood condition)
   Def: blood condition of deficient volume
9. hem/o (blood) + -lytic (pertaining to destruction)
   Def: pertaining to the destruction of blood
10. sider/o (iron) + -penia (deficiency)
    Def: deficiency of iron

Case Study: Mary Kate Knowles

1. red blood cells (RBCs)
2. sickle cell crisis
3. liver
4. spleen
5. b

Exercise 7

1. G 2. B 3. E 4. D 5. C
6. F 7. A
8. deficiency (-penia) lymph cells (lymphocyt/o)
   Term: lymphocytopenia
9. abnormal increase (-cytosis) white blood cells (leuk/o)
   Term: leukocytosis
10. inflammation (-itis) lymph vessels (lymphangi/o)
    Term: lymphangitis
11. condition (-ism) excessive (hyper-) spleen (splen/o)
    Term: hypersplenism
12. lymphaden/o (lymph gland) + -pathy (disease)
    Def: disease of the lymph gland

13. lymphangi/o (lymph vessel) + -itis (inflammation)
    Def: inflammation of the lymph vessels
14. thromb/o (clot) + cyt/o (cell) + -penia (deficiency)
    Def: deficiency of clotting cells
15. lymph/o (lymph) + -cytosis (abnormal increase of cells)
    Def: increase in lymph cells

Case Study: Christian Halvorson

1. hemostasis
2. joint
3. coagulation
4. blood
5. attraction condition

Exercise 8

1. D 2. B 3. A 4. F 5. C
6. E

Case Study: Rebekah Robbins

1. anaphylaxis
2. allergen
3. immediate-response allergy
4. edema
5. ana- (without) + -phylaxis (protection)

Exercise 9

1. G 2. I 3. B 4. D 5. F
6. H 7. A 8. E 9. C

Case Study: Cooper Billings

1. acute lymphocytic leukemia
2. immature
3. all
4. immature
5. chronic

Exercise 10

1. K   2. H   3. G   4. A
5. I   6. B   7. L   8. M
9. D 10. A 11. D 12. C
13. E 14. J 15. F
16. process of recording (-graphy) lymph vessels (lymphangi/o)
    Term: lymphangiography
17. process of recording (-graphy) artery (arteri/o) pertaining to (-ic) spleen (splen/o)
    Term: splenic arteriography
18. process of recording (-graphy) lymph gland (lymphaden/o)
    Term: lymphadenography

Case Study: Ramon Alvarez

1. microorganisms
2. prothrombin time
3. partial thromboplastin time
4. thrombocyte
5. systemic inflammatory response syndrome

Exercise 11

1. potassium level = 3.7 mEq/L
2. sodium level = 142 mEq/L
3. 15 mg/dL

Exercise 12

1. E 2. D 3. C 4. A 5. F
6. B
7. splen/o (spleen) + -ectomy (removal)
   Term: splenectomy
8. adenoid/o (adenoid) + -ectomy (removal)
   Term: adenoidectomy
9. platelet + -pheresis (removal)
   Term: plateletpheresis
10. lymphaden/o (lymph gland) + -ectomy (removal)
    Term: lymphadenectomy

Case Study: Donna LeMasters

1. sentinel
2. under the arm, armpit
3. lymph gland, lymph node
4. inflammation of a lymph vessel
5. unilateral

Exercise 13

1. mild pyrexia
2. pharyngeal inflammation
3. cervic/o (neck) + -al (pertaining to) lymphaden/o (lymph gland) + -pathy (disease)
   Def: lymph gland disease pertaining to the neck
4. splenomegaly
5. lymphocytosis
6. He produced antibodies to the Epstein-Barr viral antigen.

Exercise 14

1. J 2. C 3. E 4. I 5. B
6. A 7. H 8. G 9. F 10. D

Exercise 15

1. Epstein-Barr virus
2. hematocrit, hemoglobin
3. acquired immunodeficiency syndrome, human immunodeficiency virus
4. comprehensive metabolic panel
5. bone marrow transplant

Chapter 9 Review

Word Part Definitions

1. –cyte
2. –gen
3. –cytosis
4. –globin
5. –poiesis
6. –edema
7. –philia
8. –penia
9. –siderin

10. –emia
11. hemat/o
12. eosin/o
13. inguin/o
14. nucle/o
15. lymphangi/o
16. myel/o
17. splen/o
18. pyr/o
19. erythr/o
20. thromb/o
21. lymphaden/o
22. cyt/o
23. neutr/o
24. axill/o
25. leuk/o
26. ser/o
27. granul/o
28. plasm/o
29. thym/o
30. lymph/o
31. morph/o
32. tonsill/o

Wordshop
1. deficiency (-penia) all (pan-) cell (cyt/o)
   Term: pancytopenia
2. abnormal increase of cells (-cytosis) white (leuk/o)
   Term: leukocytosis
3. inflammation (-itis) lymph gland (lymphaden/o)
   Term: lymphadenitis
4. deficiency (-penia) clotting cells (thrombocyt/o)
   Term: thrombocytopenia
5. process of recording (-graphy) lymph gland (lymphaden/o)
   Term: lymphadenography
6. abnormal increase of cells (-cytosis) red (erythr/o)
   Term: erythrocytosis
7. removal (-ectomy) adenoids (adenoid/o)
   Term: adenoidectomy
8. swelling (-edema) lymph (lymph/o)
   Term: lymphedema
9. stopping/controlling (-stasis) blood (hem/o)
   Term: hemostasis
10. breakdown (-lysis) blood (hem/o)
    Term: hemolysis
11. substance (-in) iron (sider/o) blood (hem/o)
    Term: hemosiderin
12. deficiency (-penia) iron (sider/o)
    Term: sideropenia

13. process of recording (-graphy) lymph vessel (lymphangi/o)
    Term: lymphangiography
14. condition of (-ism) excessive (hyper-) spleen (splen/o)
    Term: hypersplenism
15. removal (-ectomy) spleen (splen/o)
    Term: splenectomy

Term Sorting
Anatomy and Physiology: agglutination, antibody, coagulation, eosinophil, hematopoiesis, hemoglobin, hemostasis, plasma, thrombocyte, thymus
Pathology: anaphylaxis, dyscrasia, edema, hypovolemia, leukocytosis, lymphangitis, mononucleosis, septicemia, sideropenia, thalassemia
Diagnostic Procedures: BMP, CBC, CMP, diff count, ELISA, Hct, lymphangiography, MCHC, monospot, Schilling test
Therapeutic Interventions: adenoidectomy, antiretrovirals, apheresis, blood transfusion, BMT, hematinic, hemostatics, plateletpheresis, splenectomy, vaccine

Translations
1. splenomegaly, splenectomy
2. pancytopenia, aplastic anemia
3. leukocytosis, blood cultures
4. anaphylaxis
5. bone marrow transplant, acute myelogenous leukemia (AML)
6. sickle cell crisis, hypersplenism
7. plateletpheresis, thrombocytopenia
8. posthemorrhagic anemia, blood transfusion
9. lymphadenopathy, mononucleosis
10. hemophilia, partial thromboplastin time (PTT)
11. pernicious anemia, Schilling test
12. purpura, septicemia
13. leukopenia, neutropenia
14. polycythemia vera

Clinical Notes
1. principal diagnosis: Sickle-Cell crisis
2. Motrin and Darvon
3. appendix

Chapter 10
Exercise 1
1. D, F   2. E   3. G   4. L
5. H   6. B   7. K   8. J
9. A, C, I
10. endo- (within) + vascul/o (vessel) + -ar (pertaining to)
    Def: pertaining to within the vessel
11. intra- (within) + ven/o (vein) + -ous (pertaining to)
    Def: pertaining to within the vein
12. peri- (around) + cardi/o (heart) + -al (pertaining to)
    Def: pertaining to around the heart

Exercise 2
1. K   2. I   3. A   4. B   5. D
6. C   7. L   8. E   9. H   10. F
11. G   12. J
13. pertaining to (-ar) between (inter-) ventricle (ventricul/o)
    Term: interventricular
14. pertaining to (-al) surrounding (peri-) apex (apic/o)
    Term: periapical
15. pertaining to (-al) before (pre-) heart (cordi/o)
    Term: precordial
16. pertaining to (-al) through (trans-) heart muscle (myocardi/o)
    Term: transmyocardial

Exercise 3
See Fig. 10-5, *B.*

Exercise 4
1. pulmonary arteries
2. tricuspid
3. mitral
4. competent
5. ejection fraction

Exercise 5
1. during
2. neck, brain
3. within
4. narrowing

Exercise 6
1. G   2. A   3. M   4. F
5. H   6. D   7. K   8. L
9. J   10. B   11. N   12. E
13. I   14. C
15. brady- (slow) + -cardia (heart condition)
    Def: slow heart condition
16. tachy- (rapid) + -cardia (heart condition)
    Def: rapid heart condition

17. cardi/o (heart) + -megaly
    (enlargement)
    Def: enlargement of the heart

Exercise 7
1. C   2. D   3. B   4. A

Case Study: Julio Montez
1. dyspnea
2. blue
3. four
4. ventricular septal defect
5. breathing

Exercise 8
1. B   2. D   3. B   4. A

Exercise 9
1. dysrhythmia
2. fibrillation
3. flutter
4. atrioventricular block
5. sick sinus syndrome
6. ventricular ectopic beats
7. ventricular tachycardia

Case Study: Cynthia Frost
1. a
2. a
3. b
4. shortness of breath
5. palpitations

Exercise 10
1. myocardial infarction
2. heart failure
3. cardiac tamponade
4. angina pectoris
5. coronary artery disease
6. inflammation (-itis) pericardium
   (pericardi/o)
   Term: pericarditis
7. inflammation (-itis)
   endocardium (endocardi/o)
   Term: endocarditis
8. disease (-pathy) heart muscle
   (cardiomy/o)
   Term: cardiomyopathy

Exercise 11
1. aneurysm
2. claudication
3. primary, essential
4. secondary
5. hemorrhoids
6. esophageal varices
7. peripheral artery occlusion
8. Raynaud disease
9. varicose veins
10. vascul/o (vessel) + -itis
    (inflammation)
    Def: inflammation of the vessels
11. hypo- (below, deficient) +
    tens/o (stretching) + -ion
    (process of)
    Def: deficient pressure

12. hyper- (excessive) + -tension
    (pressure)
    Def: excessive pressure
13. thromb/o (clot) + phleb/o
    (vein) + -itis (inflammation)
    **Def: inflammation of a clot
    in a vein**

Case Study: Anne Louise Potts
1. atheromas
2. c
3. hardening
4. cholesterol
5. claudication

Exercise 12
1. hemangioma
2. cardiac myxosarcoma
3. atrial myxoma
4. hemangiosarcoma

Exercise 13
1. heart vessels
2. normal heartbeat
3. arrhythmia
4. the upper chambers of the heart
5. enlarged
6. electrocardiogram

Exercise 14
1. MUGA scan
2. lipid profile
3. cardiac enzymes test
4. digital subtraction angiography
5. myocardial perfusion imaging
6. radiography
7. exercise stress test
8. cardiac catheterization
9. PET scan
10. incision (-tomy) vein (phleb/o)
    Term: phlebotomy
11. process of recording (-graphy)
    heart (cardi/o) vessel (angi/o)
    Term: angiocardiography
12. process of recording (-graphy)
    vein (phleb/o)
    Term: phlebography
13. process of recording (-graphy)
    electricity (electr/o) heart
    (cardi/o)
    Term: electrocardiography
14. process of recording (-graphy)
    heart (cardi/o) sound (echo-)
    Term: echocardiography

Case Study: Jennifer Cahill
1. myocardial infarction
2. myocardium
3. cardiodynia, cardialgia
4. electrocardiogram
5. cardiac enzymes test

Exercise 15
1. PACAB
2. CABG

3. CPR
4. PICC
5. commissurotomy
6. PTCA
7. MIDCAB
8. RFCA
9. LVAD
10. EVLT
11. AICD
12. phleb/o (vein) + -ectomy
    (removal)
    Def: removal of a vein
13. pericardi/o (pericardium) +
    -centesis (surgical puncture)
    **Def: surgical puncture of the
    pericardium**
14. hemorrhoid/o (hemorrhoid) +
    -ectomy (removal)
    Def: removal of a hemorrhoid
15. scler/o (hard) + -therapy
    (treatment)
    **Def: treatment (by) hardening
    (veins)**
16. valvul/o (valve) + -plasty
    (surgical repair)
    Def: surgical repair of a valve
17. ather/o (fatty plaque) +
    -ectomy (removal)
    Def: removal of plaque

Exercise 16
1. C   2. A, C, D   3. A, E
4. A, D, E 5. A, D, E   6. A, E
7. B   8. F   9. G

Case Study: Micah Sutton
1. narrowing
2. bicuspid
3. orthopnea
4. c
5. a

Case Study: Bradley Chadwick
1. heart failure
2. edema
3. diuretics
4. left ventricular assist device
5. angiotensin-converting enzyme

Exercise 17
1. H   2. J   3. D   4. F   5. A
6. B   7. I   8. C   9. E   10. G

Chapter 10 Review

Word Part Definitions
1. –cardia
2. tetra-
3. –pathy
4. brady-
5. –sclerosis
6. echo-
7. tachy-
8. –graphy

9. –um
10. –megaly
11. arteri/o
12. cardi/o or coron/o
13. pulmon/o
14. vascul/o or angi/o
15. lumin/o
16. endocardi/o
17. angi/o or vascul/o
18. pariet/o
19. myocardi/o
20. phleb/o
21. hemangi/o
22. aort/o
23. corpor/o
24. coron/o or cardi/o
25. ather/o
26. epicardi/o
27. thromb/o
28. atri/o
29. sept/o
30. isch/o
31. cyan/o
32. pericardi/o

Wordshop
1. inflammation (-itis) surrounding (peri-) heart (cardi/o)
   Term: pericarditis
2. inflammation (-itis) clot (thromb/o) vein (phleb/o)
   Term: thrombophlebitis
3. condition of (-ia) rapid (tachy-) heart (cardi/o)
   Term: tachycardia
4. process of recording (-graphy) sound (echo-) heart (cardi/o)
   Term: echocardiography
5. process of recording (-graphy) vessel (angi/o)
   Term: angiography
6. surgical repair (-plasty) vessel (angi/o)
   Term: angioplasty
7. condition of (-ia) abnormal (dys-) rhythm (rhythm/o)
   Term: dysrhythmia
8. abnormal condition of hardening (sclerosis) artery (arteri/o)
   Term: arteriosclerosis
9. pain (-dynia) heart (cardi/o)
   Term: cardiodynia
10. removal (-ectomy) fatty plaque (ather/o)
    Term: atherectomy
11. pertaining to (-ary) heart (cardi/o) lung (pulmon/o)
    Term: cardiopulmonary
12. removal (-ectomy) vein (phleb/o)
    Term: phlebectomy

13. pertaining to (-eal) outside (extra-) body (corpor/o)
    Term: extracorporeal
14. pertaining to (-al) through (trans-) heart muscle (myocardi/o)
    Term: transmyocardial
15. process of recording (-graphy) vein (phleb/o)
    Term: phlebography

Term Sorting
Anatomy and Physiology: aorta, atrium, bundle of His, capillary, diastole, endocardium, Purkinje fibers, septum, systole, ventricle
Pathology: aneurysm, arrhythmia, bradycardia, bruit, CAD, claudication, endocarditis, hemangiosarcoma, HTN, SOB
Diagnostic Procedures: angiocardiography, auscultation, BP, ECG, EST, fluoroscopy, lipid profile, MUGA scan, phlebography, phlebotomy
Therapeutic Interventions: CABG, commissurotomy, ECC, EVLT, LVAD, MIDCAB, pericardiocentesis, PTCA, TEA, valvuloplasty

Translations
1. patent ductus arteriosus (PDA), murmur
2. tetralogy of Fallot, echocardiography
3. pulmonary edema, heart failure (HF)
4. coronary artery disease (CAD), cardiodynia or angina
5. phlebography, thrombophlebitis
6. diaphoresis, tachycardia
7. cardiac enzymes test, electrocardiography
8. endovenous laser ablation (EVLT), varicose veins
9. angina pectoris, nitrate or antianginals
10. pericardiocentesis, cardiac tamponade
11. cardiac pacemaker, sick sinus syndrome (SSS)
12. percutaneous transluminal coronary angioplasty (PTCA), transmyocardial revascularization (TMR)
13. tricuspid stenosis, valvuloplasty

Discharge Summary
1. dyspnea
2. diaphoresis
3. substernal (under the breastbone)

4. no cyanosis
5. echocardiography
6. coronary artery bypass graft

Chapter 11

Exercise 1
1. T   2. N   3. S   4. V
5. E, O 6. Q   7. H   8. C
9. Z   10. AA 11. F 12. G
13. R 14. D, L 15. U 16. B
17. X 18. DD 19. J, P 20. BB
21. Y 22. K 23. CC 24. W
25. I 26. M 27. A
28. inter- (between) + cost/o (rib) + -al (pertaining to)
    Def: pertaining to between the ribs
29. in- (in) + spir/o (breathe) + -atory (pertaining to)
    Def: pertaining to breathing in
30. para- (near) + nas/o (nose) + -al (pertaining to)
    Def: pertaining to near the nose
31. endo- (within) + trache/o (trachea) + -al (pertaining to)
    Def: pertaining to within the trachea

Exercise 2
See Figs. 11-1A and 11-2.

Exercise 3
1. difficulty breathing unless in an upright position
2. a nosebleed
3. hiccup or hiccough
4. tachypnea
5. make sounds
6. apnea
7. cyanosis
8. crackles
9. pleurodynia
10. wheezing
11. clubbing
12. discharge (-rrhea) nose (rhin/o)
    Term: rhinorrhea
13. pain (-dynia) chest (thorac/o)
    Term: thoracodynia
14. spitting (-ptysis) blood (hem/o)
    Term: hemoptysis
15. good, normal (eu-) breathing (-pnea)
    Term: eupnea
16. excessive (hyper-) breathing (-pnea)
    Term: hyperpnea

Case Study: Sara McClellan
1. inflammation
2. voice box

3. dysphonia
4. aphonia

Case Study: Mario Castellanto
1. flail chest
2. thoracodynia
3. atelectasis
4. dyspnea
5. cyanosis

Exercise 4
1. coryza
2. URI
3. deviated septum
4. vocal polyps
5. pleurisy
6. croup
7. atelectasis
8. emphysema
9. asthma
10. pulmonary abscess
11. pneumoconiosis
12. cystic fibrosis
13. flail chest
14. pertussis
15. pneumon/o (lungs) + -ia (condition)
    Def: condition of the lungs
16. pneum/o (air) + -thorax (pleural cavity, chest)
    Def: air in the pleural cavity
17. py/o (pus) + -thorax (pleural cavity, chest)
    Def: pus in the pleural cavity
18. blood (hem/o) pleural cavity, chest (-thorax)
    Term: hemothorax
19. inflammation (-itis) bronchi (bronchi/o)
    Term: bronchitis
20. bronchi (bronch/o) spasm (-spasm)
    Term: bronchospasm

Case Study: Allen Roher
1. coal worker's pneumoconiosis (CWP)
2. black lung disease
3. d
4. SOB
5. asbestosis

Exercise 5
1. benign
2. chondroadenoma
3. non–small cell lung cancer
4. oat cell carcinoma

Exercise 6
1. clear to auscultation
2. no wheezes
3. no crackles (rales)
4. chest x-ray
5. atelectasis

Exercise 7
1. Mantoux skin test
2. arterial blood gas (ABG)
3. sweat test
4. lung ventilation scan
5. pulmonary angiography
6. process of viewing (-scopy) bronchi (bronch/o)
    Term: bronchoscopy
7. process of viewing (-scopy) voice box (laryng/o)
    Term: laryngoscopy
8. process of measurement (-metry) breathing (spir/o)
    Term: spirometry

Case Study: Mikasa Roven
1. oxygen
2. breathing
3. chronic obstructive pulmonary disease

Exercise 8
1. lungs
2. breathing in
3. bronchoscopy
4. lungs
5. URI

Exercise 9
1. E   2. H   3. I   4. G   5. F
6. D   7. A   8. B   9. C
10. excision (-ectomy) voice box (laryng/o)
    Term: laryngectomy
11. surgical repair (-plasty) nose (rhin/o)
    Term: rhinoplasty
12. new opening (-stomy) windpipe (trache/o)
    Term: tracheostomy

Case Study: Morgan Butterfield
1. c
2. inspiratory stridor
3. tachypnea
4. epiglottitis
5. b

Exercise 10
1. C
2. E
3. D
4. A
5. B
6. nebulizer
7. inhaler
8. ventilator

Exercise 11
1. chest x-ray, right middle lobe
2. purified protein derivative, tuberculosis
3. upper respiratory infection

4. chronic obstructive pulmonary disease, dyspnea on exertion
5. coal workers' pneumoconiosis
6. emergency department, respiratory syncytial virus

Chapter 11 Review

Word Part Definitions
1. eu-
2. hyper-
3. hypo-
4. a-
5. –pnea
6. –ptysis
7. –rrhea
8. dys-
9. –metry
10. –ectasis
11. capn/o
12. pneum/o or pulmon/o
13. steth/o, pector/o or thorac/o
14. spir/o
15. orth/o
16. pleur/o
17. rhin/o or nas/o
18. sept/o
19. thorac/o, steth/o or pector/o
20. py/o
21. pharyng/o
22. muc/o
23. ox/i
24. phren/o
25. pulmon/o or pneum/o
26. pector/o, thorac/o or steth/o
27. cost/o
28. sin/o
29. tonsill/o
30. salping/o
31. laryng/o
32. rhin/o or nas/o

Wordshop
1. difficult (dys-) breathing (-pnea)
    Term: dyspnea
2. rapid (tachy-) breathing (-pnea)
    Term: tachypnea
3. abnormal condition (-osis) dust (coni/o) lung (pneum/o)
    Term: pneumoconiosis
4. discharge (-rrhea) nose (rhin/o)
    Term: rhinorrhea
5. process (-ation) breathing (spir/o) out (ex-)
    Term: expiration
6. pus (py/o) chest (-thorax)
    Term: pyothorax
7. inflammation (-itis) pleurae (pleur/o)
    Term: pleuritis
8. surgical repair (-plasty) nose (rhin/o)
    Term: rhinoplasty

25. narc/o or somn/o
26. neur/o
27. cerebr/o
28. gnos/o
29. radicul/o or rhiz/o
30. somn/o or narc/o
31. osm/o
32. mening/o

Wordshop
1. inflammation (-itis) many (poly-) nerve (neur/o)
   Term: polyneuritis
2. inflammation (-itis) brain (encephal/o)
   Term: encephalitis
3. paralysis (-plegia) four (quadri-)
   Term: quadriplegia
4. process of recording (-graphy) brain (encephal/o) sound (echo-)
   Term: echoencephalography
5. incision (-tomy) nerve (neur/o)
   Term: neurotomy
6. condition (-ia) no, not, without (a-) recognition (gnos/o)
   Term: agnosia
7. condition (-ia) no, not, without (an-) sense of smell (osm/o)
   Term: anosmia
8. nerve (neur/o) pain (-algia)
   Term: neuralgia
9. abnormal (para-) condition of sensation (-esthesia)
   Term: paresthesia
10. process of recording (-graphy) many (poly-) sleep (somn/o)
    Term: polysomnography
11. resection (-tomy) spinal nerve root (rhiz/o)
    Term: rhizotomy
12. destruction (-lysis) nerve (neur/o)
    Term: neurolysis
13. condition (-ia) of no, not, without (a-) sense of taste (geus/o)
    Term: ageusia
14. condition (-ia) difficult (dys-) sleep (somn/o)
    Term: dyssomnia
15. slight paralysis (-paresis) four (quadri-)
    Term: quadriparesis

Term Sorting
Anatomy and Physiology: axon, cauda equina, cerebellum, CNS, CSF, meninges, neuron, neurotransmitter, synapse, ventricle

Pathology: agraphia, ALS, amnesia, fasciculation, HIVD, hydrocephalus, sciatica, spina bifida, syncope, TIA

Diagnostic Procedures: ADL, Babinski reflex, echoencephalography, EP, GARS, LP, MRI, neuroendoscopy, PSG, SPECT

Therapeutic Interventions: cordotomy, craniectomy, hypnotic, nerve block, neurolysis, neuroplasty, neurorrhaphy, rhizotomy, TENS, vagotomy

Translations
1. CVA, contralateral
2. hemiparesis, aphasia
3. hematoma, amnesia
4. vertigo, syncope
5. spina bifida, meningocele
6. hydrocephalus, ventriculoperitoneal shunt
7. tremors, hypokinesia
8. narcolepsy, MSLT
9. lumbar puncture (spinal tap), meningitis
10. polysomnography, hypersomnia
11. rhizotomy, trigeminal neuralgia
12. migraine, aura
13. neuralgia, paresthesia
14. sciatica, HIVD

Discharge Summary
1. vertigo—dizziness, sensation of movement when there is none; syncope—fainting
2. magnetic resonance angiography (imaging the carotid arteries with contrast agent)
3. within and outside the skull
4. incoordination

Chapter 13

Exercise 1
1. B 2. E, G 3. A, I 4. C
5. H 6. D, F 7. K 8. J
9. pertaining to (-ar) two (bin-) eyes (ocul/o)
   Term: binocular
10. pertaining to (-al) above (supra-) the orbit (orbit/o)
    Term: supraorbital
11. pertaining to (-ar) outside (extra-) the eye (ocul/o)
    Term: extraocular

Exercise 2
See Fig. 13-1.

Exercise 3
1. J 2. L 3. I, M 4. B
5. B 6. K 7. H 8. E

9. F 10. D 11. G 12. A
13. C
14. extra- (outside) + ocul/o (eye) + -ar (pertaining to)
    Def: pertaining to outside the eye
15. pre- (in front of) + retin/o (retina) + -al (pertaining to)
    Def: pertaining to in front of the retina
16. intra- (within) + scler/o (sclera) + -al (pertaining to)
    Def: pertaining to within the sclera

Exercise 4
See Fig. 13-2A.

Exercise 5
1. D 2. I 3. F 4. B
5. L 6. E 7. G 8. J
9. K 10. H 11. C 12. A
13. xer/o (dry) + ophthalm/o (eye) + -ia (condition)
    Def: condition of dry eye
14. eso- (inward) + trop/o (turning) + -ia (condition)
    Def: condition of turning inward
15. blephar/o (eyelid) + -chalasis (relaxation, slackening)
    Def: relaxation or slackening of the eyelid
16. dacryocyst/o (lacrimal sac) + -itis (inflammation)
    Def: inflammation of the tear sac
17. inflammation (-itis) eyelid (blephar/o)
    Term: blepharitis
18. inflammation (-itis) lacrimal gland (dacryoaden/o)
    Term: dacryoadenitis
19. drooping (-ptosis) eyelid (blephar/o)
    Term: blepharoptosis
20. process of (-ion) turning (trop/o) in (en-)
    Term: entropion

Case Study: Michael Schwartz
1. c 2. d 3. c 4. a

Exercise 6
1. J 2. I 3. F 4. G
5. K 6. B 7. L 8. A
9. E 10. D 11. H 12. C
13. M
14. nyctal/o (night blindness) + -opia (vision condition)
    Def: night blindness vision condition

15. (without) + chromat/o (color) + -opsia (vision condition)
    Def: without color vision condition
16. (lack of) + phak/o (lens) + -ia (condition)
    Def: condition of no lens
17. hemi- (half) + an- (without) + -opsia (vision)
    Def: without half vision condition
18. opt/o (vision) + -ic (pertaining to) neur/o (nerve) + -itis (inflammation)
    Def: inflammation of the nerve pertaining to vision
19. inflammation (-itis) cornea (kerat/o)
    Term: keratitis
20. vision condition (-opia) old age (presby-)
    Term: presbyopia
21. inflammation (-itis) uvea (uve/o)
    Term: uveitis
22. disease (-pathy) retina (retin/o)
    Term: retinopathy

Exercise 7
1. retinoblastoma
2. intraocular melanoma
3. choroidal hemangioma

Exercise 8
1. E   2. H   3. F   4. B   5. I
6. G   7. C   8. D   9. A   10. J
11. K

Case Study: Johanna Reynolds
1. age-related macular degeneration
2. a
3. c
4. a

Exercise 9
1. H   2. G   3. L   4. A
5. J   6. K   7. I   8. F
9. D   10. M   11. E   12. B
13. C
14. trabecul/o (little beam) + -tomy (incision)
    Def: incision of the little beam (orbital network of the eye)
15. dacryocyst/o (lacrimal sac) + rhin/o (nose) + -stomy (new opening)
    Def: new opening between the lacrimal sac and the nose
16. vitr/o (vitreous humor) + -ectomy (removal)
    Def: removal of vitreous humor

Exercise 10
1. C   2. E   3. B   4. A   5. D

Case Study: Lizzie Kawa
1. c   2. a   3. d   4. a   5. d

Exercise 11
1. cataracts
2. preoperatively (before the surgery)
3. destroyed by breaking into small pieces
4. posterior lens implant
5. topical anesthetic

Exercise 12
1. myopia
2. laser-assisted in-situ keratomileusis, photorefractive keratectomy
3. visual acuity
4. age-related macular degeneration
5. ophthalmology
6. intraocular pressure
7. visual field

Exercise 13
1. E, I   2. B   3. C   4. A
5. H   6. F   7. G, J   8. D
9. pre- (before) + auricul/o (ear) + -ar (pertaining to)
   Def: pertaining to before (in front of) the ear
10. supra- (above) + tympan/o (eardrum) + -ic (pertaining to)
    Def: pertaining to above the eardrum
11. circum- (around) + aur/o (ear) + -al (pertaining to)
    Def: pertaining to around the ear

Exercise 14
See Fig. 13-25.

Exercise 15
1. A   2. H   3. K   4. G
5. F   6. I   7. B   8. D
9. C   10. E   11. J   12. L
13. ear (ot/o) pain (-algia)
    Term: otalgia
14. condition (-ia) small (micro-) ears (ot/o)
    Term: microtia
15. abnormal condition (-osis) of hardening (-sclerosis) ear (ot/o)
    Term: otosclerosis

Case Study: Carole Hancock
1. vertigo
2. tinnitus
3. hearing

Exercise 16
1. acoustic neuroma
2. ceruminoma

Exercise 17
1. no lymphadenopathy
2. no wheezing
3. tympanic membrane
4. oropharynx
5. otitis media

Exercise 18
1. E   2. D   3. F   4. A   5. B
6. C
7. ot/o (ear) + -scopy (visual exam)
   Def: visual exam of the ear
8. tympan/o (eardrum) + -metry (process of measurement)
   Def: process of measurement of the eardrum
9. audi/o (hearing) + -metric (pertaining to measurement)
   Def: pertaining to measurement of hearing

Exercise 19
1. E   2. B   3. C   4. A   5. D

Case Study: Raheem Amari
1. otitis media
2. otoscope
3. mastoiditis
4. c
5. tympanostomy
6. mastoidectomy

Exercise 20
1. C   2. D   3. A   4. B

Case Study: Susan Zietz
1. cerumen
2. ceruminolytic
3. ceruminoma
4. b

Exercise 21
1. E   2. C   3. A   4. D   5. B

Chapter 13 Review

Word Part Definitions
1. –plasty
2. extra-
3. –itis
4. exo-
5. –cusis
6. an-
7. presby-
8. –opsia
9. macro-
10. micro-
11. lacrim/o
12. kerat/o
13. cerumin/o
14. tympan/o or myring/o
15. dacryocyst/o
16. ot/o or auricul/o
17. opt/o
18. audi/o or acous/o

Exercise 4
1. brachytherapy
2. mapping
3. sentinel
4. en bloc resection
5. margins
6. immunotherapy
7. CAM
8. 3DCRT

Case Study: Tamara Ramos
1. breast
2. a
3. b
4. c
5. a

Case Study: Akiyo Kato
1. a 2. b 3. b 4. b 5. a

Exercise 5
1. protocol
2. kill
3. replication
4. antineoplastic hormones
5. alkylating agents
6. antimetabolites
7. mitotic inhibitors

Exercise 6
1. Cancer has spread beyond breast tissue.
2. neck and liver
3. surgery and chemotherapy
4. decreased level of sodium in the blood
5. She probably will live only a few months.

Exercise 7
1. biopsy
2. grade 4
3. cancer, fecal occult blood test
4. certified tumor registrar; tumor, nodes, metastases
5. single-photon emission computed tomography

Chapter 16 Review

Word Parts
1. neo-
2. –plasia
3. –oma
4. apo-
5. dys-
6. –genesis
7. ana-
8. –blast
9. –carcinoma
10. ecto-
11. –stasis
12. –sarcoma
13. meta-
14. –plasm
15. hyper-
16. –ptosis
17. mut/a
18. blast/o
19. sarc/o
20. onc/o
21. path/o
22. nod/o
23. derm/o
24. carcin/o

Wordshop
1. tumor (-oma) of a nerve (neur/o)
   Term: neuroma
2. tumor (-oma) of a blood vessel (hemangi/o)
   Term: hemangioma
3. malignant tumor (-sarcoma) of bone (oste/o)
   Term: osteosarcoma
4. tumor (-oma) of a gland (aden/o)
   Term: adenoma
5. tumor (-oma) of embryonic (blast/o) retina [retinal cells] (retin/o)
   Term: retinoblastoma
6. treatment (-therapy) using short distance (brachy-)
   Term: brachytherapy
7. condition of formation (-plasia) apart (ana-)
   Term: anaplasia
8. falling (-ptosis) away (apo-)
   Term: apoptosis
9. process of (-tion) change (mut/a)
   Term: mutation
10. tumor (-oma) of the meninges (mening/o)
    Term: meningioma
11. star (astr/o) cell (cyt/o) tumor (-oma)
    Term: astrocytoma
12. kidney (nephr/o) tumor (-oma)
    Term: nephroma
13. dark (phe/o) color (chrom/o) cell (cyt/o) tumor (-oma)
    Term: pheochromocytoma

Term Sorting
Benign Neoplasms: acoustic neuroma, BPH, dermatofibroma, fibroids, leiomyoma, meningioma, neuroma, osteoma, pheochromocytoma, thymoma
Malignant Neoplasms: adenocarcinoma, Ewing sarcoma, hemangiosarcoma, hypernephroma, Kaposi sarcoma, leukemia, myxosarcoma, retinoblastoma, seminoma, Wilms tumor
Diagnostic Procedures: AFP, biopsy (bx), BTA, CA125, CT scan, hCG, mammogram, PET, PSA, SPECT
Therapeutic Interventions: 3DCRT, BMT, brachytherapy, chemotherapy, gamma knife surgery, immunotherapy, IMRT, lumpectomy, mastectomy, radiotherapy

Translations
1. seminoma, multiple myeloma, adenocarcinoma
2. differentiated
3. metastasis
4. Pap smear, severe dysplasia
5. lumpectomy, radiotherapy (radiation, radiation therapy), chemotherapy
6. brachytherapy
7. leukemia, chemotherapy, BMT

Discharge Summary
1. sigmoid colon cancer
2. colonoscopy
3. sigmoid colectomy, appendectomy
4. All of the nodes were negative for carcinoma.

Index